Menstrual Disorders

EDITED BY

Deborah B. Ehrenthal, MD, FACP
Matthew K. Hoffman, MD, MPH, FACOG
Paula J. Adams Hillard, MD

WOMEN'S HEALTH SERIES EDITOR

Pamela Charney, MD, FACP

AMERICAN COLLEGE OF PHYSICIANS
PHILADELPHIA

Clinical Consultant: David R. Goldmann, MD, FACP
Director, Editorial Production: Linda Drumheller
Developmental Editor: Victoria Hoenigke
Production Supervisor: Allan S. Kleinberg
Senior Production Editor: Karen C. Nolan
Editorial Coordinator: Angela Gabella
Interior Designer: Patrick Whelan
Cover Designer: Flatiron Industries

Printed in the United States of America
Composition by UB Communications
Printing/binding by Versa Press

Library of Congress Cataloging-in-Publication Data

Menstrual disorders: a practical guide / edited by Deborah Ehrenthal, Paula Adams Hillard, Matthew Hoffman.
   p. ; cm.
   Includes bibliographical references and index.
   ISBN 1-930513-66-6 (alk. paper)
      1. Menstruation disorders.   2. Primary care (Medicine)   I. Ehrenthal, Deborah.   II. Hillard, Paula Adams.   III. Hoffman, Matthew, MD.   IV. American College of Physicians.
   [DNLM: 1. Menstruation Disturbances—therapy.   2. Menstruation.
Disturbances—diagnosis. WP 550 M5487 2005]
RG163.M46 2005
618.1'72—dc22

                                                                              2005057025

The authors and publisher have exerted every effort to ensure that the drug selection and dosage set forth in this book are in accord with current recommendations and practice at the time of publication. In view of ongoing research, occasional changes in government regulations, and the constant flow of information relating to durg therapy and drug reactions, the reader is urged to check the package insert for each drug for any change in indications and dosage and for added warnings and precautions. This care is particularly important when the recommended agent is a new or infrequently used drug.

06 07 08 09 10 / 10 9 8 7 6 5 4 3 2 1

Editors

Deborah B. Ehrenthal, MD, FACP
Departments of Internal Medicine
and Obstetrics and Gynecology
Christiana Care Health Services
Newark, Delaware;
Clinical Assistant Professor of Medicine
Thomas Jefferson University
Philadelphia, Pennsylvania

Matthew K. Hoffman, MD, MPH, FACOG
Department of Obstetrics and Gynecology
Christiana Care Health Services
Newark, Delaware

Paula J. Adams Hillard, MD
Professor, Departments of Pediatrics and Obstetrics
and Gynecology
University of Cincinnati College of Medicine
Cincinnati Children's Hospital Medical Center
Cincinnati, Ohio

Women's Health Series Editor

Pamela Charney, MD, FACP
Clinical Professor of Medicine
Clinical Associate Professor of Obstetrics and Gynecology
and Women's Health
Albert Einstein College of Medicine
Bronx, New York;
Program Director
Internal Medicine Residency
Norwalk Hospital
Norwalk, Connecticut

Contributors

Jane E. Dopkins Broecker, MD
Assistant Professor of Obstetrics and
    Gynecology
Ohio University College of Osteopathic
    Medicine
Athens, Ohio

Ellen Harrison, MD, FCCM
Associate Professor of Medicine and
    Clinical Obstetrics, Gynecology and
    Women's Health
Jack D. Weiler Hospital
Bronx, New York

Susan Johnson, MD, MS
Professor of Obstetrics and Gynecology
University of Iowa Hospitals and
    Clinics
Iowa City, Iowa

Renee K. Kottenhahn, MD, FAAP
Department of Pediatrics
Division of Adolescent Medicine
Christiana Care Health Services
Newark, Deleware

Catherine LeClair, MD
Assistant Professor of Obstetrics and
    Gynecology
Oregon Health and Sciences University
Portland, Oregon

Shahab Minassian, MD
Department of Obstetrics and
    Gynecology
Drexel University College of Medicine
Co-Director, Center for Polycystic
    Ovarian Syndrome at Drexel
    University College of Medicine
Philadelphia, Pennsylvania

Sophia Ouhilal, MD
Clinical Instructor, Obstetrics and
    Gynecology and Women's Health
Albert Einstein College of Medicine
Bronx, New York

Joseph E. Patruno, MD
Director of Gynecology Services
Lehigh Valley Hospital
Allentown, Pennsylvania

Elisabeth H. Quint, MD, FACOG
Professor of Obstetrics and Gynecology
University of Michigan
Ann Arbor, Michigan

Margaret V. Ragni, MD, MPH
Professor of Medicine
University of Pittsburgh School of
    Medicine
Director, Hemophilia Center of
    Western Pennsylvania
Pittsburgh, Pennsylvania

Henry M. Rinder, MD, FACP
Associate Professor
Laboratory Medicine and Internal
  Medicine
Director, Clinical Pathology Residency
  Training
Director, Laboratory Medicine Cases
  On-Line
Yale University School of Medicine
New Haven, Connecticut

Nanette Santoro, MD
Professor and Director
Division of Reproductive
  Endocrinology/Infertility
Albert Einstein College of Medicine
Bronx, New York

Kimberly W. Schlesinger, MD
Peninsula Cancer Institute
Williamsburg, Virginia

D. Paul Shackelford, MD
Associate Clinical Professor
Greenville Women's Physicians
Greenville, North Carolina

Katherine Sherif, MD
Director, Center for Women's Health
Drexel University College of Medicine
Philadelphia, Pennsylvania

Preface

The clinical issues related to reproduction and the menstrual cycle encompass many fields of medical expertise. Like many areas of women's health, there is no single group of specialists whose training and experience gives them a broad understanding of these disorders and who can care for the whole woman. The concept for this book on menstrual issues came from editor of the ACP Women's Health series, Pam Charney. She realized, before I did, that the move to my current position as an internist teaching in an obstetrics and gynecology residency program would give me a unique window into this field. With my attention turned to office gynecology, I found a high incidence of menstrual complaints in women I was seeing for management of medical problems or simply for annual exams. Understandably, women with a menstrual complaint will generally seek the advice of a gynecologist and, in fact, primary care practitioners typically refer their patients with menstrual complaints or infertility to the gynecologist. The great irony is that the etiology of many menstrual symptoms is an underlying medical problem, which the primary care provider is best equipped to address.

Except for brief chapters in some newer women's health books, I have found few resources available to guide primary care physicians and gynecologists through the assessment and management of menstrual disorders. Gynecology textbooks typically cover menstrual disorders in a single chapter and do not discuss in great depth symptom etiology or disease management. Some very useful information can be found in endocrinology textbooks, but management of the gynecologic issue is not a priority. Reproductive endocrinology textbooks cover some of these topics well, but do not go far in addressing medical concerns. Whereas the gynecologist will look for underlying pelvic pathology and may do an endocrinologic work-up, the typical goal of management is to create a normal menstrual cycle. Although in some cases this may completely meet the patent's needs, it can at times mask symptoms and delay diagnosis of underlying medical problems, or it may not address the critical health issues. The topic of menstrual disorders looked to be an area begging for a more interdisciplinary approach.

Our goal for *Menstrual Disorders* was to blend the fields of gynecology, adolescent medicine, internal medicine, and medical subspecialties to create a comprehensive, coherent, integrated, and straightforward guide to the diagnosis and management of menstrual issues for the busy clinician. It synthesizes information for each topic in a way that has not been done in previous textbooks. The book is edited by an internist, a generalist gynecologist, and a pediatric/adolescent gynecologist to ensure a balanced perspective. Many of the chapters are written by a collaborative team of internists and gynecologists. Attention is given to the connection between the menstrual complaint and underlying medical problems as well as to addressing its impact on short- and long-term health. An evidence-based approach is taken where there are data; otherwise, expert opinion is used. Each chapter is self-contained.

The book begins with a review and discussion of the normal menstrual cycle. Special attention is paid in this chapter to the adolescent in whom cycle irregularity can be confusing for the clinician and for her. The second section of the book addresses the common menstrual complaints of women from adolescence through the menopause. The third section addresses the important areas of interplay between underlying medical problems and related menstrual issues. This includes a chapter about polycystic ovary syndrome, a chapter addressing issues for women with bleeding disorders and coagulopathies, and a discussion of menstrual issues for women with disabilities. The final chapter in this section considers women with chronic medical problems and addresses the menstrual, reproductive, and contraceptive issues in these patients. The book concludes with a chapter addressing the details of procedural options in the management of abnormal uterine bleeding..

Menstrual Disorders: A Practical Guide represents the collaborative efforts of my colleagues in internal medicine, gynecology, hematology, and pediatrics who worked together to synthesize this broad area. Tremendous thanks must go to my co-editors Paula Adams Hillard and Matthew Hoffman, whose efforts and wisdom made this book possible. Thanks also to Pam Charney and Raymond Powrie, both of whom provided much appreciated expertise and support. Finally, to all of our contributors, thank you for your hard work and patience while working with us to fulfill our vision.

Deborah B. Ehrenthal, MD, FACP

Contents

REVIEW OF THE NORMAL MENSTRUAL CYCLE

1. The Normal Menstrual Cycle 3
   Jane E. Dopkins Broecker and Paula J. Adams Hillard

COMMON MENSTRUAL COMPLAINTS

2. Abnormal Uterine Bleeding 29
   Matthew K. Hoffman

3. Amenorrhea 51
   Catherine LeClair, Deborah B. Ehrenthal, and Paula J. Adams Hillard

4. Perimenopausal Bleeding 77
   Sophia Ouhilal, Ellen Harrison, and Nanette Santoro

5. Dysmenorrhea 97
   Joseph E. Patruno

6. Premenstrual Syndrome 125
   Susan Johnson

MEDICAL ISSUES

7. Polycystic Ovary Syndrome 141
   Katherine Sherif and Shahab Minassian

8. Menstrual Issues in Women with Developmental
   Disabilities 157
   Elisabeth H. Quint

9. Bleeding Disorders 171
   Kimberly W. Schlesinger, Henry M. Rinder, and Margaret V. Ragni

10. Menstrual and Reproductive Issues in Women
    with Chronic Medical Problems 197
    Deborah B. Ehrenthal and Renee K. Kottenhahn

MANAGEMENT DETAILS

11. Procedural Management of Abnormal Uterine Bleeding . . 245
    D. Paul Shackelford and Matthew K. Hoffman

Index 253

Review of the
Normal Menstrual Cycle

The Normal Menstrual Cycle

Jane E. Dopkins Broecker, MD
Paula J. Adams Hillard, MD

The menstrual cycle has been associated with the lunar cycle since classical days, as shown by the etymology of *menstruation.* Its origins lie in the Greek *mene,* "the moon," and the Latin *mensis,* "a month" (1). Many superstitions and misconceptions about menstruation have existed throughout history, and many still exist today. Our current understanding of menstrual cyclicity is founded on extensive research dating to the 19th century when several authors published data from menstrual calendars to "prove" that the female cycle was indeed related to the length of the lunar month. For example, Clos claimed that these data definitively demonstrated statistical association of the phases of the moon and a patient's recorded menstrual dates (2). Other authors have refuted this association based on calendars collected from many women. The best data on the normal menstrual cycle comes from Treloar, who, between 1935 and 1962, collected prospective data on menstrual cycle length and cyclicity from over 2700 women totaling more than 25,000 person years and over a quarter of a million cycles (3).

Uterine bleeding is poorly understood by patients and, with the advent of hormonal manipulation, the variety of types and patterns of uterine bleeding have increased. Uterine bleeding is usually due to a normal ovulatory menstrual cycle, in which falling levels of estrogen and progesterone in the luteal phase eventually lead to ischemia and sloughing of the endometrium. However, most women do not distinguish this kind of bleeding from other causes of endometrial bleeding and refer to any bleeding as a "period." Endometrial bleeding in a woman with a structurally normal uterus may also be caused by other etiologies, such as the abnormal uterine bleeding typical of spontaneous anovulation. In addition, iatrogenic uterine bleeding is quite common in women taking hormones for management of menses, contraception, or replacement therapy. Bleeding from the endometrial lining during placebo pills in combination oral contraception, or break-through bleeding on menopausal hormone therapy, is often viewed by women as "menstruation" or a "period," although this process is hormonally and histologically quite different from a normal menstrual cycle. Normal menstruation may also be altered by intrinsic hormonal abnormalities, intrauterine structural abnormalities, or neoplastic processes. Deviation from normal patterns of flow will often provide evidence of an underlying disorder. Familiarity with normal menstrual patterns is essential for recognition of abnormal patterns and identification of underlying abnormalities.

Menstrual cycling begins at menarche, defined as a girl's first menstruation; persists throughout the reproductive years; and ends with menopause, or the cessation of menstrual cycling. The normal menstrual cycle is best understood by an examination of the endocrine changes responsible for menarche and the ways in which the ovarian hormones and the hypothalamic pituitary axis affect menstruation. Anovulation is common in girls of young gynecologic age (i.e., the early years after menarche) due to the innate immaturity of the hypothalamic pituitary axis. With increasing gynecologic age, the hypothalamic pituitary axis matures and a regular pattern is established that persists for most of a woman's reproductive years. The presence of menstrual molimina (e.g., breast tenderness, nausea, mood changes, bloating) has been associated with ovulatory cycles (4). Menstrual cycles shorten in the later reproductive years and eventually become sporadic in the years before menopause. Eventually, ovulation does not occur at all, resulting in menopause, when menstrual cycles cease all together.

Hormonal Patterns Responsible for the Normal Menstrual Cycle

Ovulatory cycles begin to occur as the hypothalamic pituitary axis matures and negative feedback mechanisms begin to function effectively. Ovulatory cycles are the norm for gynecologically mature girls and adult women of reproductive age. The ovarian cycle can be divided into two phases, the follicular and the luteal, each having characteristic histologic changes and resulting hormone levels that cause changes in the endometrium (5). In the follicular phase of the cycle, the endometrium is in the proliferative phase, and during the luteal phase the endometrium becomes secretory, with well-developed glands and mature stromal support (Fig. 1-1).

During the follicular phase, follicle-stimulating hormone (FSH) stimulates recruitment of several ovarian follicles. Estradiol levels are low at the beginning of the cycle, but as follicles are recruited, each of these follicles secretes

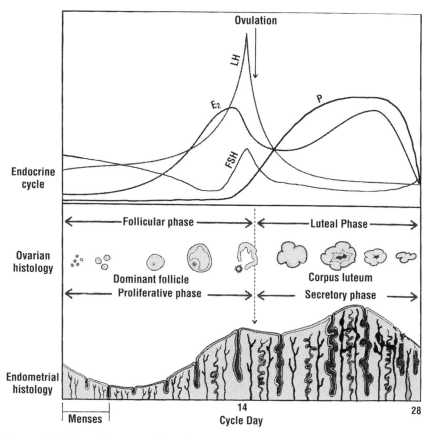

Figure 1-1   Normal menstrual cycle. (From Hillard PA, Berek JS, Novak E, eds. Novak's Gynecology, 13th ed. Philadelphia: Lippincott Williams & Wilkins; 2002;160; with permission.)

estrogen, causing serum estradiol levels to rise. During this phase, the decidua basalis undergoes mitotic growth, giving rise to the decidua functionalis with its straight endometrial glands and relatively rare vascular structures. Hormonal feedback mechanisms promote the orderly development of a single dominant follicle. Toward the end of the follicular phase, rising estrogen levels provide negative feedback on pituitary FSH secretion, while luteinizing hormone (LH) continues to rise, eventually surging with resultant ovulation 24-36 hours later.

Progesterone levels are low during the follicular phase, approximately 3 ng/mL, but after ovulation the corpus luteum secretes progesterone, causing a precipitous rise in serum progesterone after ovulation (6). Measurement of progesterone in the mid-luteal phase (cycle day 21-23) can provide presumptive evidence of ovulation if levels are at least 6.5 ng/mL but preferably over 10 ng/mL. Progesterone stimulation of the endometrium results in the development of a secretory endometrium, the hallmark of ovulation. Eosinophilic protein-rich secretory products are seen in the glandular lumens, and in the second half of the luteal phase the stroma becomes edematous and spiral arterioles form.

In the absence of conception and human chorionic gonadotropin (hCG) stimulation from a developing pregnancy, the corpus luteum regresses, and both estrogen and progesterone levels fall in preparation for the next cycle. With withdrawal of estradiol and progesterone, there is spasm of the spiral arteries, which causes ischemia of the endometrium. Release of proteolytic enzymes and breakdown of lysosomes fosters further tissue degradation, and the entire functionalis layer of the endometrium is shed efficiently in menstrual flow. Although prostaglandins are produced throughout the menstrual cycle, prostaglandin-F2α rises to peak levels at the time of menstruation, is a potent vasoconstrictor of spiral arterioles, and induces myometrial contractions: this is the etiology of primary dysmenorrhea

Menarche and Early Gynecologic Years

Normal Pubertal Development and Initiation of Menstruation

During puberty, the neuroendocrine system of the hypothalamus undergoes maturational changes. Gonadotropin-releasing hormone (GnRH) pulses produced in the hypothalamus are sensed by the anterior pituitary and lead to increased production of the gonadotropins FSH and LH. The higher levels of FSH and LH cause follicular growth, with a resulting increase in sex steroid levels. Rising levels of estrogen, pulsatile secretion of GnRH, and noctournal LH pulsations lead to initiation of menses and eventually create cyclic menstrual patterns.

There seems to be growing public perception that the age of menarche is earlier now than it was several generations ago, and along with that perception is the concern that menarche will continue to occur earlier and earlier for girls in this century. The seminal report of pubertal development came from Marshall and Tanner in 1969, who prospectively studied 192 girls of lower socioeconomic status in an orphanage in Great Britain. The average age of menarche in this report was 13.47 (7). A recent large study in the United States conducted by the Pediatrics Research in Office Settings Network assessed pubertal development in girls presenting for routine care and collected retrospective data on age at menarche (8). The study showed a younger age of pubertal development and a slightly younger age of menarche than those reported by Marshall and Tanner in 1969. The study also showed ethnic differences, with white girls having average ages of adrenarche at 10.0, thelarche at 10.5, and menarche at age 12.9. For African-American girls, development occurred slightly earlier, with the average ages of adrenarche at 8.6, thelarche at 8.9, and menarche at 12.2 years (8) (Fig. 1-2). While improvements in nutrition may account for the documented decrease in the average age of menarche from a century ago, there has been no clinically significant change in the age of menarche in the last 50 years in developed industrialized locations, nor is the age of menarche expected to fall further (9-11).

By age 14, 95% of girls will have had menarche (12). Menarche typically occurs at Tanner stage IV breast development and is rare before Tanner stage III breast development (Table 1-1 and Fig. 1-3) (7). Traditionally, primary amenorrhea has been defined as no menarche by age 16; however, many diagnosable and treatable disorders can and should be detected earlier, using the statistically derived guideline of age 14. Thus, an evaluation for primary amenorrhea should be considered for any girl who has not reached menarche by age 14 or has not done so within 2 years of obtaining Tanner stage IV breast development.

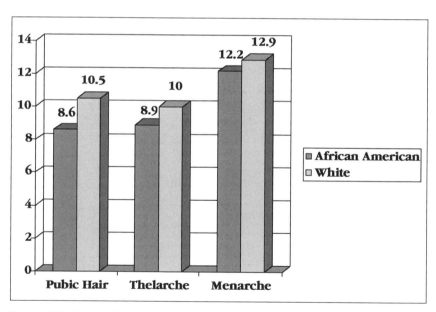

Figure 1-2   Age at adrenarche, thelarche, and menarche as stratified by race. (From Herman-Giddens ME, Slora EJ, Wasserman RC, et al. Secondary sexual characteristics and menses in young girls seen in office practice: a study from the Pediatric Research in Office Setting Network. Pediatrics. 1997;99:505-12; with permission.)

Table 1-1   Tanner Staging

Tanner Staging: Breast

Stage I
No palpable breast tissue, areola minimally pigmented and less than 2 cm, with elevation of papilla only

Stage II
Breast bud visible and palpable under the areola, with elevation of breast and papilla into a small mound

Stage III
Breast and areola enlarge further, with a continuous round contour

Stage IV
Areola and papilla enlarge and project to form a secondary mound above the remaining breast

Stage V
Mature adult breast develops, with resolution of the secondary mound to a smooth rounded contour with projection of the papilla only

Tanner Staging: Pubic Hair

Stage I
No sexually stimulated pubic hair, but some non-sexual hair may be present

Stage II
Sparse growth of coarse, long, crinkly, pigmented hair, primarily on the labia majora

Stage III
Amount of pubic hair increases with some spread to mons pubis, and hair becomes coarser, darker, and curlier

Stage IV
Adult type pubic hair on labia and mons, but not yet extending to the medial thigh

Stage V
Adult distribution of coarse hair, with some spread to the medial surface of the thighs

Adapted from Novak's Gynecology, 13th ed. Philadelphia: Lippincott Williams & Wilkins; 2002:808-9.

Because menarche is such an important milestone in a girl's development, it is important to be able to educate girls and their parents about what to expect of a first period, and about the range for normal cycle length of subsequent menses; girls who have been educated about menarche and early menstrual patterns will experience less anxiety when it does occur (13). A girl's first period is usually reported to be of medium flow, and need for menstrual products should not be excessive. Duration of a girl's first menses is usually within the range of 2-7 days (11). Knowing these parameters, it may be helpful to talk to girls who are at Tanner stage III concerning what to expect of their first period.

Many girls and parents are curious about when to expect the second menstrual period and what to expect during the early months after menarche. A

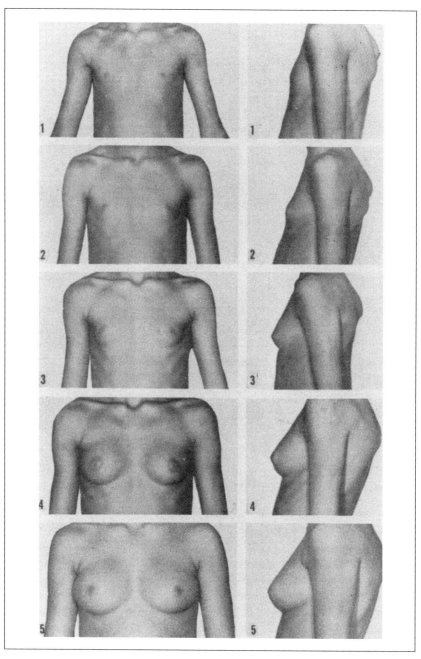

Figure 1-3 Sex maturity ratings of breast changes in adolescent girls. (Courtesy of J.M. Tanner, MD, Institute of Child Health, Department of Growth and Development, University of London, England.)

prospective World Health Organization international and multi-center study of 3073 girls documented the range of early cycle lengths for adolescent girls. Median first-cycle length after menarche was 34 days; 38% of girls had a cycle length that exceeded 40 days. As many as 5%-10% of girls had more than 60 days between first and second menses, whereas 4%-7% had a first-cycle length of less than 20 days (16).

Disorders of puberty timing in puberty development is determined in large part by genetic predisposition, but other factors are known to affect the initiation and rate of progression of pubertal development (6). Geographic, nutritional, physiologic, and psychologic factors, among others, play a role in pubertal development. Leptin, a peptide that is secreted in adipose tissue and acts on the central nervous system, plays a role in earlier onset of puberty for girls with higher composition of body fat. Conversely, anorexics and excessive exercisers often have delayed puberty and later age of menarche or have secondary amenorrhea (6).

Precocious puberty has been defined by some as pubertal development less than 2.5 standard deviations from the mean, correlating with the age of 8, but new information on pubertal development suggests that pubertal development is normal for many girls before this age (17). The recent cross-sectional study of the American Academy of Pediatrics documented racial variation, with African American girls having pubertal development earlier than white girls (18). In this study, 27% of African American and 7% of white girls had growth of pubic hair or breast development at 7 years of age. Thus, pubertal changes beginning between the ages of 6 to 8 should be assessed on an individual basis, and evaluation based on clinical presentation (6). Three quarters of precocious puberty is idiopathic, with a specific etiology (most commonly an ovarian tumor, adrenal disease, or McCune-Albright syndrome) typically identified in only one quarter. In girls 5 years and older, precocious puberty is usually idiopathic and GnRH-dependent (6).

Early Cycles and the Transition to Regular Ovulation

Cycle Length and Duration in the Early Gynecologic Years

Anovulatory cycles, or bleeding in the absence of ovulation, is typical for girls of young gynecologic age and can be differentiated from the ovulatory, menstrual, cycles in the gynecologically mature female. The early cycles are usually somewhat irregular due to the innate immaturity of the hypothalamic pituitary axis. From hormonal studies we know that it is typical for at least half of menstrual cycles to be anovulatory in the first gynecologic year (14). In an anovulatory cycle, the GnRH pulsations from the hypothalamus cause pulsitile release of FSH from the pituitary gland, which acts on follicles in the ovary with the result of estrogen production. Because the positive estrogen feedback mechanism has not yet matured, FSH and LH midcycle surges are not produced, and follicular maturation and ovulation do not occur. In the absence of ovulation, corpus luteum formation and progesterone production do not occur (15).

In the absence of ovulation, estrogen levels remain high, and progesterone levels remain relatively low (18). The endometrium attains a greater height and has little structural support. Histologically, the lining displays intense vascularity, back-to-back glandularity, and little stromal matrix (18). Because this tissue is relatively fragile, it will suffer spontaneous superficial breakage and bleeding, resulting in menstrual flow. The fragile structure of this estrogenized endometrium sheds sporadically and unevenly, resulting in variable intervals between bleeding episodes and variation in amount of blood flow (Table 1-2) (18). In anovulatory cycles, progesterone levels are relatively low. Moliminal symptoms (premenstrual symptoms, usually uncomfortable, including cramping, bloating, moodiness, and breast tenderness) are typically associated with ovulatory cycles and are typically absent with anovulatory bleeding.

Most anovulatory cycles actually come at fairly regular intervals and fall within established parameters, despite the fragile structure and uneven healing of the endometrium stimulated by unopposed estrogen. During the first 2 years after menarche, cycles may be somewhat irregular due to the high proportion of anovulatory cycles, but 90% of girls will have cycles within the range of 21-42 days, with 2-8 days of flow (14).

Cycle length is more variable for adolescents than for women aged 20-40. Treloar documented 275,947 cycles in 2702 women and reported data for

Table 1-2   Characteristics of Anovulatory Endometrium and Bleeding

Anovulatory Endometrium

- Estrogen production unopposed by progesterone
- Thick endometrium
- Very vascular endometrium
- Predominance of glandular tissue with very little stromal support
- Endometrial tissue very fragile
- Endometrium spontaneously bleeds at various sites; bleeding is random (not universal)

Anovulatory Endometrium Bleeding

- No vasoconstriction
- No tight coiling of spiral vessels
- No orderly collapse to induce stasis
- Less prostaglandin-induced uterine muscle cramping
- Bleeding may be long and heavy

menstrual norms by gynecologic year and the statistical limits of normal at the 5th percentile and 95th percentile (3). In the first gynecologic year the 5th percentile for cycle length is 23 days and the 95th percentile is 90. By the fourth gynecologic year, fewer girls are having such long cycles, but anovulation is still significant for some, with the 95th percentile at 50 days. By the seventh gynecologic year, cycles are shorter and less variable, with the 5th percentile at a 27-day cycle length and the 95th percentile at 38 days (Table 1-3). A graphic representation of another large data set demonstrates similar findings with greater variation in cycle length at the extremes of menstrual life: adolescence and peri-menopause (Fig. 1-4).

An anovulatory pattern is typical in the early gynecologic years. Although most anovulatory cycles fall within expected norms, there are times when anovulatory cycles produce excessive flow and fall outside the normal parameters. A prospectively completed menstrual calendar can help the clinician assess whether or not a girl is having a normal or abnormal bleeding pattern (Figs. 1-5 and 1-6).

Normal Maturation of the Hypothalamic Pituitary Axis and Transition to Ovulatory Cycles

As the hypothalamic-pituitary axis matures, anovulatory cycles give way to the more regular ovulatory cycles. Some girls have a high proportion of anovulatory cycles, whereas others quickly establish regular ovulatory cycles. Interestingly, girls with early menarche more quickly establish ovulatory cycles than girls who are older at menarche (19). As many as one third of

Table 1-3   Menstrual Parameters for the Adolescent and Adult

Menstrual Characteristics	Young Gynecologic Age (2-5 Years After Menarche)	Adult Ovulatory Cycles	Menopausal Transition
Cycle pattern	Somewhat irregular	Regular and predictable	Regular or more variable
Duration of flow	2-7 days	2-7 days	2-7 days
Cycle length	21-45 days	21-34 days	21 days to 11 months
Average volume flow	30 mL	30 mL	Not studied
Moliminal symptoms	Variably present	Usually present	Variably present; sometimes more pronounced

Adapted from Flug D, Largo RH, Prader A. Menstrual patterns in adolescent Swiss girls: a longitudinal study. Ann Hum Biol.1984;11:495-508; and Widholm O, Kantero RL. A statistical analysis of the menstrual patterns of 8,000 Finnish girls and their mothers. Acta Obstet Gynecol Scand. 1971;14:(Suppl):1-36.

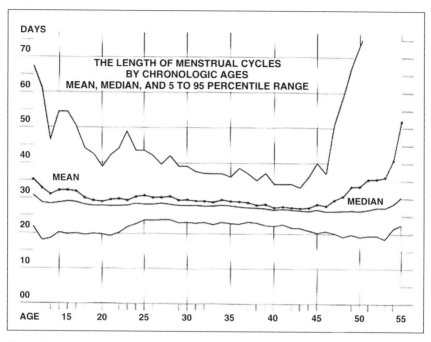

Figure 1-4   Length of menstrual cycle by age. This graph depicts the relatively longer cycles and wider variation in cycle length typical during adolescence, with evolution toward more regular cycles during the middle reproductive years, then eventual return to greater variation in cycle length in the perimenopausal stage (31,645 cycles reported by 656 women). (From Vollman RF. The menstrual cycle. In Friedman EA, ed. Major Problems in Obstetrics and Gynecology, vol. 7. Philadelphia: WB Saunders; 1977; with permission.)

adolescents willstill have anovulatory cycles in the fifth year after menarche (17). By the seventh year after menarche, more than 90% of cycles are ovulatory (20).

A prospectively recorded menstrual calendar will help both the clinician and an adolescent better understand her cycles. Many young teens expect that a "monthly" period will occur on the same date of each month. These girls will mistakenly perceive a 26-day cycle with one menses occurring at the beginning of the month and another at the end of that month as "two periods" in a month. If a girl has an anovulatory cycle and has, for example, a 40-day cycle, she may believe that she has "skipped a month" when she actually had an anovulatory cycle that fell within expected norms. Many girls describe their early cycles as having been relatively painless menses that occasionally "skip a month" but note that recently their periods have become more regular and are associated with increased cramping, breast-tenderness,

MENSTRUAL CALENDAR

YEAR:

	1	2	3	4	5	6	7	8	9	10	11	12	13	14	15	16	17	18	19	20	21	22	23	24	25	26	27	28	29	30	31
JAN																														■	■
FEB																															
MAR																															■
APR																															■
MAY																															
JUN																															
JUL																															■
AUG																															
SEP																															■
OCT																															
NOV																															
DEC																															

CODES: S = spotting
L = light flow
N = normal flow
H = heavy flow
X = menstrual flow (if just tracking flow)

Figure 1-5 Menstrual calendar.

MENSTRUAL CALENDAR

YEAR: _____

	1	2	3	4	5	6	7	8	9	10	11	12	13	14	15	16	17	18	19	20	21	22	23	24	25	26	27	28	29	30	31
JAN																				N	N	L	L								
FEB														H	N	L	L	L	H										■	■	■
MAR						N			L	H	N																				
APR		L	H	L	H		L	L																							■
MAY	L	H	L	L	L																		H			L			L	H	N
JUN	N	N	L																					N	N	L	H	N	N	L	■
JUL																		L	H	N	N	L	L								
AUG																		L	L												
SEP											H	N	N	L	H	N															■
OCT						L	H	N	N	L				L																	
NOV						L	N	L																							■
DEC				L	H																									L	N

CODES: S = spotting
  L = light flow
  N = normal flow
  H = heavy flow
  X = menstrual flow (if just tracking flow)

Figure 1-6 Menstrual calendar with a normal menstrual cycle documented.

and moodiness. These moliminal symptoms and dysmenorrhea are typical of ovulatory cycles, whereas girls who are anovulatory usually report minimal discomfort.

Parameters of Normal Menstrual Flow in the Early Years after Menarche
Because variation in cycle length and duration of flow is expected in the early years after menarche, it can be challenging to distinguish normal from abnormal patterns of flow. A detailed history and focused examination will facilitate the differentiation and identification of clinically important abnormalities. In adult women, the characterization and perception of menstrual flow as "light," "medium," or "heavy" has been shown to correlate poorly with actual measured losses (21). This may be even more true in teens who have little historical or peer information with which to compare. To more accurately characterize menstrual losses, girls should be asked for the number of pads or tampons used on the heaviest day of menses, as well as the frequency of change. Additional inquiries will better characterize the flow, including questions about the number of days of heavy flow and the use of double protection (both a tampon and a pad). Soiling of clothes is common in young teens who are not used to coping with menstrual flow, especially at schools where there are restrictions and rules on trips to the restroom. This alone does not indicate a bleeding history consistent with menorrhagia, but primarily indicates difficulties in learning menstrual hygiene. However, girls who frequently soil bed sheets at night or who pass large clots can be classified as experiencing menorrhagia.

A history of soaking a pad or tampon more frequently than every 3 hours or soaking more than the typical 3-5 pads a day for more than one day suggests excessively heavy flow. For these girls, an underlying disorder should be considered and a complete blood count is warranted to objectively document menorrhagia and to rule out anemia. An underlying coagulopathy is commonly found in adolescents with menorrhagia. The American College of Obstetrics and Gynecology recommends that adolescents with menorrhagia be screened for von Willebrand's disease (see Chapter 9).

Abnormal Bleeding Patterns in Adolescents

Reassurance may be all that is necessary for a teen who has slightly irregular cycles within the first 2 years of menarche and who is not anemic. Bleeding patterns become more predictable as mature reproductive age is approached and a normal pattern of ovulation is established. However, for patients who have bleeding patterns that are markedly irregular and outside the normal parameters for early cycling, the possibility of a significant underlying abnormality should be considered (Table 1-4).

Table 1-4   Common Causes of Abnormal Bleeding Patterns in the Adolescent

Hormonal

- Anovulation (dysfunctional uterine bleeding)
- Thyroid dysfunction
- Prolactinoma
- Side effects of hormonal contraception
- Androgen excess/polycystic ovarian syndrome
- Hypothalamic suppression in patients with female athlete triad/anorexia

Bleeding Diatheses

- Platelet disorders (ITP, Fanconi's anemia, others)
- Coagulopathy (inherited clotting factor deficiencies, vitamin K deficiency, anticoagulant therapy, consumption coagulopathy, liver or renal disease)

Local Pathology

- Sexually transmitted infection with cervicitis or endometritis
- Foreign body (such as a tampon or intrauterine device)
- Structural abnormality of the uterus or cervix (fibroid, polyp, or uterine septum)
- Trauma

Malignancy

- Leukemia
- Genital tract malignancy

Pregnancy

- Threatened spontaneous abortion or spontaneous abortion
- Ectopic pregnancy
- Incomplete elective termination
- Post-abortion endometritis

For adolescents with cycles less than 21 days, duration of menstrual flow over 7 days, or excessively heavy bleeding, a underlying cause should be sought (22). Girls with bleeding disorders such as von Willebrand's may hemorrhage and become hemodynamically unstable during their first menses, and future menses will follow the expected cyclicity but be excessively heavy (23). In contrast, girls with heavy bleeding secondary to anovulation typically present with acutely heavy menses, frequent bleeding, bleeding lasting for weeks, or an "on again, off again" type of flow. Structural causes of excessive bleeding are less common in adolescents than in older adults, but can occur. Pregnancy is an important, and not uncommon, cause of abnormal bleeding in adolescents, so a confidential history and a urine hCG is essential for any girl with abnormal bleeding.

Cycles longer than 90 days are unusual (>95th percentile, even during the first gynecologic year) and may signal significant disease with future health implications. Conditions such as eating disorders, female athlete triad, hyperprolacinoma, and even premature ovarian failure have implications for future bone health. The most common cause of oligomenorrhea and amenorrhea in adolescents is polycystic ovary syndrome (PCOS). It is important to diagnose and treat adolescents with PCOS because the syndrome has signs and symptoms that are particularly unpleasant for adolescents (acne, obesity, abnormal hair growth), as well as long-term risks such as diabetes, cardiovascular disease, and endometrial cancer (see Chapter 7) (6).

Menstruation During Mature Reproductive Age

Normal Adult Cycles and Parameters

Because disorders of menstruation are one of the most frequent reasons both adolescent girls and adult women seek medical care, a thorough understanding of normal menstrual physiology and cycle characteristics is essential. As discussed in the preceding section, cycles are typically anovulatory in the early gynecologic years, become intermittently ovulatory as the negative feedback mechanisms mature, and eventually establish a normal pattern of ovulation by the third to sixth gynecologic year (24). Normal menstruation lasts 4-7 days, results in mean blood loss of 30 mL, and most (98%) cycles are 21-35 days in length (25,26). The follicular phase varies between individuals, and may be as short as 7 days for some women and as long as 21 days for others. The normal luteal phase has a fixed length, with ovulation predictably occurring approximately 14 days before menstration (6).

Women have many more menstrual cycles today than they did several generations ago. In the past, shorter life expectancy, more term pregnancies, and longer duration of lactation limited the number of menstrual cycles women experienced. Today the average woman, with menarche at age 13 and menopause at the age of 52, will experience 39 potential years of cycling, which would correlate with 507 menses, given an average 28-day cycle. Even with three pregnancies, each followed by a year of lactation, a typical woman's total number of menstrual cycles will be 435.

Abnormal Bleeding Patterns in Adults

Knowing normal menstrual cycle parameters helps the clinician identify and describe abnormal bleeding patterns. Precise definitions vary between experts, and some terms listed below are now rarely used but are important in the older literature. The definitions are adapted from those found in *Dorland's Illustrated Medical Dictionary* (27):

- *Amenorrhea*—the absence or cessation of menses.
  - □ *Primary amenorrhea*—menstruation that has not occurred by age 14-16 or within 2 years of obtaining Tanner stage IV breast development.
  - □ *Secondary amenorrhea*—absence of menses for 3-6 months (13). The time frame is a somewhat arbitrary parameter but one that is commonly used. In fact, Vollman's extensive research on adult menstrual cycles shows that the 95th percentile for cycle length in reproductive-aged women is 42 days (2), so it is reasonable to suspect an abnormality in a woman with a cycle length over that limit.

- *Hypermenorrhea*—excessive uterine bleeding occurring at regular intervals, the period of flow being of usual duration.

- *Hypomenorrhea*—uterine bleeding of less than the normal amount occurring at regular intervals, the period of flow being of the same or less than usual duration.

- *Menometrorrhagia*—excessive uterine bleeding occurring both during the menses and at irregular intervals.

- *Menorrhagia*—regularly timed episodes of bleeding that are either excessive in amount and/or duration. Menstrual loss over 80 mL per cycle or more than 7 days of flow may lead to anemia over time; measurement of hemoglobin and hematocrit may help identify women with menorrhagia (28).

- *Metrorrhagia*—irregular bleeding episodes.

- *Oligomenorrhea*—infrequent menstrual flow, occurring at intervals of 35 days to 6 months, often irregular.
  - □ *Oligohypermenorrhea*—infrequent menstruation with excessive menstrual flow.
  - □ *Oligohypomenorrhea*—infrequent menstruation with diminished menstrual flow.

- *Polymenorrhea*—abnormally frequent menstruation, defined as that occurring at regular intervals of less than 21 days.

Ovulation

Signs and Symptoms of Normal Menstrual Cycling

Certain symptoms and signs accompany each phase of the menstrual cycle, and certain signs and symptoms are associated with particular phases of the cycle. Early in the cycle, basal body temperature is relatively low (approximately 98°F) (6) and relatively few symptoms or signs exist. After ovulation, progesterone levels rise and basal body temperature becomes elevated and remains above the baseline charted in the follicular phase until menstruation occurs. If pregnancy occurs, menstruation does not begin, and temperature remains relatively elevated. The color and consistency of cervical mucous change around ovulation and can be noticed by women who pay close attention to their vaginal discharge. Clear, stretchy, mucous is typical at midcycle, around the time of ovulation.

Symptoms of Functional Cysts

Formation of a cystic follicle is a normal ovarian function. Cystic follicles are usually asymptomatic and only 2-3 cm in size. A follicular cyst represents an exaggeration of this process and is typically defined as over 3 cm and usually less than 8 cm in diameter. On ultrasound, follicular cysts are round, simple in appearance, without septations, and are usually anechoic. Although cystic follicles are normal findings, ultrasound technicians and radiologists occasionally make special note of these follicular cysts, even when they are small. Occasionally a patient with a normal cystic follicle is told by the ultrasound technician that she has a "cyst" and she may become worried that something is wrong. Extensive education and reassurance in the office that this finding is normal is often necessary for patients who have been told they have cysts.

Although formation of cysts is part of normal ovarian function, ovulation may be accompanied by abdominal or pelvic pain. This, usually mid-cycle, ovulatory pain, termed *mittleschmirz*, is often described as unilateral, sharp, stabbing, and self-limited. *Dorland's* gives its German derivation: *mittel* mid, middle, + *schmerz* pain, suffering (27).

In the latter half of the cycle, discomfort may be caused by a corpus luteum cyst. Corpus luteum cysts are usually asymptomatic but may be associated with a sense of pressure if they become fairly large, with severe pain (with rupture into the cyst or intraperitoneal hemorrhage), and with excruciating pain (with ovarian torsion). The mechanism of pain from a corpus luteum cyst may be associated with hemorrhage within the enclosed space of the cyst.

Moliminal Symptoms

Before and during menstration, breast tenderness, a sense of bloating, headache, moodiness, and cramping can and often do occur. These symptoms are collectively referred to as *moliminal symptoms*. In 1965 *Dorland's* defined the word this way: "a natural and normal effort made for the performance of any normal function, especially the monthly effort to establish the menstrual flow" (29). Interestingly, the most recent edition (2000) of *Dorland's* gives a slightly different definition: "a laborious effort made for the performance of any normal body function, especially that manifested by a variety of mild but unpleasant symptoms preceding or accompanying the menstrual period" (27). These normal physiologic processes are often sensed by girls and women and raise awareness that menstruation will soon ensue.

Dysmenorrhea

Primary dysmenorrhea, or menstrual cramping in the absence of structural abnormality, is due to prostaglandin-mediated smooth muscle contraction. It is easily identified by history, with many describing centralized crampy discomfort low in the pelvis, typically beginning a day before or at the onset of menses, and continuing for the first 1-2 days of menstrual flow. A diagnosis of endometriosis should be considered for those who have onset of pain more than 2 days before menses and have pain that continues for the entire duration of menses. Primary dysmenorrhea is usually easily and effectively treated with adequate doses and frequency of nonsteroidal anti-inflammatory drugs (NSAIDs) and/or combination hormonal contraceptives. Patients who are refractory to both NSAIDs and oral contraceptives should be evaluated for the possibility of other etiologies of pain, including endometriosis (the most common cause of secondary dysmenorrhea in teens), structural abnormalities (leiomyomata), or infectious causes (endometritis). See Chapter 5 for further discussion.

Menopause

Symptoms, such as hot flushes or variable cycle lengths, and signs, such as elevated FSH levels, may indicate that menopause is approaching, but menopause is defined retrospectively, after a woman has had a year of amenorrhea. The average age of natural menopause is between the ages of 50 and 52 (30,31), but the average age of onset for the menopausal transition is 47 and lasts approximately 4 years (32). In recent years, increasing interest in menopause has sparked new studies on the endocrinology of menopause, the medical impact of menopause on other body systems, and the psychosocial importance of this time of transition from the reproductive years to the post-menopausal state. The term *menopause* is derived from the Greek words *men* (month) and *pauses* (cessation). *Perimenopause* literally means "about or around the menopause" and is a term with which many women are familiar.

An older term, *climacteric*, comes from the Greek word for "latter" and indicates the period of time when a woman passes from the reproductive stage of life through the perimenopausal transition and the menopause to the post-menopausal years. The American Society for Reproductive Medicine suggests that the term *perimenopause* be used only with patients and in the lay press because it does not have a scientifically based definition. A more precise scientifically based definition is the term *menopausal transition*. The menopausal transition begins with variations in menstrual cycle length in a woman who has a monotropic FSH rise and ends with the final menstrual period (33). Familiarity with these terms is important because despite the logic for using a scientifically based definition for the time surrounding menopause, *perimenopause* and *climacteric* are still used by patients and clinicians alike and are cited throughout the medical literature.

During the reproductive years, and in the absence of pathology, menstrual cycles are regular, ovulatory, and have FSH levels in the normal reproductive age range. As women age and enter the early part of the menopausal transition, FSH levels rise because of increased negative feedback effects on the hypothalamus and pituitary, which results in high-normal levels of estradiol (34,35). The actions of inhibin and activin, ovarian proteins produced by the sertoli and granulosa cells, on FSH are dynamic and play a role in the endocrine function of the pituitary and ovary. Interestingly, a study of daily serum and urinary hormone levels in perimenopausal women show increased urinary estrone compared with younger reproductive age controls (35).

The impact of changing reproductive endocrine function has variable effects on the menstrual cycles of perimenopausal women. For some women, regular cycles may occur up to the menopause, when periods then abruptly cease. For others, cycle length may be variable, with some cycles being ovulatory and others anovulatory. Cycles may become shorter, due to a shortened follicular phase, or may become longer. During these years, menopausal symptoms are noted by many women, including specific sensation of hot flashes, as well as more non-specific complaints such as irritability, fatigue, memory complaints, sleep disturbances, and increasing pre-menstrual symptoms (36).

Just before menopause it is common for women to have two or more skipped menstrual periods and at least one inter-menstrual interval of 60 days or more (32). Women with 3-11 months of amenorrhea will likely become menopausal within 4 years (32). After menopause, FSH and LH levels are high and circulating estradiol levels are low (10-20 pg/mL) compared with reproductive-age women who have levels of 40-400 pg/mL (6). Bleeding after menopause is, by definition, abnormal and often indicates pathology. Common causes of post-menopausal bleeding include genital tract neoplasm, endometrial atrophy, structural abnormalities, and iatrogenic endometrial stimulation secondary to hormone therapy.

Conclusion

Pubertal development, menstrual cycling, and menopause are normal processes that are often misunderstood. Knowing normal parameters for each phase of female development and reproductive function can help clinicians reassure patients that what they are experiencing is a normal part of reproductive changes or may lead to a diagnosis of significant pathology. Hormonal management of menses and menopause, while it may normalize abnormal patterns, may also obscure diagnosis of true underlying pathology, such as polycystic ovarian syndrome, hypothalamic amenorrhea, or bleeding disorders. In addition, hormonal management in the absence of intrinsic abnormality may actually cause abnormal bleeding patterns. For these reasons, a clear understanding of normal parameters for menstrual cycling is important because it will help prevent inappropriate treatment as well as aid in identification of abnormal patterns that do require further investigation and treatment.

REFERENCES

1. Haubrich WS. Medical Meanings, 2nd ed. Philadelphia: American College of Physicians; 2003:144.

2. Vollman RF. The Menstrual Cycle, vol 7. Philadelphia: WB Saunders; 1977.

3. Treloar AE, Boynton RE, Behn BG, Brown BW. Variation of the human menstrual cycle through reproductive life. Int J Fertil. 1967;12:77-126.

4. Magyar DM, Boyers SP, Marshall JR, Abraham GE. Regular menstrual cycles and premenstrual molimina as indicators of ovulation. Obstet Gynecol. 1979;53:411-4.

5. Palter SF, Olive DL. Reproductive physiology. In: Berek JS, ed. Novak's Gynecology. Baltimore: Williams & Wilkins; 1996:149-72.

6. Speroff L, Glass RH, Kase NG. Clinical Gynecology, Endocrinology and Infertility, 6th ed. Baltimore: Williams and Wilkins; 1999.

7. Marshall WA, Tanner JM. Variations in pattern of pubertal changes in girls. Arch Dis Child. 1969;44:291-303.

8. Herman-Giddens ME, Slora EJ, Wasserman RC, et al. Secondary sexual characteristics and menses in young girls seen in office practice: a study from the Pediatric Research in Office Settings network. Pediatrics. 1997;99:505-12.

9. Wyshak G, Frisch RE. Evidence for a secular trend in age of menarche. N Eng J Med. 1984;306:1033-5.

10. MacMahon B. Age of Menarche: United States, 1973. Hyattsville, MD: National Center for Health Statistics, 1974.

11. Zacharias L, Rand WM, Wurtman RJ. A prospective study of sexual development and growth in American girls: the statistics of menarche. Obstet Gynecol Surv. 1976;31: 325-37.

12. Mansfield MJ, Emans SJ. Adolescent menstrual irregularity. J Reprod Med. 1984;29: 399-410.

13. Frank D, Williams T. Attitudes about menstration among fifth-, sixth-, and seventh-grade pre- and post-menarchal girls. J Sch Nurs. 1999;15:25-31.

14. Borsos A, Lampe L, Balogh A, et al. Ovarian function after the menarche and hormonal contraception. Int J Gynaecol Obstet. 1988;27:249-53.

15. Speroff L, Glass RH, Kase NG. Clinical Gynecology, Endocrinology and Infertility, 6th ed. Baltimore: Williams and Wilkins; 1994.

16. World Health Organization multicenter study on menstrual and ovulatory patterns in adolescent girls. II. Longitudinal study of menstrual patterns in the early postmenarcheal period, duration of bleeding episodes and menstrual cycles. World Health Organization Task Force on Adolescent Reproductive Health. J Adolesc Health Care. 1986; 7:236-44.

17. Root AW. Precocious puberty. Pediatr Rev. 2000;21:10-9.

18. Herman-Giddens ME, Slore EJ, Wasserman RC, et al. Secondary sexual characteristics and menses in young girls seen in office practice: a study from the Pediatric Research in Office Settings network. Pediatrics. 1997;99:505-12.

19. Apter D, Vihko R. Early menarche, a risk factor for breast cancer, indicates early onset of ovulatory cycles. J Clin Endocrinol Metab. 1983;57:82-6.

20. Vihko R, Apter D. Endocrine characteristics of adolescent menstrual cycles: impact of early menarche. J Steroid Biochem. 1984;20:231-6.

21. Chimbira TH, Anderson ABM. Relation between measured menstrual blood loss and patient's subjective assessment of loss, duration of bleeding, number of sanitary towels used, uterine weight and endometrial surface area. Br J Obstet Gynaecol. 1980;87:603-9.

22. Bevan JA, Maloney KW, Hillery CA, et al. Bleeding disorders: a common cause of menorrhagia in adolescents. J Pediatr. 2001;138:856-61.

23. Claessens E, Cowell CA. Acute adolescent menorrhagia. Am J Obstet Gynecol. 1981;139:277.

24. Flug D, Largo RH, Prader A. Menstrual patterns in adolescent Swiss girls: a longitudinal study. Ann Hum Biol. 1984;11:495-508.

25. Widholm O, Kantero RL. A statistical analysis of the menstrual patterns of 8,000 Finnish girls and their mothers. Acta Obstet Gynecol Scand Suppl. 1971;14:(Suppl): 1-36.

26. Munster K, Schmidt L, Helm P. Length and variation in the menstrual cycle: a cross sectional study from a Danish county. Br J Obstet Gynaecol. 1992;99:422.

27. Dorland's Illustrated Medical Dictionary, 29th ed. Philadelphia: WB Saunders; 2000.

28. Hallberg L, Hogdahl A, Nilsson L, Rybo G. Menstrual blood-loss: a population study. Acta Obstet Gynecol Scand. 1966;45:320-51.

29. Dorland's Illustrated Medical Dictionary, 24th ed. Philadelphia: WB Saunders; 1964.

30. Gold E, Bromberger J, Crawford S, et al. Factors associated with age at natural menopause in a multiethnic sample of midlife women. Am J Epidemiol. 2001;153:865-74.

31. McKinlay SM, Bifano NL, McKinlay JB. Smoking and age at menopause in women. Ann Intern Med. 1985;103:350-6.

32. American Society for Reproductive Medicine. The Menopausal Transition: A Practice Committee Report. December 2001.

33. Soules M, Sherman S, Parrott E, et al. Executive summary: Stages of Reproductive Aging Workshop (STRAW). Fertil Steril. 2001;76:874-8.

34. Shideler S, De VG, Kalra P, Benirschke K, Lasley B. Ovarian-pituitary hormone interactions during the perimenopause. Maturitas. 1989;11:331-9.

35. Santoro N, Brown J, Adel T, Skurnick J. Characterization of reproductive hormonal dynamics in the perimenopause. J Clin Endocrinol Metab. 1996;81:1495-501.

36. Guthrie J, Dennerstein L, Hopper J, Burger H. Hot flushes, menstrual status, and hormone levels in a population-based sample of midlife women. Obstet Gynecol. 1996; 88:437-42.

Common Menstrual Complaints

2

Abnormal Uterine Bleeding

Matthew K. Hoffman, MD, MPH

A bnormal uterine bleeding affects approximately 10 million US women and accounts for almost one third of all outpatient gynecologic visits; it is the most common reason for a gynecologic visit amongst adolescents (1-4). The failure of regular menstrual cycles to occur can cause patient anxiety, social inconvenience, and sexual dysfunction. Moreover, menstrual irregularities can result in anemia and be harbingers of other serious medical conditions. It is therefore important for providers to understand the causes, evaluation, and treatment of abnormal bleeding.

Clinical observation and scientific investigation have suggested normative values for cycle interval, flow duration, and amount of menstrual blood loss for the typical ovulatory menstrual cycle. Treloar examined more than 25,000 woman years of data for over 2700 women, and Vollman reported more than 30,000 cycles recorded by 650 women. Normative parameters derived from these studies are presented in Table 2-1 (5,6).

Despite the objectivity of these definitions, volume measurements of flow are impractical. Moreover, patient perception of these characteristics remains highly variable. As many as 15% of women with a menstrual blood loss of less than 20 mL per cycle will report their cycles as excessively heavy. In contrast, a third of women with a cycle menstrual blood loss of more than 80 mL will describe their cycles as light or moderate (7-9). Although these definitions of normal and abnormal are helpful, it remains the patient's perception of her menstrual symptoms which results in the physician visit and by which the success of treatment is measured. To help better define a patient's menstrual complaints, special terminology has been developed (Table 2-2) (10).

A woman's age remains the most predictive factor for developing menstrual cycle dysfunction. Longitudinal studies have shown that women at the extremes

Table 2-1   Normative Menstrual Cycle Characteristics

Characteristic	Normal	Abnormal
Cycle interval	24-35 days	<21 days or >45 days in teens <21 days or >35 days in adults
Flow duration	4-6 days	<3 days or >7 days
Menstrual blood loss	30 mL	>80 mL

Table 2-2   Menstrual Terminology

Term	Cycle Length	Flow Duration	Amount of Blood Loss
Menorrhagia	Normal	Normal	Increased
Metrorrhagia	Irregular	Normal	Normal
Menometrorrhagia	Irregular	Variable	Increased
Polymenorrhea	<24 days	Normal	Normal
Oligomenorrhea	Increased	Normal	Variable
Amenorrhea	Increased >90 days	None	None

of reproductive age have the highest incidence of menstrual disturbances. The cycle interval tends to be more variable in the immediate 5-7 years following menarche and the 5-8 years preceding menopause. Nonetheless, 20% of women of reproductive years will experience menstrual irregularities (10).

Etiology

Abnormal uterine bleeding can herald systemic diseases and pathologic conditions. The likelihood of these conditions is similarly related to a patient's age. The following discussion presents the most common causes of abnormal uterine bleeding based on age (Table 2-3).

Birth to Menarche

Birth to First Week of Life
Uterine bleeding in newborn girls in the 2-3 days immediately after birth is exclusively the result of estrogen withdrawal of maternal estrogens. Evaluation of this condition consists solely of examination and reassurance (11,12), which should be provided by the clinicians caring for both mother and baby before discharge from the hospital.

Table 2-3   Most Common Causes of Abnormal Uterine Bleeding by Age

Birth to Menarche	Perimenarchal Adolescent	Reproductive Age	Perimenopausal	Postmenopausal
• Estrogen withdrawal • Foreign body • Infection • Genital tumors • Precocious puberty • Urethral prolapse • Trauma	• Hypothalamic immaturity • Blood dyscrasia • Inadequate luteal function • Anorexia/bulimia • Polycystic ovary syndrome	• Anovulation • Blood dyscrasia • Luteal dysfunction • Pregnancy • Contraceptive use • Uterine infection/polyps/fibroids/cancer	• Uterine infection/polyps • Fibroids/cancer • Hormone replacement therapy	• Atrophic vaginitis • Uterine infection/polyps/fibroids/cancer

From Smith RP, ed. Clinical Management of Abnormal Uterine Bleeding. Educational Series on Women's Health Issues. Boston: Jesperson & Associates; 2002; with permission.

First Week of Life to Menarche

After the first week of life, vaginal bleeding is a rare complaint. In a review series of 52 patients in a referral center, 21% of the children were found to have a neoplasm as the underlying cause of their bleeding. An additional 21% had bleeding due to isosexual precocious puberty (13). Although the incidences of neoplasm and isosexual precocious puberty are probably over-reported in that review, these important diagnoses need to be excluded as part of the evaluation of this age group. The most common cause of bleeding in prepubertal girls is vulvovaginitis. Trauma, including that caused by sexual abuse, must also be ruled out. As such, a complete examination by a provider who is experienced in pediatric gynecology is warranted.

Perimenarchal Adolescent (Approximately 8-15 Years of Age)

Puberty represents the development of secondary sexual characteristics in response to hormonal changes to prepare the body for possible pregnancy. The development of secondary sexual characteristics occur in a coordinated fashion. Breast development (thelarche) is the first sign in most girls, usually followed by pubic hair development (adrenarche), and then menarche. Whether breasts or pubic hair develops first may vary by race, with African American girls more likely to experience adrenarche before thelarche. Irregular cycles during the first 2 years following menarche is a common event, although wildly chaotic cycles are neither common nor should they be dismissed as normal. The immature hypothalamic pituitary ovarian axis is incapable of responding to estrogen with a luteinizing hormone surge. As the axis matures, regular periods will ensue (typically within 2-3 years of menarche). Cycles during this transition are typically within the parameters of 21-45 days. Bleeding less frequently than every 90 days is distinctly uncommon and should be evaluated.

Although irregular menstruation due to an immature pituitary axis is common in adolescents, it is essential that a clinician consider other secondary causes. For every patient, an examination should be performed and a pregnancy test obtained. Though often ignored by clinicians, hyperandrogenism can be found in almost one third of adolescents presenting with irregular menstruation. The evaluation of these patients should also include consideration of polycystic ovarian disease and coagulopathies (14,15). Given the associated co-morbidities, one must also consider bulimia and anorexia in the differential diagnosis. Even normal-weight girls with bulimia often have anovulatory cycles. Anorexia nervosa is an important cause of infrequent scanty periods and amenorrhea. Another comon cause of infrequent cycles in adolescents is exercise-induced amenorrhea.

An underlying coagulopathy is commonly found in adolescents presenting with menorrhagia. These adolescents typically present with regular but heavy bleeding. In one study of adolescents presenting to an emergency room with excessive uterine bleeding, 19% were found to have an underlying coagulation disorder. Of those with a hemoglobin of less than 10 g/dL, 25% were diagnosed with a bleeding disorder, and 50% of adolescents who were hospitalized for vaginal bleeding had an underlying coagulopathy (16). If an evaluation by history, physical examination, and laboratory studies does not reveal an underlying disorder and the bleeding is not clinically significant (as evidenced by a normal CBC), appropriate treatment should include reassurance and consideration of beginning a combination hormonal contraceptive for cycle control.

Women of Reproductive Age (Menarche to Perimenopause)

This category is the largest group of women presenting with the complaint of abnormal uterine bleeding. Although differential diagnosis is extensive, it should be remembered that among women of menstrual age up to 80% of those with abnormal uterine bleeding do not have an anatomic cause for their bleeding (11). Historically women without an anatomic or pathologic cause of their bleeding have been given the diagnosis of *dysfunctional uterine bleeding*. Because the majority of these cases have anovulation as an underlying root cause, the American College of Obstetricians and Gynecologists (ACOG) has recommended that the more descriptive term *anovulatory uterine bleeding* be used (11). Nonetheless, this diagnosis can only be conferred once other causes of menstrual irregularities have been eliminated.

Anovulatory Uterine Bleeding

Anovulatory bleeding can further be subdivided into three fundamental categories (17):

- Bleeding due to estrogen withdrawal
- Bleeding due to estrogen breakthrough
- Bleeding due to progesterone breakthrough

Bleeding due to estrogen withdrawal occurs because of declining levels of estrogen. This condition can occur as a result of the normal menstrual cycle when estrogen levels will typically dip during the time of ovulation. This will typically manifest itself as spotting around the time of ovulation (day 14). Other iatrogenic causes of bleeding due to estrogen withdrawal include cessation of hormonal treatment and bilateral oophorectomy.

Bleeding due to estrogen breakthrough is the result of chronic unopposed estrogen stimulation of the endometrium. This is the most common cause of anovulatory uterine bleeding. It is the type of bleeding that many women experience with the onset of menarche, the perimenopausal period, obesity, and polycystic ovarian syndrome. Without the effects of progesterone to cause the endometrium to mature and slough at a predictable interval, the endometrium will continue to proliferate. Ultimately this growth outstrips the structural support of the endometrial lining, causing unpredictable bleeding, with variable intervals between bleeding episodes and variation in amount of blood flow. Many of the patients will only experience uterine bleeding several times a year.

Progesterone breakthrough bleeding is the result of a relatively high progesterone-to-estrogen ratio. Such conditions do not occur naturally but are commonly seen in clinical practice with the use of the progestin-only pill and Depo-Provera. In the setting of a progestin-dominant environment, the endometrium becomes thin and atrophic. Typically this will result in irregular spotting until the endometrium completely atrophies.

Bleeding Due to Anatomic Lesions

Anatomic lesions cause bleeding in 20% of women. Several common anatomic causes of abnormal bleeding include uterine leiomyomas and endometrial and endocervical polyps. It is teleologically appealing to assume that anatomic lesions are associated with unpredictable bleeding because they are assumed not to be under hormonal control. Clinical studies have, however, consistently demonstrated that the most common complaint amongst women with leiomyomas and endometrial polyps is menorrhagia, not abnormal cycle intervals. This may represent the fact that fibroids and endometrial polyps can be found in a high percentage of asymptomatic women and therefore may not be the true underlying cause of the bleeding in women with such lesions. Post-coital bleeding is frequently associated with endocervical polyps.

Endocervical polyps are found in approximately 4% of gynecologic patients, particularly amongst multiparous women in their 40s and 50s (18). The cause of endocervical polyps is uncertain, but they are felt to occur in response to local irritation. Similarly, endometrial polyps are common findings, occurring in 20%-25% of reproductive women, with a peak incidence in women in their 40s (19). Endometrial polyps can range from a few millimeters to several centimeters and occasionally will prolapse through the cervix. Uterine fibroids occur in the majority of women, yet only 20%-40% ultimately result in symptoms. Treatment should be tailored towards resolution of the symptoms.

Perimenopause to Menopause

Although menopause represents the cessation of menses due to follicular exhaustion, it has been well recognized that before this event women will commonly go through a period of irregular menstruation referred to as the *perimenopause*. Due to the smaller number of follicles and their accelerated depletion, feedback inhibition to the pituitary is erratic and in turn menstrual irregularities develop. Clinically, this presents on average at age 46, lasts 5 years, and is often accompanied by other menopausal symptoms.

Unfortunately, the diagnosis of perimenopause remains a clinical diagnosis that can only reliably be made following the onset of menopause. Although evaluation of FSH is appropriate to rule out hypergonadotrophic hypogonadism, perimenopause cannot be diagnosed through laboratory evaluation. Similarly, evaluation of the endometrium is imperative to rule out significant pathology. (See Chapter 4 for further discussion.)

Postmenopause

Postmenopausal bleeding requires a thorough and prompt evaluation due to its co-association with endometrial carcinoma and endometrial hyperplasia. Among women with endometrial carcinoma, 90% will present with the complaint of abnormal or, more commonly, postmenopausal bleeding (20). Many studies have demonstrated that obesity, unopposed estrogen, and diabetes are risk factors for endometrial carcinoma. It is important to remember that exclusion of these risk factors does not exclude uterine cancer. In a study of Italian women with endometrial carcinoma, only half had an identifiable risk factor (21). Similarly, a family history of breast and colon cancer are important to elicit because these malignancies are known to co-occur (21). After a thorough evaluation, however, the most common diagnosis remains benign, such as endometrial atrophy and atrophic vaginitis. It is thus imperative that the practitioner is able to recognize the sundry causes of postmenopausal bleeding.

Few longitudinal studies have been done of the frequency of post-menopausal bleeding. In a study of 271 postmenopausal Danish women, 10.7% self-reported postmenopausal bleeding. This symptom occurred much more frequently in women who were newly postmenopausal (41%), followed by women who were more than 3 years postmenopausal (4%) (22).

In a recent study of 457 women with genital causes of bleeding who underwent histologic evaluation of the endometrium, the most common causes of bleeding were atrophy (50%), endometrial hyperplasia (10%), endometrial adenocarcinoma (8%), endometrial polyps (9%), cervical carcinoma (1%), and other causes (23).

Evaluation of Abnormal Bleeding

History

When taking a history from a woman with abnormal bleeding, there are several aspects of general and reproductive health that should be addressed. It is important to explore whether the bleeding is indeed genital in origin and rule out other sites of bleeding such as the gastrointestinal or urinary tracts (24). A history of hepatic, renal, autoimmune, vasculitic, and endocrine disease should be sought. The patient's age provides a great deal of information as to the possible causes. Symptoms of other medical conditions that can affect the menstrual cycle should be elicited (e.g., diabetes, obesity, thyroid disorders). For instance, hypothyroid patients generally report menorrhagia and hyper-thyroid patients may occasionally report amenorrhea.

A detailed menstrual history is a central element to the evaluation of abnormal bleeding. Information regarding the onset, duration, pattern, and quantity of bleeding should be obtained. Associated symptoms and interference with daily activities should be elicited. The possibility of pregnancy needs to be addressed before other diagnoses are considered.

It is imperative to explore when the abnormal uterine bleeding began and establish whether the patient has ever had a normal menstrual cycle. Ovulatory status may be clarified through history of moliminal symptoms (breast tenderness, bloating, etc.). One needs to inquire about any evidence of bleeding tendency in the patient and her relatives, particularly bleeding associated with surgical procedures. The patient should be asked about epistaxis, gum bleeding, and bruising. While they are seldom asymptomatic, clotting disorders can remain undiagnosed until the perimenopausal years. In one study of women with menorrhagia in whom no cause was found, 17% were found to have an inherited bleeding disorder that had remained undiagnosed; roughly half of these women were 40 years of age or older. Of these, von Willebrand's

disease was the most common, occurring in 13% of the women, with no difference in prevalence between women above and below 40 years of age (25).

Other elements of the history can be useful in looking for anatomic causes.
A history of post-coital bleeding suggests a cervical cause such as an endocervical polyp, ectropion, or cervical carcinoma. Intermenstrual bleeding has
been suggested as a marker of an anatomic cause. Despite the logical appeal
of this argument, objective studies of bleeding patterns have failed to corrob-
orate this. In fact, the most common complaint among women with anatomic
causes is menorrhagia.

Exclusion of Pregnancy

Complications of pregnancy remain an extremely common cause of abnormal
uterine bleeding, particularly among adolescents and women of reproductive
age. Moreover, it has long been recognized that many pregnancies detected by
urine beta-human chorionic gonadotropin (β-HCG) are not clinically recognized by women (26).

The mainstay of detection of pregnancy has become the urine β-HCG.
These tests will typically (98%) become positive 7 days after ovulation (27).
Presence of a negative urine β-HCG virtually excludes pregnancy. Additionally, age should be used with caution to eliminate the possibility of pregnancy.
Spontaneous pregnancies have been reported in women in early adolescence
and into the mid-fifties. The presence of menstruation suggests the possibility
of ovulation and in turn the potential for pregnancy. Particularly among adolescents, a pregnancy test should be performed when abnormal bleeding
occurs, even if sexual activity is denied; young women may not feel comfortable divulging this information, and the consequences of missing the diagnosis are too high.

Physical Examination

A complete physical examination is important to verify the source of bleeding,
assess the findings of acute or chronic blood loss, identify any genital pathology
that can be detectable on exam, and look for systemic diseases that might be
responsible for the clinical complaint. Vital signs, including orthostatic
changes, can provide an indication of hemodynamic state and consequences of
anemia and may shed light on the thyroid status. A skin evaluation may provide some useful clues such as hirsutism or acanthosis nigricans (suggestive
of polycystic ovarian syndrome), pallor, petechiae, or bruising. The thyroid
gland should be carefully examined and signs of thyroid dysfunction observed.

Pelvic examination should include visual inspection of the vulva to evaluate
for any lesions which may be the nidus of the bleeding. Similarly, a speculum

examination must be performed to determine the source and cause of bleeding. Testing for chlamydia and gonorrhea are imperative in sexually active women under the age of 25 or in those at high risk for sexually transmitted diseases (28). A Pap smear is useful in screening for cervical malignancy. If a cervical lesion or mass is grossly noted, biopsy or excision of the lesion should be incorporated into the evaluation. It is not uncommon for endometrial polyps, uterine fibroids, and sarcomas to present as a mass protruding through the cervix. Broad-based or highly vascular lesions may require excision in an operating room by a gynecologist; however, most lesions can be safely and simply removed by twisting. Similarly, this should be accompanied by a bimanual examination to assess the size and contour of the uterus. Women with an enlarged uterus should be suspected of having adenomyosis or fibroids.

Diagnostic Testing

Pap Smear

The Pap smear is specifically designed for examination of a squamous lesion of the ectocervix. Its use is therefore a critical part of examining women with abnormal bleeding. It should be remembered that the Pap smear is a screening test for cervical cancer with a false-negative rate that can approach 20% (29). Thus, if the cervix appears or feels grossly abnormal a cervical biopsy and/or endocervical curettage should be performed.

Although designed to screen for cervical cancer, studies have consistently demonstrated that women with endometrial carcinoma will commonly have a Pap smear demonstrating either endometrial carcinoma or atypical glandular lesions of undetermined significance. Using these criteria, the sensitivity of the Pap smear approaches 50% for endometrial cancer and may be higher with liquid-based cytology (30,31). Given the relative insensitivity of this test in comparison to other methods of endometrial evaluation, more definitive and directed endometrial evaluation is required in women at risk.

BENIGN ENDOMETRIAL CELLS ON POSTMENOPAUSAL PAP SMEAR

In 2001, the Bethesda system of Pap smear classification system recommended that benign endometrial cells be reported in women who are over the age of 40. This finding was felt to represent a surrogate for irregular bleeding depending on the woman's hormonal status and portion of the menstrual cycle when the smear was obtained (32). Despite the universality of this recommendation, the clinical significance of this finding remains controversial and unclear. In a meta-analysis by Mount et al, it was found that 1.1% of postmenopausal women had this finding and that the minority had actual endometrial pathology (33). In this series, 5.2% of women with this finding had underlying endometrial pathology (hyperplasia, polyps, carcinoma). It is interesting to note that amongst the women with endometrial carcinoma all but one (who did not report her symptoms) had either postmenopausal spotting or bleeding. It is this finding that has brought into question the clinical utility of reporting benign endometrial cells on routine Pap smears.

ATYPICAL GLANDULAR CELLS

In conformity with the 2001 Bethesda system, the cytologic findings of both squamous and glandular abnormalities are to be reported. These glandular abnormalities are categorized as "atypical glandular cells, either endocervical, endometrial, or 'glandular cells' not otherwise specified (AGC NOS); atypical glandular cells, either endocervical or 'glandular cells' favor neoplasia (AGC 'favor neoplasia'); and endocervical adenocarcinoma in situ (AIS)" (34). Amongst all three of these groups, significant numbers of both premalignant disease and existing cancer are found. It is thus imperative that these women undergo immediate colposcopy; additionally, if they are over the age of 35, have atypical endometrial cells, or have a history of unexplained vaginal bleeding, they should undergo endometrial evaluation. If this evaluation fails to yield an explanation of disease, it is recomended that women with AIS or AGC 'favor neoplasia' undergo excision of the cervix with cold-knife conization (34).

HISTIOCYTES ON POSTMENOPAUSAL PAP SMEAR

Histiocytes have in the past been viewed as a potential marker for endometrial pathology. This loose association has spurred providers to perform endometrial evaluation in otherwise asymptomatic women. More recent studies have demonstrated that there is little utility in this strategy (35-37). Amongst women who were found to have significant endometrial pathology when their Pap smear showed histiocytes, almost all had symptoms of either postmenopausal bleeding or atypical glandular cells on Pap smear. Thus women with histiocytes on their Pap smears without other abnormalities or history of postmenopausal bleeding should not undergo endometrial evaluation.

Endometrial Evaluation

The need to undergo endometrial evaluation is contingent upon patient age and duration of symptoms. Most cases of endometrial carcinoma arise due to unopposed estrogen for a prolonged period of time. Although age greater than 35 serves as a marker for this duration of exposure (Fig. 2-1), cases of endometrial carcinoma and hyperplasia have been detected in women in their teens and 20s (38). These case reports are consistent in that they include women who are obese and/or have a history of chronic anovulation for 2 to 3 years. Thus, an evaluation of the endometrium must be undertaken in all women over the age of 35, those who have failed hormonal therapy, or

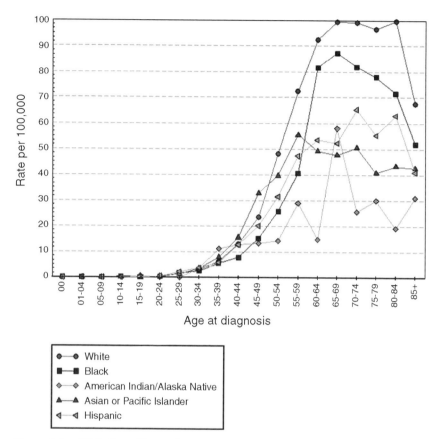

Figure 2-1   SEER (Surveillance, Epidemiology, and End Results Program) crude incidence rates of endometrial carcinoma and hyperplasia by race.

those who have a history of prolonged chronic anovulation or unopposed estrogen exposure (39).

The method of evaluation partly depends on the practitioner's experience and skills. Methods to evaluate the endometrium include endometrial sampling using a piston suction device, ultrasonography, sono-hysterography, and D&C with hysteroscopy. Each of these methods has its own utility and limitations. A comparison of the different methods is presented in Table 2-4.

PISTON SUCTION DEVICES

Piston suction devices have gained popularity because of their ease of use, relative safety, tolerability, and low cost. The fundamental technique involves threading a thin flexible catheter through the cervix using a speculum and then applying suction. To sample the endometrium the device needs to be

Table 2-4   Comparison of Endometrial Assessment Technologies

Assessment Technology	Sensitivity for Endometrial Cancer/Hyperplasia	Sensitivity for Benign Disease	Specificity	Technically Unable
Endometrial biopsy	83-100%	44.6-51%	98.5-100	4-10%
Ultrasound for endometrial stripe	94-96%	23.5-60%	60%	10%
Sonohysterography	94-100%	96-100%	66-80%	1%
D&C/Hysteroscopy	97-98%	97-98%	93-100	0%

From Smith RP, ed. Clinical Management of Abnormal Uterine Bleeding. Educational Series on Women's Health Issues. Boston: Jesperson & Associates; 2002; and Cooper J. Contemporary Management of Abnormal Uterine Bleeding. Obstet Gynecol Clin North Am. 2000;27:xi-xiii; with permission.

inserted through the internal cervical os, which for most women is at least 4 cm deep. Commonly a small amount of resistance is encountered at this point, which is usually resolved with either gentle pressure or by using a single-tooth tenaculum on the anterior cervical os to straighten the curvature of the cervix. Failure to go beyond the internal cervical os will result in an inadequate sample. (Air should not be introduced into the uterus.) The device is then withdrawn from the uterus, obtaining a tissue sample.

There are many piston suction products (Pipelle, Tis-U-trap, Novak curette, etc.), all of which have similar effectiveness (11). Complications from these devices can include cervical stenosis (4%-10%), intrauterine infection (approximately 1 per 500), and uterine perforation (approximately 1 per 2000) (1). The limitation of these devices are that they only sample the minority (4.5%-15%) of the endometrial cavity (11). Despite this limitation, their ability to detect endometrial carcinoma remains very good, ranging from 84% to 100% (1). Failure to detect these lesions is often associated with the carcinoma having a small surface area or being located within an endometrial polyp. Thus, persistent symptoms or an inadequate biopsy require additional investigation (40). Although exclusion of endometrial carcinoma and atypical hyperplasia is clearly the primary objective, evaluation of benign disease remains the more common clinical situation. Unfortunately, these devices are limited in their ability to detect other diseases (44.6% and 51%) (1).

If an inadequate sample is obtained, this cannot be seen as a sign of atrophy. Farrell et al, in a study of 141 cases of "insufficient" sample on initial Pippelle biopsy, found that 20% of the samples on further evaluation had significant uterine pathology, including four cases of cancer (40). Other authors have found significant pathology in almost half of all women with an insufficient sample (41). It would thus seem prudent to pursue futher workup in cases of insufficient biopsy.

ULTRASONOGRAPHY AND SONOHYSTEROGRAPHY

The use of ultrasonography to determine the endometrial thickness in the evaluation of postmenopausal bleeding for the exclusion of endometrial carcinoma has become a well-accepted technique. It has the advantages of being inexpensive and noninvasive. Moreover, uterine fibroids are easily visualized, although whether they impinge upon the endometrial cavity causing bleeding is less clear (42). If the endometrial thickness is less than 5 mm in the postmenopausal woman, one can be 96% certain that endometrial carcinoma is excluded (43). The utility of this technique has been extended to menstruating women by performing the ultrasound during the 4th, 5th, or 6th day of a woman's cycle (44). If a woman's stripe is greater than or equal to 5 mm or unable to be visualized, the patient will require further evaluation. The diagnostic accuracy of transvaginal ultrasound to detect endometrial polyps and submucous fibroids is limited (45,46). Another limitation of this technique is that approximately 10% of women have an inadequate study, which limits applicability (1).

Sonohysterography consists of injecting normal saline into the uterine cavity as an adjunct to transvaginal sonography. By providing a contrast media one can delineate other intrauterine pathology such as polyps and or submucous fibroids. This technique is performed by placing a catheter transcervically and injecting small amounts of normal saline. A transvaginal ultrasound is performed simultaneously. Because of the invasive nature of this procedure, it should not be used in women who are potentially pregnant or have cervical/uterine infections (47). Using sonohysterography, the ability to detect focal lesions is comparable to that of hysteroscopy (46). Moreover, this technique can be used to make a technically unsatisfactory measurement of endometrial stripe satisfactory. Several caveats should be remembered. The value of this technology remains in its negative predictive value. That is to say, if a focal lesion is detected or an endometrial thickness greater than 4 mm is noted, the patient still requires an invasive procedure for complete evaluation. Moreover, in women with a large uterus or stenotic cervix this technique may not be feasible (48). Similarly, success with performing this technique is greater in premenopausal women than in postmenopausal women (49).

D&C WITH HYSTEROSCOPY

D&C has long been held as the "gold standard" in the evaluation of abnormal uterine bleeding; more recently, direct visualization with hysteroscopy has refined the technique. Without the benefits of hysteroscopy, D&C has been shown to detect only 62.5% of intrauterine disorders (1). This D&C with hysteroscopy couples direct visualization of focal lesions with histologic sampling. Additionally, it can be therapeutic if a focal lesion is removed or an endometrial ablation is performed. If neither a focal lesion is resected nor an endometrial ablation performed, the procedure should be regarded as diagnostic. Further treatment will then be predicated upon the histology obtained. Although still performed in the operating room for the majority of patients, office hysteroscopy using different instrumentation can be well tolerated and is associated with minimal complications.

Other Laboratory Testing

COMPLETE BLOOD COUNT

Complete blood count is always indicated in a woman with complaints of abnormal uterine bleeding. This will also allow the detection of platelet disorders and consideration of whether an existing anemia is microcytic or macrocytic.

THYROID TESTING

It has long been known that thyroid disease can be associated with menstrual irregularities. Hypothyroid patients tend to report menorrhagia and hyperthyroid patients amenorrhea. Clinical guidelines for when to initiate routine screening remain conflicted, and few studies have specifically looked at the cost effectiveness of thyroid screening in otherwise asymptomatic women with abnormal uterine bleeding. Clearly, in women who are symptomatic or have physical evidence of thyroid disease, screening with a TSH remains appropriate. In women over the age of 40, almost 10% of women with menstrual irregularities will have a form of thyroid dysfunction (50). Whether successful treatment of these women results in return to normal menstrual function remains unclear. Nonetheless, based upon these data, it is probably reasonable to consider screening asymptomatic women with menstrual disorders over the age of 40.

STUDIES OF COAGULATION

The ACOG has suggested that evaluation for von Willebrand's disease be considered in the following groups of women: adolescents with severe menorrhagia, women with significant menorrhagia with no other defined cause, and women who are to undergo hysterectomy for menorrhagia (25). It should be remembered that many women with an inherited coagulopathy are not diagnosed until perimenopause or later.

Treatment

General Principles

Once an appropriate evaluation has been completed, treatment should be geared towards control of acute bleeding, prevention of future abnormal cycles, and reducing the risk of endometrial hyperplasia/carcinoma. Medical management remains the first line of therapy assuming anatomic causes are not found. Surgical management is reserved for those patients with anatomic causes or for whom medical management has failed. It is important to weigh each patient's desire for cycle control, contraceptive needs, and medical risks and benefits in selecting the optimal therapy. Women with abnormal uterine bleeding may experience substantial anemia and may benefit from iron supplementation. Occasionally, bleeding may become heavy enough that hospitalization and/or transfusion are required.

Ovulating Patients with Menorrhagia

Patients who ovulate with menorrhagia often benefit from non-steroidal anti-inflammatory drugs (NSAIDs) (51). NSAIDs favorably affect prostaglandins, which play an important role in vasoconstriction and platelet aggregation in the endometrium. By altering these prostaglandins, NSAIDs have been shown to effectively decrease the amount of menstrual bleeding by up to 40%. Among the NSAIDs, mefenamic acid, ibuprofen, naproxen, and indomethacin have been shown to be effective in treating women with menorrhagia (52). Combination oral contraceptives, continuous progesterone as administered through Depo-Provera, and progesterone-containing IUD are also effective options.

Antifibrinolytics, such as tranexamic acid, have been shown more effective than NSAIDs in reducing blood loss (50% decrease versus approximately 20% decrease) (53-55). Nonetheless, antifibrinolytics are not available in the United States.

Anovulatory Uterine Bleeding

Women with anovulatory bleeding require periodic progestin administration to prevent the endometrium from developing hyperplasia. Progestins may be administered as cyclic oral norethindrone/medroxyprogesterone acetate, combination oral contraceptive, or via a levonorgestrel-containing intra-uterine device (IUD). Although cyclical progestin administration is useful for anovulatory bleeding, such regimens have actually been shown to worsen vaginal bleeding in ovulatory women (53,56,57). Various dosages and durations of cyclic protestins have been suggested. Recently, a review indicated that progestin therapy was most effective when given for at least 21 days per month. Alternatively, progestin-containing IUDs provide daily progesterone exposure and are associated with an 85% reduction of blood loss (57,61). Oral contraceptives are the most commonly prescribed form of progestin medication for anovulatory bleeding. These have the advantage of providing effective contraception, and their use may be extended safely to the perimenopausal patient if she is a non-smoker and has no contraindications to oral contraceptives.

To control acute vaginal bleeding, oral contraceptive pills are a very effective option. Traditionally, these are given in a high dose to provide acute estrogenic support to the endometrium. One popular regimen is to give a 30-µg pill three times a day for 3 days, twice a day for 2 days, then daily.

If medical treatment fails, surgical treatment is appropriate. In considering the different options, one should keep in mind that an abnormal bleeding problem will generally resolve when a woman reaches menopause. Surgical options include endometrial ablation, uterine artery embolization, and hysterectomy. Therapy should be individualized depending on the risk-benefit ratio and patient-specific characteristics. The patient should be referred to a gynecologist for surgical assessment.

Bleeding Due to Anatomic Causes or Failed Medical Therapy

The procedural approach to patients with anatomic causes of uterine bleeding or who fail medical therapy is discussed at length in Chapter 11.

Endocervical Polyps

Standard treatment of endocervical polyps consists of simple excision by twisting and is generally therapeutic. If the lesion is broad-based or there is concern about risk for significant bleeding, surgery is appropriate. It is imperative that the specimen be sent for pathology because these lesions occasionally are endometrial in origin and can contain significant pathology. Rarely do they recur after removal.

Endometrial Polyps

Hysteroscopic resection or removal at the time of D&C are appropriate treatment options for women with endometrial polyps. Hysteroscopic resection is the preferred method because this allows complete visualization and excision of the polyp, particularly if the polyps are multiple. In symptomatic women, resolution of symptoms are seen in approximately 80% of cases (62,63).

Uterine Fibroids

The traditional resolution of hysterectomy is increasingly being challenged by more conservative modalities such as hysteroscopic resection, myomectomy, and uterine artery embolization. Short-term data suggest dramatic improvements in symptoms for the majority of women with these options; however, long-term data, including the need for subsequent surgery, are lacking.

Postmenopausal Bleeding

As with pre-menopausal bleeding, treatment should be guided by the previous evaluation. Several common and specific cases are discussed in the following sections.

Endometrial Hyperplasia

The risk associated with endometrial hyperplasia is clearly dependent upon the absence or presence of atypia. The finding of atypical hyperplasia carries a 25%-29% risk of ultimately developing endometrial carcinoma (64,65). In contrast, women with either simple or complex endometrial hyperplasia without atypia are much more likely to regress spontaneously (simple hyperplasia, 80%; complex hyperplasia, 79%) and have a very low risk of going on to develop endometrial carcinoma (1-3%) (66). Interestingly, the risk of endometrial carcinoma with atypical endometrial hyperplasia is further increased in elderly women (older than age 35, 11%; age 36-55, 12%; older than age 55, 28%) (67).

Women with hyperplasia without atypia can thus be managed by long-term follow up after D&C. If abnormal bleeding recurs, repeat endometrial sampling is warranted. Additionally, it is prudent to hormonally withdraw premenopausal women who are anovulatory with monthly Provera (10 mg for 10 days of each month), a progestin-containing IUD, or combination oral contraceptives.

In contrast, management of atypical endometrial hyperplasia is driven by the patient's age, medical condition, and desire to retain fertility. In young women who desire to retain fertility, it is appropriate to offer progestin therapy in the form of Provera (10 mg for 10 days of each month), Megace Provera (20-40 mg per day), a progestin-containing IUD, or combination oral contraceptives. If conservative medical management is to be considered, it must be accompanied by regular endometrial sampling of no longer than 6 months duration. Alternatively, definitive surgical treatment in the form of hysterectomy is appropriate for older women and those not desiring pregnancy due to the high risk of relapse and progression to endometrial carcinoma. These cases are best managed by a gynecologist comfortable with this group of patients.

Endometrial Carcinoma

Upon diagnosis of endometrial carcinoma, the patient should be referred to a gynecologist or gynecological oncologist capable of addressing the issue.

Treatment options include surgery, radiation, and/or hormonal therapy, but surgery has become the mainstay of treatment. Each option must be individualized to the patient's desires and medical condition.

Atrophy of the Endometrium

Treatment of atrophy remains a highly individualized choice. As a general rule endometrial atrophy will result in amenorrhea with time and no further intervention. The decision to initiate hormonal therapy should be predicated on the presence of symptomatic vaginal atrophy (discharge and dyspareunia) and desire for regular cycles versus watchful waiting. Women with a uterus require the addition of a progesterone and a discussion of the risks and benefits of hormone replacement therapy.

Recurrent Postmenopausal Bleeding

Because all investigative methods of postmenopausal bleeding can produce false-negatives, it is important to re-evaluate patients who experience recurrent postmenopausal bleeding. Few studies have specifically addressed the optimal method of re-evaluation, but D&C with hysteroscopy should be strongly considered. Some practitioners have advocated that hysterectomy be considered. The few studies examining re-evaluation have found high rates of benign pathology (45%) and variable rates of endometrial hyperplasia and carcinoma (0%-20%) (66,67). Thus the decision to proceed with hysterectomy must be highly individualized.

REFERENCES

1. Cooper J. Contemporary management of abnormal uterine bleeding. Obstet Gynecol Clin North Am. 2000;27:xi-xiii.
2. Awwad JT, Toth TL, Schiff I. Abnormal uterine bleeding in the perimenopause. Int J Fertil. 1993;38:261-9.
3. Demir SC, Kadayyfcy TO, Vardar MA, Atay Y. Dysfunctional uterine bleeding and other menstrual problems of secondary school students in Adana, Turkey. J Pediatr Adolesc Gynecol. 2000;13:171-5.
4. Deligerogloe D. Dysfunctional uterine bleeding. Ann N Y Acad Sci. 1997:816:158.
5. Treloar AE, Behn BG, Brown BW. Variation of the human menstrual cycle through reproductive life. Int J Fertil. 1967;12:77-126.
6. Vollman R. The degree of variability of the length of the menstrual cycle in correlation with age of woman. Gynaecologia. 1956; 142:310-4.
7. Cole SK, Thomson AM. Sources of variation in menstrual blood loss. J Obstet Gynaecol Br Commonw. 1973;78:933-9.
8. Fraser IS, Hutton B, Macey D. Endometrial blood flow measured by xenon-133 clearance in women with normal menstrual cycles and dysfunctional uterine bleeding. Am J Obstet Gynecol. 1987;156:158-66.

9. Haynes PJ, Anderson AB, Turnbull AC. Measurement of menstrual blood loss in patients complaining of menorrhagia. Br J Obstet Gynaecol. 1977;84:763-8.

10. Speroff L. Clinical Gynecologic Endocrinologic and Infertility, 6th ed. Baltimore: Williams & Wilkins; 1999.

11. Smith RP, ed. Clinical Management of Abnormal Uterine Bleeding. Educational Series on Women's Health Issues. Boston: Jespersen & Associates; 2002.

12. Sanfiippo JS, Dewhurst J, Lee PA. Pediatric and Adolescent Gynecology. Philadelphia: WB Saunders; 1994.

13. Hill NC, Morton KE. The aetiology of vaginal bleeding in children: a 20-year review. Br J Obstet Gynaecol. 1989;96:467-70.

14. Schwayder J. Pathophysiology of abnormal uterine bleeding. Obstet Gynecol Clin North Am. 2000;27:219-34.

15. Hilliard P. Menstruation in young girls: a clinical perspective. Obstet Gynecol. 2002;99: 655-62.

16. Claessens EA. Acute adolescent menorrhaghia. Am J Obstet Gynecol. 1981;139:277-80.

17. Schrager S. Abnormal uterine bleeding. Am Fam Physician. 1999;60:1371-82.

18. Farrar HK Jr. Benign tumors of the uterine cervix. Am J Obstet Gynecol. 1961;81:124-37.

19. Woodruff ENJ. Novak's Gynecologic and Obstetric Pathology with Clinical and Endocrine Relations, 8th ed. Philadelphia: WB Saunders; 1979.

20. Berek JS. Practical Gynecologic Oncology, 3rd ed. Philadelphia: Lippincott Williams & Wilkins; 1994.

21. Parazzini F, La Vecchia C, Bruzzi P, Decarli A. Population attributable risk for endometrial cancer in northern Italy. Eur J Cancer Clin Oncol. 1989;25:1451-6.

22. Astrup K. Frequency of spontaneously occurring postmenopausal bleeding in the general population. Acta Obstet Gynecol Scand. 2004;83:203-7.

23. Gredmark T, Havel G, Mattsson LA. Histopathological findings in women with postmenopausal bleeding. Br J Obstet Gynaecol. 1995;2:133-6.

24. Munro M. Abnormal uterine bleeding in the reproductive years. Part I: pathogenesis and clinical investigation. J Am Assoc Gynecol Laparosc. 1999;6:393-416.

25. Von Willebrand's Disease in Gynecologic Practice. ACOG Committee Opinion. 2001; Washington, DC.

26. Wilcox AJ, O'Connor JF, Baird DD, et al. Incidence of early loss of pregnancy. N Engl J Med. 1988;319:189-94.

27. Chard T. Pregnancy tests: a review. Hum Reprod. 1992;7:701-10.

28. Sexually transmitted diseases treatment guidelines. MMWR. 2002;51(RR-6):2.

29. Stenchever M, Herbst A, Mishell D. Comprehensive Gynecology, 4th ed. St. Louis: Mosby; 2001;869-98.

30. Gu M, Barakat RR, Thaler HT, Saigo PE. Pap smears in women with endometrial carcinoma. Acta Cytol. 2001;45:555-60.

31. Schorge JO, Hynan L, Ashfaq R. ThinPrep detection of cervical and endometrial adenocarcinoma: a retrospective cohort study. Cancer. 2002;96:338-43.

32. Solomon D, Kurman R, Moriarty A, et al. The 2001 Bethesda System: terminology for reporting results of cervical cytology. JAMA. 2002;287:2114-9.

33. Mount SL, Eltabbakh GH, Olmstead JI, Drejet AE. Significant increase of benign endometrial cells on Papanicolaou smears in women using hormone replacement therapy. Obstet Gynecol. 2002;100:445-50.

34. Wright TC Jr, Massad LS, Twiggs LB, Wilkinson EJ. ASCCP-Sponsored Consensus Conference. 2001 Consensus Guidelines for the management of women with cervical cytological abnormalities. JAMA. 2002;287:2120-9.

35. Nassar A, Nasuti JF. Value of histiocyte detection in Pap smears for predicting endometrial pathology: an institutional experience. Acta Cytol. 2003;47:762-7.

36. Wen P, Wang N, Knop N, et al. Significance of histiocytes on otherwise-normal cervical smears from postmenopausal women: a retrospective study of 108 cases. Acta Cytol. 2003;47:135-40.

37. Nguyen TN, Ferenczy A, Franco EL. Clinical significance of histiocytes in the detection of endometrial adenocarcinoma and hyperplasia. Diagn Cytopathol. 1998;19:89-93.

38. Ries LAG, Kosary CL, Hankey BF, et al. SEER Cancer Statistics Review, 1975-2000. National Cancer Institute: Bethesda, Maryland.

39. Management of Anovulatory Bleeding. ACOG Technical Bulletin. 2000;14.

40. Farrell T, Owen P, Baird A. The significance of an 'insufficient' Pipelle sample in the investigation of post-menopausal bleeding. Acta Obstet Gynecol Scand. 1999;78:810-2.

41. Gordon SJ. The incidence and management of failed Pipelle sampling in a general outpatient clinic. Aust N Z J Obstet Gynaecol. 1999;39:115-8.

42. Nanda S, Chadha N, Sen J, Sangwan K. Transvaginal sonography and saline infusion sonohysterography in the evaluation of abnormal uterine bleeding. Aust N Z J Obstet Gynaecol. 2002;42:530-4.

43. Smith-Bindman R, Kerlikowske K, Feldstein VA, et al. Endovaginal ultrasound to exclude endometrial cancer and other endometrial abnormalities. JAMA. 1998;280: 1510-7.

44. Goldstein SR, Zeltser I, Horan CK, et al. Ultrasonography-based triage for perimenopausal patients with abnormal uterine bleeding. Am J Obstet Gynecol. 1997;177:102-8.

45. Kamel HS, Darwish AM, Mohamed SA. Comparison of transvaginal ultrasonography and vaginal sonohysterography in the detection of endometrial polyps. Acta Obstet Gynecol Scand. 2000;79:60-4.

46. Farquhar C, Ekeroma A, Furness S, Arroll B. A systematic review of transvaginal ultrasonography, sonohysterography and hysteroscopy for the investigation of abnormal uterine bleeding in premenopausal women. Acta Obstet Gynecol Scand. 2003;82: 493-504.

47. Breitkopf D, Goldstein SR, Seeds JW. Saline infusion sonohysterography. Obstet Gynecol. 2003;102:659-62.

48. Bradley LD, Magen AB. Radiographic imaging techniques for the diagnosis of abnormal uterine bleeding. Obstet Gynecol Clin North Am. 2000;27:245-76.

49. de Kroon CD, Dieben SW, Jansen FW. Saline contrast hysterosonography in abnormal uterine bleeding: a systematic review and meta-analysis. Br J Obstet Gynaecol. 2003; 110:938-47.

50. Sowers M, Perdue C, Araujo KL, et al. Thyroid stimulating hormone (TSH) concentrations and menopausal status in women at the mid-life: SWAN. Clin Endocrinol (Oxf). 2003;58:340-7.

51. Archer D. Medical management of menorrhagia in pre- and perimenopausal women. Perimenopause, Serono Symposia USA. New York: Springer-Verlag; 1997:271-80.

52. Munro M. Abnormal uterine bleeding in the reproductive years. Part II: medical management. J Am Assoc Gynecol Laparosc. 2000;7:17-35.

53. Preston JT, Adams EJ, Smith SK. Comparative study of tranexamic acid and norethisterone in the treatment of ovulatory menorrhagia. Br J Obstet Gynaecol. 1995;102:401-6.

54. Bonnar J. Treatment of menorrhagia during menstruation: randomised controlled trial of ethamsylate, mefenamic acid, and tranexamic acid. BMJ. 1996;313:579-82.

55. Andersch B, Rybo G. An objective evaluation of flurbiprofen and tranexamic acid in the treatment of idiopathic menorrhagia. Acta Obstet Gynecol Scand. 1988;67:645-8.

56. Conyngham R. Norethisterone in menorrhagia. N Z Med J. 1965;64:697-701.

57. Fraser I. Treatment of ovulatory and anovulatory dysfunctional uterine bleeding with oral progestogens. Aust N Z J Obstet Gynaecol. 1990;30:352-6.

58. Irvine GA, Lumsden MA, Heikkila A, et al. Randomised comparative trial of the levonorgestrel intrauterine system and norethisterone for treatment of idiopathic menorrhagia. Br J Obstet Gynaecol. 1998;105:592-8.

59. Crosignani PG, Mosconi P, Oldani S, et al. Levonorgestrel-releasing intrauterine device versus hysteroscopic endometrial resection in the treatment of dysfunctional uterine bleeding. Obstet Gynecol. 1997;90:257-63.

60. Barrington JW, Bowen-Simpkins P. The levonorgestrel intrauterine system in the management of menorrhagia. Br J Obstet Gynaecol. 1997;104:614-6.

61. Lahteenmaki P, Puolakka J, Riikonen U, et al. Open randomised study of use of levonorgestrel releasing intrauterine system as alternative to hysterectomy. BMJ. 1998; 316:1122-6.

62. Tjarks M, Van Voorhis BJ. Treatment of endometrial polyps. Obstet Gynecol. 2000;96:886-9.

63. Cravello L, et al. Hysteroscopic resection of endometrial polyps: a study of 195 cases. Eur J Obstet Gynecol Reprod Biol. 2000;93:131-4.

64. Ferenczy A. The biologic significance of cytologic atypia in progestogen-treated endometrial hyperplasia. Am J Obstet Gynecol. 1989;160:126-31.

65. Kurman RJ, Norris HJ. The behavior of endometrial hyperplasia: a long-term study of "untreated" hyperplasia in 170 patients. Cancer. 1985;56:403-12.

66. Fung Kee Fung M, Faught W. Does persistent postmenopausal bleeding justify hysterectomy? Eur J Gynaecol Oncol. 1997;18:26-8.

67. Twu NF. Five-year follow-up of patients with recurrent postmenopausal bleeding. Zhonghua Yi Xue Za Zhi (Taipei). 2000;63:628-33.

3

Amenorrhea

Catherine LeClair, MD
Deborah B. Ehrenthal, MD
Paula J. Adams Hillard, MD

For women of reproductive age, a normal menstrual cycle is a marker of general good health. Changes or abnormalities in the menstrual cycle can be an early sign of illness or disease. For this reason, obtaining a menstrual history is essential. Menstrual changes may indicate problems related to the reproductive system, such as premature ovarian failure, or may be an early sign of an important underlying disorder such as hypothyroidism, an eating disorder, or chronic liver disease. When the menstrual cycle is found to be abnormal, the underlying cause must be sought.

Cyclic hormonal rhythm is indicated by a predictable menstrual flow that occurs between 21 and 35 days in reproductive-aged women; two thirds of women menstruate every 28 ± 3 days (1). *Amenorrhea* is defined as the absence or cessation of menses. Absence of menses for 3 months occurs in approximately 5% of reproductive-aged women each year (2,3). *Oligomenorrhea* is defined as irregular or infrequent menses with cycle lengths usually longer than 35-40 days.

Amenorrhea has classically been divided into primary and secondary categories. *Primary amenorrhea* is when menstruation has not occurred by age 16 years in the presence of other secondary sexual characteristics *or* when menstruation has not occurred by age 14 in the absence of secondary sexual characteristics. *Secondary amenorrhea* is when menstruation has not occurred in 3-6 months after a previously established normal menstrual pattern.

Amenorrhea is not a definitive diagnosis but an indication that a definitive illness or disorder must be sought. When regular menstruation fails to occur, either at an appropriate time in pubertal development or after the establishment of regular cycles, further diagnostic evaluation for cause is necessary. If evaluation is not pursued, major morbidity and even mortality may result. Amenorrhea can be associated with an increased risk of osteopenia/osteoporosis, especially with wrist or hip fracture; it may indicate an underlying syndrome associated with an increased risk of cardiovascular morbidity and diabetes; or it can be associated with declining or absent fertility and impending ovarian failure.

Pregnancy is the most common cause of amenorrhea among reproductive-aged women. Because over half of all pregnancies occurring in the United States are unintended, a pregnancy test should always be performed as an initial study, even in teens who are unable or unwilling to acknowledge sexual activity. *The subsequent discussions of amenorrhea will assume that pregnancy has been ruled out by a sensitive urine or serum pregnancy test.*

Amenorrhea may be caused by hormonal contraception, including oral contraceptive pills, and is more common among long-term users of depot medroxyprogesterone acetate and the levonorgestrel intrauterine system. In the presence of hormonal contraception, amenorrhea, or lack of withdrawal bleeding, does not have the same pathologic implications as does spontaneous amenorrhea, and does not merit further evaluation, other than perhaps ruling out pregnancy if contraception compliance is suspect. Combination contraceptives may, however, mask an underlying abnormality.

In the absence of pregnancy or hormonal contraception, regular menses is generally a sign of adequate estrogen and/or progesterone production in response to appropriate hypothalamic and pituitary stimulation. Amenorrhea or oligomenorrhea can occur as a result of the failure of hypothalamic or pituitary stimulation of the ovary, resulting in insufficient estrogen production or the failure of ovulation. Ovarian dysfunction can result in lack of menses or scanty menses despite adequate hypothalamic and pituitary secretion. Amenorrhea with normal ovarian, pituitary, and hypothalamic function may result if there is an obstruction in the lower genital outflow track (cervical or vaginal) or if there is scarring of the endometrium.

Primary Amenorrhea and Menstruation in the Adolescent

More than 95% of girls will have initiated menarche by age 14. Early cycles are usually irregular because more than half of menstrual cycles are anovulatory in the first year after menarche due to the innate immaturity of the hypothalamic-pituitary axis (Figure 3-1). However, most anovulatory cycles occur at fairly regular intervals and fall within known parameters (4). During the first 2 years after menarche, cycles may be somewhat irregular, but 90% of girls will have cycles within the range of 21-42 days, with 2-8 days of flow (5,6). Evaluating a completed menstrual calendar can help the clinician assess whether a girl is having a normal or abnormal bleeding pattern.

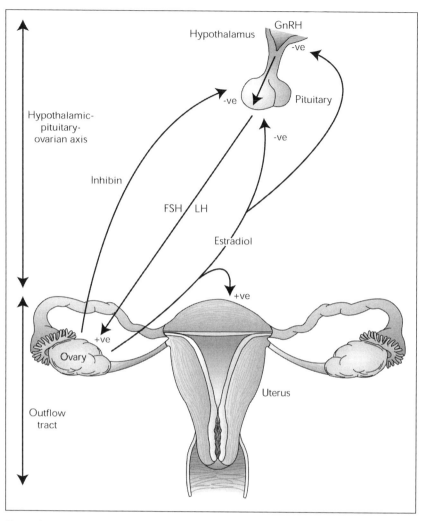

Figure 3-1   Hypothalamic-pituitary axis. (From Stovall TG, Ling FW, eds. Gynecology for the Primary Care Physician. Philadelphia: Current Medicine; 1999; with permission.)

Though early cycles are often anovulatory, there is usually a progression to more regular ovulatory cycles as the hypothalamic-pituitary axis matures. The pituitary gland, under the direction of the pulsatile release of gonadotropin-releasing hormone (GnRH) from the hypothalamus, begins to secrete the gonadotropin follicle-stimulating hormone (FSH) and luteinizing hormone (LH). These gonadotropins signal follicular development in the ovary. It is this sequence that is responsible for the normal production and secretion of estrogen and progesterone and thus the advent of puberty.

Some girls (often those with relatively early menarche) quickly establish regular ovulatory cycles, but up to one third of adolescents still have anovulatory cycles in the fifth year after menarche (7,8). By the seventh year after menarche, over 90% of cycles are ovulatory. Girls who are having ovulatory cycles will typically describe regular menses with associated moliminal symptoms such as breast tenderness, mood changes, and bloating (9). Dysmenorrhea is typical of an ovulatory cycle, whereas girls who are anovulatory report minimal discomfort during menstrual flow.

As already mentioned, most girls will have initiated menarche by age 14. Traditionally, primary amenorrhea has been defined as no menses by age 16; however, many diagnosable and treatable disorders can and should be detected earlier, using the statistically derived guideline of age 14. Lack of initiation of breast development by age 12 is found in girls with ovarian dysgenesis or other disorders that result in failure of estrogen production (10). Menarche typically occurs approximately 2 years after the initiation of breast development and typically at the attainment of Tanner stage 4 breast development. An evaluation for primary amenorrhea should be considered for any girl who has not begun to have breast development by age 12-13 or who has not reached menarche by age 14 or within 2 years of obtaining Tanner stage 4 breast development. Thus, attention to pubertal milestones, growth, and development are essential. Adrenarche occurs normally in girls with ovarian insufficiency; however, breast development and the pubertal growth in height do not occur or are delayed.

Etiology of Amenorrhea

Pathologic causes of primary and secondary amenorrhea may occur anywhere in the endometrial-ovarian-pituitary-hypothalamic axis (see Figure 3-1). The differential diagnosis is extensive, and there is great overlap between the primary and secondary causes. The discussion below organizes the causes of primary and secondary amenorrhea into three groups: 1) outflow tract abnormalities, 2) ovarian failure, and 3) chronic anovulation (Table 3-1). Simple physiologic causes of amenorrhea, however, including pregnancy, lactation, and menopause, need to be ruled out before this broad differential is considered (1,11). Ovarian failure (hypergonadotropic hypogonadism) is the most common cause of primary amenorrhea (12).

Outflow Tract Abnormalities

Outflow tract abnormalities exist when there is absence of a patent genital tract or when there are abnormalities of the endometrium that make it unable to respond to hormonal stimulation. These are much more common as causes

Table 3-1   Causes of Amenorrhea and Oligomenorrhea (Excluding Pregnancy, Lactation, and Menopause)

Outflow tract abnormalities	
Primary	Imperforate hymen, transverse vaginal septum, müllerian agenesis, androgen-insensitivity syndrome
Secondary	Asherman's syndrome (uncommon), tuberculosis of the endometrium (rare)
Ovarian failure (hypergonadotropic hypogonadism)	
Primary	Turner's syndrome, Swyer's syndrome, other chromosomal abnormalities, radiation- or chemotherapy-induced ovarian failure, premature ovarian failure
Secondary	Radiation- or chemotherapy-induced ovarian failure, chromosomal abnormalities, autoimmune or idiopathic premature ovarian failure
Chronic anovulation	
Hyperandrogenism	Polycystic ovary syndrome (PCOS), congenital adrenal hyperplasia (rare), androgen-secreting tumor (rare)
Hyperprolactinemia	Prolactinoma, medications, hypothyroidism, other
Hypothalamic hypogonadism	Eating disorders, athletics, functional/psychological and physiological stress
Pituitary insufficiency	
Thyroid disease	Hyperthyroidism, hypothyroidism
Cushing's syndrome	Rare but not to be missed
Medications	Hormonal
	Cytotoxic
	Others

of primary amenorrhea and are rarely causes of secondary amenorrhea. Physical exam will identify most outflow tract abnormalities. Hormone levels, when tested, will usually be normal.

Presenting as Primary Amenorrhea

An imperforate hymen or a transverse vaginal septum results in amenorrhea. *Imperforate hymen* is at the extreme of a spectrum of variations in hymenal configuration (13). Variations in the embryologic development of the hymen are common and result in fenestrations, septa, bands, microperforations, anterior displacement, and differences in rigidity and/or elasticity of the hymenal tissue. If an imperforate hymen is confirmed during the examination of a young girl, the ideal timing for the surgical correction is after the onset of puberty with its associated estrogen stimulation but before the anticipated onset of menses (see Treatment secton later in this chapter). Unfortunately, an imperforate hymen is most often not suspected until several months of cyclic abdominal pain with uterine and vaginal distension indicate possible outflow tract obstruction. Urinary obstruction, retrograde menses, and endometriosis with subsequent potential impact on fertility may be the consequence. *Transverse vaginal septa* occur less commonly than imperforate hymen but require careful diagnosis and surgical management by an experienced gynecologic surgeon.

Müllerian agenesis is the congenital absence of the female genital tract. Mayer-Rokitansky-Küster-Hauser syndrome is the cumbersome eponym used to describe this condition; it is the second most common etiology of primary amenorrhea (12). The condition typically involves vaginal and uterine agenesis. Müllerian agenesis may involve the presence of a rudimentary uterine horn, with or without a functioning endometrium. Because the embryologic development of the genital tract and renal collecting system are so closely tied, 15%-40% of patients with müllerian agenesis have renal tract abnormalities. In addition, 12% of girls have skeletal abnormalities, most commonly in the cervical spine. Thus, radiographic evaluation of the urinary tract and spine should be performed on girls diagnosed with müllerian agenesis (14). Gonadal development is independent of outflow tract development, so ovarian function is intact with normal secondary sexual characteristics. These patients should be evaluated by gynecologists experienced with this condition. Although surgical and nonsurgical options for creation of a neovagina exist, most gynecologists today strongly favor a nonsurgical technique that involves the use of progressively larger Lucite dilators at a time when the young woman is motivated to do so. Alternatively, a neovagina can be surgically created by a variety of techniques, often with the use of a skin graft (15).

Androgen-insensitivity syndrome, formerly known as "testicular feminization," is an X-linked enzyme defect in the androgen receptor that leads to testosterone insensitivity. Although the genotype is 46,XY, phenotypically patients are female. The lack of sensitivity to testosterone prevents development of male genitalia, an androgen-dependent process. Müllerian-inhibiting substance is still successfully secreted, and its effect on the growing fetus is to inhibit the development of the müllerian tract. Thus the uterus, uterine cervix, and upper vagina do not develop. The result is a phenotypic female with scant or absent axillary and pubic hair, normal breast development, absent uterus and a blind vaginal pouch. The rudimentary testes may be present in the abdomen, inguinal canal, or labia majora (the last being the analogous structure in the female to the scrotal sac in the male) and require removal because of the high risk of malignant transformation. Testosterone levels are usually elevated. Careful and sensitive discussion is warranted (16).

Presenting as Secondary Amenorrhea

Structural abnormalities of the uterus and endometrium acquired after puberty can result in secondary amenorrhea but are a very rare cause of amenorrhea in adults (3). These rare causes include Asherman's syndrome and tuberculosis infection of the endometrium. Asherman's syndrome may occur if there is a past history of pregnancy-related curettage for postpartum hemorrhage or endometritis. Uterine scarring and synechiae lead to an abnormal endometrial surface that does not respond normally to sex steroids. Hysterosonogram, hysterosalpingogram, or hysteroscopy can show the presence of webs of scar tissue and/or synechiae in an otherwise normal cavity. The evaluation and management of this condition requires surgical expertise from an experienced gynecologist. Tuberculosis infection of the uterine cavity is a rare cause of secondary amenorrhea (3).

Hypergonadotropic Hypogonadism (Premature Ovarian Failure)

Hypergonadotropic hypogonadism is defined as primary or secondary amenorrhea in women younger than 40 who have elevated gonadotropin levels. It is found in up to 10% of women with secondary amenorrhea (11). Given the significance of this diagnosis, abnormal studies should be reported at least 30 days apart for verification. The most common underlying etiologies of hypergonadotropic primary and secondary amenorrhea differ, as discussed below. Women with hypergonadotropic hypogonadism will have low estrogen levels. In addition to addressing fertility issues, management must address their risk for developing long-term complications of estrogen deficiency such as osteoporosis.

Presenting as Primary Amenorrhea
Young women with Turner's syndrome (karyotype 45,X) typically manifest certain physical characteristics such as short stature, webbed neck, shield chest, multiple nevi, and cubitus valgus. They show little or no breast development, and the genital tract appears hypoestrogenic. A similar clinical picture is found with 46,XXiq karyotype and in some mosaic karyotypes. Some girls will have spontaneous breast development or menses. In addition, these girls may show signs of cardiac and renal abnormalities and a tendency for thyroid dysfunction. A thorough work-up of these systems is important and usually includes laboratory and radiographic studies. Prevention of the various health conditions caused by hypoestrogenism, namely osteoporosis, is a key component of treatment with hormone replacement therapy and calcium supplementation.

Pure gonadal dysgenesis is rare. A normal karyotype (46,XX) is found, yet there is no gonadal function. These girls do not manifest the typical somatic traits of Turner's syndrome but share prepubertal sexual characteristics. They are usually of normal stature. Because there can be a link to neurosensory deafness, auditory evaluation is necessary. A girl with a 46,XY karyotype without signs of androgen-insensitivity syndrome has Swyer's syndrome, another rare cause of gonadal dysfunction that is otherwise known as vanishing testes syndrome. These patients have an intact müllerian system (uterus, uterine cervix, and upper vagina) but no secondary sexual traits. Although girls with Swyer's syndrome share a common karyotype with those with androgen-insensitivity syndrome (see Outflow Tract Abnormalities section), they differ in that there is the presence of a female genital tract. Due to the presence of the Y chromosome, these girls must also have the gonadal tissue removed because of the possibility of malignant transformation. Trisomies 13 and 18 are associated with ovarian dysgenesis and failure.

Presenting as Secondary Amenorrhea

The cessation of ovarian function typically begins in the fourth decade of a woman's reproductive life, 51 years being the average age of menopause. Premature ovarian failure is defined as failure of ovarian function before age 40 and occurs in 1% of the population (17). It is suspected when a woman presents with typical menopausal symptoms such as hot flushes, night sweats, mood instability, vaginal dryness, and secondary amenorrhea, although these symptoms are not always present. When gonadotropins are measured, the FSH is characteristically elevated, usually two standard deviations above the normal range.

Causes of premature ovarian failure include chemotherapy, radiation therapy, chromosomal abnormalities (usually in the X chromosome), and autoimmunity. Up to 30% of cases are felt to be the result of autoimmunity (18). In most cases a specific cause cannot be identified. While fertility is generally significantly reduced, there are reports of pregnancy in women who have been diagnosed with premature ovarian failure due to occasional spontaneous ovarian follicular activity (19,20).

Ovarian failure that develops before the age of 30 should prompt testing for chromosomal abnormalities. Women with Turner's syndrome, especially those with mosaicism, have been known to display early ovarian function and menstruation but with subsequent premature ovarian failure and amenorrhea. Fragile X syndrome, partial X chromosomal deletions, and milder degrees of X chromosome mosaicism have been associated with ovarian failure as well (17).

Premature ovarian failure can be seen in association with autoimmune disorders such as diabetes, autoimmune thyroid disease, systemic lupus erythematosus, rheumatoid arthritis, and Addison's disease. Screening for diabetes and thyroid disease is indicated in women with idiopathic premature ovarian failure. Testing for other autoimmune processes such as adrenal insufficiency may be recommended based on clinical indications (21). Recent data suggest that screening for adrenal autoantibodies may be an effective test for Addison's disease in this population (22).

Chronic Anovulation

Chronic anovulation is the most common nonphysiologic cause of secondary amenorrhea and is identified in the absence of ovarian failure or outflow tract abnormalities. It is also a common cause of oligomenorrhea and abnormal vaginal bleeding and thus may present with a variety of clinical pictures. Some patients with anovulation are hypoestrogenemic and at risk for osteoporosis; others have normal or high levels of unopposed estrogen and are at risk for endometrial hyperplasia and endometrial cancer. Early diagnosis of the underlying disorder is key in avoiding the medical and social sequelae that may develop, especially if they persist unidentified for years. The causes of chronic anovulation can be sorted into several major groups: hyperandrogenism, hyperprolactinemia, hypogonadism caused by functional abnormalities of the hypothalamus and the pituitary, thyroid diseases, and (rarely) Cushing's syndrome.

Hyperandrogenism

Hyperandrogenic anovulation is one of the most common causes of amenorrhea and is usually due to polycystic ovary syndrome (PCOS). Present in 6%-10% of reproductive-aged women, the characteristic features include androgen excess with or without skin manifestations, ovulatory dysfunction (anovulation or oligo-ovulation), and absence of another cause of androgen excess. A conference including the European Society of Human Reproduction and Embryology and the American Society for Reproductive Medicine met in 2003 to develop consensus diagnostic criteria for PCOS (23). Per these Rotterdam criteria, PCOS is diagnosed in the presence of two of the three following criteria: oligo-ovulation or anovulation, clinical and/or biochemical signs of hyperandrogenism, and polycystic ovaries on ultrasound. Other etiologies, such as congenital adrenal hyperplasia, androgen-secreting tumors, or Cushing's syndrome, must be excluded.

Originally thought to be a primary ovarian disorder, PCOS is now understood to be an endocrine disorder caused by androgen excess and associated with chronic anovulation. The underlying abnormality in the process is thought to be insulin resistance. Menstrual symptoms usually date to the time of menarche. Significant weight gain may induce the clinical picture in women with previously normal cycles. Physical findings may include evidence of hyperandrogenism, including acne, hirsutism, and alopecia. Signs of virilization are usually absent but may be seen occasionally. Obesity, especially truncal obesity, is common, although lean women may also exhibit other clinical characteristics. Acanthosis nigricans may be present and is a sign of insulin resistance. Women with PCOS are anovulatory but have normal estrogen levels, thus they are not at risk for the consequences of estrogen deficiency.

However, exposure to unopposed estrogens over time leads to an increased risk of endometrial hyperplasia and endometrial cancer. These women are also at greater risk for cardiovascular disease and diabetes, so they benefit from screening and lifestyle modification to reduce such risk.

Although PCOS is the most common cause of hyperandrogenic anovulation, other causes of elevated androgens should be considered (24). Adrenal or ovarian tumors and ovarian hyperthecosis can result in elevated androgen levels. This is more likely in women who have hirsutism of recent onset or who have signs of virilization on physical examination. Signs of virilization include temporal balding, deepening of voice, decreased breast size, increased muscle mass, loss of female body contours, and clitoral enlargement. Clitoral length over 10 mm is considered abnormal; diameter of less than 7 mm is normal. A better test is the clitoral index (the product of the width and length of the glans clitoris), which, if it is greater than 35 mm^2, is abnormal and correlates statistically with androgen excess (25). Late-onset or mild congenital adrenal hyperplasia may present as hyperandrogenic anovulation and is rare.

Testing for hyperandrogenic anovulation will reveal normal gonadotropin levels (although sometimes with an abnormally elevated LH/FSH ratio) and a normal thyroid-stimulating hormone (TSH). Prolactin (PRL) may be mildly elevated in association with hyperandrogenism. Total estrogen levels are normal, and the progesterone challenge, if done, will usually be positive. Androgen levels are generally elevated with elevated levels of total testosterone and/or free or percent-free testosterone, along with variably elevated levels of DHEAS. Normal levels of 17-hydroxyprogesterone (17-OHP) will rule out late-onset congenital adrenal hyperplasia.

Hyperprolactinemia

Hyperprolactinemia is seen in up to a third of women with secondary amenorrhea; its diagnosis should be sought in all women presenting with oligomenorrhea and amenorrhea. Clinical history can be helpful, but galactorrhea is present in only one third of women with elevated prolactin levels (3). Because adenomas are usually small at the time of presentation, headache and neurologic symptoms are rare. Elevated levels of prolactin inhibit GnRH pulsatility and cause failure of the positive feedback response to gonadotropin secretion induced by estrogen. This can lead to clinical symptoms of a luteal phase defect and a relatively normal menstrual cycle, or to more significant symptoms of amenorrhea with or without galactorrhea (26). It can also increase adrenal androgen production and thus present with signs of hyperandrogenism.

A variety of processes can lead to hyperprolactinemia. It may be the result of a prolactin-secreting adenoma, the most common pituitary tumor. These may be microadenomas (up to 10 mm) or macroadenomas (>10 mm). Prolactin levels may be elevated in the setting of other pituitary adenomas as well as empty sella syndrome and other structural lesions of the hypothalamus and pituitary stalk. Primary hypothyroidism can cause hyperprolactinemia and, once recognized, is easily treated. Estrogens and many other commonly used medications can cause elevations in prolactin levels, usually in the range of 25-100 µg/L, although the levels of estrogens in currently available oral contraceptives rarely do (1,25-28). Commonly used non-hormonal medications that may cause elevated prolactin levels include serotonin reuptake inhibitors, verapamil, phenothiazines, risperidone, monoamine oxidase inhibitors, tricyclic antidepressants, and opiates (Table 3-2). Nipple stimulation can lead to an elevation in the prolactin level, as can chest wall lesions such as those

Table 3-2   Causes of Elevated Prolactin Levels

Pituitary disease	Prolactinoma, acromegaly, Cushing's syndrome, empty sella syndrome, lymphocytic hypophysitis	
Hypothalamic disease	Primary and metastatic neoplasms, encephalitis, sarcoidosis, pseudo-tumor cerebri, eosinophilic granuloma, irradiation, vascular compromise, pituitary stalk compression or section	
Neurogenic	Breast stimulation, chest wall stimulation, chest surgery, chest wall lesions (herpes zoster), spinal cord lesions, rare ectopic production from distant neoplasms	
Metabolic	Pregnancy, lactation, hypothyroidism, hyperandrogenemia (PCOS), adrenal insufficiency, chronic renal failure, cirrhosis, pseudocyesis	
Medications		
Neuropsychiatric	Metaclopramide, phenothiazines, butyrophenones, risperidone, monoamine oxidase inhibitors, tricyclic antidepressants	Levels may be over 100 µg/L
	Selective serotonin reuptake inhibitors	Levels usually stay in normal range
Antihypertensives	Verapamil	Not other calcium channel blockers
	Reserpine and methyldopa	
Hormones	Estrogen	May cause mild elevation, but rare with today's low-dose combination oral contraceptives
Other	Opiates, narcotics, amphetamines	

caused by herpes zoster. Upper spinal cord lesions and ectopic prolactin-producing syndromes are possible but rare. Mild elevations can be seen with physical and psychological stress (27).

Diagnosis is made with measurement of serum prolactin levels. Normal prolactin levels are usually less than 20 ng/mL but may be up to 50 ng/mL due to transient physiologic processes. Because prolactin levels show a diurnal variation and are lowest between 8 a.m. and noon, any abnormal level should be repeated in an 8 a.m. specimen before further evaluation proceeds. Thyroid testing should be done as well because prolactin levels rise in the setting of primary hypothyroidism. Prolactin levels greater than 100 ng/mL are-typically seen with microadenomas; levels over 200 ng/mL are seen with stalk compression. However, up to 15%-20% of macroadenomas produce levels under 100 ng/mL. Women with a repeatedly elevated prolactin level should consider pituitary imaging with computed tomography or magnetic resonance imaging (26).

Hypogonadotropic Hypogonadism

A *hypothalamic disorder* is a common cause of amenorrhea and anovulation. It usually presents as abrupt onset of amenorrhea in a woman with a previously normal menstrual history, less commonly as a cause of primary amenorrhea. Hypothalamic amenorrhea is most often the result of global physiologic changes that disrupt the normal pulsatile secretion of GnRH from the hypothalamus and results in low levels of FSH and LH leading to anovulation and hypoestrogenemia. Chronic medical conditions, such as renal failure, liver disease, inflammatory bowel disease, AIDS, and obesity, can lead to hypothalamic suppression through a variety of mechanisms. Destructive or infiltrative processes in the hypothalamus, such as lymphoma, sarcoidosis, or hemochromatosis, can rarely lead to hypothalamic amenorrhea.

Elements of a patient's medical history, social history, and physical exam often suggest the diagnosis of idiopathic functional hypothalamic amenorrhea early in the evaluation process. Specific attention must be paid to weight history, dietary history, exercise history, and evidence of medical or emotional stress. A specific diet history and evidence of significant weight loss should be sought, with attention to the possibility of an eating disorder and of resulting nutritional deficiencies. Vigorous exercise can result in suppression of the hypothalamic gonadotropins and lead to amenorrhea. This may be related to exercise alone or be part of the female athlete triad (which includes disordered eating, amenorrhea, and osteoporosis, as discussed in Chapter 10). The amount of exercise required to cause amenorrhea is not defined and seems to vary among individuals (29).

Physical and emotional stress can also lead to functional hypothalamic amenorrhea, and elements in the patient's history and physical exam may suggest stress-induced disorder, but it is a diagnosis of exclusion and laboratory testing should be completed. It has been hypothesized that functional hypothalamic amenorrhea can be precipitated by a combination of psychosocial stressors and metabolic challenge; cognitive behavioral therapy has been shown to be an effective treatment resulting in recovery of ovarian function (30,31). Although women with hypothalamic amenorrhea do not commonly experience hot flushes, evidence of estrogen deficiency may be present on vaginal exam. Kallman's syndrome or isolated gonadotropin deficiency (familial hypogonadotropic hypogonadism) with anosmia should be considered in young women presenting with primary amenorrhea and minimal sexual development.

Laboratory testing will reveal low or normal LH and FSH. TSH and prolactin level will be normal. Serum estradiol levels, if measured, will be low, and the progesterone challenge will be negative. Radiologic imaging of the brain with magnetic resonance imaging should be considered in women whose clinical scenario does not provide an explanation, whose amenorrhea develops suddenly, or in women who have abnormal neurologic symptoms or findings.

Pituitary Insufficiency

If the pituitary gland is unable to respond to hypothalamic stimulation, then gonadotropin levels will be low and unable to stimulate ovulation. Sheehan's syndrome, infarction, and damage to the pituitary gland after obstetric hemorrhage can cause *pituitary insufficiency or failure* and lead to anovulation. Simmond's syndrome is similar but occurs in non-obstetric hemorrhage. Pituitary failure can also be caused by the toxic effects of bilirubin (kernicterus), iron (thalassemia major), and galactose (galactosemia). Pituitary disorders can be caused by tumor, infarction, infection, and, less commonly, toxic effects of biochemicals.

Thyroid Disease

Thyroid disease commonly causes changes in menstrual function (32). Hypothyroidism can lead to menorrhagia, amenorrhea, and infertility; hyperthyroidism can lead to oligomenorrhea, amenorrhea, and infertility. Both are easily diagnosed with the super-sensitive test for TSH, which is widely available and should always be used during evaluation.

Cushing's Syndrome

Though Cushing's syndrome is uncommon, the diagnosis should be sought in women with suggestive symptoms because of the dire consequences of missing the diagnosis. Cushing's syndrome is characterized by a constellation of signs and symptoms, including amenorrhea, weight gain with truncal obesity, easy bruising, moon facies, buffalo hump, cervical fat pad, hypertension, weakness and fatigue, proximal muscle weakness, hirsutism, personality changes, ecchymoses, purplish abdominal striae, edema, and hyperglycemia. It is caused by the increased production of cortisol by the adrenal glands. It is most commonly caused by bilateral adrenal hyperplasia due to hyper-secretion of ACTH by a pituitary adenoma or by a non-endocrine tumor. The diagnosis should be sought in patients presenting with amenorrhea in the setting of many of the classic symptoms. Screening for Cushing's syndrome can be done by an overnight dexamethasone suppression test or by a 24-hour urine collection for free cortisol. If either screening test is abnormal, the patient should be referred to an endocrinologist for further evaluation and definitive diagnosis and management (25).

Medications and Drug Interactions

Hormonal Medications

Amenorrhea can be the expected result of some hormone medications, such as combination hormonal contraceptives (CHCs), depot medroxyprogesterone acetate (DMPA, Depo Provera), GnRH antagonist, and depot leuprolide (Depo Lupron). Typically, women on CHCs have predictable cyclic bleeding. However, a fraction of women will present with persistent or occasional lack of withdrawal bleeding. In women who are amenorrheic on CHCs, it is essential to rule out pregnancy and establish consistent use. Lack of withdrawal bleeding is not of itself pathologic. Women who use continuous CHCs, either for the management of endometriosis or to manage menstrual symptoms, may become amenorrheic as well. Menstrual suppression with extended and continuous combination pills is becoming more widespread for women with lifestyle and quality-of-life issues; in this situation, amenorrhea is the desired outcome. This option is attractive to some women with menstrual symptoms such as dysmenorrhea, menstrual headaches, and heavy bleeding (33). While studies of long-term outcomes are ongoing, experience with the induction of amenorrhea suggest that this is not a medical concern, and women can be reassured of the lack of evidence for harmful effects of therapeutic amenorrhea.

Use of DMPA as a contraceptive typically leads to a variety of menstrual abnormalities, including irregular bleeding, oligomenorrhea, and amenorrhea (34). Irregular bleeding is most common during the first 3-12 months of use; at the end of 1 year, approximately 50% of women have achieved amenorrhea, with an increasing percentage achieving amenorrhea over additional months (35). DMPA has been used to induce therapeutic amenorrhea, although the outcome cannot be guaranteed. After an injection, menstrual irregularities may persist beyond the 13 weeks of expected effect. Upon discontinuation of DMPA, it may take over a year to resume ovulation. One study found the average return of ovulation was 8.5 months from the last injection. There is no evidence of detrimental effect on fertility (36). Amenorrhea that persists more than 1 year after stopping DMPA should be further evaluated (37).

Depot leuprolide is a GnRH analogue that disrupts pulsatile frequency of hypothalamic secretion, resulting in decreased production of FSH and LH, which causes ovarian suppression and secondary amenorrhea during use. Benefit is seen by women with endometriosis, uterine leiomyomata, and problematic menstruation (caused by severe anemia, chronic illness, and chemotherapy) (38). There are emerging data suggesting that the use of depot leuprolide may help to preserve ovarian function when chemotherapeutic agents pose risk of ovarian failure (39).

Cytotoxic Drugs

Cyclophosphamide, chlorambucil, busulphan, methotrexate, and other chemotherapeutic agents lead to amenorrhea through their cytotoxic effects and can cause ovarian failure.

Other Drugs

Glucocorticosteroids, antibiotics (sulfasalazine and cotrimoxazole), thyroid supplements, spironolactone, cimetidine, colchicine, marijuana, opiates, and neuroleptic agents can be associated with menstrual irregularities and amenorrhea. The induction of hyperprolactinemia is the mechanism by which antipsychotic agents induce amenorrhea (see earlier discussion of hyperprolactinemia in this chapter).

Evaluation and Diagnosis of Primary Amenorrhea

A careful medical history will often suggest specific causes of primary amenorrhea, such as excessive exercise or eating disorders. The constellation of irregular periods, significant acne, and obesity should not be attributed solely to "adolescence"; the diagnosis of hyperandrogenism/PCOS should be considered as a possible cause of primary amenorrhea. Pubertal milestones should be ascertained.

A careful inspection of the external genitalia can suggest obstructing anatomy. In making the diagnosis of imperforate hymen, care must be taken that more complex anomalies are not misdiagnosed, because inappropriate surgical treatment can cause serious complications. A pelvic ultrasound can confirm the presence or absence of müllerian structures and associated renal abnormalities. Magnetic resonance imaging may be required to clarify complex anatomic abnormalities such as uterine duplications or obstructing vaginal septa. Laboratory evaluation should include measurement of gonadotropins because gonadal dysgenesis must be considered as a cause of primary amenorrhea. Prolactin and TSH should also be measured. Further testing is dictated by findings on physical examination. Measurement of androgens can bolster a clinical diagnosis of PCOS. Although less commonly a cause of primary amenorrhea, history of an eating disorder and excessive exercise should be sought. Documentation of hypoestrogenism with the measurement of an estradiol can be helpful in an effort to convince young women that lifestyle modification is imperative. A karyotype will be required to confirm androgen insensitivity or other chromosomal anomaly when suggested by elevated gonadotropins. Pregnancy should always be ruled out with a sensitive urine or serum pregnancy test, even with primary amenorrhea and a negative sexual history.

Evaluation and Diagnosis of Secondary Amenorrhea

History

The possibility of pregnancy should be addressed, along with the patient's current and previous methods of contraception, to identify simple physiologic causes of amenorrhea. A complete medical history will identify a chronic illness that may lead to hypothalamic amenorrhea or premature ovarian failure. A thorough past surgical and obstetrical history can help identify women with outflow tract abnormalities. A complete list of medications and use of illicit drugs is essential because many can alter the normal menstrual cycle.

The history should explore the patient's menstrual cycles since menarche to determine whether there is any history of regular ovulatory menstruation. The presence of associated moliminal symptoms of breast tenderness, fluid retention, and cramping can be useful in identifying menstrual bleeding as ovulatory. Duration of amenorrhea and specifics about oligomenorrhea should be defined. Symptoms of flushing and vaginal dryness suggest ovarian failure. Women with excess hair growth should be further queried for the chronicity and rate of hair growth, in addition to other signs of androgen excess such as acne, balding, and deepening of the voice. Use of depilatories and other forms of hair removal should be ascertained explicitly because these measures may mask significant hirsutism. The presence of galactorrhea, headaches, or visual field defects will suggest a prolactinoma. Eliciting symptoms of Cushing's syndrome such as easy bruising, weight gain with truncal obesity, weakness and fatigue, personality changes, and new purplish abdominal striae are crucial. Symptoms of thyroid disease should be sought. A social history should be taken to identify evidence of eating disorders, excessive exercise, and social and psychological stress.

Physical Examination

A thorough physical exam, including a breast and pelvic exam, should be performed. General appearance may suggest an eating disorder; typical findings of short stature and webbed neck may suggest Turner's syndrome; Cushingoid features may be present. Vital signs will include blood pressure, pulse, height, and weight; a body mass index should be calculated. A skin exam will assess for the presence of acne, hair loss or hirsutism, acanthosis nigricans, pathological striae, and bruising. Tanner staging should be done in young women. The thyroid gland should be examined and other signs of thyroid disease sought. Breast exam should assess nipple discharge. A thorough pelvic exam can suggest the presence of an adnexal mass. Clitoral size should be measured (normal is less than 1 cm) to identify indicators of virilization; atrophic vaginitis should be noted as sign of estrogen deficiency. In an adolescent, the extent of a gynecologic exam is determined by age, maturity, and sexual history, and can be supplemented by a pelvic ultrasound examination.

Diagnostic Testing

Further evaluation of secondary amenorrhea will follow the algorithm in Figure 3-2. The clinician may choose to proceed in a stepwise approach as described below, thus minimizing the extent of testing, or to group more tests to arrive at an answer faster and with fewer trips to the laboratory (Table 3-3). Some patients will present with a history and physical exam that strongly suggests a specific diagnosis, which will lead to specific testing earlier.

In the patient with a normal physical exam and a negative office-based urine pregnancy test, the first step is to check serum TSH and prolactin (40). A woman with a long history of oligomenorrhea who has evidence of hirsutism and insulin resistance on exam probably has PCOS and serum androgens could be drawn with her initial labs. If the TSH is abnormal, thyroid disease is the culprit; further evaluation of the thyroid will lead to a diagnosis and management plan. If the prolactin is elevated, the next step will be to repeat the prolactin level at 8 a.m. to verify the elevated level is not due to the normal diurnal variation of prolactin. If the level remains elevated, the patient's history and medications need to be reviewed for multiple causes of an elevated PRL (see Table 3-2). If no cause is found, pituitary imaging should be considered for identification of a pituitary adenoma. Once the thyroid and the prolactin disorders have been treated, the menstrual cycle should return to normal. If diagnosis is still not possible, futher evaluation must ensue.

When a woman has clinical symptoms and signs suggesting Cushing's syndrome, a screening test should be considered with the first round of testing. Random morning cortisol levels are of little value in making this diagnosis. A

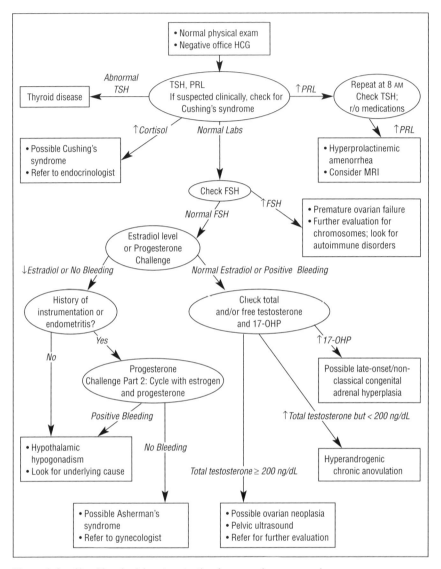

Figure 3-2   Algorithm for laboratory testing for secondary amenorrhea.

24-hour urinary free cortisol is a good screening test. Normal is less than 220-330 nmol depending upon the assay used. An alternative test is the overnight dexamethasone suppression test, which has high sensitivity and low specificity. A 1 mg dose of dexamethasone is taken by the patient at 11 p.m. or midnight, and at 8-9 a.m. the next morning a serum cortisol level is drawn. A normal cortisol level is less than 140 nmol/L (25). Any patient with an abnormal

Table 3-3   Basic Laboratory Testing for Amenorrhea

Step 1 Office HCG, TSH, prolactin
Step 2 FSH
Step 3 Progesterone challenge (Part 1, possibly Part 2) or serum estradiol level

If clinically indicated:
• Overnight dexamethasone suppression test or 24-hour urinary-free cortisol
• Total and free testosterone
• 17-alpha-hydroxyprogesterone

HCG = human chorionic gonadotropin; TSH = thyroid-stimulating hormone; FSH = follicle-stimulating hormone.

screening test should be referred to an endocrinologist for further evaluation and management.

With a normal exam and normal TSH and PRL, the next step is to check the FSH to diagnose premature ovarian failure. If the FSH is elevated, it should be re-checked because the implications of premature ovarian failure can be considerable. If it is again elevated, the diagnosis of hypergonadotropic hypergonadism (ovarian failure) is made. In women under 30, chromosome studies should be performed to look for uncommon mosaic abnormalities; symptoms and signs of other autoimmune disorders including thyroid disease (which has already been assessed), Addison's disease, systemic lupus erythematosus, and rheumatoid arthritis should be sought if karyotype is normal.

If this point is arrived at without a diagnosis, it is evident that the premenopausal woman has anovulation not caused by ovarian failure. The next step in the evaluation is to determine whether she has normal or low estrogen levels. This can be done using the progestational challenge or by measurement of serum estradiol levels. The progestational challenge test has been around for years and is a classic part of this evaluation. It gives information about the patient's endogenous estrogen levels as well as the patency of her outflow tract. The test consists of the administration of oral medroxyprogesterone acetate 10 mg daily for 10 days. This will precipitate a withdrawal bleed in a woman with an endometrium that is adequately proliferated from the effects of endogenous estrogens. Bleeding should occur with 10-14 days of the medication. If no bleeding occurs, this indicates a negative result, which may be due to an outflow tract that is not intact or to a poorly estrogenized endometrium caused by low endogenous estrogen levels. Some authors have argued against the use of this test because it may be falsely positive in up to 50% of women with impending ovarian failure (41), preferring instead to measure estradiol levels.

Part two of the progestin challenge test may be done at this point if there is concern about the normalcy of the outflow tract (i.e., if there is a history of instrumentation or endometritis suggesting Asherman's syndrome). This consists of administration of conjugated equine estrogen 2.5 mg orally daily for 25 days followed by medroxyprogesterone acetate 10 mg orally daily for days 16-25. This should induce a withdrawal bleed in women with low endogenous estrogens but with a functioning outflow tract. It is assumed that the outflow tract is intact and responsive to stimulation of estrogen and progesterone if a withdrawal bleed occurs. If there is no bleeding (negative test), the diagnosis of Asherman's syndrome should be considered and the woman should be referred to a gynecologist for further evaluation and management.

A negative progestin challenge test or low estradiol level and low levels of LH and FSH leads to the diagnosis of hypothalamic hypogonadism. Underlying causes must be sought. As discussed earlier in this chapter, there are many clinical scenarios that can lead to hypothalamic hypogonadism. However, if an explanation cannot be found, magnetic resonance imaging of the brain should be considered to rule out an infiltrative or mass lesion as the cause.

Women with adequate endogenous estrogen levels will have a positive progestin challenge or normal serum estradiol levels. Caution is urged in the interpretation of estradiol levels, however, because the measurement represents only a snapshot in time. For example, in girls and women with exercise-induced amenorrhea, estradiol levels may be low during track season; during the "off-season," menses and estradiol levels can be normal.

Consideration should be given to assessing androgen levels at this point if there are any signs or a family history of hyperandrogenism. It is important to remember that not all women with elevated androgen levels will manifest obvious hirsutism, so testing should be considered in everyone. Testing should include total testosterone levels with or without free testosterone levels (in younger women with PCOS, free testosterone may better reflect androgen levels than the total testosterone level) as well as an 8 a.m. 17-OHP level. A total testosterone level above 50 is considered elevated (42). Women with elevated 17-OHP levels should be referred to an endocrinologist for evaluation for late-onset congenital adrenal hyperplasia. Women with total testosterone levels above 200 should have a pelvic ultrasound performed, and referral for further testing should be considered to rule out an ovarian neoplasm.

Treatment of Primary Amenorrhea

In almost all cases of primary amenorrhea, young women should be referred to an obstetrician/gynecologist or a reproductive endocrinologist. If a Y chromosome is present, the patient requires gonadectomy to prevent the possibility of malignant transformation. In addition, hormone replacement with estrogen is important in order to prevent the long-term effects of hypoestrogenism, namely osteoporosis. Calcium supplementation should also be urged.

When müllerian agenesis is diagnosed, a discussion regarding creation of a neovagina must occur. The young woman should be referred to the nearest tertiary care center for management by clinicians experienced in the medical and surgical options for therapy. Because these women maintain ovarian function, estrogen replacement is not necessary. Information about reproductive options, including egg retrieval, surrogate motherhood, and adoption, should be addressed by the specialist (44).

Androgen insensitivity syndrome also requires estrogen replacement. Gonadectomy should occur, the gonads being found in the abdomen, pelvis, inguinal canal, or labia majora. Often these women have development of a vaginal pouch but may need further dilation in order to have comfortable intercourse. As with müllerian anomalies, an experienced gynecologist should address the nonsurgical or surgical creation of a neovagina. The emotional stigmata of carrying a male karyotype should also be addressed with sensitivity and counseling.

The two anatomic abnormalities described previously, imperforate hymen and transverse vaginal septum, lead to painful, cyclic abdomino-pelvic pain from menstrual obstruction. These adolescents will require surgical correction to relieve the pain associated with this condition. This is a relatively minor procedure but should be performed by a gynecologist with experience in diagnosing genital anomalies. Inadvertent attempts at surgical correction when other anomalies such as vaginal agenesis are present can result in significant scarring that hampers subsequent efforts at surgical repair and can involve surgical injury to the rectum or urinary tract. Care must be taken in evaluation to ensure that other, more complex anomalies are not misdiagnosed. These patients also benefit from management by clinicians most experienced with complex genital anomalies.

Turner's syndrome also requires further work-up. Because of the high association of renal anomalies, ultrasound of the collecting system should be performed. Echocardiogram will verify a structurally normal heart. Thyroid dysfunction is also highly associated with Turner's syndrome, and these women should be appropriately monitored with TSH. Cervical spine skeletal abnormalities are seen in 12% of Turner's patients, and thus a C-spine x-ray is warranted.

Treatment of Secondary Amenorrhea

Outflow Tract Abnormalities

Women whose history and evaluation are consistent with outflow tract abnormalities should be referred to a gynecologist for definitive diagnosis and management. If Asherman's syndrome is confirmed through further testing, which may include a hysterosalpingogram or hysteroscopy, the condition can be corrected by surgically removing the synechiae. This is usually done in the operating room using an operative hysteroscope.

Ovarian Failure

When ovarian failure has been diagnosed, chromosomal analysis should be performed in all women under 30, and women with abnormal chromosomes should be referred for genetic counseling. A search for autoimmune disorders such as systemic lupus erythematosus, rheumatoid arthritis, Addison's disease, and autoimmune thyroid disease should be considered based on clinical grounds. Women desiring future childbearing should be referred to an infertility specialist to learn their options. Early menopause increases the risk of the development of osteoporosis and women with premature ovarian failure may benefit from estrogen replacement to prevent osteoporosis (45,46).

Chronic Anovulation

Women with hyperprolactinemia can be treated with a dopamine agonist, usually bromocriptine. Once corrected, ovulatory function is restored in the majority of women (31). One study found that 80% of women treated had ovulatory cycles after 6 months of therapy (47). Surgical correction may be needed in some women with macroadenomas that affect vision, have mass effect, or fail to respond to medical treatment. Hyperprolactinemia due to the use of medications, especially psychotropic drugs, requires a collaborative and individualized approach because alternative drugs may or may not be available or effective. Hypothyroidism is easily treated with oral thyroid replacement, restoring normal ovulatory function. Women with Cushing's syndrome, Sheehan's syndrome, or adult-onset congenital adrenal hyperplasia should be promptly referred to an endocrinologist for management. Most women with androgen excess will have PCOS. See Chapter 7 for full discussion.

In the case of hypothalamic hypogonadism, the underlying cause must be addressed. Women with eating disorders generally require a multidisciplinary management team. Although causality is still an issue, women with anorexia nervosa are certainly at significant risk for osteopenia and osteoporosis. It is unclear whether replacement with estrogens diminishes bone loss, and expert recommendation is divided on the role of hormone replacement therapy and oral contraceptives in the management of this group (48). Athletes with excessive exercise should be encouraged to decrease their level of exercise to the point that normal menstrual cycles resume. Nevertheless, eating disorders can be associated with persistent anovulation even after weight stabilization.

Because eating disorders can be associated with pregnancy-related complications, recovery or complete remission is imperative before attempting pregnancy. Calcium and vitamin D should be recommended in both groups.

Amenorrhea Caused by Medications

When amenorrhea seems to be caused by specific medications, alternative drugs should be considered. This requires consultation among medical specialists about other medications available and the risk of switching medical therapy. When alternative therapies are not available or advisable, management should be individualized.

Conclusion

Amenorrhea itself is not a definitive diagnosis but rather is a sign indicating the need to identify an underlying disorder. In managing patients with amenorrhea, the clinician is faced with a challenging situation that requires careful and in some cases timely deduction of the underlying disorder in an effort to manage associated symptoms and to prevent serious sequelae. This often includes the involvement of an obstetrician/gynecologist or reproductive endocrinologist.

REFERENCES

1. Speroff L, Glass RH, Kase NG. Clinical Gynecologic Endocrinology and Infertility, 6th ed. Philadelphia: Lippincott Williams & Wilkins; 1999:421-85.

2. Treloar AE, Boynton RE, Behn BG, Brown BW. Variation of the human menstrual cycle through reproductive life. Int J Fertil. 1967;12:77-126.

3. Nelson LM, Bakalov V, Pastor C. Amenorrhea. eMedicine [serial online]. September 25, 2002. Available at: http://www.emedicine.com/med/topic117.htm. Accessed December 2002, 2002.

4. Hillard P. Menstruation in young girls: a clinical perspective. Obstet Gynecol. 2002; 99:655-62.

5. Treloar AE, Boynton RE, Behn BG, Brown BW. Variation of the human menstrual cycle through reproductive life. Int J Fertil. 1967;12:77-126.

6. Vollman RF. Assessment of the fertile and sterile phases of the menstrual cycle. Int Rev Nat Fam Plan. 1977;1:40.

7. Apter D, Vihko R. Early menarche, a risk factor for breast cancer, indicates early onset of ovulatory cycles. J Clin Endocrinol Metab. 1983;57:82-6.

8. Metcalf MG. Incidence of ovulation from the menarche to the menopause: observations of 622 New Zealand women. N Z Med J. 1983;96:645-8.

9. Magyar DM, Boyers SP, Marshall JR, Abraham GE. Regular menstrual cycles and premenstrual molimina as indicators of ovulation. Obstet Gynecol. 1979;53:411-4.

10. Reindollar RH, Byrd JR, McDonough PG. Delayed sexual development: a study of 252 patients. Am J Obstet Gynecol. 1981;140:371-80.

11. Reindollar RH, Novak M, Tho SPT, McDonough PG. Adult-onset amnorrhea: a study of 262 patients. Am J Obstet Gynecol. 1986;155:531-43.

12. Timmreck LS, Reindollar RH. Contemporary issues in primary amenorrhea. Obstet Gynecol Clin North Am. 2003;30:287-302.

13. Hillard P. Imperforate hymen. eMedicine Journal [serial online]; 2002.

14. Spence J, Gervaize P, Jain S. Uterovaginal anomalies: diagnosis and current management in teens. Curr Womens Health Rep. 2003;3:445-50.

15. Laufer MR. Congenital absence of the vagina: in search of the perfect solution. When, and by what technique, should a vagina be created? Curr Opin Obstet Gynecol. 2002; 14:441-4.

16. Patterson MN, McPhaul MJ, Hughes IA. Androgen insensitivity syndrome. Baillieres Clin Endocrinol Metab. 1994;8:379-404.

17. Nelson LM, Bakalov V, Pastor C. Ovarian insufficiency in eMedicine. Revised Jan 2, 2004. Accessed September 23, 2004.

18. Yan G, Shoenfeld, D, Penney C, et al. Identification of premature ovarian failure patients with underlyng autoimmunity. J Womens Health Gender-Based Med. 2000;9: 275-87.

19. Nelson, et al. The development of luteinizing graafian follicles in patients with karyotypically normal spontaneous premature ovarian failure. J Clin Endo Metab 1994;79: 1470-5.

20. Taylor AE, Adams JM, Mulder JE, et al. A randomized, controlled trial of estradiol replacement therapy in women with hypergonadotropic amenorrhea. J Clin Endocrinol Metab. 1996;81:3615-21.

21. Kim TJ, et al. Routine endocrine screening for patients with karyotypically normal spontaneous premature ovarian failure. Obstet Gynecol. 89:777-9.

22. Bakalov VK, et al. Adrenal autoantibodies detect asymptomatic auto-immune adrenal insufficiency in young women with spontaneous premature ovarian failure. Human Reprod. 2002;27:2096-3.

23. Rotterdam ESHRE/ASRM-Sponsored PCOS Consensus Workshop Group. Revised 2003 consensus on diagnostic criteria and long-term health risks related to polycystic ovary syndrome. Fertil Steril. 2004;81:19-25.

24. Polycystic ovary syndrome. ACOG Practice Bulletin. 2002;41.

25. Larsen P, Kronenberg HM, Polansky KS, et al. Williams Texbook of Endocrinology, 10th ed. Philadelphia: WB Saunders; 2002.

26. Yazigi, RA, Quintero CH, Salemeh WA. Prolactin disorders. Fertil Steril. 1997;67:215-25.

27. Schlechte JA. Prolactinoma. N Engl J Med. 2003;349:2035.

28. Molitch ME. Disorders of prolactin secretion. Endocrinol Metab Clin North Am. 2001;30:585-610.

29. Fagan KM. Pharmacologic management of athletic amenorrhea. Clin Sports Med. 1998;17:327-41.

30. Marcus MD, Loucks TL, Berga SL. Psychological correlates of functional hypothalamic amenorrhea. Fertil Steril. 2001;76:310-6.

31. Berga SL, Marcus MD, Loucks TL, et al. Recovery of ovarian activity in women with functional hypothalamic amenorrhea who were treated with cognitive behavior therapy. Fertil Steril. 2003;80:976-81.

32. Koutras DA. Disturbances of menstruation in thyroid disease. Ann N Y Acad Sci. 1997; 816:280-4.

33. Kaunitz AM. Menstruation: choosing whether...and when. Contraception. 2000;62:277-84.

34. Kaunitz AM. Injectable depot medroxyprogesterone acetate contraception: an update for U.S. clinicians. Int J Fertil Womens Med. 1998;43:73-83.

35. Kaunitz AM. Long-acting injectable contraception with depot medroxyprogesterone acetate. Am J Obstet Gynecol. 1994;170:1543-9.

36. Schwallie PC, Assenzo JR. Contraception. 1974;10:181-202.

37. Davis A. A 21-year-old woman with menstrual irregularity. JAMA. 1997;277:1308-14.

38. Plosker GL, Brogden RN. Leuprorelin: a review of its pharmacology and therapeutic use in prostatic cancer, endometriosis and other sex hormone-related disorders. Drugs. 1994;48:930-67.

39. Blumenfeld Z. Ovarian rescue/protection from chemotherapeutic agents. J Soc Gynecol Invest. 2001;8(1 Suppl Proceedings):S60-4.

40. Laufer MR, Floor AE, Parsons KE, Barbieri RL. Hormone testing in women with adult-onset amenorrhea. Gynecol Obstet Invest. 1995; 40:200-3.

41. Rebar RW, Connolly HV. Clinical features of young women with hypergonadotropic amenorrhea. Fertil Steril. 1990;53:804-10.

42. Luthold WW, Borges MF, Marcondes JA, et al. Serum testosterone fractions in women: normal and abnormal clinical states. Metab Clin Exp. 1993;42:638-43.

43. Speroff L, Glass RH, Kase NG. Clinical Gynecologic Endocrinology and Infertility. 6th ed. Philadelphia: Lippincott Williams & Wilkins; 1999:505-11.

44. Timmreck LS, Reindollar RH. Contemporary issues in primary amenorrhea. Obstet Gynecol Clin North Am. 2003;30:287-302.

45. Anasti JN, Kalantaridou SN, Kimzey LM, et al. Bone loss in young women with karyotypically normal spontaneous premature ovarian failure. Obstet Gynecol. 1998;91:12-5.

46. Ohta H, Sugimoto I, Masuda A, et al. Decreased bone mineral density associated with early menopause progresses for at least ten years: cross-sectional comparisons between early and normal menopausal women. Bone. 1996;18:227-31.

47. Vance ML, Thorner MO. Prolactinomas. Endocrinol Metab Clin North Am. 1987;16: 731-53.

48. Bruni V, Dei M, Vicini I, et al. Estrogen replacement therapy in the management of osteopenia related to eating disorders. Ann N Y Acad Sci. 2000;900:416-21.

4

Perimenopausal Bleeding

Sophia Ouhilal, MD
Ellen Harrison, MD
Nanette Santoro, MD

The age at which a woman presents with a menstrual bleeding disorder greatly influences differential diagnosis, testing, and treatment. To recognize and address abnormal uterine bleeding in a perimenopausal woman, the clinician needs to understand the physiological state of a healthy perimenopausal woman and the normal range of altered bleeding patterns. Because women of perimenopausal age have a higher risk of serious genital tract pathology than younger women, diagnosis and treatment of bleeding abnormalities requires awareness of differential diagnoses and strategies for their evaluation. This chapter will summarize the features of perimenopause, review physiologic and pathologic causes of bleeding, and discuss diagnostic approaches and options for treatment.

Menopausal Transition (Perimenopause) Defined

Menopausal transition is a gradual process that occurs over years. The World Health Organization (WHO) defines *menopausal transition*, or *perimenopause*, as the 2 to 8 years that precede menopause and the first year after cessation of menses (1). It is a period during which oocytes undergo rapid depletion and ovulation and menses cease. Hormonal and menstrual pattern changes may occur in a woman's 30s, but perimenopause more typically begins in the late 40s (2). *Early perimenopause* is defined as at least one menses within the past 3 months associated with increased variability of cycles of more than 7 days or skipped cycles; *late perimenopause* is defined by amenorrhea of 3 to 11 months (3).

Epidemiology

The epidemiological study of perimenopause is complex: there is no gold standard test; duration is variable; and it is largely based on subjective judgments of the woman, whose perspective may be culturally and/or psychologically influenced. In other words, perimenopause is not determined by biological factors alone.

One way to approach the epidemiology of perimenopause numerically is to make estimations based on census data, with the assumption that perimenopause lasts an average of 5 years. The 2000 United States census reported approximately 21.5 million women aged 40 to 49 (4). Thus there are roughly 11 million women in the United States in perimenopause. Racial distribution is as follows: white women in their 40s, approximately 8 million; African Americans, 1.2 million; American Indians, 150,000; Asians, 450,000; Pacific Islanders, 25,000; and other races, approximately 500,000 (4,5). Average age of onset is 46, with 95% of women entering perimenopause between ages 39 and 51. Average duration is 5 years; duration is 2-8 years for 95% of women.

Cultural Attitudes Towards Menstruation

Women's perspective on perimenopause influences their clinical presentation and expectations of care. A questionnaire has been developed to measure attitudes towards menstruation and menstrual symptoms (6). The WHO has evaluated perceptions in various cultures through examining bleeding pattern change with oral contraceptive use. It found that aversion to amenorrhea was culture dependent (7). Women in western countries had fewer negative attitudes about amenorrhea than women in undeveloped countries. A study of Dutch women on preferred frequency and characteristics of menstrual bleeding in relation to reproductive and hormonal status found that over 50% of women aged 45-49 (perimenopausal but still menstruating) would prefer to be amenorrheic. Preference for amenorrhea increased with age. These preferences contrast sharply with the everyday practice of prescribing oral contraceptives to mimic monthly bleeding and switching of oral contraceptive to reverse amenorrhea (8).

The Historical Perspective

Perimenopausal bleeding may be more common in our modern age than in the distant past (9-13). Evidence in contemporary hunter-gatherer populations suggests that prehistoric women may have had far fewer periods than modern women because of later menarche, earlier and more frequent pregnancies, and more prolonged lactational amenorrhea (14-16). Evidence from contemporary hunter-gatherers suggests that our prehistoric ancestors had only about 160 periods per lifetime compared with about 450 for modern women. Shorter life expectancy would also have affected frequency of perimenopause in prehistory.

Normal Hormonal Changes with Aging

Aging leads to a progressive change in menstruation. Normal menstruation requires an exquisitely timed and coordinated sequence of hypothalamic-pituitary-ovarian events, which are disrupted as the once-abundant supply of ovarian follicles nears exhaustion. Signaling by products of developing follicles is disrupted as the follicles decrease in number, and their depletion is concomitantly accelerated.

Higher levels of follicle-stimulating hormone (FSH) and lower levels of inhibin, with often normal or elevated levels of estradiol and luteinizing hormone (LH), usually characterize perimenopausal menstrual cycles (17-23). Higher FSH levels reflect lower inhibin production by ovarian granulosa cells. FSH may fluctuate widely during perimenopause and thus is not a useful tool for predicting onset of menopause (24). Estradiol levels fluctuate widely, and extreme elevations may occur during the perimenopausal period (23).

Because hormone levels are erratic, menses may become erratic. One common change is an increasing number of anovulatory cycles. The first change that occurs is a shortening of menstrual cycles followed by an increase in cycle frequency and amount of bleeding. (Perimenopausal cycles may be shorter by up to 3 to 7 days, probably because of earlier ovulation.) Skipped cycles subsequently occur. A period of prolonged amenorrhea of 3-11 months or a range of more than 42 days is a good predictor of menopause within the next 4 years (25). In late perimenopause, the interval between menses increases as fewer normal cycles occur. These changes are normal results of aging.

Because there may be variations in hormonal change in women from different racial and cultural backgrounds, much remains to be learned about the exact mechanisms by which perimenopausal transition takes place.

Risk Factors

As women age, the prevalence of organic pathologies increases, and increased risk of endometrial hyperplasia and cancer is associated with hypertension, obesity, and diabetes in perimenopausal women (26). In women younger than

Table 4-1   Causes of Perimenopausal Abnormal Bleeding

- Anovulation
- Obesity
- Thyroid disorders (hyperthyroidism, hypothyroidism)
- Fibroids

age 40, the risk of endometrial cancer remains extremely low, and bleeding is more likely due to anovulation or intracavitary lesions such as polyps or submucous fibroids. The incidence of fibroids is extremely high in African American women and may occur in up to 40% of perimenopausal African American women. This does not, however, mean that 40% of African American women will have bleeding abnormalities caused by their fibroids. Causes of perimenopausal abnormal bleeding are listed in Table 4-1.

Etiology

Evaluating changes in the pattern of bleeding during perimenopause presents special challenges to the clinician. Bleeding pattern changes are a common finding in healthy perimenopausal women and frequently occur in the absence of any pathologic conditions. However, vigilance is necessary because the prevalence of organic pathologies is higher in perimenopausal women with abnormal bleeding compared with their younger counterparts. The causes of perimenopausal bleeding can be hormonal or nonhormonal, benign, premalignant, or malignant.

Benign lesions such as polyps and submucous fibroids are more prevalent in perimenopausal women and are risk factors for abnormal bleeding. Although the mechanisms are not well understood, anatomic lesions such as polyps and fibroids are believed to cause abnormal bleeding by distorting the endometrial cavity.

Obesity, hyperthyroidism, and hypothyroidism are also risk factors for abnormal bleeding that more frequently occur in perimenopausal women than in younger menstruating women. As already mentioned, mechanisms of hormonal change may vary among women from different racial or cultural backgrounds.

High body mass index (BMI) seems to influence menstrual cycle function adversely in women in the early menopause transition (27). Women with even a modest elevation in their BMI to 26 kg/m^2 have been found to be less likely to ovulate, to have more variability in follicular phase length, and to excrete fewer LH, FSH, and progesterone metabolites when daily urinary sampling was done.

Table 4-2   Abnormal Menstrual Patterns

Menstrual Pattern	Definition
Intermenstrual bleeding	Bleeding between menstrual cycles
Metrorrhagia	Irregular bleeding
Menorrhagia	Excessive bleeding at regular intervals
Polymenorrhea	Menstrual cycle interval less than 21 days
Oligomenorrhea	Menstrual cycle interval longer than 37 days

Recognizing Abnormal Bleeding Patterns

The several kinds of abnormal menstrual patterns are listed in Table 4-2 (28). Perimenopausal patterns are extremely variable; almost any pattern is possible (29). Patients may experience regular menstrual cycles, occasional spotting, or alternate between skipping a few cycles and return to normal menstruation. Some women may have longer intermenstrual intervals (26,30-32).

Some changes in menstrual pattern are more likely to represent important pathology than others, but all abnormal bleeding must be evaluated. Infrequent cycles, cycles of variable length, or a single late and copious period will likely warrant no, or minimal, intervention, whereas intermenstrual bleeding or excessive bleeding requires diagnostic and therapeutic intervention.

Diagnosis

When diagnosing abnormal bleeding in perimenopausal women, the normal changes of the menstrual cycles associated with aging should be kept in mind. However, it is important to rule out local uterine pathologies, pregnancy, and thyroid abnormalities before diagnosing onset of perimenopause, and the physician should not allow the wide range of physical symptoms occurring with variable menstrual patterns to cloud his or her diagnosis, whether the diagnosis is of pathology or of normal perimenopause (2).

The clinician must be more watchful for a malignant process when evaluating menstrual irregularities in perimenopausal women compared with younger women. As women age, concomitant medical conditions such as hypertension, obesity, and diabetes become more prevalent, and these are associated with a higher risk of endometrial hyperplasia and cancer in perimenopausal women (26). The physiologic changes naturally occurring with age can themselves increase risk for malignant disease; anovulatory cycles during perimenopause not pathologic in themselves are characterized by unopposed estrogenic stimulation of the endometrium, which predisposes to endometrial hyperplasia, a premalignant pathology, and endometrial carcinoma. In women younger than 40 years of age, the risk of endometrial cancer remains extremely low (risk increases after age 40).

Clinical Presentation

Women in perimenopausal transition will often present for consultation about menstrual irregularities. Common presenting complaints are changes in menstrual cyclicity, changes in the quantity of bleeding, or symptoms of anemia. The presentation may be asymptomatic anemia incidentally found by laboratory testing or a serious episode of acute blood loss with volume depletion. Menstrual cycles as short as 17 days have been reported in normal populations of women traversing menopause (33). For other patients, bleeding patterns may not be a complaint but rather elicited upon questioning as part of an annual examination. How long and how often before these perimenopausal bleeding patterns are reported to the physician depend on the severity of the symptomatology and how much it interferes with activities of daily living. Associated conditions such as hot flashes, premenstrual symptoms, or symptoms of anemia may also influence when the patient will consult. Furthermore, there may be related cultural issues, age, and racial variations in how and when symptoms are reported.

History

The detailed menstrual history is a central element when evaluating the perimenopausal-bleeding patient. Information regarding the onset, duration, pattern, and quantity of bleeding should be obtained. Associated symptoms and interference with daily activities should be elicited. The possibility of pregnancy needs to be addressed. Ovulatory status may be clarified by the history.

Several aspects of general and reproductive health should be addressed by history taking with the perimenopausal-bleeding patient. It is important to explore whether the bleeding is indeed genital in origin and rule out other sites of bleeding such as the gastrointestinal or genitourinary tracts (34). A history of hepatic, renal, autoimmune, vasculitic, and endocrine disease should also be sought. Perimenopause coincides with the age at which many unrelated conditions appear, which may indirectly influence bleeding patterns. Examples of such conditions include diabetes, obesity, and thyroid disorders. Hypothyroid patients may report amenorrhea and menorrhagia, and hyperthyroid patients may occasionally report amenorrhea. Changes may be subtle but ultimately lead to significant dysfunction if they go undetected and untreated.

It is imperative to explore whether abnormal bleeding began during perimenopause or was a consistent feature of menses earlier in life. One must inquire about any evidence of abnormal bleeding patterns in the patient and her relatives. Previous experience with trauma, delivery, surgery, and dental extractions should also be sought.

A history suggestive of clotting disorders should be elicited. The patient should be asked about epistaxis, gum bleeding, and bruising. A positive family history, a history of lengthy, excessive menstrual bleeding, and a history of bruising or bleeding after procedures should raise the level of suspicion sufficiently to warrant testing. Most inherited clotting disorders have manifested themselves before a woman reaches perimenopause; however, although they are seldom asymptomatic, clotting disorders can remain undiagnosed until the perimenopausal years. In one study of women with menorrhagia in whom no cause was found, 17% were found to have an inherited bleeding disorder that had remained undiagnosed; roughly half of these women were 40 years of age or older. Of these disorders, von Willebrand's disease was the most common, occurring in 13% of the women, with no difference in the prevalence in women above and below 40 years of age. Factor XI deficiency was the next most frequent disorder (35). Key elements of history taking are listed in Table 4-3.

Physical Examination

A complete physical examination must be performed in a woman with perimenopausal bleeding abnormalities to verify the source of bleeding, assess the findings of acute or chronic blood loss, confirm genital pathology detectable on exam, and to look for systemic diseases that might be responsible for the clinical complaint. Vital signs including orthostatic changes can provide an indication of hemodynamic state and consequences of anemia and may shed light on the thyroid status. A skin evaluation may provide some useful clues such as hirsutism or acanthosis nigricans (suggestive of polycystic ovarian syndrome), pallor, petechiae, or bruising. The thyroid gland should be carefully examined and signs of thyroid dysfunction observed. The gynecological examination should evaluate non-uterine causes of genital tract bleeding and should include a careful inspection of the vulva, vagina, and cervix. A Papanicolaou test with sampling of the exocervix with a spatula and the endocervix with a cytobrush should also be done. A bimanual examination including a rectovaginal exam should then be performed to assess the uterus and ovaries. Particular attention should be paid to the size and contour of the uterus as well as the presence of tenderness. The gynecological examination might yield important information in a perimenopausal, bleeding patient. A cervical ectropion or polyp might explain postcoital bleeding, and an enlarged uterus might suggest fibroids, possible neoplasia, or even pregnancy.

Table 4-3   Key Elements of History Taking for Patient with Perimenopausal Bleeding

Bleeding history	• Age of menarche • Last menstrual period • Menstrual patterns • Bleeding: quantity, duration, timing, precipitants • Symptoms of anemia, fever, weight loss • Interference with activities of daily living
Vasomotor symptom history	• Presence of hot flashes (36-38) • Description of the quality of the flash: intensity, timing, location, alleviating and worsening conditions, interference with activities of daily living and quality of life (39-44)
Medical history	• Platelet and clotting disorders: bruising, epistaxis, gum bleeding, bleeding following delivery, dental and surgical procedures, trauma • Chronic hepatic disease • Renal insufficiency • Autoimmune and vasculitides • Thyroid disorders • Diabetes, hypertension
Screening history	• Date and outcome of last Pap test • Date and outcome of last breast examination and mammogram
Pregnancy and contraception	• Sexual activity • Contraception: last menstrual period, intrauterine device, oral contraceptive pill
Medications	• Anticoagulants • Hormone replacement therapy (45,46) • Corticosteroids • Chemotherapeutic agents
Family history	• Breast cancer • Osteoporosis • Cardiovascular disease • Coagulopathies/thromboembolism

Differential Diagnosis

Examples of pathologies that may manifest as perimenopausal bleeding abnormalities and associated causes are listed in Table 4-4.

Medical Workup

All patients with abnormal bleeding should have a complete blood count to assess the hemoglobin, hematocrit, and platelets. Objective evidence of anemia can clarify the extent of blood loss in many cases. Patients can accommodate

Table 4-4   Differential Diagnosis for Perimenopausal Bleeding

Abnormal uterine bleeding	• Anovulation • Uterine fibroids • Uterine polyps • Clotting dyscrasias • Endometrial hyperplasia • Neoplasias (e.g., cervical or endometrial carcinoma) • Pregnancy
Amenorrhea	• Pregnancy • Hypothalamic amenorrhea related to excess diet including anorexia nervosa or bulimia • Excessive exercise
Thyroid abnormalities	• Hyperthyroidism: frequent, light bleeding • Hypothyroidism: infrequent, heavy bleeding
Iatrogenic causes	• Contraceptives (progestin-only agents and intrauterine devices) • Anticoagulants
Systemic diseases	• Hepatic failure: clotting abnormalities • Renal disease: irregular bleeding

large volumes of menstrual blood loss over time and may be chronically anemic without ever providing a history of repeated excessive menstruation.

To rule out hypothyroidism or hyperthyroidism, perimenopausal women should be screened for thyroid dysfunction with an initial TSH measurement. If TSH is abnormal, further thyroid testing is warranted (47). It should be appreciated that secondary and tertiary hypothyroidism, which are rare, will not be adequately detected by a TSH level alone.

On an individual basis, other tests, such as tests of clotting, synthetic function of the liver, renal function, or alternative causes of anemia, may be useful based on information obtained from the history and physical exam.

A workup for clotting abnormalities should be individualized. In patients with a history suggestive of a clotting disorder, a basic workup should include a complete blood count, including hemoglobin, hematocrit, white blood cell count, differential, mean cell volume, platelet count, prothrombin time, activated thromboplastin time, a peripheral smear, and testing for von Willebrand's disease (34). If surgery or an invasive procedure is being contemplated, one should keep in mind that approximately one in six women with menorrhagia unexplained by any anatomic disease has a previously undiagnosed clotting disorder (48). Some physicians may recommend testing in these circumstances, but one should consider the practice environment and the patient's individual circumstances in deciding what workup is warranted (49). For fuller discussion, see Chapter 9.

A luteal phase progesterone may be measured if ovulatory status is uncertain, although ovulatory status can change from month to month in perimenopausal women. Cervical cytology and sexually transmitted disease screening for chlamydia and gonorrhea should be considered. A pregnancy test should be routinely performed in cases of perimenopausal bleeding.

Laboratory Testing and Clinical Judgment

Although FSH and LH are typically elevated and estradiol is typically low in postmenopausal patients, this is not necessarily the case in perimenopausal patients. In fact, FSH, LH, and estradiol measurements are not helpful in menstruating women because their levels may fluctuate widely during the perimenopausal transition. Furthermore, a single result that falls outside the normal range for reproductive-aged women cannot be relied upon to predict cessation of menses. In fact, three worldwide population studies failed to confirm the value of FSH testing (50-52). FSH testing is indicated for ruling out hypogonadotropic hypogonadism. Currently, tests for inhibins, activins, müllerian-inhibiting substance, and various other hormonal combinations are being investigated. What is certain is that no laboratory test can replace clinical judgment.

In general, a diagnosis of perimenopause is based on the patient's history of symptoms, such as irregular bleeding and hot flashes, after having first ruled out other etiologies for these symptoms.

Endometrial Evaluation

The evaluation of abnormal bleeding in the perimenopausal patient should include an assessment of the endometrial cavity. Even though abnormal bleeding may simply be anovulatory or dysfunctional, these are diagnoses of exclusion, and pathologic etiologies such as polyps, submucous fibroids, hyperplasia, and carcinomas should be ruled out first.

Endometrial polyps are benign growths in the uterus that should be removed by a gynecologist because they may lead to bleeding by disturbing the endometrial cavity (removal is usually uncomplicated). Upon removal, polyps are sent for pathological analysis to rule out rare neoplastic changes. Submucous fibroids are benign tumors of the uterus that protrude in the endometrial cavity. They too lead to abnormal bleeding, which often prompts their removal. Endometrial hyperplasia is an abnormal thickening of the endometrial cavity that, if left untreated, may lead to endometrial cancer. (One should remember that a thickened endometrium in a premenopausal woman does not necessarily mean that pathology is present [53]). If any of these pathological changes are found, the patient should be referred to a gynecologist for further management.

Organic pathologies can be differentiated by several diagnostic techniques (Table 4-5). Choice of approach should be individualized and discussed with

Table 4-5   Perimenopausal Bleeding Diagnostic Techniques

• Endometrial biopsy	• Hysteroscopy
• Ultrasonography	• Dilatation and curettage
• Sonohysterography	• Magnetic resonance imaging

each patient after an evaluation of the risks and benefits involved. If under-lying neoplastic or hyperplastic process is suspected, a Pipelle endometrial biopsy should be performed. If biopsy is negative, saline infusion sonohys-terography is a minimally invasive way of identifying polyps or submucous fi-broids (54). If polyps or submucous fibroids are diagnosed, the patient may undergo a hysteroscopy-guided resection in the operating room.

Endometrial Biopsy
The Pipelle biopsy is the standard for office endometrial sampling (55). Simple and widely used to rule out endometrial hyperplasia and carcinoma, it is a quick office procedure; it causes mild cramping but is usually well tolerated by patients and yields rapid results on the status of the endometrium (55). Stovall assessed 40 women with known carcinoma and performed Pipelle biopsies before per-forming a total abdominal hysterectomy. Neoplasia was diagnosed in 39 of 40 patients, with an accuracy of 97.5% (56). Although the pain associated with en-dometrial biopsy is usually tolerable, some women may occasionally experience severe pain, particularly if they have cervical stenosis (34). The discomfort asso-ciated with endometrial biopsy can be minimized with routine use of oral anal-gesia, which may be combined with local anesthesia (34). A negative endometrial biopsy in a patient who has persistent abnormal vaginal bleeding merits further evaluation because a blind biopsy procedure cannot completely rule out a focal neoplasic or hyperplastic pathology. Endometrial biopsy may miss focal structural abnormalities such as fibroids or polyps (55). Patients with persistent symptoms, despite a normal endometrial biopsy, should be further assessed.

Ultrasonography
Noninvasive options for investigating abnormal uterine bleeding in peri-menopausal women include endovaginal ultrasound and sonohysterogram. Endovaginal ultrasound is inexpensive and minimally invasive. It allows for visualization of the uterus and adnexa and can assess endometrial thickness and the myometrium. Endovaginal ultrasound studies for vaginal bleeding have been mostly performed on women with postmenopausal bleeding. A threshold of 5 mm for endometrial thickness by transvaginal ultrasound had a negative predictive value of 99% in ruling out carcinoma and is generally considered a reasonable standard of care for the postmenopausal woman (57). Conclusive data for perimenopausal women are lacking.

Sonohysterography

A sonohysterogram may yield helpful additional information that may not be seen on regular transvaginal ultrasound. Fluid enhancement of the endometrial image leads to a dramatically improved ability to delineate uterine polyps or submucous fibroids. The principle of the sonohysterogram is to instill fluid in the uterine cavity, usually normal saline, to enhance the vaginal ultrasound assessment of the endometrial detail. The sonohysterogram technique is as follows: An endovaginal ultrasound is first performed to assess the uterus and adnexa. The ultrasound probe is then removed, a sterile (one-armed) speculum is inserted, and the cervix cleansed. A catheter is then threaded past the cervix into the uterine cavity, the speculum is removed, and the ultrasound probe placed, taking care to maintain the intrauterine position of the catheter. Balloon catheters can be used, as they are less likely to become dislodged, but they have the disadvantage of causing uterine cramping. Fluid is then instilled under low pressure, with direct sonographic visualization and the uterus viewed in its longitudinal and transverse axes from cervix to fundus.

Significant polyps or submucous myomas should be readily visualized by sonohysterogram. For evaluating abnormal uterine bleeding, the sonohysterogram is superior to transvaginal ultrasound alone because of its ability to detect focal lesions. In one study, transvaginal ultrasound had a rate of detection of 23.5% for focal intrauterine pathology compared with the sonohysterogram rate of 94.1% (58). In another study, transvaginal ultrasound failed to diagnose 20% of polyps, whereas sonohysterogram identified almost all abnormalities (59).

Hysteroscopy

Patients with persistent symptoms, despite a normal endometrial biopsy, should be further assessed. Hysteroscopy may be performed instead of sonohysterography depending on the physician's preference and the individual's condition. Hysteroscopy has the advantage of direct visualization of the cavity with possibility for directed biopsies. A diagnostic hysteroscopy can be performed in an office setting with minimal patient discomfort and a very low incidence of complications. It may also be combined with an operative hysteroscopy if a polyp or submucous myoma is diagnosed and needs to be resected. Because it is a costly procedure and requires specific equipment and a skilled operator, operative hysteroscopy should be performed in the operating room.

Dilation and Curettage

If one is unable to enter the uterine cavity for an endometrial biopsy or a sonohysterography, one should stop the procedure. It may be that the cervix is stenotic, that the uterus is very deviated, or that there is a lesion obstructing entry into the uterine cavity. Continuing the procedure might result in uterine perforation and bleeding. An MRI can be performed in such circumstances to obtain an enhanced view of the interior of the uterus. However, in most clinical settings, a dilatation and curettage by a gynecologist should then be performed under anesthesia. Intra-operative ultrasound may be a helpful guide when entering the cavity. If there is a high index of suspicion for neoplasia, the patient may be referred to a gynecologic oncologist for sampling.

Magnetic Resonance Imaging

MRI is a noninvasive procedure that can precisely localize fibroids and help distinguish between myomas and adenomyosis (60). The overall diagnostic potential of MRI appears comparable to sonohysterogram and hysteroscopy, with a sensitivity near 100% for submucous myomas and a specificity of 91% compared with a specificity of 90% for endovaginal ultrasound and 87% for hysteroscopy (61).

Treatment

Treatment of abnormal perimenopausal bleeding should be geared towards control of acute bleeding and prevention of future abnormal bleeding, as well as minimization of endometrial hyperplasia and endometrial cancer risks. Initial management should be medical. Surgical management can be offered if medical management fails. The etiology of the bleeding, the individual patient's risk-benefits ratio, and the desired outcome are all factors in selecting the most appropriate treatment.

Prolonged intervals of amenorrhea are common in perimenopausal women, and no treatment is usually required if the patient ovulates periodically (2). Furthermore, because any menstrual pattern is possible, perimenopausal women are not protected from pregnancy and should be informed of this. If a woman is sexually active, contraceptive methods should be discussed and offered. If abnormal uterine bleeding is present, one has to effectively rule out any organic pathology. If fibroids, polyps, hyperplasia, neoplasia, or vaginal and cervical abnormalities are found, the patient should be referred to a gynecologist for further management. One should also keep in mind that not all fibroids are the cause of bleeding and not all polyps need to be removed: if there are no underlying organic reproductive tract pathologies, medical treatment may be preferable for anovulatory bleeding.

Women with perimenopausal bleeding may experience substantial fatigue due to anemia and may benefit from iron supplementation. Antifibrinolytics such as tranexamic acid have been evaluated and shown to be effective in reducing blood loss by about 50% compared with nonsteroidal anti-inflammatories (NSAIDs), which lead to an approximately 20% decrease in blood loss (62-64). However, these medications are not available in the United States. Ovulating patients with menorrhagia may benefit from anti-inflammatory drugs that reduce heavy bleeding (65). Cyclooxygenase (COX) is involved in the conversion of arachidonic acid into prostaglandins within the endometrium, and anti-inflammatory drugs such as NSAIDs act by inhibiting COX. Effective NSAIDs for menorrhagia include mefenamic acid, ibuprofen, naproxen, and indomethacin (66). Patients who do not respond to one preparation may be tried on several others before this approach is abandoned. Progestins, such as medroxyprogesterone acetate or norethinedrone may be administered monthly or as a levonorgestrel intra-uterine device (IUD). Although cyclical progestins may be useful for anovulatory bleeding, trials have shown little benefit of cyclical progestin treatment for ovulatory abnormal bleeding (62,67-70).

A recent systematic review indicated that progestin therapy was most effective when given for at least 21 days per month. Progestin IUDs are associated with a dramatic reduction of blood loss of approximately 85% and high patient satisfaction (68,70-73). Oral contraceptives are the most commonly prescribed medication for abnormal uterine bleeding in women of reproductive age (particularly for anovulatory bleeding) and may be given to a perimenopausal patient if she is a non-smoker and has no contraindications. If a woman is also experiencing vasomotor symptoms and has no other source of contraception, oral contraceptive pills can provide multiple benefits. Perimenopausal women may tolerate the 7-day/free-week pill poorly, with a resurgence of bothersome vasomotor symptoms. For these women, and for women troubled by menorrhagia, continuous oral contraceptives can be tried and titrated to the woman's convenience. Danazol has been shown to effectively reduce blood loss at doses of 200-400 mg per day (66,74-76). Its use, however, is limited because of its many unpleasant side effects, which may include deepening of the voice, acne, and near-universal weight gain (66).

If medical treatment fails, surgical treatment may be offered for abnormal uterine bleeding. In considering the different options, one should remember that the bleeding problem will resolve soon, as the woman reaches menopause. If fertility is not desired, temporary measures versus definitive measures need to be considered. Modalities include endometrial ablation (temporizing), and in some cases uterine artery embolization (temporizing) versus hysterectomy (definitive). Therapy should be individualized depending on the risk-benefit ratio and patient-specific characteristics. The patient should be referred to a gynecologist for a pre-surgical assessment. For a complete discussion of surgical options, see Chapter 12.

Managing Bleeding on Hormone Replacement Therapy

Perimenopausal women on hormone replacement therapy (HRT) who present with abnormal bleeding are difficult to manage. Most studies on breakthrough bleeding have been performed on postmenopausal women, so data on peri-menopausal women using HRT are lacking. Therefore, even though one may consider prescribing HRT to perimenopausal women, cases should be individualized and the risk-benefit ratio thoroughly discussed. The main reason to prescribe HRT to perimenopausal women is for relief of vasomotor symptoms. One small study of vasomotor symptoms in perimenopausal women in need of contraception entailed treatment with low doses of transdermal estradiol (0.05 mg/day for 21 days) and different oral progestins. These women had an improvement in hot flashes and night sweats, and the regimen appeared to have contraceptive efficacy (77). Another study treating symptomatic peri-menopausal women with 0.02 mg ethinyl estradiol and 1 mg norethinedrone acetate showed a decrease in the incidence and severity of hot flashes (78).

It is not known whether or not the doses of hormone used in HRT regimens, which are often 2-3 times lower than those used in oral contraceptives, will cause anovulation and therefore provide contraception. There are insufficient data to assume that HRT will protect a perimenopausal woman from an unwanted pregnancy. Breakthrough ovulation may also be a source of irregular bleeding for a woman on HRT, and this complicates the diagnosis. Often, the fastest way to get to the underlying diagnosis is to stop the hormones and observe menstrual cycle function (if any) for a few months.

Transitioning from Oral Contraceptives to Hormone Replacement Therapy

Perimenopausal women who require contraception and do not smoke may be easily managed on oral contraceptives. Oral contraceptives have the dual benefit of providing contraception while regularizing menstruation and providing relief for hot flashes. A question that often arises among clinicians is: When should a perimenopausal patient on oral contraceptives be transitioned to HRT? Furthermore, in light of the recent Women's Health Initiative findings, it is possibly preferable to not prescribe HRT at all, take the patient off the contraceptive pill, reassess vasomotor symptoms, then decide on any need for further treatment. The timing of the switch is hampered by the reality that cessation of menses, the hallmark of menopause, will not be observed in women taking oral contraceptives. There is no foolproof strategy for finding the physiologically perfect time to safely switch from oral contraception to HRT. Clinicians may choose the arbitrary age of 51, which is the median age of menopause, to make the switch, or they may tailor the timing to the woman's contraceptive needs. The FDA has approved oral contraceptive use up to the time of menopause. Importantly, despite the increased risk of myocardial infarction associated with oral contraceptive use, there is clearly no increased risk of breast cancer in women who have taken oral contraceptives

(79). Hormone use prior to a woman's last menstrual period does not pose the same risks as it does to postmenopausal women (80).

When to Refer

The decision on when to refer a perimenopausal patient with bleeding depends on the individual circumstances and one's level of comfort with the management of gynecological and endocrinological disease. Medical pathologies, such as thyroid dysfunction or coagulopathies, would warrant referral to an internist, endocrinologist, or hematologist. The presence of abnormal perimenopausal bleeding warrants a gynecological workup to rule out causes of bleeding such as fibroids, polyps, hyperplasia, or neoplasia, any of which may require surgical intervention.

Conclusion

The menopausal transition is a period in a woman's life about which much remains to be learned. Several disease conditions may first appear that may indirectly cause the irregularities discussed in this chapter. Perimenopause is often coupled with problematic vaginal bleeding, and it is important to identify abnormally heavy bleeding that can cause anemia. It is crucial to rule out systemic abnormalities, such as thyroid dysfunction, and pathologies of the reproductive tract, such as vaginal and cervical disease, as well as uterine abnormalities, such as polyps, fibroids, hyperplasia, and neoplasia. Once those abnormalities have been excluded, treatment should be individualized and depends upon a proper assessment of the risks and benefits involved. Clearly, an approach to perimenopausal bleeding that includes a proper evaluation and understanding of the different issues involved will help optimize the care of perimenopausal women.

REFERENCES

1. World Health Organization. Research on the Menopause in the 1990's: Report of a WHO Scientific Group. Geneva: WHO Technical Report Series 866; 1996.
2. Clinical challenges of perimenopause: consensus opinion of the North American menopause society. Menopause. 2000;7:5-13.
3. Santoro N. Hormonal Consequences and Treatments for the Perimenopause. Advanced Tutorial in Women's Health: Healthy Transitions from Peri- to Postmenopause. 17-19 May 2002, New York.
4. Bureau of the Census, Current Population Reports, by Sex, Age and Race; 2000.
5. Bureau of the Census, Current Population Reports. Projections of the Population of the United States: 1977 to 2050, Report No. Series P25-704, 1993.

6. Brooks-Gunn J, Ruble DN. The menstrual attitude questionnaire. Psychosom Med. 1980;42:503-12

7. World Health Organization Task Force on Psychosocial Research in Family Planning. Special Program of Research, Development and Research Training in Human Reproduction. A cross-sectional study of menstruation: implications for contraceptive development and use. Stud Fam Plan. 1981;12:3-16

8. Den Tonkelad I, Bjorn JO. Preferred frequency and characteristics of menstrual bleeding in relation to reproductive status, oral contraceptive use, and hormone replacement therapy use. Contraception. 1999;59:357-62

9. Magner LN. A History of Medicine. New York: Marcel Dekker; 1992.

10. Golub S. Periods, from Menarche to Menopause. Newbury Park, CA: Sage Publications; 1992.

11. Crawford R. Superstitions of menstruation. Lancet. 1915;2:1331.

12. Pliny the Elder. Historia Naturalis. Carbondale: Southern Illinois University Press; 1962.

13. Speroff L, Glass RH, Kase NG. Clinical Gynecologic Endocrinology and Infertility. 6th ed. Philadelphia: Lippincott Williams & Wilkins; 1999:518.

14. Eaton SB, Pike MC, Short RV, et al. Women's reproductive cancers in evolutionary context. Q Rev Biol. 1994;69:353-67.

15. Djerassi C. The Politics of Contraception. Vol 1. Stanford, CA: Stanford Alumni Association; 1979.

16. Thomas SL, Ellertson C. Nuisance or natural and healthy: should monthly menstruation be optional for women? Lancet. 2000;355:922-4

17. Lenton EA, Landgren BM, Sexton L, Harper R. Normal variation in the length of the follicular phase of the menstrual cycle: effect of chronological age. Br J Obstet Gynaecol. 1984;91:681-4.

18. Metcalf MG, Livesey LH. Gonadotropin excretion in fertile women: effect of age and the onset of the menopausal transition. J Endocrinol. 1985;105:357-62.

19. Lee SJ, Lenton EA, Sexton L, Cooke ID. The effect of age on the cyclical patterns of plasma LH, FSH, estradiol and progesterone in women with regular menstrual cycles. Hum Reprod. 1988;3:851-5.

20. Burger HL, Dudley EC, Hopper JL, et al. The endocrinology of the menopausal transition: a cross-sectional study of a population-based sample. J Clin Endocrinol Metab. 1995;80:3537-45.

21. Lenton EA, Sexton L, Lee S, Cooke ID. Progressive changes in LH and FSH and LH:FSH ratios in women throughout reproductive life. Maturitas. 1988;10:35-43

22. Metcalf MG, Donald RA, Livesey JH. Pituitary-ovarian function before, during and after menopause: a longitudinal study. Clin Endocrinol. 1982;17:489-94.

23. Santoro N, Brown JR, Adel T, Skurnick JH. Characterization of reproductive hormonal dynamics in the perimenopause. J Clin Endocrinol Metab. 1996;81:1495-501.

24. Stellato RK, Crawford SL, McKinlay SM, Longcope CL. Can follicle-stimulating hormone be used to define menopausal status? Endocr Pract. 1998;4:137-41.

25. Taffe JR, Dennerstein L. Menstrual patterns leading to the final menstrual period. Menopause. 2002;9:32-40.

26. Greendale GA, Sowers MF. The menopause transition. Endocrinol Metab Clin North Am. 1997;26:261-77.

27. Santoro N, and the Swan Daily Hormone Study Writing Group. Entry into the menopausal transition and high BMI are associated with decreased luteal function [Abstract]. 84th Annual Meeting of the Endocrine Society. San Francisco, 21-24 June 2002.

28. Goldstein SR, Santoro N. Textbook of Perimenopausal Gynecology. New York: Parthenon; 2002:69-76.

29. McKinley SM, Brambilla PJ, Posner JG. The normal menopause transition. Maturitas. 1992;14:103-15.

30. Sherman BM, Korenman SG. Hormonal characteristics of the human menstrual cycle throughout reproductive life. J Clin Invest. 1975;55:699-706.

31. Van Look PF, Lothian H, Hunter W, et al. Hypothalamic-pituitary-ovarian function in perimenopausal women. Clin Endocrinol. 1977;7:13-31.

32. Treolar AE, Bonton RE, Behn BG, et al. Variation of the human menstrual cycle throughout reproductive life. Int J Fertil. 1967;12:77-127.

33. Treolar AE. Menstrual cyclicity and the premenopause. Maturitas. 1981;3:249-64.

34. Munro MG. Abnormal uterine bleeding in the reproductive years. Part I—Pathogenesis and clinical investigation. J Am Assoc Gynecol Laparosc. 1999;6:393-416.

35. Kadir RA, Economides DL, Sabin CA, et al. Frequency of inherited bleeding disorders in women with menorrhagia. Lancet. 1998;351;485-9.

36. McKinley SM, Jeffrys M. The menopausal syndrome. Br J Prev Soc Med. 1974;28:108-15.

37. Thompson B, Hart SA, Durno D. Menopausal age and symptomatology in a general practice. J Biosoc Sci. 1973;5:71-82.

38. Lock M. Menopause in cultural context. Exp Gerontol. 1994;29:307-17.

39. Kronenberg F. Hot flashes: epidemiology and physiology. Ann N Y Acad Sci. 1990;592: 52-86; discussion 123-33.

40. Freedman RR, Woodward SW. Behavioral treatment of menopausal hot flushes: evaluation by ambulatory monitoring. Am J Obstet Gynecol. 1992;167:436-9.

41. Israel D, Youngkin EQ. Herbal therapies for perimenopausal and menopausal complaints. Pharmacotherapy. 1997;17:970-84.

42. Hirata JD, Swiersz LM, Zell B, et al. Does dong quai have estrogenic effects in postmenopausal women? A double-blind, placebo-controlled trial. Fertil Steril. 1997;68:981-6.

43. Wyon Y, Lindgren R, Lundeberg T, Hammar M. Effects of acupuncture on climacteric vasomotor symptoms, quality of life, and urinary excretion of neuropeptides among postmenopausal women. Menopause. 1995;2:3-12.

44. Washburn S, Burke GL, Morgan T, Antony M. Effect of soy protein supplementation on serum lipoproteins, blood pressure and menopausal symptoms in perimenopausal women. Menopause. 1999;6:7-13.

45. Ouhilal S, Santoro N. Update: weighing the merits of hormone replacement. Emerg Med. 2002;10:30-45.

46. Pham KTC, Freeman EW, Grisso JA. Menopause and hormone replacement therapy: focus groups of African-American and Caucasian women. Menopause. 1997;4:71-9.

47. Screening for thyroid disease. In: Guide to Clinical Preventive Services. Report of the US Preventive Services Task Force. Baltimore: Williams & Wilkins; 1989:71-5.

48. ACOG Committee on Gynecologic Practice. Obstet Gynecol. 2001;98:1185.

49. Kouides PA. Obstetrical and gynaecological aspects of von Willebrand disease. Best Pract Res Clin Haematol. 2001;1492:381.

50. Burger HG, Dudley EC, Hopper JL, et al. Prospectively measured levels of serum follicle-stimulating hormone, estradiol, and the dimeric inhibins during the menopausal transition in a population based cohort of women. J Clin Endocrinol Metab. 1999;84: 4025-30.

51. Brambilla D, McKinlay SM. A prospective study of factors affecting age of menopause. J Clin Epidemiol. 1989;42:1031-9.

52. Rannevik G, Jeppsson S, Johnell O, et al. A longitudinal study of the perimenopausal transition: altered profiles of steroid and pituitary hormones, SHBG and bone mineral density. Maturitas. 1995;21:103-13.

53. De Waay DJ, Syrop CH, Nygaard IE, et al. Natural history of polyps and leiomyomata. Obstet Gynecol. 2002;100:3-7.

54. Goldstein SR, Zeltser I, Horan CK, et al. Ultrasonography-based triage for perimenopausal patients with abnormal uterine bleeding. Am J Obstet Gynecol. 1997;177:102-8.

55. Oriel KA, Schrager S. Abnormal uterine bleeding. Am Fam Physician. 1999;60:1371-82.

56. Stovall TG, Ling FW, Morgan PL. A prospective randomized comparison of the pipelle endometrial sampling device with the novack curette. Am J Obstet Gynecol. 1991;165: 1287-90.

57. Postmenopausal estrogen/progestin intervention study. 1997;337:1792.

58. Krampl E, Bourne T, Hurlen-Solbakken H, Istre O. Transvaginal ultrasonography sonohysterography and operative hysteroscopy for the evaluation of abnormal uterine bleeding. Acta Obstet Gynecol Scand. 2002;80:616-22.

59. Dueholm M, Forman A, Jensen ML, et al. Transvaginal sonography combined with saline contrast sonohysterography in evaluating the uterine cavity in premenopausal patients with abnormal uterine bleeding. Ultrasound Obstet Gynecol. 2002;18:54-61.

60. Bradley LD, Falcone T, Amgen AB. Radiographic imaging techniques for the diagnosis of abnormal uterine bleeding. Obstet Gynecol Clin North Am. 2000;27:245-76.

61. Dueholm M, Lundorf E, Hansen ES, et al. Evaluation of the uterine cavity with magnetic resonance imaging, transvaginal sonography, hysterosonographic evaluation and diagnostic hysteroscopy. Fertil Steril. 2001;76:350-7.

62. Preston JT, Cameron IT, Adams EJ, Smith SK. Comparative study of tranexamic acid and norethisterone in the treatment of ovulatory menorrhagia. Br J Obstet Gynaecol. 1995;102:401-6

63. Andersch B, Milsom I, Rybo G. An objective evaluation of flurbiprofen and tranexamic acid in the treatment of idiopathic menorrhagia. Acta Obstet Gynecol Scand. 1988.67: 645-8.

64. Bonnar J, Sheppard BL. Treatment of menorrhagia during menstruation: randomized controlled trial of ethamsylate, mefenamic acid, and tranexamic acid. BMJ. 1996;313: 579-82.

65. Archer DF. Medical management of menorrhagia in pre- and perimenopausal women. In: Lobo RA, ed. Perimenopause. New York: Springer-Verlag: Serono Symposia USA; 1997:271-80.

66. Munro MG. Abnormal uterine bleeding in the reproductive years. Part II-medical management. J Am Assoc Gynecol Laparosc. 2000;7:19-32.

67. Conyngham RB. Norethisterone in menorrhagia. NZ Med J. 1965;64:697-701.

68. Fraser IS. Treatment of ovulatory and anovulatory dysfunctional uterine bleeding with oral progestogens. Aust N Z J Obstet Gynecol. 1990;30:352-6.

69. Cameron IT, Leask R, Kelly RW, et al. The effects of danazol, mefenamic acid, norethisterone and a progesterone-impregnated coil on endometrial prostaglandin concentrations in women with menorrhagia. Prostaglandins. 1987;34:99-110.

70. Irvine GA, Campbell-Brown MB, Lumsden MA, et al. Randomized comparative trial of the levonorgestrel intrauterine system and norethisterone for treatment of idiopathic menorrhagia. Br J Obstet Gynaecol. 1988;105:592-8.

71. Crosignani PG, Vercellini P, Mosconi P, et al. Levonorgestrel-releasing intrauterine device versus hysteroscopic endometrial resection in the treatment of dysfunctional uterine bleeding. Obstet Gynecol. 1997;90:257-63.

72. Barrington JW, Bowen-Simpkins P. The levonorgestrel intrauterine system in the management of menorrhagia. Br J Obstet Gynaecol. 1997;104:614-6.

73. Lahteenmaki P, Haukkamaa M, Puolakka J, et al. Open randomized study of use of levonorgestrel releasing intrauterine system as alternative to hysterectomy. BMJ. 1998;316:1122-6.

74. Higham JM, Shaw RW. A comparative study of danazol, a regimen of decreasing doses of danazol, and norethinedrone in the treatment of objectively proven unexplained menorrhagia. Am J Obstet Gynecol. 1993;169:1134-9.

75. Bonduelle M, Walker JJ, Calder AA. A comparative study of danazol and norethisterone in dysfunctional uterine bleeding presenting as menorrhagia. Postgrad Med J. 1991;67:833-6.

76. Dockeray CJ, Sheppard BL, Bonnar J. Comparison between mefenamic acid and danazol in the treatment of established menorrhagia. Br J Obstet Gynaecol. 1989;96:840-4.

77. De Leo V, Lanzetta D, Morgante G, et al. Inhibition of ovulation with transdermal estradiol and oral progestogens in perimenopausal women. Contraception. 1997;55:239-43.

78. Casper RF, Dodin S, Reid RL. The effect of 20 micrograms ethinyl estradiol/1 mg norethinedrone acetate (Minestrin), a low dose oral contraceptive on vaginal bleeding patterns, hot flashes and quality of life in symptomatic perimenopausal women. Menopause. 1997;4:139-47.

79. Tanis BC, van den Bosch MA, Kemmeren JM, et al. Oral contraceptives and the risk of myocardial infarction. N Engl J Med. 2001;345:1787-93.

80. Steinberg KK, Thacker SB, Smith SJ, et al. A meta-analysis of the effect of estrogen replacement therapy on the risk of breast cancer. JAMA. 1991;265:1985-90.

5

Dysmenorrhea

Joseph E. Patruno, MD

Dysmenorrhea is defined as pelvic pain that occurs before and during a woman's menstrual cycle. The word is derived from Greek origin [*dys-* + *rhein*], meaning "painful monthly flow." Dysmenorrhea, one of the most common gynecologic complaints, is estimated to affect 60% to 90% of reproductive-age females (1,2). Although common, only a minority of females actually seek medical attention for the symptom. Nonetheless, the dysmenorrhea's effects on a woman's physical and emotional health can be significant, particularly as underlying disorders may go untreated in those who do not seek medical care. To maximize treatment options, it is critical that the clinician not assume that dysmenorrhea is "only a normal part of menses." The primary care physician is in an ideal position to identify patients with dysmenorrhea and in most cases effectively evaluate and treat them.

Dysmenorrhea has traditionally been divided into two basic types; primary and secondary. *Primary dysmenorrhea* presents soon after menarche, which is typically the time a woman starts to ovulate. By definition, primary dysmenorrhea is not associated with an organic pelvic process. In contrast, *secondary dysmenorrhea* is attributable to pathology in the pelvis. Dysmenorrhea may develop acutely or be a chronic process and can occur at any time in the reproductive life of the patient. Although the trademark of dysmenorrhea is pain, associated symptoms include nausea, vomiting, diaphoresis, tachycardia, diarrhea, lethargy, dizziness, breast tenderness, bloating, edema, headaches, and mood alterations. Some combination of these symptoms are identified in more than 50% of women with dysmenorrhea (3).

Pain with dysmenorrhea by definition occurs or is exacerbated on or around the time of menses. Patients with cyclic pelvic pain that exceeds a 6-month period may also be classified as having chronic pelvic pain in addition to dysmenorrhea (4). It is important to recognize that a variety of non-gynecologic and gynecologic conditions can cause perimenstrual pain. Common non-gynecologic systems to consider as a potential source of pelvic pain include the gastrointestinal, urological, and musculoskeletal systems. Organic gynecologic explanations, or causes of secondary dysmenorrhea, include endometriosis, adenomyosis, chronic infection, and structural lesions of the uterus. Non-gynecologic and organic gynecologic causes of pelvic pain will be discussed later in this chapter within the section on Secondary Dysmenorrhea.

Primary Dysmenorrhea

Primary dysmenorrhea is a condition that affects mostly adolescents in the first several years after menarche. Although not life threatening, primary dysmenorrhea can be debilitating and has significant ramifications in regard to physical symptoms, adverse effects on family, and financial cost to society.

Epidemiology and Risk Factors

Dysmenorrhea is common and affects women of varied races, cultures, and socio-economic backgrounds. Among young women, 59.7% reported some element of menstrual pain. Forty-nine percent of these described the pain as mild, whereas 51% characterized the pain as moderate or severe. In this review, dysmenorrhea led to school absenteeism in 14% to 25% of female students (5). Various reviews have shown prevalence rates for dysmenorrhea ranging from 52% to 93% (2,6-9).

Prevalence of dysmenorrhea increases in women of early reproductive years and reaches a peak during early adulthood. There is a 36.2% incidence of symptoms during the first gynecologic year compared with 64.7% in the fifth gynecologic year after menarche (10). It is common for early menstrual cycles to be painless because in this age group cycles are commonly anovulatory. Primary dysmenorrhea often improves after the age of 25 (10).

Dysmenorrhea is a significant problem from an individual and a public health perspective. It has been estimated that 140 million work and school hours are lost annually due to menstrual-related symptoms and that the financial cost of dysmenorrhea, in terms of lost productivity alone, exceeds two billion dollars every year in the United States (11).

There are few absolute risk factors for primary dysmenorrhea. Family and genetic history may be pertinent because a woman is more likely to suffer from severe dysmenorrhea if her mother or sisters has experienced it (2,12). Social factors may influence the occurrence of dysmenorrhea. Women who are more physically active report less dysmenorrhea (13), and in physically active women who do experience dysmenorrhea, the pain is less severe (14).

The use of tobacco and its effects on dysmenorrhea are under debate (2,15). Similarly, the effect of alcohol on dysmenorrhea remains unclear, with most data showing that use of alcohol has little influence on the severity or duration of menstrual pain (10). There is no clear association between dietary intake and dysmenorrhea (16). Supplementation with omega-3 fatty acid containing fish oil resulted in a marked reduction of menstrual pain in adolescents with dysmenorrhea (17).

The gynecologic and menstrual histories of individual women influences symptoms of dysmenorrhea. Gynecologic parameters protective against dysmenorrhea include later menarche, previous vaginal delivery, short menstrual periods, and the use of oral contraceptive pills (2). Although dysmenorrhea is thought to be more prevalent after tubal ligation, this has not been established in the scientific literature (18,19). Worsened menstrual pain, in these cases, may be a result of discontinuing hormonal contraception rather than the actual sterilization procedure.

Etiology and Pathophysiology

The true etiology of primary dysmenorrhea may still not be completely understood. Historically, cervical obstruction or incomplete passage of menstrual effluvium from the uterus were theorized to be the primary causes of pain. Today, the primary pathogenesis of dysmenorrhea is thought to primarily involve an excessive or imbalanced production of prostaglandins. Prostaglandins are potent substances produced in a number of tissues in the body. It is postulated that some regulatory interplay exists between ovarian hormonal changes, the production of prostaglandins, and their effects on intrauterine pressure. Ovarian hormones and prostaglandins have both local and systemic effects. In addition to causing menstrual pain, they are thought to cause undesirable perimenstrual symptoms such as headaches and diarrhea. A variety of synthetic prostaglandins, used clinically as abortifacients and as uterotonics, produce physiologic effects similar to endogenous prostaglandins.

Pickles, in the 1950s, isolated a substance from menstrual fluid that he identified as a smooth muscle stimulant (20). This material was identified as prostaglandin E and F and was found to be abundant in the endometrium of reproductive aged women. Levels of the prostaglandins have been found to be higher in the luteal phase of the menstrual cycle, and women with dysmenorrhea have been shown to have higher baseline levels of prostaglandins than have controls without menstrual pain (3,21).

The specific sequence of prostaglandin production can be traced in the prostaglandin cascade (Figure 5-1). Ovulation triggers the production of progesterone, which is thought to be the primary activator of phospholipase

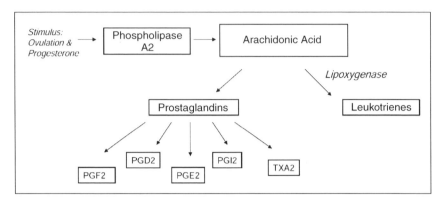

Figure 5-1   Prostaglandin synthesis cascade.

A2 and stimulator of the prostaglandin cascade. Phospholipase A2 converts phospholipids to arachidonic acid, which is subsequently broken down into either prostaglandins or leukotrienes. Leukotrienes promote inflammation, vasoconstriction, and uterine contractions, leading to symptoms that include dysmenorrhea. Prostaglandins derived from arachidonic acid include prostaglandin E2a, prostaglandin F2a, thromboxane a2, and prostacyclin. These agents have different biological effects on tissue. It is believed that a high level of these substances, or perhaps an imbalance between various prostaglandins, is the underlying cause of dysmenorrhea.

Prostaglandin F2a is a major contributor to the symptoms of dysmenorrhea. It is a potent vasoconstrictor and uterotonic and is found in abundance in the menstrual fluid of dysmnenorrheic women. Additionally, plasma concentrations of the substance correlate well with menstrual pain (3). In contrast, prostacyclin may be protective against dysmenorrhea because those with painful menses have been shown to have lower levels of this metabolite. This may be because prostacyclin is a vasodilator and promotes relaxation of the uterus (22).

Other mechanisms are thought to contribute to dysmenorrhea. Women who experience dysmenorrhea show enhanced pain perception for a variety of gynecologic and non-gynecologic stimuli compared with non-dysmenorrheaic women (23,24). Altered pain processing may be secondary to a baseline enhanced neural sensitivity to prostaglandins, or perhaps, an effect of persistent stimulation from noxious stimuli. Vasopressin, a hormone produced endogenously in the posterior pituitary, has also been postulated to cause myometrial hyperactivity, reduced uterine blood flow, and pain. Biochemical data show increased circulating vasopressin levels in women with painful menses (25). As mentioned, leukotrienes, as potent mediators of inflammation, have also been suspected as possible metabolic contributors to dysmenorrhea (26).

It has been speculated that a number of other clinical symptoms and conditions may exacerbate (although they may perhaps be the result of) dysmenorrhea. For instance, psychiatric diagnoses such as depression and anxiety disorders are found more commonly in women with dysmenorrhea than in controls (27). Similarly, women with dysmenorrhea are more apt to have sleep deprivation thought to worsen the effect of pain on daytime functioning (28). Whether these alterations are a product of the pain, or contributors to the pain, is difficult to decipher.

Evaluation

Dysmenorrhea should be approached as a symptom and not a diagnosis. To be considered or defined as dysmenorrhea, pain must be related to the menstrual cycle; structural and anatomical issues that require further management are perhaps also related to the menstrual cycle. A careful pain history should include information about the timing and duration of pain (e.g., pain occurring 1 day before onset of menstrual flow or pain occurring throughout the menstrual period), severity of the pain (using a scale), and alleviating and exacerbating factors of the pain. In addition to a complete history, a detailed physical examination is recommended at the time of initial presentation to rule out pathologic causes of pain (Figure 5-2). Clinical signs and symptoms suggesting secondary dysmenorrhea should be considered, and these are discussed later in this chapter.

Laboratory and radiographic studies are rarely helpful in the diagnosis of primary dysmenorrhea. In cases of secondary dysmenorrhea, imaging and laboratory studies may be more fruitful. Standardized pain scoring tools and menstrual diaries may also objectively measure pain severity and confirm a cyclic component to the pain.

History
In the evaluation of any reproductive-aged female, a menstrual history is critical. If the patient describes significant menstrual pain, the symptom should be explored in greater detail. A temporal association of the pain with both menarche and menses should be established. Information on the quality, distribution, intensity, and radiation pattern of the pain are important to obtain. Associated symptoms should also be identified.

Primary dysmenorrhea typically begins with the onset of menses or shortly before menstrual flow. Secondary dysmenorrhea, on the other hand, may begin several days to a week before menstrual bleeding. While secondary dysmenorrhea often persists throughout the menstrual cycle, primary dysmenorrhea typically abates within the first few days of flow. Dysmenorrhea pain is typically described as "sharp" or "crampy" and is often most pronounced in

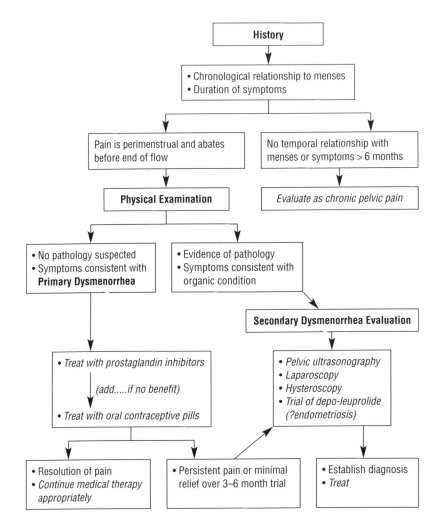

Figure 5-2   Algorithm for the diagnosis and treatment of dysmenorrhea.

the central lower quadrants or suprapubic region (3). The pain commonly radiates to the back, upper thighs, and legs.

Associated pain symptoms should be explored. Dyspareunia, which is pain during intercourse, suggests an organic cause for menstrual pain; consider a diagnosis of secondary (as opposed to primary) dysmenorrhea and an etiological investigation. The physician should assess associated symptoms such as depression, fatigue, menstrual irregularities, and systemic complaints. A history of sexual abuse may be uncovered as a contributing factor to menstrual pain

(29). Additionally, attention should be given to evaluation of coinciding pain complaints that may affect the musculoskeletal, neurologic, urologic, or gastrointestinal systems. Conditions involving these systems, such as irritable bowel syndrome (IBS), interstitial cystitis, and migraine headaches are known to affect primarily women and to have cyclic exacerbations with menses. Other aspects of the history to review include past surgery, previous pelvic infections, infertility, and unusual obstetric events. Once again, findings in any of these areas may point toward a secondary cause of dysmenorrhea.

Objective pain measurement tools, such as a pain rating scale of 1-10, are valuable in assessing patients with pelvic pain and dysmenorrhea. Pain diaries allow for qualification and quantification of pain symptoms and confirm the critical cyclic pattern of the patient's symptoms. Other forms allow for an organized and comprehensive evaluation of the pain and associated symptoms. For example, charting headache or nausea frequency in relation to menstrual flow will help to link these symptoms to the pathophysiology of dysmenorrhea.

Physical Examination

A complete physical examination, in most cases, should be performed at the time of initial assessment in any patient with dysmenorrhea. Patients with primary dysmenorrhea by definition should have a normal, essentially benign, examination. Those with secondary dysmenorrhea may or may not have significant physical findings to explain their symptomatology.

An abdominal examination should localize the point of pain sites and regions where the pain radiates. Palpation of the abdomen should be performed to assess for possible organomegaly, fluid shift, or signs of acuity.

The pelvic examination should include an evaluation of the external genitalia that focuses on the escutcheon, inguinal masses, and the labia. Speculum examination should allow for close visualization of the vaginal vault and the cervix. Specifically, the cervix should be assessed for lesions, or purulent discharge. Bimanual examination is performed to evaluate the upper genital tract. Size, contour, and focal tenderness of the uterus and adnexa should be noted. Reproducible pain should be documented and isolated to specific parts of the pelvis if possible. The presence of cervical motion tenderness, adnexal masses, parametrial thickening, and uterosacral ligament nodularity all suggest organic gynecologic pathology. Pain in the area of the anterior vagina or bladder may be suggestive of interstitial cystitis (IC) or other bladder conditions. Tenderness and nodularity posterior to the uterus or a laterally deviated cervix are associated with endometriosis. Finally, rectovaginal examination should be performed, assessing sphincter tone, the presence or absence of masses, tenderness, or fullness along the rectovaginal septum. Significant findings on this part of the exam, once again, may be indicative of pelvic or bowel pathology.

There is some controversy regarding the timing of complete pelvic examination of virginal teenagers presenting with typical primary dysmenorrhea. An increasing number of clinicians utilize a trial of conservative medical therapy before performing an exam. Other practitioners insist initially on a first pelvic exam or imaging. For virginal teenagers where the clinical history is unclear, or in those who do not respond to conservative medical therapy, a pelvic examination is essential. Ultrasound evaluation may also be helpful in young patients who are anxious or in acute pain.

Laboratory and Imaging Studies

Rarely, lab tests are helpful in evaluating the patient with primary dysmenorrhea. The patient's history and clinical findings will dictate which lab tests to consider. In sexually active, fertile women, a urine pregnancy screen may be considered to rule out ectopic pregnancy or miscarriage. In those at risk for, or with characteristic symptoms of gonorrhea, cervical testing for *N. gonorrhea* and chlamydia should also be considered. A complete blood count may be ordered to assess for possible anemia or infection, whereas a urinalysis should be considered in those with bladder symptoms or suprapubic pain

Ultrasound of the pelvis may also provide important information in the evaluation. This is especially true in those with risk factors for upper genital tract pathology, and in those with inadequate, inconclusive, or abnormal pelvic examinations. Other radiographic studies, such as abdominal X-rays, computed tomography (CT), and magnetic resonance imaging (MRI), rarely contribute to the work-up of the patient with simple dysmenorrhea.

Treatment

A number of modalities exist for the treatment of dysmenorrhea. First-line therapy is geared towards blocking the production of, and decreasing the effects of, prostaglandins. Many over-the-counter and prescription-strength prostaglandin inhibitors are available (Table 5-1). Other medical therapies effective in the treatment of dysmenorrhea include hormonal regimens (see Figure 5-2); hormonal therapy with a combination oral contraceptive is the second-line treatment. Finally, in refractory or severe cases of primary dysmenorrhea, surgical evaluation and management may be necessary. Evaluation for surgical management is often necessary for patients with organic pathology or secondary dysmenorrhea.

Prostaglandin Synthetase Inhibitors/Nonsteroidal Anti-Inflammatory Drugs

Prostaglandin synthetase inhibitors (PGSIs) are well studied and proven in the treatment of primary dysmenorrhea (30). These agents inhibit cyclo-oxygenase, a precursor to noxious prostaglandins. Biochemical studies confirm lower

Table 5-1   Prostaglandin Inhibitor Therapy for Dysmenorrhea

Agent	Dosing	Maximum Daily Dose
First-line Therapy		
Ibuprofen (Motrin, Excedrin)	200-800 mg orally 3 to 4 times daily as needed	3200 mg
Naproxen (Naprosyn)	250-500 mg orally twice daily; XL: 750-1000 mg orally once daily	1375 mg
Mefenamic acid (Ponstel)	500 mg load orally, then 250 mg every 6 hours	1500 mg
Other NSAIDs		
Diclofenac (Voltaren, Cataflam)	50 mg orally 2 to 3 times daily; 75 mg orally twice daily; or 100 mg XR orally once or twice daily	225 mg (200 mg XR)
Diflunisal (Dolobid)	500-1000 mg initially, then 250-500 mg orally every 8 to 12 hours	2500 mg
Etodolac (Lodine)	200-400 mg orally 2 to 3 times daily; XL: 400-1200 mg once daily	1200 mg
Flurbiprofen (Ansaid)	200-300 mg/day in 2 to 4 divided doses	300 mg
Ketoprofen (Orudis)	25-75 mg orally 3 to 4 times daily (XL-Oruvail): 200 mg once daily	300 mg
Ketorolac (Toradol)	10 mg orally every 4 to 6 hours	40 mg
Nabumetone (Relafen)	1000 mg orally once or twice daily	2000 mg
Oxaprozin (Daypro)	1200 mg orally once daily (600 mg tablets)	1800 mg
Piroxicam (Feldene)	20 mg orally once daily	20 mg
Sulindac (Clinoril)	150–200 mg orally twice daily	400 mg
COX-2 Inhibitor		
Celecoxib (Celebrex)	400 mg load followed by 200 mg orally, twice daily	400 mg

levels of prostaglandins in menstrual fluid and lower uterine tone in women treated with these medications (31). In a meta-analysis reviewing 51 PGSI trials which reviewed data on 1649 women, it was shown that, overall, 72% of dysmenorrheic women reported pain relief with prostaglandin-blocking medications alone (32). These agents also have a broader spectrum of benefit in that they relieve other prostaglandin-induced symptoms such as headaches, bloating, diarrhea, and breast tenderness.

Several classes of prostaglandin synthetase inhibitors exist. These include aspirin, fenemates, and nonsteroidal anti-inflammatory drugs (NSAIDs). Although many agents are available for dysmenorrhea, there are few data comparing these medications. In choosing an ideal agent, the physician should consider cost, dosing schedules, and side effects of the medications. which differ between agents.

Many prescription-strength non-steroidal agents are available to treat the dysmenorrheic patient. In the fenemate class, mefenamic acid has been clinically proven to decrease pain, reduce menstrual blood loss, and improve nausea, backache, and headache. A specific benefit of this agent includes short duration of onset and long duration of action. In controlled trials mefenamic acid was found to be more effective than placebo and completely resolved pain in 87% of dysmenorrhea sufferers (32). Other prescription NSAIDs used in the treatment of dysmenorrhea are listed in Table 5-1 with their recommended dosing. Based on good clinical data, ibuprofen, naproxen, and mefenamic acid are all excellent, well-tolerated, first-line therapeutic options in the treatment of the dysmenorrheic woman (30). There is little evidence substantiating better efficacy with newer, more expensive agents, but they may offer more favorable dosing and side effect profiles (30,32-35).

Once started on NSAIDs, most women with primary dysmenorrhea notice a fairly rapid benefit. The full efficacy of these agents, however, may take several months to achieve. When starting these agents it is recommended that the patient initiate therapy when symptoms actually begin. In women who have predictable menses or who have premenstrual symptomatology, there may be a benefit to starting therapy prophylactically before the start of symptoms (36). Chan et al demonstrated that the introduction of therapy on cycle day one was as effective as beginning therapy 3 days prior to the expected onset of menses (37). Scheduled use of the NSAIDs around the clock may be beneficial, compared with dosing only with symptoms, because a more consistent serum level of the medication is maintained.

In females who do not respond to recommended starting doses of these medications, increasing the initial starting dose of the drug, without altering the maintenance dose, is a reasonable option (38). In principle, patients should be managed on the lowest dose of the agent that is tolerated and provides relief. Dosing should not exceed the maximum daily recommended dose of the drug. When appropriate, a trial of different agents may be necessary to identify which medication is best tolerated, most effective, and best suited for the individual patient.

Although most prostaglandin inhibitors are effective in ameliorating dysmenorrhea, there are exceptions of which the clinician should be aware. For instance, aspirin is only effective in high doses, and indomethacin, in standard doses, has been shown to be less effective, with more side effects, than other NSAIDs in the treatment of dysmenorrhea (32,33). Acetominophen, also a commonly used over-the-counter analgesic, does not have anti-prostaglandin properties and is also less effective than NSAIDs in the treatment of dysmenorrhea (33,34).

COX-2 Inhibitors

COX-2 inhibitors block the conversion of arachidonic acid to prostaglandins earlier in the prostaglandin cascade than do traditional prostaglandin inhibitors. They are associated with fewer adverse gastric side effects than NSAIDs and can be taken on a once-a-day basis (39). Currently, only celecoxib (Celebrex) is indicated for the treatment of primary dysmenorrhea and cyclic pain associated with endometriosis (40). These agents are costly and should be reserved for patients who do not respond to NSAIDs, have contraindications to them, or are intolerant of traditional NSAIDs. Recent data linking COX-2 inhibitors to cardiac events should also be considered when prescribing them (41).

Oral Contraceptive Pills

When a dysmenorrheic patient does not respond to NSAIDs or has a suboptimal response, hormonal therapy is often the next step in management. Combination oral contraceptive pills (OCPs) are the agents most often used for this purpose. OCPs have been advocated as treatment for primary dysmenorrhea since they were first introduced in the 1960s. In a recent review of the literature, Proctor concluded that standard OCPs were more effective than placebo in relieving menstrual pain (42). Similar data have shown that OCPs improve dysmenorrhea in 80% to 90% of users (43). OCPs reduce menstrual pain by suppressing ovulation, decreasing the thickness of the endometrium, and consequently lessening the duration of menstrual flow. It is speculated that the thinner endometrial cavity promotes the production of fewer prostaglandins, which results in less cramping and pain.

There are numerous birth control pills and hormonal birth control methods available. In the treatment of dysmenorrhea, an ideal agent or a dosing schedule is not established. A recent review demonstrated that newly available low-dose agents (20-µg pills) are as effective as traditional pills in decreasing both menstrual flow and pain (44). The efficacy of newer, combined hormonal contraceptive delivery systems like the vaginally placed NuvaRing and Ortho-Evra dermal patch currently have no clinical evidence supporting their use specifically for dysmenorrhea. Early data regarding the Ortha-Evra patch suggests that when used in a cyclic manner this transdermal agent may offer less benefit than traditional pills in preventing and treating dysmenorrhea (45).

Continuous dosing, or the prolonged use of of active birth control pills beyond typical 21-days, has become fashionable in recent years. Such dosing is thought to benefit those with adverse menstrual symptoms. A number of non-contraceptive benefits have been established with this continuous dosing protocol, including decreased menorrhagia, decreased perimenstrual symptoms, and improved cyclic pain (46). However, use of the extended-cycle OCP regimens is associated with a significant incidence of unscheduled bleeding, particularly in the first few months. Additionally, the long-term safety of such regimens has not been well established.

Birth control pills have a number of side effects, contraindications, and limitations that need to be considered by the clinician. The most common side effects of these agents are nausea, headache, and breast tenderness. Contraindications to the use of estrogen-containing agents include undiagnosed abnormal bleeding, pregnancy, past thromboembolism, liver disease, or history of estrogen-sensitive tumor. Women older than 35 years who smoke should not be prescribed OCPs because of the increased risk of thromboembolism and associated morbidity.

OCPs may be used alone in conjunction with prostaglandin synthetase inhibitors in patients with dysmenorrhea. Although the use of these agents together has not been evaluated clinically, they offer complementary benefits in the treatment of dysmenorrhea. A majority of women with primary dysmenorrhea will respond to a combination of NSAIDs and OCPs. Lack of response to these medications should prompt a more thorough evaluation of the pain for potential secondary etiologies.

Unlike prostaglandin inhibitors, which can be taken acutely, OCPs must be taken on a daily basis in order to suppress ovulation and be effective. Patients may find this inconvenient, and compliance in taking the pill daily may not be optimal. Once again the complete benefit of hormonal management may not be seen for several months after starting the medication. Naturally, in women with dysmenorrhea who are trying to conceive oral contraceptive pills are not acceptable. Conversely, in those with cyclic mentrual pain needing contraception, birth control pills offer dual benefit.

Progestational Agents

Several progesterone-containing agents are available for clinical use in this country. Like combination OCPs, progestins may treat dysmenorrhea by suppressing ovulation and altering endometrial growth and prostaglandin levels. At present there are no progestational agents approved specifically for the treatment of primary dysmenorrhea. Several agents have been clinically evaluated, however, and have shown benefit in the treatment of cyclic pelvic pain (47). For instance, depo-medroxyprogesterone acetate (Depo-Provera), a long-acting, intramuscularly administered progestin, has clinically been demonstrated to be effective in the treatment of dysmenorrhea secondary to endometriosis (48).

Benefits of progestins are often outweighed by side effects. Common adverse effects of these agents include breakthrough bleeding, amenorrhea, weight gain, depression, and edema. Additionally, resumption of menses may be delayed in users of Depo-Provera. Because it is an effective contraceptive, Depo-Provera is of course not recommended for use in patients trying to conceive or desirous of fertility within the coming year.

Progesterone-containing intrauterine devices (IUDs) offer hormonal benefits with little systemic absorption and thus fewer adverse effects. Currently, the only progesterone-containing IUD available in the United States is the Mirena intrauterine system (IUS). This apparatus, which is fortified with levonorgestrel, provides patients with excellent contraception and a number of non-contraceptive benefits, including relief of menstrual pain (49). In clinical trials the Mirena IUS has been shown to decrease the prevalence of dysmenorrhea from 60% to 29% in those using the agent over a 3-year period (50). Traditional copper-containing IUDs, on the other hand, are apt to aggravate or worsen dysmenorrhea and should therefore not be used in women with significant menstrual pain. Newer progestine-releasing systems that offer better side-effect profiles are being investigated and may prove beneficial both as contraceptives and in the management of dysmenorrhea (51).

Other Hormonal Agents

Other hormonal agents are available and can be used off-label for the treatment of dysmenorrhea. GnRH analogs (goseralin acetate, leuprolide acetate, naferalin acetate) suppress ovulation and induce a state of medical menopause. In general, these agents are expensive, poorly tolerated, and can have significant long-term health implications. If used for dysmenorrhea, they should be prescribed by a specialist completely familiar with their risks.

Other Medical Therapies: Past and Future

A variety of other medications, with different mechanisms of action, have also been evaluated and used in the treatment of dysmenorrhea. Most of these agents have little clinical evidence to support their use and safety for this indication, however. Nonetheless, in certain refractory cases of primary dysmenorrhea their use, under appropriate supervision, may be reasonable.

Calcium antagonists, including nifedipine and verapamil, have direct relaxing effects on the uterus, both in clinical and in laboratory studies (52,53). Nifedipine is beneficial in young females with primary dysmenorrhea but failed in patients confirmed to have organic or secondary causes for pain. The authors publishing this data propose the short-term administration of calcium channel blockers to help differentiate those with primary versus secondary dysmenorrhea (54).

Beta-adrenergic receptor agonists, such as terbutaline, have been looked at as a potential treatment for primary dysmenorrhea. These agents also work through directly relaxing the myometrium. Studies have shown little benefit, however, in the management of dysmenorrheic patients (55,56).

Antispasmodics, such as hyoscine and butylbromide, have been empirically prescribed in the past for dysmenorrhea, though clinical studies supporting the use of such agents for menstrual pain are lacking.

Narcotics can play a role in the treatment of primary dysmenorrhea. Because of side effects and addictive potential, however, these agents must be used cautiously and judiciously. There have been no head-to-head comparisons between narcotics and NSAIDs. In patients who are unresponsive to NSAIDs and have pain requiring the use of narcotics, the diagnosis of primary dysmenorrhea should be questioned. Newer agents combining narcotics with NSAIDs are currently being marketed. Vicoprofen is a combination of the narcotic hydrocodone with the NSAID ibuprofen. These agents may be valuable in the short-term management of patients with severe primary dysmenorrhea or, for longer-term use, in those with secondary processes causing menstrual pain.

Novel medical treatment options may become available for dysmenorrhea in the future. Research is being focused on the development of agents that specifically inhibit leukotrienes in the prostaglandin cascade (56,57). Similarly, the importance of vasopressin as a potentiator of dysmenorrhea is being explored more fully. Should this endogenous hormone prove to play a factor in the symptom, a vasopressin blocker may be fruitful as an adjunctive treatment for dysmenorrhea (58,59).

Surgical Therapy

Surgery has traditionally been an important means of diagnosing and treating pelvic pain. In most cases of primary dysmenorrhea, surgical intervention is unnecessary as a diagnostic modality and therapy. Surgical evaluation and treatment should be reserved for those with severe or atypical symptoms and in those who fail to respond to traditional therapies. It also may be warranted in those with abnormal findings on examination or radiographic studies suggesting secondary causes for pain.

In the past, cervical stenosis was thought to be the major precipitator or cause of dysmenorrhea. As such, cervical dilation was advocated and commonly performed. There is no evidence to support this treatment for women with primary dysmenorrhea, and today this procedure is rarely performed.

Laparoscopy may offer benefit in both the diagnosis and the treatment of those with atypical or severe dysmenorrhea. By definition, those with primary dysmenorrhea should have a normal pelvis at the time of laparoscopy. The procedure is used by the surgeon to not only diagnose but to treat pathology. Conditions and causes of secondary dysmenorrhea amenable to laparoscopic treatment include endometriosis, pelvic adhesions, and ovarian cysts. Even when laparoscopy reveals no organic explanation for dysmenorrhea, the procedure should not be considered superfluous: knowledge that there are no abnormalities on laparoscopy is likely to provide the patient with reassurance and a sense of well being. Additionally, it will provide the physician with valuable information for counseling and for customizing further treatment.

A number of conservative laparoscopic surgical techniques have been advocated as treatment for primary dysmenorrhea. Laparoscopic uterosacral nerve ablation (LUNA) involves the surgical interruption of sympathetic nerve fibers at the level of the cervix. The procedure should only be considered in the 20% to 25% of patients who fail medical management. LUNA has been shown to be most beneficial in patients with severe or refractory dysmenorrhea and in those with central pelvic pain due to endometriosis. A review conducted by Proctor et al concluded, however, that LUNA did not offer additional benefit over conservative laparoscopic surgical management alone in the treatment of endometriosis (60). Presacral neurectomy (PSN), also through the denervation of the pelvis, similarly has been performed as a surgical therapy for dysmenorrhea, dyspareunia, and pelvic pain (61,62). Small studies have quoted a 75% to 80% effectiveness rate in alleviating dysmenorrhea pain (61). Complications from such procedures include bleeding, ureteral transection, and sympathetic bladder and bowel dysfunction. The true benefit and long-term efficacy of these operations remain uncertain.

Hysterectomy is a commonly performed surgery for chronic pelvic pain. It should only rarely be considered as an option in the patient with primary dysmenorrhea. This is, in part, because many with primary symptoms are young and still desirous of fertility. Definitive surgery should be considered only when conservative therapeutic efforts have failed and the practitioner is convinced it will relieve the patient's pain.

Alternative Treatments

A number of alternative therapies have been evaluated for the treatment of dysmenorrhea. Behavioral therapy and relaxation training has been used successfully in the management of spasmodic pain associated with menstruation (63). In addition, certain activity modification and relaxation techniques have been shown to reduce pain severity (64). This therapeutic approach combines systematically increasing activity levels while limiting pain medications and increasing social reinforcement. Behavioral treatments such as biofeedback may have some utility in the treatment of dysmenorrhea, but large clinical studies are lacking (65,66).

Transcutaneous electrical nerve stimulation (TENS) has been found to be an effective and safe method of relieving pain with primary dysmenorrhea (67). The TENS procedure involves placing electrodes on the skin and then using an electric current, at different frequencies and intensities, to stimulate tissue and alleviate pain. The apparatus is thought to decrease pain by two likely mechanisms: 1) impeding the propagation of pain impulses along neural sensory fibers, and 2) activating the release of endogenous endorphins. The use of TENS has also been shown to reduce the occurrence of diarrhea, fatigue, and menorrhagia (68). Side effects from the procedure are rare but include muscle vibrations, tightness, headache, and mild skin irritation at the site of application (69).

Acupuncture is a non-traditional medical practice that may offer benefit in a variety of medical conditions. It is believed that the nervous system may be activated by acupuncture, promoting the activation of the endogenous opioid system. Helms recently reported that 10 of 11 dysmenorrheic subjects treated with genuine acupuncture showed improvement in symptoms, compared with only 4 of 11 women treated with placebo acupuncture (70). Acupuncture techniques also improve systemic symptoms of nausea, headache, backache, fluid retention, and breast tenderness in cycling females.

The use of heat to treat dysmenorrhea has a long history and is supported by both anecdotal and clinical evidence. The mechanism by which heat controls dysmenorrhea is not well understood, however. Alteration in pain thresholds, direct effects on uterine contractility, and a general sense of well being are theories behind effectiveness of heat therapy. It has been evaluated in the scientific literature, and a review by Akin et al showed that continuous, low-level, topical heat offered similar benefit to oral ibuprofen for the management of menstrual pain (71). This study also documented that heat complimented the effects of ibuprofen, offering better and quicker pain relief than either of these treatment modalities alone. Ideal dosing schedule and optimal temperature for heat therapy in the treatment of dysmenorrhea has not been well established.

Secondary Dysmenorrhea

A number of organic conditions can present with dysmenorrhea as a major symptom. Secondary dysmenorrhea may develop any time between menarche and menopause and not uncommonly presents during a woman's fourth and fifth decade of life. History and physical examination are critical to evaluation of the patient with suspected secondary dysmenorrhea (Table 5-2). Further diagnostic testing, unlike with primary dysmenorrhea, is often helpful to firmly establish the cause of the patient's pain. Studies to consider are CT, MRI, or pelvic ultrasound. Occasionally, invasive laparoscopy may be needed to establish a diagnosis and provide the patient with appropriate therapy. The characteristics of secondary dysmenorrhea (e.g., its duration, at what point in the cycle it begins) and typical physical findings on examination have been described earlier in this chapter.

For women with persistent symptoms, or in those found to have a secondary cause of dysmenorrhea, prompt referral to a gynecologist for consideration of a diagnostic laparoscopy, or to an appropriate subspecialist, is recommended (Table 5-3).

Table 5-2   Clinical Signs and Symptoms Suggesting Secondary Dysmenorrhea

Clinical History	Secondary Dysmenorrhea Etiology
Dysmenorrhea occurring in first 1-2 menstrual cycles	Uterine anomaly, cervical stenosis, outflow obstruction
Dysmenorrhea presenting after 25 years of age	Endometriosis, adenomyosis, uterine fibroids, ovarian cyst/neoplasia, complication of pregnancy (ectopic pregnancy, abortion)
Dysmenorrhea with dyspareunia	Endometriosis, adenomyosis, ovarian cyst/neoplasia, pelvic inflammatory disease
Dysmenorrhea with irregular/heavy bleeding	Endometriosis, adenomyosis, uterine fibroids, pelvic inflammatory disease
Dysmenorrhea with prior pelvic surgery	Cervical stenosis, pelvic adhesive disease
Dysmenorrhea with bowel complaints	Irritable bowel syndrome
Dysmenorrhea with bladder complaints	Interstitial cystitis, bacterial cystitis
Dysmenorrhea with fatigue and myalgia	Fibromyalgia
Dysmenorrhea with abnormal pelvic examination (enlarged uterus, pelvic mass, cervical motion tenderness, uterosacral nodularity, etc.)	Uterine anomaly, endometriosis, adenomyosis, uterine fibroids, ovarian cyst/neoplasia, pelvic inflammatory disease

Table 5-3   Indications for Referral to an Obstetrician/Gynecologist

- Abnormal pelvic or ultrasound study suggestive of organic gynecologic condition
- Dysmenorrhea in conjunction with other gynecologic or peri-menstrual symptoms suggesting organic gynecologic condition
- Primary dysmenorrhea unresponsive to treatment over 3-6 months with prostaglandin inhibitors and/or oral contraceptive pills
- Severe or acute pain suggesting other organic processes or uncertain diagnosis

Secondary dysmenorrhea may be a result of gynecologic pathology such as cervical obstruction, endometriosis, adenomyosis, chronic infection, or pelvic congestion syndrome. However, the physician should not overlook the possibility of non-gynecologic etiologies of pain. It has been estimated that 50% of diagnostic laparoscopies performed for pelvic pain, in patients with normal radiographic studies, demonstrate no obvious gynecologic pathology (72). As with the gynecologic assessment, the practitioner should consider and approach the non-gynecologic organ systems in an organized and a complete manner.

Endometriosis

Endometriosis is the most common secondary cause of dysmenorrhea. The incidence of the condition ranges from 5% to 15% of all women, and endometriosis is responsible for 70% to 80% of cases of chronic pelvic pain (3). The clinician should always consider the possibility of endometriosis in any woman who presents with dysmenorrhea.

Endometriosis is characterized by the growth of glands or stroma found normally in the uterus in aberrant or heterotopic locations. Patients with endometriosis may be asymptomatic (one third) or present with symptoms such as dyspareunia, menorrhagia, constipation, diarrhea, dysuria, or increased urinary frequency. The most common symptom of endometriosis, however, is cyclic pain or dysmenorrhea. The pain typically presents 36 to 48 hours before menses and may persist throughout flow. Over time the pain will often become more chronic and affect patients at times other than menses.

Classic physical findings in those with endometriosis include uterosacral nodularity, cervical stenosis, lateral deviation of the cervix, and a fixed tender retroverted uterus. Typically, however, pelvic examination is completely unremarkable, with the exception of nonfocal tenderness. The gold standard for diagnosing endometriosis is via biopsy, thus requiring either laparoscopy or exploratory laparotomy. In cases involving endometriotic cysts or endometriomas, radiographic studies will demonstrate the abnormality. Recent studies have advocated empirically treating patients thought to have endometriosis with GnRH agonists to avoid laparoscopy. If the patient responds to the therapy the diagnosis may be inferred. If there is no improvement, diagnostic and, perhaps, therapeutic laparoscopy by a gynecologic specialist is indicated (73,74).

The treatment of endometriosis is focused on inhibiting ovulation, the ovarian production of estrogen, and inducing amenorrhea. Medical agents which accomplish this purpose include OCPs, danazol, GnRH agonists, and depo-medroxyprogesterone acetate. Unlike patients with primary dysmenorrhea, endometriosis sufferers will often have a suboptimal response to PGSI therapy alone. PGSIs may provide adjunctive benefit in treating the condition, however. Surgical management of endometriosis includes laparoscopic ablation or excision of lesions and adhesions and, at times, hysterectomy. Often surgeons will remove the ovaries during this procedure to alleviate further hormonal stimulation of implants.

Adenomyosis

Adenomyosis, like endometriosis, may present with cyclic, suprapubic, or pelvic pain. In this condition, endometriotic lesions penetrate the uterine myometrium. Unlike patients with endometriosis, who typically present in their 20s and 30s, those with adenomyosis are typically diagnosed one to two decades later in life.

Physical findings of adenomyosis may be subtle and may include a mildly enlarged, tender, "boggy" uterus on bimanual examination. Diagnosis in the past was based on clinical suspicion and confirmed pathologically only after hysterectomy. Both transvaginal ultrasound and MRI have been found to be effective noninvasive methods of diagnosing adenomyosis preoperatively (75). Conservative treatment for adenomyosis relies on cyclic hormones and prostaglandin inhibitors. Because women with the condition tend to be older and have completed childbearing, definitive surgery by hysterectomy is often the treatment chosen.

Pelvic Infection

Chronic pelvic infection has also been implicated as a cause of chronic pelvic pain, which may be worse during menstrual cycles. In patients with risk factors for infection, or with past histories of upper genital tract infection, the diagnosis should be considered. The evaluation of such patients may reveal focal adnexal tenderness or masses. Treatment with antibiotics may provide improvement in symptoms in more acute cases. Ultrasound may demonstrate enlarged, fluid-filled fallopian tubes or adnexal masses. Laparoscopy may further confirm the diagnosis with findings of abnormal tubes or adnexal or perihepatic adhesions, suggesting past infection. The prevalence of chronic infection as a cause of dysmenorrhea and pelvic pain is presumed low, however, with a laparoscopic series finding chronic infection alone in only 3 of 170 patients with pelvic pain (72).

Pelvic Congestion Syndrome

Like chronic infection, pelvic congestion syndrome is a controversial and rare cause of dysmenorrhea and pelvic pain. The presence of dilated veins in the pelvis has been observed for nearly half a century, but the significance of this finding remains unclear (76). The diagnosis requires pelvic veins measuring more than 1 cm in diameter. The etiology of pelvic congestion is not certain. Procedures including ovarian vein ligation and embolization have provided some benefit of pain symptoms in small study groups of patients diagnosed with the finding (77). Traditionally, hysterectomy has been the definitive treatment for pelvic congestion syndrome.

Uterine Anomalies and Cervical Stenosis

Uterine anomalies and cervical stenosis rarely cause dysmenorrhea. A variety of mullerian anomalies (congenital developmental defects of the uterus) have been identified, many of which lead to obstructed or incomplete passage of materials from the menstrual tract. These defects may affect the upper or lower genital tract. Patients with these conditions will often present with cyclic pelvic pain and primary amenorrhea. Uterine abnormalities and cervical stenosis should be considered in adolescents who are perimenarchal. Like uterine anomalies, cervical stenosis or narrowing of the cervical canal may prevent menstrual flow from exiting the uterus and passing through the vagina. Cervical stenosis may lead to increased pressure in the uterus due to hematometra, resulting in cyclic pain and retrograde menstrual flow. This retrograde flow is thought to be a predisposer to the development of endometriosis. Cervical stenosis is generally rare and may be congenital in nature or caused by surgical trauma such as conization or cryotherapy of the cervix.

Post-ablation syndrome is becoming a more common cause of secondary dysmenorrhea. This condition occurs in women who undergo incomplete ablation of the endometrial cavity. The syndrome presents with cyclic pain coinciding with the time women might expect menses and is more apt to occur in those who have undergone tubal ligation where menstrual effluvian subsequently gets trapped in the uterus (78,79). Diagnosis of either of these conditions requires a careful examination and at times adjunctive radiologic studies such as ultrasound. MRI continues to be an excellent, non-invasive means of assessing the upper genital tract and diagnosing uterine abnormalities.

Obstructive, symptomatic genital tract lesions are managed in most cases through surgery. This intervention is focused on establishing a functional outflow tract to allow for free passage of menstrual blood. Patients with post-ablation pain syndromes often require hysterectomy to alleviate pain.

Non-Gynecologic Considerations

Gastrointestinal Pain
A number of gastrointestinal conditions may contribute to or manifest themselves through pelvic pain. Because the bowel is situated near, and shares neural innervation with the gynecologic organs, distinguishing gastrointestinal from gynecologic pain can be difficult. Specific conditions of the gastrointestinal tract that should be considered in the patient with pelvic pain include inflammatory bowel disease (IBD), diverticulitis, chronic appendicitis, and, especially, irritable bowel syndrome (IBS).

IBS is considered the most common non-gynecologic cause of pelvic pain. Eighty percent of those diagnosed with the condition are women. Symptoms of IBS include altered bowel function (constipation and diarrhea), abdominal distention, and pain lasting at least 3 months in duration (80). The pathophysiology of IBS probably involves abnormal gastrointestinal motility with augmented sensation of visceral stimuli (81). Bowel symptoms can vary with a woman's menstrual cycle, making it difficult to distinguish between gynecologic and bowel dysfunction. Compounding these diagnostic difficulties is the fact that 61% of women with dysmenorrhea meet diagnostic criteria for IBS

(82). It is likely that women with dysmenorrhea and IBS may share a common physiologic basis for their pain.

The diagnosis of IBS relies on a characteristic history. Non-specific findings on physical examination include mild abdominal distention, hyperactive bowel sounds, and focal tenderness on rectal exam. Although many patients with the condition undergo gastrointestinal evaluation, barium enemas and endoscopy are unremarkable. CT may be helpful in ruling out other colonic processes such as cancer and diverticulitis.

In women diagnosed with IBS, treatment is based on symptomatology. Recommended therapies include fiber supplementation, anticholinergics, and newer serotonin receptor agonists, along with behavioral therapy for stress reduction.

Urologic Conditions

A number of conditions affecting the urinary tract may similarly manifest with pelvic pain. Urologic conditions should be considered, especially in those with midline or suprapubic discomfort or tenderness. Infectious cystitis, urethral syndrome, renal calculi, and interstitial cystitis (IC) all may cause pelvic pain. IC may be exacerbated by hormonal alterations and menses. Because IC is rarely considered as a cause of secondary dysmenorrhea, the diagnosis is often not made at an early stage when it is most treatable.

Interstitial cystitis remains an enigmatic cause of chronic pelvic pain; its prevalence is estimated at 52 to 450 per 100,000 individuals (83,84). Ninety percent of IC sufferers are female. The pathophysiology behind the condition has been speculated to involve damage to the uroepithelial layer in the bladder, altered pain processing, and perhaps immunologic insult, resulting in mast cell degranulation. The true etiology of the condition, however, is unknown, and treatment is empiric. Symptoms vary greatly among patients and usually include a combination of cyclic pelvic pain (which may radiate), perineal pain, urinary frequency, dyspareunia, nocturia, and urgency. The typical IC symptoms get worse the week before menses and may persist into early flow, somewhat similarly to dysmenorrhea.

Cystoscopy, after bladder distention under anesthesia, remains the gold standard for diagnosis. Therapy for IC advocates dietary and behavioral modification and multimodal medical therapy involving uroepethelial layer protectors, or re-builders, such as pentosyn polysulfate (Elmiron). Tricyclic antidepressants and antihistamines also have been used to treat symptoms associated with IC.

Musculoskeletal Disorders

A variety of musculoskeletal abnormalities have been associated with pelvic pain or may present as dysmenorrhea. Specifically, the physician should consider hernias, spinal column disorders, and fibromyalgia, which is a common condition. Abdominal wall pain has been described as a frequently missed cause of abdominal and pelvic pain; the presence of abdominal wall trigger points (without other sites that would qualify for a diagnosis of fibromyalgia) should be sought and considered in the list of possible causes of pain.

Fibromyalgia is a chronic condition broadly classified as a pain-processing disorder. The etiology of the condition is uncertain, but it afflicts 2% to 6% of the population, 80% of whom are women (85). The diagnosis of fibromyalgia is based on criteria established by the American College of Rheumatology. Diagnosis requires the presence of pain in four quadrants of the patient's body with focal tender or painful points on palpation in at least 11 of 18 anatomic locations (86). Other conditions that present with pelvic pain that are more common in patients with fibromyalgia include IBS, IC, chronic headaches, and primary dysmenorrhea (87). The symptom of pelvic pain with fibromyalgia may therefore result from stimuli originating from a variety of organs and systems.

A number of medical and behavioral therapies have proven efficacious in treating the symptoms of fibromyalgia, such as tricyclic antidepressants, muscle relaxants, hypnotics, exercise, stress reduction, improved sleep hygiene, physical therapy, and cognitive behavioral therapy (88).

Conclusion

Dysmenorrhea is a common condition with which the obstetrician-gynecologist and primary care physician should be familiar. Few women with dysmenorrhea seek medical attention or are familiar with available management options to treat the pain. But when dysmenorrhea is ignored, underlying medical problems and gynecologic diseases may be left untreated, leading to potential long-term disability. In the assessment of any woman, a review of systems should include questions related to menstrual function and pain.

Treatment of primary dysmenorrhea is primarily medical. First-line therapy includes prostaglandin inhibitors. Hormonal therapy with combination oral contraceptives has traditionally been the second-line treatment for dysmenorrhea. Behavioral modification and non-traditional therapeutic options like acupuncture may offer adjunctive benefits in certain sufferers. Similarly, heat therapy is a simple, relatively safe, and effective adjunctive treatment for women with dysmenorrhea. Surgical intervention, although an important means of evaluating for secondary causes of dysmenorrhea, is rarely ideal therapy for the patient with primary dysmenorrhea. Conservative surgical therapies may prove beneficial in patients with severe symptoms or in those refractory to established medical management

The patient with primary dysmenorrhea should be seen initially every few months to evaluate symptoms and effectiveness of therapy. These visits will also facilitate a doctor-patient rapport that is essential in the treatment of this chronic problem. Consideration of both gynecologic and non-gynecologic etiologies of pain are important. Certain diagnostic studies may provide critical information in those patients with non-gynecologic symptoms or severe or atypical pain.

REFERENCES

1. Jamieson DJ, Steege JF. The prevalence of dysmenorrhea, dyspareunia, pelvic pain, and irritable bowel syndrome in primary care practice. Obstet Gynecol. 1996;87:55-8.

2. Andresch B, Milsom I. An epidemiologic study of young women with dysmenorrhea. Am J Obstet Gynecol. 1982;144:655-60.

3. Daewood MY. Dysmenorrhea. Clin Obstet Gynecol. 1990;33:168-78.

4. ACOG technical bulletin. Chronic pelvic pain. Number 223—May 1996 (replaces No. 129, June 1989). American College of Obstetricians and Gynecologists. Int J Gynaecol Obstet. 1996;54:59-68.

5. Klein JR, Litt IF. Epidemiology of adolescent dysmenorrhea. Pediatrics. 1981;68;661-4.

6. Harlow SD, Park M. A longitudinal study of risk factors for the occurrence, duration and severity of menstrual cramps in a cohort of college women. Br J Obstet Gynaecol. 1996;103:1134-42.

7. Campbell MA, McGrath PJ. Use of medication by adolescents for the management of menstrual discomfort. Arch Pediatr Adolesc Med. 1997;151:905-13.

8. Robinson JC, Plichta S, Weisman CS, et al. Dysmenorrhoea and the use of oral contraceptives in adolescent women attending a family planning clinic. Am J Obstet Gynecol. 1992;166:578-83.

9. Pedron-Neuvo N, Gonzalez-Unzaga LN, De Celis-Carrillo R, et al. [Incidence of dysmenorrhoea and associated symptoms in women aged 12-24 years.] Ginecol y Obstet Mex. 1998;66:492-4. Spanish.

10. Widholm O. Dysmenorrhea during adolescence. Acta Obstet Gynecol Scand. 1979;87 (Supplement):61-6.

11. Svennurud S. Dysmenorrhea and absenteeism. Acta Obstet Gynecol Scand. 1959;38 (Supplement):1-88.

12. Whitehead WE, Crowell MD, Heller BR, et al. Modeling and reinforcement of the sick role during childhood predicts adult illness behavior. Psychosom Med. 1994;56:541-50.

13. Izzo A, Labbriola D. Dysmenorrhea and sports activities in adolescents. Clin Exp Obstet Gynecol. 1991;18:109-16.

14. Golomb LM, Solidum AA, Warren MP. Primary dysmenorrhea and physical activity. Med Sci Sports Exercise. 1998;30:906-9.

15. Hornsby PP, Wilcox AJ, Weinberg CR. Cigarette smoking and disturbance of menstrual function. Epidemiology. 1998;9:193-8.

16. Balbi C, et al. Influence of menstrual factors and dietary habits on menstrual pain in adolescent age. Eur J Obstet Gynecol Reprod Biol. 2000;91:143-8.

17. Harel Z, Biro FM, Kottenhahn RK, Rosenthal SL. Supplementation with omega-3 polyunsaturated fatty acids in the management of dysmenorrhea in adolescents. Am J Obstet Gynecol.1996;174:1335-8.

18. DeStefano F, Perlman JA, Peterson HB, et al. Long-term risk of menstrual disturbances after tubal sterilization. Am J Obstet Gynecol. 1985;152:835.

19. Harlow BL, et al. Does tubal sterilization influence the subsequent risk of menorrhagia or dysmenorrhea? Fertil Steril. 2002;77:754-60.

20. Pickles VR, Hall WJ, Best FA, Smith GN. Prostaglandins in the endometrium and menstrual fluid from normal and dysmenorrheic subjects. J Obstet Gynecol Br Commonwealth. 1965;72:185-92.

21. Halbert DR, Demers LM, Fontana J, Jones DED. Prostaglandin levels in endometrial jet wash specimens before and after indomethacin therapy. Prostaglandins. 1975;10: 1047-56.

22. Zahradnik HP, Breckwoldt M. Contribution to the pathogenesis of dysmenorrhea. Arch Gynecol. 1984;236:99-108.

23. Giamberardino MA, Berkeley KJ, Iezzi S, et al. Pain threshold variations in somatic wall tissues as a function of menstrual cycle, segmental site, and tissue depth in non-dysmenorrheic, dysmenorrheic women, and men. Pain. 1997;71:187-97.

24. Bajaj P, Madsen H, Arendt-Neilsen LA. Comparison of modality-specific somatosensory changes during menstruation in dysmenorrheic and non-dysmenorrheic women. Clin J Pain. 2002;18:180-90.

25. Haukttsson A, Akerlund M, Forsling ML, et al. Plasma concentrations of vasopressin and a prostaglandin F2-alpha metabolite in women with primary dysmenorrhea before and during treatment with combined oral contraceptives. J Endocrinol. 1987;115: 355-61.

26. Abu JI, Konje JC. Leukotrienes in gynaecology: the hypothetical value of anti-leukotrien therapy in dysmenorrhea and endometriosis. Hum Reprod Update. 2000;6:200-5.

27. Sigmon ST, Dorhofer DM, Rohan KJ, et al. Psychophysiological, somatic, and affective changes across the menstrual cycle in women with panic disorder. J Consult Clin Psychol. 2000;68:425-31.

28. Baker FC, Driver HS, Rogers GC, et al. High nocturnal body temperatures and disturbed sleep in women with primary dysmenorrhea. Am J Physiol. 1999;277:E1013-21.

29. Golding JM, Wilsnack SC, Learman LA. Prevalence of sexual assault history among women with common gynecologic symptoms. Am J Obstet Gynecol. 1998;179:1013-9.

30. Proctor ML, Sinclair OJ, Farquhar CM, et al. Non-steroidal anti-inflammatory drugs for primary dysmenorrhoea (Protocol for a Cochrane Review). In: The Cochrane Library, Issue 4, 2001. Oxford: Update Software.

31. Lundstrom V, Green K, Wiqvist N. Prostaglandins, indomethacin, and dysmenorrhea. Prostaglandins. 1976;11:893-907.

32. Owen PR. Prostaglandin synthetase inhibitors in the treatment of primary dysmenorrhea: outcome trials reviewed. Am J Obstet Gynecol. 1984;148:96-103.

33. Zhang WY, Li Wan Po A. Efficacy of minor analgesics in primary dysmenorrhoea: a systematic review. Br J Obstet Gynaecol. 1998;105:7809.

34. Milsom I, Minic M, Dawood MY, et al. Comparison of the efficacy and safety of non-prescription doses of naproxen, and naproxen sodium with ibuprofen, acetaminophen, and placebo in the treatment of primary dysmenorrhea: a pooled analysis of five studies. Clin Ther. 2002;24:1384-400.

35. Sande HA, Salvesen T, Izu A. Treating dysmenorrhea with anti-inflammatory agents: a double blind trial with naproxen sodium. Int J Gynaecol Obstet. 1978;16:240-1.

36. Pedron-Nuevo N, Gonzalez-Unzaga M, Medina-Santillan R. [Preventive treatment of primary dysmenorrhea with ibuprofen.] Gynecol Obstet Mex. 1998;66;248-52. Spanish.

37. Chan WY, Fuchs F, Powell AM. Effects of naproxen sodium on menstrual prostaglandins and primary dysmenorrhea. Obstet Gynecol. 1983;61: 285-91.

38. Owen PP. Dysmenorrhea. In: Stovall TG, Ling FW, eds. Gynecology for the Primary Care Physician. Philadelphia: Current Medicine; 1999:315-9.

39. Hayes EC, Rock JA. COX-2 inhibitors and their role in gynecology. Obstet Gynecol Surv. 2002;57:768-80.

40. Alsalameh S, Burien M, Mahr G, et al. The pharmacologic properties and clinical use of valdecoxib, a new cyclooxygenase-2-selective inhibitor. Aliment Pharmacol Ther. 2003; 17:489-501.

41. Davies NM, Jamali F. COX-2 selective inhibitors cardiac toxicity: getting to the heart of the matter. J Pharm Pharm Sci. 2004;29;7:332-6.

42. Proctor ML, Roberts H, Farquhar C. Combined oral contraceptives for primary dysmenorrhoea. In: The Cochrane Library, Issue 4, 2001. Oxford, Update Software. Search date 1999; Primary sources: Medline, Embase, Cinahl, Cochrane Controlled Trials Register, and hand-searched citation lists.

43. Muse KN. Cyclic pelvic pain. Obst Gynecol Clin N Am. 17:427-440.

44. Larsson G, Milsom I, Lindstedt G, et al. The influence of low-dose combined oral contraceptive on menstrual blood loss and iron status. Contraception. 1992;46:327-34.

45. Sicat BL. OrthoEvra, a new contraceptive patch. Pharmacotherapy. 2003;23:472-80.

46. Sulak PJ, Cressman BE, Waldrop E, et al. Extending the duration of active oral contraceptive pills to manage hormone withdrawal symptoms. Obstet Gynecol. 1997;89:179-83.

47. Kaunitz AM. Injectable depot-medroxyprogesterone acetate contraception: an update for U.S. clinicians. Int J Fertil Womens Med. 1998;43:73-83.

48. Vercellini P, De Giorgio O, Oldani S, et al. Depo-medroxyprogesterone acetate versus an oral contraceptive combined with very-low-dose danazol for long-term treatment of pelvic pain associated with endometriosis. Am J Obstet Gynecol. 1996;176:396-401.

49. Jensen JT. Noncontraceptive applications of the levonorgestrel intrauterine system. Curr Womens Health Rep. 2002;2:417-22.

50. Baldaszti E, Wimmer-Puchinger B, Loschke K. Acceptibility of long-term contraceptive levonorgestrel-releasing intrauterine system (Mirena): a 3-year follow-up study. Contraception. 2003;67:87-91.

51. Wildemeersch D, Schacht E, Wildemeersch P. Treatment of primary and secondary dysmenorrhea with a novel 'frameless' intrauterine levonorgestrel releasing drug delivery system: a pilot study. Eur J Contracept Reprod Health Care. 2001;6:192-8.

52. Andersson DE, Ulmsten U. Effect of nifedipine on myometrial activity and lower abdominal pain in women with primary dysmenorrhea. Br J Obstet Gynecol. 1978;85: 142-8.

53. Sandahl B, Ulmsten U, Andersson KE. Trial of calcium antagonist nifedipine in the treatment of primary dysmenorrhoea. Arch Gynceol. 1979;227:147-51.

54. Ulmsten U. Calcium blockade as a rapid pharmacologic test to evaluate primary dysmenorrhea. Gynceol Obstet Invest. 1985;29:78-83.

55. Akerlund M, Andersson KE, Ingemarsson J. Effects of terbutaline on myometrial activity, uterine blood flow, and lower abdominal pain in women with primary dysmenorrhea. Br J Obstet Gynecol. 1976;19:303-12.

56. Ylikorkala O, Dawood MY. New concepts in dysmenorrhea. Am J Obstet Gynecol. 1978;130:833-47.

57. Abu JI, Konje JC. Leukotrienes in gynaecology: the hypothetical value of anti-leukotriene therapy in dysmenorrhoea and endometriosis. Hum Reprod Update. 2000;6:200-5.

58. Serradeil-Le Gal C, Wagnon J, Valette G, et al. Nonpeptide vasopressin receptor antagonists: development of selective and orally active V1a, V2 and V1b receptor ligands. Prog Brain Res. 2002;139:197-210.

59. Brouard R, Bossmar T, Fournie-Lloret D, et al. Effect of SR49059, an orally active V1a vasopressin receptor antagonist, in the prevention of dysmenorrhoea. BJOG. 2000; 107:614-9.

60. Proctor ML, Farquhar CM, Sinclair OJ, et al. Surgical interruption of pelvic nerve pathways for primary and secondary dysmenorrhoea. In: The Cochrane Library, Issue 4, 2001. Oxford: Update Software. Search date 1998.

61. Kwok A, Lam A, Ford R. Laparoscopic presacral neurectomy: retrospective series. Aust N Z J Obstet Gynaecol. 2001;41:195-7.

62. Chen FP. Laparoscopic presacral neurectomy for chronic pelvic pain. Changgeng Yi Xue Za Zhi. 2000;23:1-7.

63. Denny DR, Gerrard M. Bahavioral treatments of primary dysmenorrhea: a review. Behav Res Ther. 1981;19:303-12.

64. Sigmon ST, Nelson RO. The effectiveness of activity scheduling and relaxation training in the treatment of spasmodic dysmenorrhea. J Behav Med. 1988;11:483-95.

65. Balick L, Elfner L, May J, Moore JD. Biofeedback treatment of dysmenorrhea. Biofeedback Self Regul. 1982;7:499-520.

66. Bennink CD, Hulst LL, Benthem JA. The effects of EMG biofeedback and relaxation training on primary dysmenorrhea. J Behav Med. 1982;5:329-41.

67. Proctor ML, Farquhar C, Kennedy S, Jin X. Transcutaneous electrical nerve stimulation and acupuncture for the treatment of primary dysmenorrhoea (Protocol for a Cochrane Review). In: The Cochrane Library, Issue 4, 2001. Oxford: Update Software.

68. Dawood MY, Ramos J. Transcutaneous electrical nerve stimulation (TENS) for the treatment of primary dysmenorrhea: a randomized crossover comparison with placebo TENS and ibuprofen. Obstet Gynecol. 1990;75:656-60.

69. Lundeberg T, Bondesson L, Lundstrom V. Relief of primary dysmenorrhea by transcutaneous electric nerve stimulation. Acta Obstet Gynecol Scand. 1985;64:491-7.

70. Helms JM. Acupuncture for the management of primary dysmenorrhea. Obstet Gynecol. 1987;69:51-6.

71. Akin MD, Weingand KW, Hengehold DA, et al. Continuous low-level topical heat in the treatment of dysmenorrhea. Obstet Gyncol. 2001;97:343-9.

72. Koninckx PR, Lessaffre E, Meuleman C, et al. Suggestive evidence that pelvic endometriosis is a progressive disease, whereas deeply infiltrating endometriosis is associated with pelvic pain. Fertil Steril. 1991;55:759-65.

73. Ling FW. Randomized controlled trial of depot leuprolide in patients with chronic pelvic pain and clinically suspected endometriosis. Pelvic Pain Study Group. Obstet Gynecol. 1999;93:51-8.

74. Schattman GL. When endometriosis is the most likely diagnosis. OBG Management. 2000;Feb(Supplement):14-8.

75. Arnold LL, Ascher SM, Schruefer JJ, Simon JA. The non-surgical diagnosis of adenomyosis. Obstet Gynecol. 1995;86:461-5.

76. Duncan CH, Taylor HC. Psychosomatic study of pelvic congestion. Am J Obstet Gynecol. 1952;64:1.

77. Tarazov PG, Prozorovski KV, Ryzhkov VK. Pelvic pain syndrome caused by ovarian varices: treatment by transcatheter embolization. Acta Radiol. 1997;38:1023-5.

78. Townsend DE, et al. Postablation sterilization syndrome. Obstet Gynecol. 1993;82;422-4.

79. Webb JC, Bush MR, Woode MD, Park GS. Hemtosalpinx with pelvic pain after endometrial ablation confirms the postablation-sterilization syndrome. J Am Assoc Gynecol Laparosc. 1996;3:419-21.

80. Drossman DA, Thompson WG, Talley NJ, et al. Identification of subgroups of functional gastrointestinal disorders. Gastroenterol Int. 1990;3:159-72.

81. Lenbo T, Munakata J, Mertz H, et al. Evidence for hypersensitivity of lumbar splanchnic afferents in irritable bowel syndrome. Gastroenterology. 1994;107:1686-96.

82. Crowell MD, Dubin NH, Robinson JC, et al. Functional bowel disorders in women with dysmenorrhea. Am J Gastroenterol. 1994;89:1973-7.

83. Curhan GC, Speizer FE, Hunter DJ, et al. Epidemiology of interstitial cystitis: a population-based study. J Urol. 1999;168:549-52.

84. Leppilahti M, Tammela TL, Huhtala H, et al. Prevelence of symptoms related to interstitial cystitis in women; a population-based study in Finland. J Urol. 2002;168:139-43.

85. Croft P, Rigby AS, Boswell R, et al. The prevalence of chronic widespeard pain in the general population. J Rheumatol. 1993;20:710-3.

86. Wolfe F, Smythe HA, Yunus MB, et al. The American College of Rheumatology. 1990 classification of fibromyalgia. Report of the multicenter criteria committee. Arthritis Rheum. 1990;33:160-72.

87. Yunus MB, Masi AT, Aldag JC. A controlled study of primary fibromyalgia syndrome: clinical features and associations with other functional syndromes. J Rheumatol Suppl. 1989;9:62-71.

88. Russell IJ, ed. Clinical overview and pathogenesis of the fibromyalgia syndrome, myofascial pain syndrome, and other pain syndromes. New York: Haworth Medical Press; 1996.

6

Premenstrual Syndrome

Susan Johnson, MD, MS

The symptoms of premenstrual syndrome may be mild and merely annoying or severe enough to cause impairment. They fall into two broad categories: psychological/emotional (e.g., irritability) and physical (e.g., breast tenderness). Most women who seek treatment have mood symptoms; however, some patients present with physical symptoms as their primary complaint. Every primary care physician who cares for women should be familiar with the diagnostic approach to this complaint, as well as the most common differential diagnoses and the most effective approaches to therapy.

Terminology

Most women who ovulate experience one or more potentially adverse symptoms that recur in the late luteal (premenstrual) phase of the cycle. The most common symptoms are irritability, mood lability, breast tenderness, food cravings, sleep disturbance, fatigue, headache, and bloating. The majority of women experience three or four mild symptoms for a only few days, and there is no great effect on their life; these common, nonproblematic symptoms are referred to as the *molimina*. The clinically relevant luteal phase syndromes discussed in this chapter, on the other hand, are typically characterized by a larger number of symptoms that last longer and are more intense.

A variety of diagnostic labels have been used for these clinically relevant luteal phase symptoms over the past century (1). In the early part of the 20th century, a syndrome called *premenstrual tension* was first described, and that label was most often used in the United States until the 1970s, when *premenstrual syndrome* emerged as the more common term. In the 1980s the American Psychiatric Association added to the appendix of DSM-III diagnostic criteria for severe luteal phase symptoms, labeling this condition *late luteal phase dysphoric disorder*. In DSM-IV-R, these criteria were slightly revised, and the name was changed to *premenstrual dysphoric disorder* (PMDD) (2). Although the existence of a less severe syndrome, *premenstrual syndrome* (PMS), is mentioned in the discussion section for PMDD, specific diagnostic criteria were not defined except to say that in PMDD the salient symptoms are the mood problems, whereas in PMS physical symptoms play a larger role.

For the clinician, the distinction between PMS and PMDD (if there is one!) is not particularly important. The PMDD label is used to describe severe luteal phase symptoms that lead to impairment, but many women with less severe symptoms, who are merely annoyed but not impaired, also seek treatment. The diagnostic approach is the same for all levels of problematic symptoms, and the same range of treatments should be considered (3). Thus, in this chapter, PMS/PMDD is used when the discussion is relevant to all levels of severity.

Clinical Criteria

Women with PMS/PMDD experience a cluster of symptoms that recur in the luteal phase and remit in the follicular phase of the menstrual cycle; these symptoms cannot be explained by another psychiatric or medical disorder (4). PMS/PMDD are distinguished from molimina by the fact that the woman experiences some level of discomfort (≥ 1 week) (PMS) and/or impairment (PMDD) as a result. Thus the key diagnostic criteria are the presence of symptoms that are typical for this syndrome, the prospective verification that symptoms are confined to the luteal phase, and the presence of impairment or discomfort.

The symptoms associated with PMS/PMDD are affective (irritability, mood swings, depression, and hostility), somatic (bloating, mastalgia, appetite changes, hot flashes, insomnia, headache, and fatigue), cognitive (confusion and poor concentration), and behavioral (social withdrawal, hyperphagia, and arguing). Ovulation, which is the event that initiates the luteal phase, typically occurs 2 weeks before the onset of menstrual flow, and symptoms typically begin 1 to 2 weeks before menses. Because the symptoms are not unique to PMS/PMDD, psychiatric disorders (e.g., depression, anxiety) or medical disorders (e.g., migraine, irritable bowel syndrome, hypothyroidism) must be differentiated from it.

The timing of symptoms should be confirmed with a prospective symptom record (charting) kept by the patient for at least two menstrual cycles. In the classic pattern, symptoms begin at or after ovulation and begin to resolve with the onset of menstrual flow. Charting is required by the DSM-IV criteria for PMDD because of data suggesting that more than half of the women who present with a specific complaint of "PMS" are found not to have a pure luteal phase pattern based on prospective charting and thus have some other explanation for all or some of their symptoms. In addition, the charting period is an excellent time to introduce self-help strategies independently of other therapy. Because as many as 30% of women will respond to these approaches, deferring the decision about pharmacological therapy for two months is acceptable to most patients.

There is no standardized method of measuring symptom severity. For the diagnosis of either PMS or PMDD to be plausible, there must be at least a 30% increase in severity of symptoms during the luteal phase as compared with the follicular phase. Problems with relationships at home and at work, parenting, and work performance can be assessed to determine the extent to which the patient's life is disrupted. The sole fact that a woman seeks treatment implies a certain level of severity.

Epidemiology

Prevalence

Symptoms that occur repetitively during the luteal (premenstrual) phase of the cycle are nearly universal among women who ovulate. The number, severity, and duration of these symptoms determine whether an individual woman has a clinically definable syndrome (PMS or PMDD) for which she may seek treatment or has symptoms that she simply considers part of her normal menstrual experience.

Based on several large cross-sectional epidemiological studies, it appears that 80% or more of ovulating women experience some level of adverse luteal phase symptoms. For the majority, the symptoms are mild, last only a few days, and are not bothersome; as mentioned previously, these symptoms are sometimes referred to as the *molimina* (5). At the other end of the spectrum, for 5%-10% of ovulating women the symptoms are numerous, severe, and last nearly the entire luteal phase of approximately 2 weeks per cycle; this group would now be characterized as having *premenstrual dysphoric disorder* (PDD) as defined in the DSM-IV appendices. The third group, in the middle, might best be described as having a week or more of the same sort of symptoms, annoying but not the cause of significant disruption of relationships, work, or other life activities; this group would now be described as having *premenstrual syndrome* (PMS).

Risk Factors

Luteal phase symptoms are found among women of all ages, but in clinical practice the majority of women who seek care are over 30 years of age. Usually they describe having had symptoms for several years, so it is not clear if

PMS/PMDD worsen with age or if older women are simply more likely to ask for help for this kind of problem.

No difference in prevalence has been found based on racial/ethnic, socioeconomic, or marital status. Women in developing cultures and women in developed countries have similar rates of severe symptoms.

Comorbidity

There is a higher rate of major depressive disorder and, probably, of postpartum depression among women with PMDD. These syndromes have not been associated with any other reproductive history characteristics, such as menstrual cycle length, amount of flow, presence or absence of dysmenorrhea, previous use of oral contraceptives, or tubal sterilization.

Pathophysiology

Based on studies of the effect of ovulation suppression, ovulation is a prerequisite for the occurrence of PMS/PMDD. The exact sequence of events from ovulation to the emergence of symptoms is not known. The practical implication of this finding is that women who are post-menopausal, amenorrheic or anovulatory, or who have had their ovaries removed by definition cannot have PMS/PMDD.

Substantial evidence suggests that many women with PMDD experience a decline in serotonin during the luteal phase; this is supported by the effectiveness of the SSRI drugs in treating these syndromes (6). Other central transmitters may be involved as well, such as MSH and endorphins.

Some investigators have speculated that PMS/PMDD is simply a variant of major depressive disorder, but this view is not the prevalent theory based on the fact that there are several important differences between these syndromes (7).

Differential Diagnosis

The symptoms of PMS/PMDD are not unique, and clinicians must be familiar with the differential diagnoses in the woman who presents with a constellation of complaints that may be PMS/PMDD.

Menstrual Magnification of a Mood Disorder

Of women who seek treatment in specialty clinics for premenstrual disorders, the majority are found to have some other mood disorder, predominately depression. The confusion is caused by the fact that many women with a mood disorder (major depressive disorder, dysphoric disorder, bipolar disorder, and depression not otherwise specified; or an anxiety disorder) commonly experience a worsening of symptoms just before or during menses, a phenomenon often referred to as *menstrual magnification* (8). The key to identifying this problem is the presence of symptoms in the follicular phase of the cycle (i.e., in the week after menses). Another common clinical presentation is a woman who is being treated with serotonin reuptake inhibitors for a diagnosis of depression and is doing well except during the late luteal/menstrual phase, when her symptoms re-emerge each month.

Medical Conditions

Many medical conditions can become "entrained" in the menstrual cycle, such that the symptoms specific to these conditions are manifested exclusively or more commonly in the late luteal or menstrual phase. The most common example is migraine headaches; 5% of women with migraines experience them exclusively in the late luteal phase (so-called "menstrual migraines"), and many more women report that their migraines increase in frequency or severity at that time. Many other conditions have been reported during the late luteal phase, including herpes, diabetes, asthma, and even coronary heart disease.

The key to diagnosis in these cases is to recognize that the symptoms are characteristic of the specific condition, not of PMS/PMDD. *The initial treatment approach should be whatever is usual for the condition.* For example, for menstrual migraine, the usual abortive therapies are the first step, with the usual prophylactic medications as needed (9). If, however, the usual therapies are not sufficient to eliminate late luteal phase symptoms, ovulation suppression may need to be considered (10).

Diagnosis

Making a diagnosis and devising a treatment plan for most women with probable PMS/PMDD is usually straightforward (11,12). The diagnostic evaluation should involve two clinic appointments separated by two menstrual cycles (Table 6-1). At the first visit, the presenting symptoms (Table 6-2) are evaluated and a differential diagnosis is developed. During the next two cycles, the woman is asked to keep a daily symptom record (charting), and the physician obtains any indicated referrals or diagnostic test results. At the second visit, all information is reviewed, and a management plan is formulated.

As mentioned earlier, because PMS/PMDD symptoms are not unique to this syndrome, other disorders must be considered. Charting should demonstrate

Table 6-1   Diagnostic Evaluation of PMS/PMDD

At the first visit:
1. Determine the range of symptoms and decide if consistent with PMS.
2. Based on the history and physical examination, decide if some other diagnosis should also be considered.
3. Obtain any laboratory tests or consultations needed to assess additional diagnoses under consideration.

Refer: Severe mood symptoms (vegetative symptoms, suicidal ideation, unable to function)

Between the first and second visit:
4. Have the patient, over a two-month period, record daily the presence or absence of the relevant symptoms, as well as the dates of her menstrual periods.
5. Recommend that the patient try lifestyle and nutritional interventions.

At the second visit:
6. Assess the symptoms pattern on the menstrual calendar and determine if consistent with PMS. If not, pursue other diagnoses. If consistent with PMS, and nonpharmacological therapy has not been effective, proceed to drug therapy.

Refer: Failure to respond to Level 1 and 2 therapies (Fig. 6-1) or if hysterectomy is being considered

Table 6-2   Common Symptoms of PMS/PMDD

• Irritability	• Breast tenderness	• Fatigue
• Mood lability	• Food cravings	• Difficulty concentrating
• Anxiety	• Headaches	• Mental "fuzziness"
• Depression	• Bloating	
• Unprovoked crying	• Aches and pains	
• Hostility	• Sleep disturbance (middle-of-night awakening)	

that symptoms occur during the luteal phase only; another symptom pattern would suggest a different cause for the symptoms. Another diagnosis should be entertained in women who are postmenopausal, anovulatory, or amenorrheic.

There are no laboratory tests that confirm the diagnosis of PMS/PMDD—it is a clinical diagnosis. Specifically, there is no value in obtaining levels of any of the reproductive hormones (estradiol, progesterone, FSH, LH, testosterone, etc.), because these levels do not vary between women with and without PMS/PMDD.

If the clinical picture suggests that a medical condition may explain the cyclic symptoms in an individual woman, appropriate tests should be performed.

Treatment

In the last decade, the pharmacological treatment of PMS has undergone a revolution because of the development of uniform operational diagnostic criteria and the use of placebo-controlled randomized clinical trials. Commonly used therapies, such as "natural" progesterone, vitamin B₆, vitamin E, evening primrose oil, and diuretics, have been shown to be ineffective, and oral contraceptives have been shown primarily helpful for physical symptoms. The remainder of this chapter describes therapeutic strategies that have been found effective.

Once an accurate diagnosis is made, appropriate interventions should be based on two principles. First, PMS is a chronic problem that typically does not resolve until menopause, making both cost and side effects important components of the treatment choice. Second, women experience different degrees of symptom severity, and the intensity of the treatment approach should be matched to the symptoms. For example, for women with mild symptoms, lifestyle and nutritional supplement therapies are a more appropriate starting place than SSRI therapy.

An overview of the treatment approach to PMS is shown in Figure 6-1.

Most women seek treatment as a result of problems with mood (irritability, mood lability, etc.), and the following treatment approaches are targeted primarily at these symptoms. For most of these treatments, however, there is a concomitant improvement in physical symptoms as well. The problem of isolated (or remaining) physical symptoms is addressed later in this chapter.

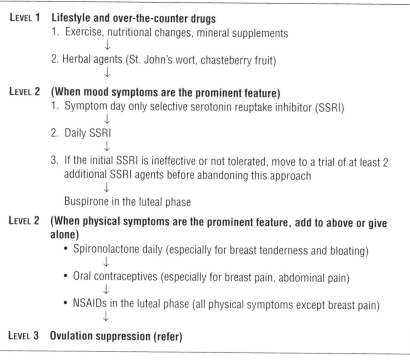

Figure 6-1 Hierarchical treatment approach to premenstrual syndrome. Move to the next level, or the next method within a level, if the current approach is ineffective over 2 to 3 cycles.

For most women it is reasonable to recommend exercise, dietary changes, and nutritional supplements as initial therapy. With this approach, approximately one third of women seeking treatment improve enough to not need prescription drug therapy.

Exercise

Regular moderate aerobic exercise has been shown in epidemiological studies to be associated with less severe premenstrual symptoms. In the single randomized trial, a group of sedentary women with PMS were randomly assigned to regular walking or continuation of usual activity for 6 months (13). The active group reported fewer symptoms at the end of the trial. A reasonable initial regimen for sedentary women is 30 minutes of brisk walking five times a week.

Diet

An increase in complex carbohydrate intake during the luteal phase has been shown in two randomized trials to reduce the severity of premenstrual mood symptoms (14). The commonly given advice to avoid sugar is the inverse of this advice, but there are no data to support it.

The role of caffeine in premenstrual symptoms is unclear. Observational studies have found that women who report the most severe premenstrual symptoms also report the highest caffeine intake, but it is unclear whether the caffeine is causative, aggravates existing symptoms, or is actually being used as self-treatment for the common symptoms of fatigue and reduced concentration. A trial of reducing or eliminating caffeine for several cycles is reasonable.

The role of sodium is purely anecdotal and probably derives from the belief that the symptoms of bloating and weight gain are due to salt or at least can be improved by reducing its intake. As with caffeine, it may be reasonable to have women experiment with reducing dietary salt, but to continue this practice only if improvement is noted.

Nutritional Supplements

Mineral Supplements
Calcium and magnesium supplements have each been shown to reduce emotional and luteal phase symptoms. Most of the data are with calcium. In the largest randomized trial, 497 symptomatic women were randomized to either placebo or 1200 mg of calcium carbonate taken daily (15). Forty percent of the women were taking oral contraceptives. After 3 months, there was an overall 48% reduction in total symptom scores from baseline in the active therapy group compared with a 30% reduction in the placebo group. Calcium has never been compared directly to SSRI therapy, but most experts believe

that calcium supplements are probably most effective in women with mild-to-moderate symptoms.

Magnesium (as magnesium pyrrolidine carboxylic acid 360 mg) has been studied in one small randomized trial with similar results (16). Calcium is the preferred choice because of the concomitant bone benefit, but for women who do not tolerate calcium, daily magnesium 400 mg is an alternative.

Herbal Remedies and Other Supplements

Girman et al. have written an excellent review of all the herbal preparations that have been used for premenstrual symptoms (17), to which interested readers are referred. To summarize their findings, based on an extensive literature review these authors conclude that evening primrose oil and vitamin B_6 are unlikely to be of significant benefit for luteal phase symptoms. Black cohosh, ginko, and kava may be of benefit, but they have not been adequately tested in placebo-controlled trials. Of these, kava (hepatotoxicity), St. John's wort (drug-drug interaction), and ginko (drug-drug interaction) can be associated with potentially severe side effects.

St. John's wort (SJW), whose active ingredient is thought to be hyperceium, is a logical therapeutic candidate because of its SSRI-like effects, and it is used by many women for PMS. However, it has been evaluated in only one open, uncontrolled, observational study (18). Thirty women with well-documented luteal phase symptoms were randomized to either placebo or SJW 80 mg bid for 3 months. Women on the active regimen reported a 50% reduction in symptoms after 2 months, which is on the same order of magnitude as calcium. However, until a placebo-controlled trial verifies these results, this therapy cannot be considered proven.

Chasteberry fruit (Vitex agnus-castus) has been shown in two randomized trials to be superior to placebo (19,20). In each trial, participants who met DSM-III criteria for luteal phase syndrome were randomized to chasteberry 20 mg or placebo. At the end of three cycles, the active therapy groups reported 50%-60% reductions in luteal phase symptoms as compared with a 25%-35% reduction among placebo users. Chasteberry fruit has few side effects and can be found in health food stores.

SSRI Therapy

For women who do not have an adequate response to exercise, dietary change, or nutritional supplements after two or three cycles, SSRI therapy is indicated (21). Numerous randomized placebo-controlled trials of fluoxetine (22), sertraline (23), paroxetine (24), and citalopram (25) have shown clear benefit compared with placebo for women with PMDD. The effect is not a general antidepressant effect; agents with different mechanisms of action are not effective (26-28).

Because there is no evidence to suggest that any specific agent is clearly superior, drug choice can be based on cost, patient preference, and the woman's response and side effect experience. It appears that lack of response to one SSRI does not predict response to other agents in this class, so trying at least three different drugs before moving to a different form of therapy has been suggested (25).

The effect of SSRIs—even fluoxetine, with its long half-life—on PMS/PMDD is usually immediate, with symptom improvement seen in 24 to 28 hours. This is quite different than when using these drugs for the treatment of depression or anxiety, where the full effect may take 4 to 6 weeks. This feature of SSRI response allows many women to use SSRIs intermittently rather than continuously.

Several randomized trials of luteal phase only or symptom day only treatment (approximately the 14 days before the onset of menses) have shown that this regimen is clearly superior to placebo (29-35). In a trial of citalopram, luteal phase therapy was found to be equivalent to daily therapy (36). A weekly dose of fluoxetine has been shown to be superior to placebo but does not appear to be as effective as luteal phase or continuous therapy (37).

Intermittent therapy has clear advantages, including lesser cost and fewer days at risk for side effects (including sexual symptoms). Thus women with PMS/PMDD and no evidence of co-existing mood disorder may begin with symptom day therapy. The initial dose for fluoxetine is 20 mg (usual range, 10-40 mg); for sertraline, 50 mg (usual range, 25-150 mg). Treatment should begin as soon as typical symptoms start. The drug should be discontinued either on the first day of menses or 1 to 3 days later, depending on the usual day that symptoms spontaneously resolve.

If intermittent therapy is insufficient, a trial of a daily SSRI therapy for at least 2 months is appropriate. At least three different agents should be tried before SSRI therapy is abandoned, since the side effect profile may differ, and, women may respond to one but not all agents in the class (25).

If the SSRI class of agents is not tolerated or not effective, an anxiolytic can be considered. Luteal phase alprazolam was found in several small trials to be superior to placebo. Luteal phase buspirone has been reported in one small clinical trial to be also superior to placebo. Because buspirone has less addictive potential and fewer side effects than alprazolam (38), the former is preferred when an anxiolytic is desirable.

Isolated Physical Symptoms

The majority of women who seek treatment for luteal phase symptoms have mood symptoms (irritability, mood lability, depressive symptoms). However, some women present with a physical symptom as their primary complaint, or, continue to have problems with a physical symptom after successful therapy with another approach (12). *Spironolactone* (50 to 200 mg as a single daily dose) may offer benefit for breast tenderness, bloating, luteal phase weight gain, and, possibly, mood symptoms. *Oral contraceptives* have been shown to reduce luteal phase physical symptoms, but they do not appear to improve, and may even worsen, mood symptoms. *Nonsteroidal anti-inflammatory agents,* given in a modestly high dose in the luteal phase (e.g., naproxen sodium 600 mg three times daily), have been shown in several small randomized trials to improve all physical symptoms *except* breast tenderness, and they may also modify mood symptoms.

Ovulation Suppression Therapy

Patients who do not respond to any of the above regimens are candidates for a trial of ovulation suppression. Oral contraceptives would seem to be a logical choice for this purpose. However, there are only two randomized clinical trials, and the results have either found no benefit for mood symptoms (39) or a insignificant improvement (40). Thus women should be referred to a specialist (ideally to a gynecologist, or possibly a psychiatrist, with a special interest in PMDD) for this form of therapy.

The "gold standard" is gonadotropin-releasing hormone agonist. The problems with long-term use of this agent are high cost and the need for "add back" estrogen therapy to prevent or minimize bone loss. Danazol, a synthetic androgen, is also effectively in suppressed ovulation and PMDD symptoms. However, because of significant side effects (weight gain, androgen side effects, and, of most concern, predictable suppression of HDL), danazol can only be used short term and is thus rarely prescribed. An inexpensive, relatively safe, and side effect free alternative is continuous medroxyprogesterone acetate given orally (20-40 mg daily) or as the depot injection (typical dose, 150 mg every three months).

Bilateral oophorectomy has been studied in two nonrandomized trials and appears to be beneficial (41,42). However, it should rarely be necessary to resort to this method given the array of effective pharmacological options. A reasonable approach is to restrict consideration of oophorectomy to women who have benefited only from gonadotropin-releasing hormone agonist therapy and who are likely to need several more years of therapy. These women should be referred to a specialist with expertise in this issue.

Summary

Our understanding of the diagnosis and treatment of PMS/PMDD has progressed greatly over the last two decades. The diagnosis is generally straightforward, with the diagnostic evaluation typically accomplished after two office visits. Therapy is based on the symptom severity of the individual patient. Because of the progress made in the understanding of PMS/PMDD treatment, most women with premenstrual symptoms, whether mild and merely bothersome or severe and disabling, can be offered effective therapy.

REFERENCES

1. Endicott J. History, evolution, and diagnosis of premenstrual dysphoric disorder. J Clin Psychiatry. 2000;61(Suppl):12:5-8.

2. Diagnostic and Statistical Manual of Mental Disorders, 4th ed. Washington, DC: American Psychiatric Association; 1994.

3. Clinical management guidelines for obstetricians-gynecologists: premenstrual syndrome. American College of Obstetricians and Gynecologists Practice Bulletin. April 2000; No. 15.

4. Freeman EW. Premenstrual syndrome and premenstrual dysphoric disorder: definitions and diagnosis. Psychoneuroendocrinology. 2003;28(Suppl 3):25-37.

5. Halbreich U, Borenstein J, Pearlstein T, Kahn LS. The prevalence, impairment, impact, and burden of premenstrual dysphoric disorder (PMS/PMDD). Psychoneuroendocrinology. 2003;28(Suppl 3):1-23.

6. Steiner M, Pearlstein T. Premenstrual dysphoria and the serotonin system: pathophysiology and treatment. J Clin Psychiatry. 2000;61(Suppl 12):17-21.

7. Endicott J, Amsterdam J, Eriksson E, et al. Is premenstrual dysphoric disorder a distinct clinical entity? J Womens Health Gend Based Med. 1999;8:663-79.

8. Hartlage SA, Brandenburg DL, Kravitz HM. Premenstrual exacerbation of depressive disorders in a community-based sample in the United States. Psychosom Med. 2004; 66:698-706.

9. Kornstein SG, Parker AJ. Menstrual migraines: etiology, treatment, and relationship to premenstrual syndrome. Curr Opin Obstet Gynecol. 1997;9:154-9.

10. Murray SC, Muse KN. Effective treatment of severe menstrual migraine headaches with gonadotropin-releasing hormone agonist and "add-back" therapy. Fertil Steril. 1997;67:390-3.

11. Kessel B. Premenstrual syndrome: advances in diagnosis and treatment. Obstet Gynecol Clin North Am. 2000;27:625-39.

12. Johnson SR. Premenstrual syndrome, premenstrual dysphoric disorder, and beyond: a clinical primer for practitioners. Obstet Gynecol. 2004;104:845-59.

13. Prior JC, Vigna Y, Sciarretta D, et al. Conditioning exercise decreases premenstrual symptoms: a prospective, controlled 6-month trial. Fertil Steril. 1987;47:402-8.

14. Freeman EW, Stout AL, Endicott J, Spiers P. Treatment of premenstrual syndrome with a carbohydrate-rich beverage. Int J Gynaecol Obstet. 2002;77:253-4.

15. Thys-Jacobs S, Starkey P, Bernstein D, Tian J. Calcium carbonate and the premenstrual syndrome: effects on premenstrual and menstrual symptoms. Premenstrual Syndrome Study Group.[Summary for patients in Can Fam Physician. 2002;48:705-7.] Am J Obstet Gynecol. 1998;179:444-52.

16. Facchinetti F, Borella P, Sances G, et al. Oral magnesium successfully relieves premenstrual mood changes. Obstet Gynecol. 1991;78:177-81.

17. Girman A, Lee R, Kligler B. An integrative medicine approach to premenstrual syndrome. Am J Obstet Gynecol. 2003;188(5 Suppl):S56-65.

18. Stevinson C, Ernst E. A pilot study of *Hypericum perforatum* for the treatment of premenstrual syndrome. BJOG. 2000;107:870-6.

19. Huddleston M, Jackson EA. Is an extract of the fruit of *Vitex agnus castus* (chaste tree or chasteberry) effective for prevention of symptoms of premenstrual syndrome (PMS)? J Fam Pract. 2001;50:298.

20. Schellenberg R. Treatment for the premenstrual syndrome with *Vitex agnus castus* fruit extract: prospective, randomised, placebo controlled study. BMJ. 2001;322:134-7.

21. Born L, Steiner M. Current management of premenstrual syndrome and premenstrual dysphoric disorder. Current Psychiatry Reports. 2001;3:463-9.

22. Steiner M, Steinberg S, Stewart D, et al. Fluoxetine in the treatment of premenstrual dysphoria [see Comment]. Canadian Fluoxetine/Premenstrual Dysphoria Collaborative Study Group. N Engl J Med. 1995;332:1529-34.

23. Yonkers KA, Halbreich U, Freeman E, et al. Symptomatic improvement of premenstrual dysphoric disorder with sertraline treatment: a randomized controlled trial [see Comment]. Sertraline Premenstrual Dysphoric Collaborative Study Group. JAMA. 1997;278:983-8.

24. Yonkers KA, Gullion C, Williams A, et al. Paroxetine as a treatment for premenstrual dysphoric disorder. J Clin Psychopharmacol. 1996;16:3-8.

25. Freeman EW, Jabara S, Sondheimer SJ, Auletto R. Citalopram in PMS patients with prior SSRI treatment failure: a preliminary study. J Womens Health Gend Based Med. 2002;11:459-64.

26. Eriksson E, Hedberg MA, Andersch B, Sundblad C. The serotonin reuptake inhibitor paroxetin is superior to the noradrenaline reuptake inhibitor maprotiline in the treatment of premenstrual syndrome. Neuropsychopharmacology. 1995;12:167-76.

27. Freeman EW, Rickels K, Sondheimer SJ, Wittmaack FM. Sertraline versus desipramine in the treatment of premenstrual syndrome: an open-label trial. J Clin Psychiatry. 1996;57:7-11.

28. Pearlstein TB, Stone AB, Lund SA, et al. Comparison of fluoxetine, bupropion, and placebo in the treatment of premenstrual dysphoric disorder. J Clin Psychopharmacology. 1997;17:261-6.

29. Halbreich U, Bergeron R, Yonkers KA, et al. Efficacy of intermittent, luteal phase sertraline treatment of premenstrual dysphoric disorder. Obstet Gynecol. 2002;100:1219-29.

30. Alpay FB, Turhan NO. Intermittent versus continuous sertraline therapy in the treatment of premenstrual dysphoric disorders. Int J Fertil Womens Med. 2001;46:228-31.

31. Jermain DM, Preece CK, Sykes RL, et al. Luteal phase sertraline treatment for premenstrual dysphoric disorder: results of a double-blind, placebo-controlled, crossover study. Arch Fam Med. 1999;8:328-32.

32. Freeman EW, Rickels K, Arredondo F, et al. Full- or half-cycle treatment of severe premenstrual syndrome with a serotonergic antidepressant. J Clin Psychopharmacol. 1999;19:3-8.

33. Young SA, Hurt PH, Benedek DM, Howard RS. Treatment of premenstrual dysphoric disorder with sertraline during the luteal phase: a randomized, double-blind, placebo-controlled crossover trial. J Clin Psychiatry. 1998;59:76-80.

34. Halbreich U, Smoller JW. Intermittent luteal phase sertraline treatment of dysphoric premenstrual syndrome. J Clin Psychiatry. 1997;58:399-402.

35. Steiner M, Korzekwa M, Lamont J, Wilkins A. Intermittent fluoxetine dosing in the treatment of women with premenstrual dysphoria. Psychopharmacol Bull. 1997;33: 771-4.

36. Wikander I, Sundblad C, Andersch B, et al. Citalopram in premenstrual dysphoria: is intermittent treatment during luteal phases more effective than continuous medication throughout the menstrual cycle? J Clin Psychopharmacol. 1998;18:390-8.

37. Miner C, Brown E, McCray S, et al. Weekly luteal-phase dosing with enteric-coated fluoxetine 90 mg in premenstrual dysphoric disorder: a randomized, double-blind, placebo-controlled clinical trial. Clin Ther. 2002;24:417-33.

38. Rickels K, Freeman E, Sondheimer S. Buspirone in treatment of premenstrual syndrome. Lancet. 1989;1:777.

39. Graham CA, Sherwin BB. A prospective treatment study of premenstrual symptoms using a triphasic oral contraceptive. J Psychosom Res. 1992;36:257-66.

40. Freeman EW, Kroll R, Rapkin A, et al. Evaluation of a unique oral contraceptive in the treatment of premenstrual dysphoric disorder[see Comment]. J Womens Health Gend Based Med. 2001;10:561-9.

41. Casson P, Hahn PM, Van Vugt DA, Reid RL. Lasting response to ovariectomy in severe intractable premenstrual syndrome. Am J Obstet Gynecol. 1990;162:99-105.

42. Casper RF, Hearn MT. The effect of hysterectomy and bilateral oophorectomy in women with severe premenstrual syndrome. Am J Obstet Gynecol. 1990;162:105-9.

Medical Issues

7

Polycystic Ovary Syndrome

Katherine Sherif, MD
Shahab Minassian, MD

Polycystic ovary syndrome (PCOS) is one of the most common causes of menstrual irregularities in the United States and a leading cause of infertility. Estimates of PCOS prevalence range between 6% and 10% in adult women. This may change as more women who are obese are screened. Most adults with PCOS report that their symptoms began during adolescence, and thus prevalence in adolescents is likely similar to that in adults. Regardless of the exact prevalence, PCOS is at least as common as type 2 diabetes, which affects 6% of the U.S. population. PCOS has been viewed as a collection of primarily reproductive disorders, including polycystic ovaries, anovulation, infertility, and possibly early pregnancy loss, along with hirsutism, acne, and obesity. More recently, PCOS has been observed to be associated with cardiovascular risk factors, including elevated blood pressure, dyslipidemia, abnormal glucose metabolism, and coagulopathies. PCOS is a paradigm of a women's health issue: the interaction of sex hormones with the vascular endothelium has extended the health concerns beyond the realm of reproductive issues and may have profound implications in the evolution of cardiovascular disease in women.

Definition and Presentation

The 2003 Rotterdam conference of the European Society of Human Reproduction and Embryology/American Society for Reproductive Medicine developed consensus statements on PCOS diagnosis, nomenclature, and long-term health risks (1). The ESHRE/ASRM diagnostic criteria for PCOS are listed in Table 7-1.

Table 7-1   ESHRE/ASRM Diagnostic Criteria for Polycystic Ovarian Syndrome

Two of three of the following:
  1. Oligo-ovulation or anovulation
  2. Clinical and/or biochemical signs of hyperandrogenism
  3. Polycystic ovaries on ultrasonography

and

Exclusion of other etiologies, including congenital adrenal hyperplasia, androgen-secreting tumors, and Cushing's syndrome

Menstrual dysfunction may take any of several forms. Most commonly, menses are irregular since the onset of menarche, with varying frequency; bleeding patterns may include infrequent menses (less than every 35 days) and excessively heavy flow, or frequent bleeding. Both frequent and infrequent menses may signal an anovulatory cycle (2). In some women, menses may be regular after menarche for a year or two, and then become irregular. Other women may be somewhat regular but frequently skip periods. While irregular menses in adolescents are frequently ascribed to the "normal" variation in cycle length before maturation of the hypothalamic-pituitary-ovarian axis, the most common cause of markedly irregular cycles (>90 days in length) is hyperandrogenism/PCOS. PCOS may present with primary amenorrhea. Many women have secondary amenorrhea, with no menses for at least 3 months. It is not unusual for a physician to see women who have not menstruated for more than 1 year.

Hyperandrogenemia refers to elevated serum concentrations of total testosterone and/or free testosterone. Hyperandrogenemia causes clinical hyperandrogenism, which presents as hirsutism, diffuse alopecia, and cystic acne. The clinical response to hyperandrogenemia may vary by race, with Asian women being less likely to exhibit hirsutism than Caucasians or African-Americans. Dehydroepiandrosterone sulfate, often elevated in PCOS, is a weak androgen and probably does not contribute as much as testosterone does to clinical hyperandrogenism.

Pathophysiology

The pathophysiology of PCOS is not completely understood. The etiology is probably multifactorial. Genetic abnormalities are actively being researched. Of the three main etiologic theories, the most widely accepted is that insulin resistance is a central feature (3). Although insulin resistance is a common feature of obesity, studies comparing obese PCOS women with obese non-PCOS women reveal insulin-receptor defects, with a higher prevalence of insulin resistance and impaired glucose tolerance in PCOS women (4). Insulin is a potent growth hormone, and hyperinsulinemia is associated with numerous effects:

- Insulin binds to insulin receptors on ovarian theca cells, causing increased sex hormone production, including testosterone.

- Hyperinsulinemia is associated with endothelial dysfunction.

- Hyperinsulinemia causes the formation of increased free fatty acids and triglycerides.

- Hyperinsulinemia is toxic to pancreatic beta cells, thereby decreasing insulin production and setting the stage for hyperglycemia.

- Hyperinsulinemia causes central obesity. Unfortunately, obesity, in turn, increases insulin resistance, which compounds the problem.

A significant proportion of women with PCOS are slender or of normal body weight. The role of insulin resistance is less clear in non-obese PCOS women, although some studies have shown that thin women are also insulin resistant. More research is in progress.

A second theory postulates that abnormally elevated luteinizing hormone results in hyperandrogenemia and anovulation (5). A third theory posits that the ovary is the source of abnormal steroidogenesis. It has been shown that ovarian theca cells grown in vitro produce increased testosterone, although it is not clear if the ovaries are abnormal or have been affected by the previous metabolic milieu (6).

Almost all experts would agree that elevated serum testosterone (either total or free testosterone), or increased receptor sensitivity to testosterone, results in androgenization. The most obvious manifestations are hirsutism, moderate-to-severe acne, and diffuse alopecia. Hyperandrogenemia interferes with the hypothalamic-pituitary axis and results in anovulation. The absence of a dominant follicle prevents atresia of non-dominant follicles, resulting in the formation of multiple peripheral cysts. Androgens also affect metabolic parameters; for example, testosterone is associated with lowered high-density lipoprotein (HDL) cholesterol concentrations (7).

Diagnosis

The most common etiology of menstrual irregularities is PCOS. Pregnancy should always be ruled out first in women with amenorrhea or a missed cycle. This is especially true in a woman who has had regular menses for years who subsequently develops menstrual irregularities. If she is not pregnant, the differential diagnosis includes hypothyroidism, prolactin-producing pituitary adenoma, late-onset (non-classical) congenital adrenal hyperplasia (CAH), and androgen-secreting tumor (ovarian or adrenal). (The differential is broader than that given here; see Chapters 2 and 3 for further discussion of evaluation.) These diagnoses should be excluded before the diagnosis of PCOS is made.

There are historical clues that may lead to accurate diagnoses. Galactorrhea may signal a prolactin-producing pituitary adenoma or thyroid dysfunction, although mild elevations of prolactin can be seen in conjunction with PCOS. Hypothyroidism may be associated with typical symptoms. The rarest of these, an androgen-secreting tumor, is accompanied by a relatively rapid onset of virilizing symptoms such as hirsutism. A history of precocious puberty and Ashkenazi Jewish or Italian heritage are suggestive of late-onset CAH.

PCOS can mimic and co-exist with late-onset CAH, a variety of adrenal enzyme deficiencies that range from mild to moderate in the steps leading to glucocorticoid production. The most common enzyme deficiency is 21-hydroxylase, which interrupts cortisol production to varying degrees depending on the degree of enzyme impairment. Because adrenal enzyme deficiencies may result in elevated adrenal androgens, the symptoms often mimic those of PCOS (8). Certain ethnic groups have a higher prevalence of late-onset CAH, including Ashkenazi Jews, Greeks, Italians, Latinas, and Slavs.

Conditions that are closely related to PCOS include elevated blood pressure, hypothyroidism, diabetes, and dyslipidemia. PCOS is common enough in women with type 2 diabetes that some experts recommend screening for PCOS in all women with type 2 diabetes. Reproductive conditions include endometrial cancer in middle age secondary to chronic anovulation.

History

The typical history reveals menarche at the average age of 12-13 years. Almost immediately, menses occur at irregular intervals. Often, teenagers will be told that irregular menses are a normal part of development and that they will grow out of it. At this point, girls are often prescribed oral contraceptive pills to initiate regular menses before the establishment of a diagnosis. Oral contraceptives result in lower serum androgen levels, decreased ovarian androgen production, and improvements in menstrual cyclicity, hirsutism, and acne, and in fact form a mainstay of therapy. However, this will often delay diagnosis and does not allow the teen to learn that she has a chronic medical condition with major reproductive and cardiovascular health risks. After a period of some years, these women often discontinue the oral contraceptive, perhaps to conceive, and resume a pattern of irregular menses. It is at this point that they often turn to a gynecologist, perhaps blaming the oral contraceptives for their menstrual irregularity and infertility rather than addressing the underlying condition that led to the requirement for oral contraceptive pills initially. A history of premature adrenarche is associated with PCOS, as is severe peri-pubertal acne, often beginning before menarche.

Women with PCOS generally do not consult internists for infertility. In fact, they may not have even tried to conceive. However, it is possible to elicit a history of infertility by asking patients if they have ever had sexual intercourse without using contraception and were surprised that they did not get pregnant.

Although women will consult a gynecologist about the irregular menses, they may not mention other troublesome symptoms. These symptoms include rapid weight gain, extreme difficulty losing weight, fatigue, hirsutism, acne, and alopecia. Patients often note that they have central obesity. Central obesity is associated with increased risk of developing diabetes. It has been postulated that eating disorders, especially bulimia, are more common in PCOS, but no clinical trials have addressed this issue.

Hair and skin changes are often noted. Women complain of hirsutism in the following areas: chin, cheek/sideburns, neck, chest and between breasts, in the periareolar area, on the upper arms and from the umbilicus to the pubic triangle. Women should be questioned about hair removal using depilatories, shaving, waxing, bleaching, laser, or electrolysis; body hair in women is culturally unacceptable in many western countries, and women go to considerable efforts to hide it. One of the most distressing symptoms reported by patients is diffuse (or androgenic) alopecia, not to be confused with patchy alopecia. Acne can be mild to severe and may occur in areas more commonly associated with men, including the upper arms, upper back and buttocks.

There is often a history of family members with irregular periods, severe acne, excess hair growth, infertility in a female relative, or few children. Type 2 diabetes is often present in parents, aunts, and uncles. PCOS is felt to be autosomal dominant in inheritance, but with variable manifestations. A family history of premature balding may be elicited in male family members.

Physical Examination

After the history, the next most important component in the diagnosis of PCOS is the physical examination.

Vital Signs

It is not unusual to find elevated blood pressure, with systolic pressure as high as 130-135 mmHg and diastolic pressure in the high 80s mmHg to low 90s mmHg range, even in young women. Most women with PCOS are obese, and in particular, have central obesity consisting of fat deposition in the abdomen, upper arms, and upper back. BMI should be determined, although up to one-third of women with PCOS are *not* obese.

Hair and Skin

Hirsutism may or may not be present on the chin, neck, cheeks, chest, peri-areolar area, upper arms, back, or abdomen. Even if there are only a few terminal hairs on the chest, between the breasts, or on the lower abdomen, hair in these areas are indicative of elevated serum androgens. Quantification of hirsutism can be done using the Ferriman-Gallway score, although this is more useful as a research than as a clinical tool (9). Hirsutism may also be relative to other family members. Women of some ethnic groups, e.g., Asians, may not display any hirsutism in the setting of hyperandrogenemia. A history of relatively rapid onset of hirsutism accompanied by severe hirsutism on the trunk is suspicious for an androgen-secreting tumor. Acne may be non-existent, mild, or severe, and may be present on the face, neck, upper arms, upper chest, back, or buttocks. Diffuse alopecia, as opposed to patchy alopecia, is not rare, and is usually mentioned by the patient if present. What may appear as a normal head of thick hair to the practitioner may not be normal to the patient.

Signs of hyperinsulinemia include acanthosis nigricans, which are hypertrophied skin in areas that crease, such as the posterior neck, axillae, elbows, under the breasts, between abdominal fat folds or in the groin. It is important to remember that hypertrophic skin does not necessarily have to be deeply hyperpigmented; the deepness of the color is dependent on the degree of pigmentation in the patient. Typical textbooks show severe acanthosis nigricans in persons with dark skin. However, those with less pigmented skin may have more subtle findings (Figures 7-1 and 7-2). Hyperinsulinemia is associated

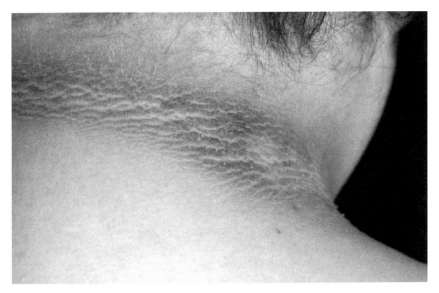

Figure 7-1   Deeply pigmented acanthosis nigricans.

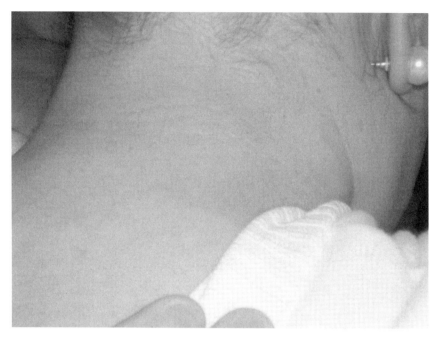

Figure 7-2   Subtle acanthosis nigricans.

with skin tags as well as acanthosis nigricans. Skin tags are commonly found around the neck, upper chest, and axillae.

Extensive abdominal striations, a buffalo hump, facial plethora and very thin limbs in contrast to abdominal obesity should prompt a work up for Cushing's disease.

Late-onset CAH may result in more severe signs of hyperandrogenism, including not only hirsutism but also signs of virilization such as disproportionately small, underdeveloped breasts; clitoromegaly; and underdeveloped labia due to early exposure to elevated androgens in precocious puberty. However, these physical findings are not unusual in PCOS.

Pelvic Exam
Inspection of the external genitalia should be completed with specific attention to the clitoris, looking for signs of enlargement that would raise suspicion of an androgen-secreting tumor. Clitoromegaly, although multiple definitions exist, is defined as a clitoral diameter greater than 1 cm or a clitoral index (width × length of clitoris) greater than 35 mm^2.

It is critical to remember that not all women with PCOS have all of the above symptoms. The phenotypic presentations are variable because the etiology is probably multifactorial. For example, some women may not have the testosterone receptors in skin that cause hirsutism, especially Asian women. Other women may have a normal BMI of less than 25 and still have PCOS. Many women do not have acne or alopecia. A very small minority will have regular menses (which may be anovulatory) but have most of the other features of hyperandrogenism and polycystic ovaries. The absence of all classically described symptoms should not automatically exclude PCOS.

Laboratory Values

Laboratory testing in the evaluation of a patient with a clinical picture suspicious for PCOS involves obtaining tests to support the diagnosis as well as those that rule out other serious causes of symptoms. The most useful lab test in the work-up of PCOS is a total testosterone; measurement of a calculated free testosterone may be an even more sensitive measure, especially in adolescents. An ultrasensitive TSH, a prolactin level, and a 17-alpha-hydroxyprogesterone level should also be obtained to rule out other etiologies. In women with symptoms suggestive of Cushing's syndrome, a 24-hour urinary cortisol level should be obtained.

It is important to note that blood values obtained while a patient is on the oral contraceptive pill (OCP) are not useful when attempting to diagnose PCOS. Pharmacologic doses of estrogen, such as are present in OCPs, decrease total and free testosterone, and elevate SHBG, HDL cholesterol, and triglycerides. Luteinizing hormone (LH) and follicle-stimulating hormone (FSH) are suppressed with OCPs. In order to obtain true hormonal measurements, patients should be off the OCP for a minimum of 4-6 weeks. The desirability of such testing to confirm a diagnosis should be weighed against the significant contraceptive and noncontraceptive benefits of OCPs in managing PCOS.

Although LH and FSH levels are usually drawn on day 3 of the menstrual cycle for an infertility evaluation, it is not necessary to do so when evaluating for PCOS. The only exception to the need to assess timing FSH and LH values occurs when a level reveals an elevated LH, which is not only a hallmark of PCOS, but also normally present immediately prior to ovulation. This can be ruled out by determining whether a menstrual period followed the day of phlebotomy by approximately 14 days. An LH and FSH may show a greater than 2-3 to 1 ratio and help confirm the diagnosis. However, the absence of this ratio does not rule out PCOS.

A total testosterone above 50 ng/dL is considered elevated (7). Most labs in the United States list a reference range between 14 and 70 ng/dL as "normal," but it is important to remember that reference ranges refer to the mean ±2 standard deviations, not to "normal" or optimal. It is unknown what an "optimal" range of serum testosterone is, but most women with a level above 50 ng/dL will have irregular menses and clinical hyperandrogenism. Free (unbound) testosterone is also usually elevated. Often in teens, only the free testosterone is elevated, and this may be true in adults (7). Because women with chronic anovulation are at higher risk of endometrial hyperplasia and endometrial carcinoma, one must consider evaluation of the endometrium in patients who fail to respond to therapy, have a history of prolonged anovulation, or are older than 35 years. For women with excessive or frequent bleeding, consideration needs to be given to other causes of bleeding.

Once a diagnosis of PCOS is made, testing should be done to assess for underlying insulin resistance and diabetes. There are many approaches to the evaluation and little evidence to support one over the other. Many investigators will diagnose impaired glucose tolerance resulting from insulin resistance using the 2-hour oral glucose tolerance test. Insulin is often tested but requires a frozen specimen for the assay to be done correctly, and insulin values often return falsely low in the office setting. The reference range for insulin is usually designated as between 5 and 25 or 30 IU; however, most experts agree that an insulin greater than 10 IU is consistent with insulin resistance. Other investigators consider the clinical utility of measuring a fasting glucose and insulin ratio to be the desired screening test; a ratio of glucose to insulin less than 4.5 IU is considered abnormal, indicating developing insulin resistance. A normal fasting glucose can also be used to rule out diabetes. This is particularly helpful in young women who are less likely to exhibit impaired glucose tolerance than are older women.

A fasting lipid profile is useful for assessing cardiovascular risk, and the typical pattern is elevated triglycerides and low HDL cholesterol. Other useful tests include sex-hormone–binding globulin, which is low in hyperandrogenemic and hyperinsulinemic states, as well as in obesity (10).

Other tests to help rule out PCOS include

- *Dehydroepiandrosterone sulfate*—DHEA-S is often elevated above 200-300 ng/dL in PCOS. However, levels above 700 ng/dL should prompt a search for an androgen-secreting tumor. Dehydroepiandrosterone (DHEA) should not be ordered because it is widely variable and unhelpful. DHEA-S measurement is useful if a patient presents with sudden onset of virilizing symptoms.

- *17-α-hydroxyprogesterone*, if elevated in an 8 a.m. measurement, may indicate late-onset CAH. However, if there is a high suspicion of CAH, a provocative test should be performed. After a baseline measurement of 17-α-hydroxyprogesterone, Cortrosyn (250 μg) is given intravenously or intramuscularly. Samples at 15, 30, and 60 minutes are drawn. If the 17-α-hydroxyprogesterone increases four-fold, the test is diagnostic of 21-hydroxylase deficiency and the patient should be referred to an endocrinologist.

- *Cortisol* should be measured in a patient with Cushingoid features. One method to measure cortisol is a 24-hour urine collection; if the cortisol is elevated, the patient should be referred to an endocrinologist. An alternative screening test is the overnight dexamethasone suppression test: 1 mg of dexamethasone is given at 11 p.m., and an 8 a.m. serum cortisol is measured. See Chapter 3 for discussion of laboratory values.

Transvaginal Sonography

Many clinicians, especially in Europe, consider transvaginal sonography (TVS) essential to diagnosis of PCOS. TVS may be necessary for infertility evaluation and management. However, if a patient does not wish to conceive, and if she has a classic history and signs of PCOS, a TVS without evidence of polycystic ovaries probably would not change management. The classic PCOS finding on TVS is a "string of pearls," which describes typical cysts that are peripheral, multiple, and less than 10 mm in diameter. There is a large body of literature in reproductive endocrinology that attempts to classify PCOS according to ovarian morphology.

Treatment

The most important strategy to address all symptoms of PCOS is to increase physical activity and to decrease calories. The role of proper nutrition and adequate physical activity cannot be overemphasized. Patients need to be encouraged to exercise, and it may help to prescribe specific activities. Patients may also benefit from education (including patient literature) on healthy diets, with emphasis on fruits and vegetables and chicken and fish, and eating fewer processed foods. Referral to a nutrition counselor may be helpful.

Treatment beyond lifestyle changes must be guided by the patient's goals and desire for fertility or need for contraception. In addition, comorbidities such as commonly associated hypertension, diabetes, dyslipidemia, and obesity must be addressed.

Combined Hormonal Contraception

Traditional treatment has focused on restoring regular menses with OCPs, which contain supraphysiologic doses of estrogens. In addition to causing monthly menstrual cycles, OCPs increase SHBG production by the liver, which binds free (unbound) testosterone. Acne may improve dramatically, and hirsutism and alopecia often decrease. However, OCPs may not cause sufficient improvement in metabolic parameters and may increase insulin resistance in some cases (11). One approach to treatment involves the use of OCPs for initial therapy coupled with lifestyle changes: weight loss and increased exercise. If insulin resistance persists or worsens with this regimen, other therapy, often in the form of metformin, can be added to or substituted for OCPs.

Metformin

Although some patients do exercise and eat well, many still have such a high degree of insulin resistance that they are unable to lose weight or ovulate. At this point, the addition of metformin may help to surmount the obstacle created by hyperinsulinemia by decreasing insulin resistance. There are no guidelines on dosage and duration, but most clinicians aim for metformin 1000 mg twice a day. This dose is similar to that of treatment of type 2 diabetes. There are currently few studies reporting the use of metformin, or its long-term effects, in adolescents with PCOS, although they are currently being prescribed for this population based on the theoretical benefits of lowering long-term cardiovascular risk. Compliance is an issue, and careful ongoing discussions of potential side effects coupled with very gradual increases in dosage are required.

Metformin is a relatively safe medication that is available in several doses and formulations. Because metformin is commonly associated with gastrointestinal effects such as nausea, bloating, and diarrhea, it is prudent to titrate up slowly. Metformin is contraindicated in renal insufficiency and the elderly, and it should be used with caution in those with liver disease or significant alcohol use. Baseline creatinine should be obtained to rule out renal disease. Lactic acidosis is a severe but rare complication that is usually seen in those with renal failure. Metformin should be started at the lowest dose (500 mg) and titrated up slowly. It should be taken once a day after the evening meal.

- *Immediate-release* metformin (Glucophage) is given three times a day after meals.

- *Extended-release metformin* (Glucophage XR) is given once or twice daily after meals.

- *Long-acting metformin* (Fortamet) is given once daily after dinner.

The dose is usually titrated by doubling the starting dose after 1-2 weeks, given that the patient does not have adverse effects that warrant discontinuation of the medication. The maximum dose is 2500 mg daily, although most clinicians titrate up to 2000 mg per day. In studies of type 2 diabetics, 2000 mg has been established as the optimal dose (12). As long as the baseline creatinine is normal, and the patient is not on other medications that affect renal function, there is no need to recheck the serum creatinine.

Ovulation and spontaneous menses usually occur by 3 months, especially in combination with improved diet and exercise. There are hundreds of case reports of patients conceiving while on metformin, and no fetal abnormalities have been reported. Some obstetricians advocate the use of metformin during the first trimester to prevent miscarriage, and a few are comfortable using metformin during the entire pregnancy. Metformin should not be used during breastfeeding. Caution should be used in prescribing metformin as sole therapy for PCOS in adolescents and young adults because of the increase in fertility. Metformin causes previously anovulatory women to ovulate, thus leading to an increased risk of unintended pregnancy if alternative contraception is not used. Adolescents may find it difficult to divulge or admit their sexual activity to clinicians, and typically do not seek medical contraception until many months after first initiating intercourse. The high risk of pregnancy also must be emphasized in post-adolescent women starting metformin. Often, they are unconcerned about pregnancy because they have been infertile for so long that they may not believe they could conceive. Sometimes conception occurs before the onset of the first spontaneous menses.

A meta-analysis of the use of metformin in PCOS concludes that metformin is effective for inducing ovulation and increasing pregnancy rates (13). Metformin was shown to decrease androgens, decrease blood pressure, and LDL cholesterol. There was no evidence supporting a weight-loss effect, or improvement in hirsutism, alopecia, or acne.

Metformin frequently causes gastrointestinal side effects such as bloating, loose stools/diarrhea, and nausea. Many patients report that if they eat refined carbohydrates with metformin, they develop diarrhea.

Hirsutism and Alopecia

In addition to OCPs, androgen-receptor antagonists, such as spironolactone, may be effective in diminishing hirsutism and alopecia (14). In the past, spironolactone has been believed to be of little value, but the doses used then were 25-50 mg a day. More recently, doses as high as 100 mg once or twice a day have been effectively utilized. Higher-dose spironolactone diminishes hirsutism both in the frequency of new terminal hair growth, and in the return of hair that has been removed. A recent systematic review of the literature concluded that a 6-month treatment with 100 mg spironolactone compared with placebo was associated with a statistically significant subjective improvement in hair growth (16). Diffuse alopecia may respond dramatically to 100 mg spironolactone once or twice a day. Other antiandrogens include flutamide (250 mg twice a day) and finasteride (5 mg daily); both drugs require monitoring with liver function tests. *All antiandrogens are contraindicated in pregnancy*. Eflornithine is a topical hair growth retardant that is applied twice a day to hirsute areas. Response rates, indicating diminished but not absent growth, are around 30%.

Acne

Acne improves with reduction of serum testosterone, and subsequent reduction of sebum production. Thus oral contraceptives are effective in managing mild-to-moderate acne by virtue of their effect on minimizing androgen production as well as decreasing free testosterone by increasing SHGB; there are no data to suggest that any one OCP formulation is more effective than another in this effect. Cystic acne should be referred to dermatologists for possible accutane use, although oral contraceptives are indicated during accutane use because of its teratogenicity. The combination of oral and topical antibiotics will improve acne, especially in conjunction with the reduction of serum androgens.

Ovulation and Infertility

Ovulation may be restored with the use of medications in patients with PCOS. With the discovery that insulin plays an important role in PCOS, and that the ovaries contain receptors that respond to insulin to upregulate production of androgens, clinicians began experimenting with insulin-sensitizing medications in the mid-90s. A large body of data supports the use of metformin in restoring ovulation, as mentioned earlier in this chapter, presumably by decreasing testosterone production indirectly by lowering serum insulin. Other insulin sensitizers used include pioglitazone and rosiglitazone; troglitazone was used before it was removed from the market. One systematic review concludes that metformin is significantly more effective than placebo in restoring ovulation (14). If a woman has not had spontaneous or induced menses for the last 3 months, a menstrual bleed should be induced with either medroxyprogesterone acetate (5-10 mg daily for 5-10 days), or oral micronized progesterone (400 mg before bed for 10 days). If she does not have an induced bleed, she may have endometrial atrophy, which could be treated by use of an OCP (containing at least 30 mcg ethinyl estradiol) for 2 months.

The recent explosion of research on the association of PCOS and insulin resistance has added a welcome new dimension in the treatment of PCOS-associated infertility, allowing for more treatment options for patients (15). As already discussed, PCOS causes anovulation or oligo-ovulation by interfering with normal follicle growth. Anovulation undoubtedly reduces fertility by reducing the number of ovulatory cycles per year in women. Cycles that happen to be ovulatory are probably more likely to be suboptimal for fertility. It is now well known that most women with PCOS, if not the vast majority, are insulin resistant, and many are obese. Thus, insulin-sensitizing agents and lifestyle modifications have been studied as treatment options for infertile patients with PCOS and have yielded acceptable results.

In the past, treatment options for PCOS-associated infertility were limited to oral or injectable ovulation-inducing medications. Clomiphene, an oral agent, has been used as first-line therapy, and injectable gonadotropins (FSH/LH or FSH alone) were used in failure to ovulate with clomiphene

Ovulation induction may be treated conservatively with the lifestyle alterations of diet modification and exercise. Realistically, this is successful in only a small number of patients, and cannot be offered to patients with PCOS of normal weight. It requires strict adherence to a program that may be difficult to complete, and may take too long for patients interested in conception immediately. Insulin sensitizers have become an excellent option for the conservative treatment of PCOS-associated infertility. Those studied have included metformin, troglitazone (which has since been removed from the market), and D-chiro-inositol (a complex carbohydrate that has not cleared phase 2 trials). Of these, metformin has been the most thoroughly studied. Metformin may be used alone as monotherapy and has been shown to allow for regular ovulation to occur. One of its advantages is its induction of monofollicular ovulation, as opposed to exogenous fertility drugs that have side effects of multiple births and ovarian hyperstimulation. The monitoring costs (ultrasound, serum hormonal assays) associated with these medications can also be avoided. Metformin does not induce cervical mucus abnormalities. Some patients experience some weight loss with metformin, an advantage prior to their pregnancy.

Diet and exercise plans may be used along with metformin to enhance the response and take advantage of its initial effect. Results have been very encouraging. Ovulation rates of 77% to 82% have been reported when doses ranging from 1500-1700 mg per day were given over 3-4 months. Pregnancy rates on metformin alone have not been reported in multiple studies. However, it may be reasonable to consider that these strong rates of ovulation could result in respectable pregnancy rates. Metformin monotherapy as a first-line treatment may be used in younger reproductive-aged patients, for those who prefer to reduce their costs or risk of multiple gestations with fertility medications, and for obese patients who prefer to lose weight before conceiving. If regular ovulation does not occur in 6-8 weeks, clomiphene treatment may be added. Preliminary studies have reported a lower risk of first-trimester miscarriage and gestational diabetes with metformin use, but further research is needed to confirm these findings.

Patients taking clomiphene and metformin alone for ovulation induction may not ovulate while on their respective medications. Metformin, given to clomiphene-resistant women as an adjunct in a multicenter study, appears to have utility as an adjunctive medication by increasing clomiphene's ovulation and pregnancy rates. There has been one report of metformin versus placebo pre-treatment of clomiphene-resistant patients undergoing injectable FSH treatment (16). A tendency to reduce the risk of ovarian hyperstimulation (and perhaps multiple gestations) was noted. Metformin may have promise as an adjunctive treatment for in vitro fertilization in women with PCOS. One study has reported that low-dose metformin treatment increases oocyte maturity and fertilization rates, and enhances embryo numbers.

Summary

Polycystic ovary syndrome, a leading cause of menstrual irregularities and infertility, is also associated with obesity, hirsutism, and cardiovascular risk factors such as elevated blood pressure, dyslipidemia, and impaired glucose tolerance. Diagnosis is based on history of menstrual dysfunction and evidence of hyperandrogenemia. Insulin resistance appears to play a central role in the pathophysiology. Treatment consists of physical activity, proper nutrition, and weight loss. OCPs induce monthly menstrual cycles and improve acne and hirsutism. Insulin sensitizers, such as metformin, induce ovulation and improve some metabolic parameters. Insulin sensitizers play an important role in PCOS-associated infertility. Additional treatment options for infertility are tailored to the patient's individual needs and may include ovulation-inducing medications in combination with insulin sensitizers.

REFERENCES

1. Rotterdam ESHRE/ASRM-Sponsored PCOS Consensus Working Group. Revised 2003 consensus on diagnostic criteria and long-term health risks related to polycystic ovary syndrome. Fertil Steril. 2004;81:19-25.

2. Balen A, Michelmore K. What is polycystic ovary syndrome? Hum Repro. 2002;17:2219-27.

3. Dunaif A. Insulin resistance and the polycystic ovary syndrome: mechanism and implications for pathogenesis. Endocr Rev. 1997;18:774-800.

4. Dunaif A, Segal KR, Futterweit W, Dobrjansky A. Profound peripheral insulin resistance, independent of obesity, in polycystic ovary syndrome. Diabetes. 1989;38:1165-74.

5. Rebar R, Judd HL, Yen SS, et al. Characterization of the inappropriate gonadotropin secretion in polycystic ovarian syndrome. J Clin Invest. 1976;57:1320-9.

6. Nelson VL, Legro RS, Strauss JF, McAllister JM. Augmented androgen production is a stable steroidogenic phenotype of propagated theca cells from polycystic ovaries. Mol Endocrinol. 1999;13:946-57.

7. Luthold WW, Borges MF, Marcondes JA, et al. Serum testosterone fractions in women: normal and abnormal clinical states. Metab Clin Exper. 1993;42:638-43.

8. Deaton MA, Glorioso JE, McLean DB. Congenital adrenal hyperplasia: not really a zebra. Amer Fam Physician. 1999;59:1190-6.

9. Ferriman D, Gallwey JD. Clinical measurement of body hair growth in women. J Clin Endocrinol Metab. 1961;21:1440.

10. Sherif K, Kushner H, Falkner BE. Sex hormone-binding globulin and insulin resistance in African-American women. Metab Clin Experim. 1998;47:70-4.

11. Sherif K. Benefits and risks of oral contraceptives. Am J Obstet Gynecol. 1999;180: S343-8.

12. Garber AJ, Duncan TJ, Goodman AM, et al. Efficacy of metformin in type 2 diabetes: results of a double-blind, placebo-controlled, dose-response trial. Am J Med. 1997; 103:491-7.

13. Lord JM, Flight IHK, Norman RJ. Metformin in polycystic ovary syndrome: systematic review and meta-analysis. BMJ. 2003;327:951.

14. Farquhar C, Lee O, Toomath R, Jepson R. Spironolactone versus placebo or in combination with steroids for hirsutism and/or acne. Cochrane Database of Systematic Reviews. 2001;4:CD000194.

15. Hull MGR. Epidemiology of infertility and polycystic ovarian disease: endocrinological and demographic studies. Gynecol Endocrinol. 1987;1:233-45.

16. George SS, George K, Irwin C, et al. Sequential treatment of metformin and clomiphene citrate in clomiphene-resistant women with polycystic ovary syndrome: a randomized, controlled trial Human Repro. 2003;18:299-304.

8

Menstrual Issues in Women with Developmental Disabilities

Elisabeth H. Quint, MD

Menstrual issues, sexuality, and contraception in women with developmental disabilities are often challenging management dilemmas for patients, parents and caregivers, and care providers. The onset of the menstrual cycle means significant change in the life of the patient, but also in the lives of the parents, school, and other caregivers. For some patients, the onset of menstruation is an easy transition, while for others it can be a trying time. The menstrual issues of the patient with developmental disabilities should in general be approached in the same manner as in the general population and be regarded as a normal and healthy process.

Epidemiology

There are not many data on the epidemiology of menstrual cycles in women with developmental disabilities. Some studies have looked at the age of menarche in women with developmental delay, but the results are mixed, with some studies finding earlier and some later menarche than in the general population (1-3). A more recent study measured follicle-stimulating hormone (FSH) and luteinizing hormone (LH) responses to gonadotropin-releasing hormone (GnRH) stimulation in teenagers with and without developmental disabilities and found an impaired response of the FSH-secreting pituitary cells in initial pubertal stages. This difference disappeared during further sexual development (4). There is some evidence that the ovarian sensitivity to FSH is blunted in patients with Down's syndrome, possibly due to lower growth hormone concentrations in these patients (5). Looking at cycle regularity, one study found that in women with Down's syndrome with regular cycles, ovulatory events were less frequent and often characterized by luteal phase defects (6). But that was not found in an older study that just examined basal body temperature charts (7). Overall, there are no data to suggest that the cycles of women with developmental disabilities are different; however, there are more women in this group with other factors that may contribute to menstrual irregularities. These factors include the use of certain medications, the prevalence of thyroid disease, and weight issues.

Women with epilepsy have an increased incidence of reproductive endocrine disorders (8). The anticonvulsants (except valproic acid) increase the activity of the cytochrome P450 hepatic microsomal oxidative enzymes. This results in more rapid clearance of steroid hormones. Neuroleptics and metoclopramide can cause hyperprolactinemia, which leads to irregular bleeding and occasionally a hypoestrogenic state, which then leads to amenorrhea. Women with Down's syndrome have a higher incidence of thyroid disease, which can disturb the normal menstrual cycle (9,10). Low food intake or swallowing problems with placement of gastric tubes is seen frequently in the mentally disabled, often leading to low weight and hypothalamic amenorrhea, leading to oligomenorrhea or amenorrhea.

Reproductive Health Evaluation

Menarche and Health History

Menarche is a time of transition and often will bring the patient and her parents to the care provider with requests to eliminate or "fix" the periods. It is very important to understand the reasoning as to why treatment is requested for each individual patient. This can include issues about the heaviness, irregularity, or discomfort of the cycle; menstrual hygiene issues; fear of pregnancy; or a feeling from the parents that the inconvenience of cycles is too much to handle. The first 2 years after menarche are often anovulatory and can cause erratic cycles (11,12). Education about the amount of irregular cycling that is normal in teenagers and how it changes over time can be very helpful to the family. Menstrual hygiene should be discussed and instruction given on the use of sanitary napkins and other suggestions for care. All caregivers and sometimes the school become involved in helping the patient manage her cycles. Experience has taught that most patients who can manage their own toileting should be able to understand the principles of menstrual hygiene.

The extent to which a medical history is available varies greatly. This depends on the level of handicap of the patient as well as the knowledge of the caregivers. If a patient can voice her own complaints or concerns, it is important for the clinician to use basic language when speaking with the patient. If the client comes with a parent or guardian, a full past medical history ought to be available. Sometimes the patient will come without any information on the cycles, and it is therefore recommended that a letter be sent to the group home before the visit addressing the importance of having this information and on the need for menstrual calendars. The importance of having an appropriate caregiver accompany the patient should also be stressed.

Sexuality needs to be discussed at every visit; patients with disabilities are often viewed as asexual and therefore frequently have limited access to appropriate services and counseling. The ability to reproduce is not necessarily affected by a mental or physical disability, so reproductive concerns must be addressed, including assessing the patient's risk for abuse as well as her ability to have a consensual sexual relationship (13,14).

Gynecological Examination

Several general principles apply to the gynecological examination of the woman with mental disabilities, and the exam may be complicated by several factors (Table 8-1). Exams may have been forceful in the past or there could be a history of abuse, which increases the patient's level of anxiety (15-17). Verbal relaxation techniques may not be as successful in this population. Patients often have multiple physical handicaps, complicating positioning and access to the vagina and abdomen; as many as 45% to 55% of patients with mental retardation have neurological abnormalities, and 21% have orthopedic problems (18). To clearly identify the caregivers and to distinguish medical care from inappropriate sexual touching, a white coat is recommended. The patient may benefit from the presence of a trusted caregiver or family member. Multiple visits are sometimes needed before the patient is comfortable and will allow an exam. The patient should be allowed to participate as much as

Table 8-1   Pelvic Examinations in Women with Developmental Disabilities

Complicating Factors
- Extreme anxiety secondary to multiple physician encounters
- Possible history of sexual abuse (10%-30%, average teens)
- Multiple physical handicaps (neurologic, 45%-55%; orthopedic, 21%)

Recommendations
- Explain the examination and allow practice (e.g., gowns) before the exam
- Wear a white coat to clearly identify self as a caregiver
- Avoid use of stirrups
- Never use force or restrain patient, only support legs gently
- Do a pelvic exam only if clearly indicated
- Try different positions

possible in the exam (for example, by touching instruments). A slow and sensitive approach will lead to a good experience for the patient. Perform a pelvic exam only if it is clearly going to benefit the patient and will add to the information gained through the medical history and the general physical examination. If an exam is indicated, the approach needs to be individualized.

The patient will often allow inspection of the external genitalia. Look for moles, hygiene, bruises, or tearing. If there are concerns about adequate hygiene, these issues should be discussed with the caregiver in a non-threatening fashion. Patients may be reluctant to allow help with hygiene or changing clothing. Bruising may be an indication of falls, self-mutilation, or abuse. Ask the caregiver for an explanation of any bruising, and assess the safety of the client. Positioning the legs for a gynecological evaluation may be quite difficult if there are physical handicaps. Stirrups may be threatening and in general are not used, as with a young child.

Options for positioning include

- Frog-leg position, with heels together in the midline and knees bent out to the sides

- V-position, with both legs extended and slightly opened

- Lying on the side with the legs bent but not separated

- Legs elevated with knees slightly bent or straight, without abduction of the hips; this position often works well because spreading the legs may evoke a strong reaction

Performing the exam in these positions may be somewhat more difficult or challenging but is likely to be more successful than the traditional lithotomy position using stirrups (19). The use of a speculum may cause a strong negative reaction. If it is important to inspect the cervix or to obtain a Pap smear, a regular length narrow Huffman speculum should be used rather than the shorter, "pediatric" speculum, which will be too short to allow cervix visualization in adolescents and adult women. If it appears that a speculum exam is not possible and a Pap smear is indicated, use the finger-directed blind Pap smear technique. One finger is placed in the vagina and the cervix is located. A moistened cotton-tipped swab or plastic brush with soft end (if using liquid-based cytology) is slid inside the vagina over the finger and placed inside the cervix. Although the results may be suboptimal, it may be the only option that can be performed without anesthesia (20). A bimanual examination may also be difficult, due to lack of cooperation and difficulty in positioning; however, the patient may allow a single-finger bimanual exam more readily than the traditional "two-finger" approach.

Patients may also have difficulty relaxing the abdominal muscles, making it difficult to feel the uterus and ovaries. Verbal guidance, the encouragement of slow deep breathing, and asking the patient to keep her head on the table will often be helpful. If a vaginal exam is not tolerated due to a tight hymen or discomfort, a recto-abdominal exam can often be performed. If bowel elimination is a problem for the patient, an extremely distended rectum may make even this exam impossible or suboptimal; a laxative or enema prior to an exam at a later date can be helpful. If the patient is clearly unable to tolerate the exam, as expressed by either verbal or non-verbal communication, her wishes should be respected. The initiation of Pap smear screening in this population should be in accordance with American Cancer Society guidelines: Pap smear at age 21 if there has been no sexual activity or within 3 years of the start of sexual activity (21).

An exam with sedation can be helpful and has been advocated by some; however, this approach has not been evaluated in a systematic fashion (22). Moreover, there are some concerns about the ethics of this approach (23). Review of data from a ketamine sedation program revealed that 14% of a study population of women with mental disabilities underwent sedation. Of these women, 25% still could not be examined (20). One of the main side effects from ketamine sedation was nausea and vomiting, which could potentially lead to aspiration in this vulnerable population. There are no data on the emotional side effects of a pelvic exam in a sedated state. Therefore the use of a sedated pelvic exam for the sole indication of routine care is probably not indicated. If a patient needs a Pap smear because of a previous abnormal result or a high-risk situation, the individual practitioner can consider the option of sedation with oral agents versus an examination under anesthesia in consultation with the patient's primary care provider.

When another procedure requires a general anesthetic (for example, a dental procedure or magnetic resonance imaging), a gynecologic exam, including a Pap smear and bimanual exam, can be performed at the same time.

Abnormal Uterine Bleeding

Diagnosis

Irregular anovulatory bleeding during the first 2 post-menarchal years is very common and needs often no further testing (12). If there is excessive bleeding, a thorough work-up is indicated, including a search for bleeding disorders.

The initial approach to abnormal uterine bleeding focuses on the documentation of the problem, including a menstrual calendar to document the regularity and heaviness of the cycles. In women with developmental disabilities, the question may become whether the bleeding is primarily a problem of menstrual hygiene or whether there is truly a medical abnormality; anemia as documented with a complete blood count will suggest the need for further evaluation. The criteria for evaluating abnormal bleeding in a woman with developmental disabilities are similar to the criteria that one would use to initiate an evaluation in a patient without disabilities. If laboratory values are needed, all labs should be ordered at the same time in a patient in whom a needlestick is difficult. Because the physical exam is often suboptimal, an ultrasound may be useful. If endometrial biopsy or dilatation and curettage are indicated, an anesthetic may be required. Because of the risks of general anesthesia, the indications for the procedure need to be well documented and compelling.

Menstrual calendars and documentation of abnormal bleeding will help to ensure that treatment is initiated for solid medical reasons and not for the convenience of caregivers. Later the calendars will help to assess the effectiveness of treatment because patient ability to communicate may be limited.

Treatment

In general, the treatment of bleeding abnormalities in women with developmental disabilities should be similar to that in the general population. If there is a clear medical indication for treatment, such as endometrial hyperplasia or anemia, or if the cycles truly interfere with the patient's daily life and are limiting participation in usual activities, treatment should be offered. Before prescribing hormonal therapies, it is important to realize that life-long treatment may be required. The long-term effects of continuous use of hormones for 30-40 years are not well-established.

For patients in whom nonsteroidal anti-inflammatory drugs (NSAIDs) are considered for the treatment of dysmenorrhea and menorrhagia, dosing intervals should be scheduled during the entire menstrual flow period rather than treatment on an "as needed" basis because the patient's ability to communicate her needs for pain medication or the heaviness of flow may be limited. If low-dose oral contraceptives are considered, a daily reminder may be needed for the patient who lives independently with some supervision.

If a patient cannot tolerate her cycles, has behavior clearly documented to occur only at the time of her periods, and has cycles that limit her daily activities, complete cessation of the cycles may be desired. This can be achieved either by continuous combined oral contraceptives, continuous oral progesterones, or depot medroxyprogesterone acetate (DMPA). The dosing for the DMPA is usually 150-250 mg every 9-12 weeks, with 50% amenorrhea reported after one year (24). Occasionally a regimen of monthly injections for 3 months, then with longer intervals, has been used. For patients using DMPA, concerns include weight gain, which can be up to 5-10 lb per year on a cumulative basis, and bone loss, especially in long-term users (25,26).

Although some data suggest that bone loss may be reversible after cessation of treatment, for women who already have limited activity due to wheelchair use or difficulty ambulating, bone loss can be an important issue. In addition, continuous ongoing therapy is often desired for menstrual management in this patient population if the periods are impossible to handle by the patient, thus obviating the theoretical reversal of osteopenia. Adequate calcium and vitamin D intake is thus important. Significant weight gain may severely affect the life of women who are dependent on others for their transfers in and out of wheelchairs. The levonorgestrel intrauterine system (Mirena) may become an alternative treatment for women with heavy cycles, although it has not been studied in this patient population.

Surgical alternatives include endometrial ablation; however, this does not always cause amenorrhea and may therefore be less desirable (27). Hysterectomy is only indicated for medical reasons, because abdominal surgery in women with mental disabilities has been associated with significant morbidity (28). In some countries vaginal hysterectomy for menstrual hygiene has been used, but this is not felt to be appropriate in the United States (29). A multidisciplinary approach is needed, with the inclusion of members of the healthcare team, the patient, the parents, and sometimes the school, workplace, or other caregivers, to find the solution that is in the best interest of the individual patient.

Amenorrhea

Diagnosis

Primary amenorrhea is fairly unusual in this population and is usually genetic or caused by structural abnormalities. Secondary amenorrhea has a long differential diagnosis and includes anovulation, hyperprolactinemia, premature ovarian failure, or hypothalamic amenorrhea. In women with developmental disabilities, some special circumstances may contribute to secondary amenorrhea. A review of medication use may reveal the use of neuroleptics or metoclopramide, leading to hyperprolactinemia, subsequent hypoestrogenemia, and amenorrhea. Weight fluctuations can lead to cessation of cycles. Patients with epilepsy may be more likely to have polycystic ovarian syndrome; the use of valproate has been suggested as a contributing factor. A detailed history, physical exam, including pelvic ultrasound in the case of primary amenorrhea, to assess the anatomy, and a basic laboratory evaluation, including thyroid-stimulating hormone (TSH), prolactin, FSH, and estradiol, will quickly lead to a diagnosis. If the prolactin level is significantly elevated, brain imaging should be considered. Although computed tomography or magnetic resonance imaging is recommended, many disabled women cannot tolerate these exams without anesthesia, and only a coned-down view of the sella can be obtained. This will rule out large space-occupying lesions in the brain.

Treatment

If a new large brain lesion has been ruled out, the treatment considerations are mostly dictated by the low estrogen levels and the prevention of osteoporosis (30). The decision to start estrogen replacement therapy requires careful consideration with input from the patient, caregivers and, if indicated, a guardian. An important consideration is the length of time the woman has been without menstrual cycles or estrogen. Breast tenderness and the reintroduction of any vaginal bleeding by hormonal therapy can be traumatic to the patient. If estrogen is indicated, a very low dose of conjugated estrogens may be started and gradually increased to a full dose; this should be combined with continuous progesterone to prevent any bleeding if possible. A low-dose oral contraceptive can be substituted.

If the patient has premature ovarian failure, indicated by a high gonadotropin level and a low estrogen level, or if she has hypothalamic amenorrhea, indicated by low gonadotropin levels and a low estrogen level, estrogen/progesterone therapy to help prevent osteoporosis may be appropriate (31). If amenorrhea or oligomenorrhea is felt to be due to anovulation, with normal estrogen and gonadotropin levels, cyclical progestins to induce bleeding every other or every third month can be used. Alternatively, cyclical or continuous oral contraceptives can be used for treatment of anovulatory bleeding and prevention of endometrial hyperplasia.

Contraception

Contraception is an issue that is often brought up, either from the patient or the caregivers. If the patient raises the issue, it needs to be addressed with her privately, if possible. The care provider has to assess whether this request is a result of the patient's desire for consensual sexual activity or is a result of coercion or abuse. It is important to assess whether the patient is able to grasp the concept of consensual sexual relations and whether she could fully consent to such a relationship. This requires an evaluation of the patient's knowledge and the understanding of the process of sexual activity; frequently sexuality education is required. The help of an expert interviewer such as a psychologist or social worker may be required. If the patient is contemplating or already engaged in a consensual sexual relationship, concrete and explicit discussions about sexually transmitted diseases and the use of condoms for safer sex are needed.

If the request is made by parents or other caregivers, the patient's safety needs to be assessed. The request may be initiated due to a crisis situation in which something has happened to the patient or to other patients in the group home or work situation. This situation may have made everyone acutely aware of the risk of abuse and pregnancy. An open discussion with the patient, caregivers, and/or family is indicated, and the caregivers' fears and the patient's actual risk for abuse or pregnancy needs to be determined. The patient's safety is obviously the foremost concern.

When the determination has been made that the patient needs contraception, safety, efficacy, and ease of use must be considered. The potential risks and benefits for each individual patient should also be assessed. Special considerations in the developmentally delayed patient are listed in Table 8-2.

Oral contraceptives are often used in women with developmental disabilities, because they are generally safe and have minimal side effects for otherwise healthy individuals. They reduce menstrual flow and cramping and provide reliable contraception, providing they are taken as indicated. Failure to comply with daily dosing may be a problem and may require daily supervision, as mentioned before. Patients with Down's syndrome can have significant cardiac abnormalities, with increased risk for thrombus formation. Immobility, resulting

Table 8-2   Contraception in Women with Developmental Disabilities

Oral Contraceptive Pill
- Daily intake; patient may need reminders or supervision
- Caution is advised in wheelchair-bound patients or those with limited mobility due to increased risk of VTE/DVT
- Down's syndrome: cardiac flow abnormalities with increased risk for VTE/DVT
- Anticonvulsants may increase metabolism of steroid hormones causing lower serum levels and the potential for contraceptive failure

Contraceptive Patch
- Limited data on patients with medical or developmental disabilities
- Monitor detachment closely
- Self-mutilating behaviors may result in picking off the patch

Intramuscular Depot Medroxyprogesterone Acetate (DMPA)
- Weight gain can lead to more difficult transfers
- Bone loss in immobilized patients or those with limited mobility may be more problematic or pronounced

Barrier Methods
- Need manual dexterity, initiative, consistent and correct use
- Patient may need help communicating with partner regarding condom use

IUD
- Difficult to assess signs of infection
- May require anesthetia for insertion
- Copper IUD: increase in flow and cramps
- Levonorgestrel IUD: decrease in flow or amenorrhea may be therapeutic or beneficial

Sterilization
- Controversial when patient cannot give consent

in increased risk of venous thromboembolism, is another theoretical concern, especially in women in wheelchairs, but there are no data addressing this issue. Although some data suggest that the risk may be slightly higher in preparations with third-generation progestins, this is controversial (32). It may therefore be advisable to use a low dose (30 μg or less) of ethinyl estradiol in combination with a first- or second-generation progestin. However, in individuals with severely limited mobility, progestin-only contraceptives may be preferable to combination oral contraceptives. Clients on anticonvulsants, with the exception of valproic acid, may need an adjustment of the estrogen dose in the oral contraceptives because these agents increase the activity of the cytochrome P450 hepatic micrososmal oxidative enzymes, resulting in a more rapid clearance of steroid hormones, lower serum levels, and possibly less effective contraception. Persistent breakthrough bleeding can signal the need for an increase in estrogen content of the oral contraceptive (33). Progestin-only oral contraceptives are a good alternative, but their contraceptive effectiveness is slightly lower than the combined oral contraceptives, they can cause more irregular bleeding, and greater attention to perfect use is required.

The contraceptive patch has not been specifically studied in this population but is clearly an attractive alternative in those patients without skin disorders and in whom the urge to pull off the patch is not a concern. Partial or total detachment of the patch occurs at an overall rate of 3.8% in the non-disabled population; therefore, this needs to be monitored closely by caregivers in women with disabilities (34). The contraceptive patch frequently results in a transient increase in breast tenderness; this may be difficult to assess in non-verbal patients. The contraceptive efficacy is similar to that of oral contraceptives but is decreased in clients over 198 lb (35).

Intramuscular DMPA has been extensively used both for contraception and for menstrual suppression, as mentioned before. An initial month-long trial of oral progestins may be used as a diagnostic trial before administering the intramuscular dose, to assess for side effects or mood changes.

Because barrier methods of contraception, including the diaphragm and cervical cap, require personal initiative, understanding, and a physical location in which to insert them privately, they are usually not an optimal option. Condoms require a great deal of communication with a partner; role-playing or other concrete recommendations may be required in order to enable protection from sexually transmitted infections.

The intrauterine device (IUD) has traditionally not been recommended in women with developmental disabilities due to the increase in bleeding and cramping that has been associated with the traditional copper-containing IUD. There has also been a concern about difficulty in communicating or reporting symptoms of infection. Anesthesia may be required for insertion. However, the availability of the levonorgestrel intrauterine system, which significantly decreases menstrual flow and is associated with 20% to 40% rates of amenor-rhea after 6 months, necessitates a re-evaluation of clinicians' long-standing views about this option, which may be appropriate for selected candidates (36).

Post-coital contraception should be discussed with all clients and care-givers, which can be very useful in cases of contraceptive failure or rape (37).

Sterilization in the mentally disabled woman is a controversial topic. The American College of Obstetrics and Gynecology presented a Committee Opin-ion on this issue in 1999 (38). It states: "The initial premise should be that nonvoluntary sterilization is ethically not acceptable, because of the violation of privacy, bodily integrity and reproductive rights." The parents, guardians, and care providers of women with mental retardation may not agree with that sentiment, and in difficult cases a hospital ethics committee may provide useful perspectives (39). There are also widely varying federal, state, and local laws and regulations to be taken into consideration, if the patient is not her own legal guardian.

A sterilization procedure should be considered, after extensive counseling, if the patient is mentally competent and is requesting it voluntarily (40).

Conclusion

Providing gynecological care for women with developmental disabilities can be a challenging task. Patience, persistence, and adaptation of the usual tech-niques will lead to a thoughtful assessment of the patient. Routine care can be changed to fit the unique needs of the individual; education of the patient and her caregivers in the areas of sexuality, safety, and abuse prevention are a vital part of the gynecological health care of these patients.

REFERENCES

1. Lindgren GW, Katoda H. Maturational rate of Tokyo children with and without mental retardation. Am J Ment Retard. 1993;98:128-34.
2. Goldstein H. Menarche, maturation, sexual relations and contraception of adolescent females with Down syndrome. Eur J Obstet Gynecol Reprod Biol. 1988;27:343-9.
3. Evans AL, McKinleay IA. Sexual maturation in girls with severe mental handicap. Child Care Health Dev. 1988;14:59-69.
4. Cento RM, Ciampelli M, Proto C, et al. Neuroendocrine features of pubertal develop-ment in females with mental retardation. Gynecol Endocrinol. 2001;15:178-83.
5. Cento RM, Ragusa L, Proto C, et al. Ovarian sensitivity to follicle stimulating hormone is blunted in normo-ovulatory women with Down's syndrome. Hum Reprod. 1997;12: 1709-13.
6. Cento RM, Ragusa L, Proto C, et al. Basal body temperature curves and endocrine pat-tern of menstrual cycles in Down syndrome. Gynecol Endocrinol. 1996;10:133-7.

7. Scola PS, Pueschel SM. Menstrual cycles and basal body temperature curves in women with Down syndrome. Obstet Gynecol. 1992;79:91-4.

8. Bauer J, Isojarvi JL, Herzog AG, et al. Reproductive dysfunction in women with epilepsy: recommendations for evaluation and treatment. J Neurol Neurosurg Psychiatry. 2002;73:121-5.

9. Prasher VP. Down's syndrome and thyroid disorders: a review. Downs Syndr Res Pract. 1999;6:25-42.

10. Koutras DA. Disturbances of menstruation in thyroid disease. Ann N Y Acad Sci. 1997;816:280-4.

11. McDonough PG, Gantt P. Dysfunctional bleeding in the adolescent. In: Barwin BN, Belisle S, eds. Adolescent Gynecology and Sexuality. New York: Masson Publishing; 1982.

12. Falcone T, Desjardins C, Bourque I, et al. Dysfunctional uterine bleeding in adolescents. J Reprod Med. 1994;39:761.

13. Sulpizi LK. Issues in sexuality and gynecologic care of women with developmental disabilities. J Obstet Gynecol Neonatal Nurs. 1996;25:609-14.

14. Haefner H, Elkins T. Contraceptive management for female adolescents with mental retardation and handicapping disabilities. Curr Opin Obstet Gynecol. 1991;3:820.

15. Westcott H. The abuse of disabled children: a review of the literature. Child Care Health Dev. 1991;17:243.

16. Blackburn M. Sexuality, disability and abuse: advice for life not just for kids! Child Care Health Dev. 1995;21:351.

17. Chamberlain A, Rauh J, Passer A, et al. Issues in fertility control for mentally retarded female adolescents: sexual activity, sexual abuse, and contraception. Pediatrics. 1984;73:445.

18. Minihan PM, Dean DH. Meeting the needs for health services of persons with mental retardation living in the community. Am J Public Health. 1990;80:1043.

19. Elkins TE, McNeeley SG, Rosen DA, et al. Clinical observation of a program to accomplish pelvic exams in difficult to manage patients with mental retardation. Adolesc Pediatr Gynecol. 1988;1:195-8.

20. Quint EH, Elkins TE. The dilemma of cervical cytology in women with mental retardation. Obstet Gynecol. 1997;89:123.

21. Saslow D. Runowicz CD, Solomon D, et al. American Cancer Society guideline for the early detection of cervical neoplasia and cancer. Cancer J Clin. 2002;52:342-62.

22. Rosen DA, Rosen KR, et al. Outpatient sedation: an essential addition to gynecologic care for persons with mental retardation. Am J Obstet Gynecol. 1991;164:825.

23. Brown D, Rosen D, Elkins TE. Sedating women with mental retardation for routine gynecological examination: an ethical analysis. J Clin Ethics. 1992;3:68.

24. Kaunitz AM. Long-acting injectable contraception with depot medroxyprogesterone acetate. Am J Obstet Gynecol. 1994;170:1543-9.

25. Scholes D, LaCroix AZ, Ichikawa LE, et al. Injectable hormone contraception and bone density: results from a prospective study. Epidemiology. 2002;13:581-7.

26. Cromer BA, Stager M, Bonny A, et al. Depot medroxyprogesterone acetate, oral contraceptives, and bone mineral density in a cohort of adolescent girls. J Adolesc Health. 2004;35:434-41.

27. Wingfield M, McClure N, Marners PM, et al. Endometrial ablation: an option for the menstrual problems in the intellectually disabled. Med J Aust. 1994;160:533.

28. McNeeley SG, Elkins TE. Gynecologic surgery and surgical morbidity in mentally handicapped women. Obstet Gynecol. 1989;74:155.

29. Sheth S, Malpani A. Vaginal hysterectomy for the management of menstruation in mentally retarded women. Int J Gynecol Obstet. 1991;35:319.

30. Zhang-Wong JH, Seeman MV. Antipsychotic drugs, menstrual regularity and osteoporosis risk. Arch Womens Mental Health. 2002;5:93-8.

31. Laml T, Schulz-Lobmeyr I, Obruca A, et al. Premature ovarian failure: etiology and prospects. Gynecol Endocrinol. 2000;14:292-302.

32. Girolami A, Spiezia L, Rossi F, Zanon E. Oral contraceptives and venous thromboembolism: which are the safest preparations available? Clin Appl Thromb Hemost. 2002; 8:157-62.

33. Back DJ, Orme MLE. Pharmacokinetic drug interactions with oral contraceptives. Clin Pharmacokinet. 1990;18:472.

34. Burkman RT. The transdermal contraceptive patch: a new approach to hormonal contraception. Int J Fertil Womens Med. 2002;47:69-76.

35. Gallo MF, Grimes DA, Schulz KF. Skin patch and vaginal ring versus combined oral contraceptives for contraception. Cochrane Database of Systematic Reviews. (1):CD003552, 2003.

36. French RS, Cowan FM, Mansour D, et al. Levonorgestrel-releasing (20 microgram/day) intrauterine systems (Mirena) compared with other methods of reversible contraceptives. BJOG. 2000;107:1218-25.

37. Grimes DA, Raymond EG. Emergency contraception. Ann Intern Med. 2002;137:180-9.

38. American College of Obstetrics and Gynecology. Sterilization of women, including those with mental disabilities. ACOG Committee Opinion 216. Washington, DC; 1999.

39. Bambrick M, Roberts GE: The sterilization of people with mental handicap: the views of parents. J Ment Defect Res. 1991;35:353.

40. Herr SS, Hopkins BL. Health care decisions for persons with disabilities. JAMA. 1994; 271:1017.

9

Bleeding Disorders

Kimberly W. Schlesinger, MD
Henry M. Rinder, MD
Margaret V. Ragni, MD, MPH

Bleeding during the menstrual cycle is regulated by normal hemostatic mechanisms. Monthly sloughing of the vessel-rich endometrium activates normal hemostasis, with subsequent clot formation and gradual cessation of bleeding. Hemostasis is accomplished by vasoconstriction of endometrial vessels, formation of the platelet plug (primary hemostasis) (Figure 9-1), and subsequent fibrin clot (secondary hemostasis) (Figure 9-2) at the sites of vessel injury (sloughing). Thus, menorrhagia can be a significant symptom in women with congenital or acquired bleeding disorders, where hemostatic mechanisms are deficient. In order to recognize when bleeding disorders underlie menorrhagia, it is important to understand the physiology and pathology of hemostasis and its constituents, the vascular endothelium, platelets, and the soluble coagulation factors that lead to fibrin clot formation.

Bleeding disorders in women often go undiagnosed, increasing their morbidity and reducing the quality of life for women (1). In the menorrhagia patient, obtaining a personal and family bleeding history, performing a thorough physical examination, and measuring coagulation screening tests may be sufficient to make the diagnosis of a bleeding disorder; proper therapy may avert unnecessary invasive procedures. To that end, the American College of Obstetrics and Gynecology has recently recommended that the following groups of women be screened for von Willebrand's disease (vWD): adolescents with menorrhagia, women with menorrhagia without another cause, and women who are undergoing hysterectomy for excessive menstrual bleeding (2).

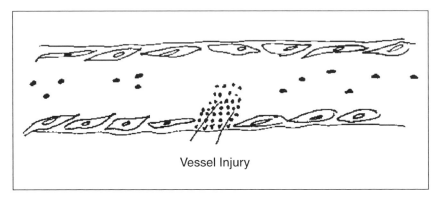

Vessel Injury

Figure 9-1   Primary hemostasis. When vessel injury occurs, von Willebrand factor (vWf) adheres to exposed subendothelial collagen and serves as the major site for platelet adhesion. Platelets are activated by shear and by thrombin formed through activation of the coagulation system on the platelet and endothelial surface; the latter is initiated through the interaction of tissue factor-VIIa. Activated platelets release serotonin, calcium, and ADP, which activate and recruit additional platelets to cause early hemostasis through platelet plug formation.

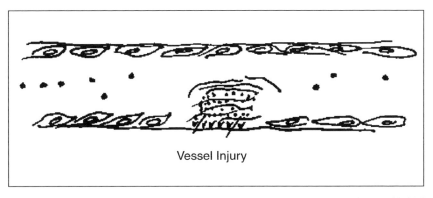

Vessel Injury

Figure 9-2   Secondary hemostasis. The sequence of events following injury and initial formation of the platelet plug and activation of the coagulation cascade is characterized by formation of cross-linked fibrin polymers on the platelet surface, lending strength to the temporary platelet plug structure. Once the fibrin clot is further strengthened by XIIIa, secondary hemostasis is achieved.

Overview of Menorrhagia and Bleeding Disorders

Menorrhagia is a major public health problem, with as many as 10%-15% of women experiencing menorrhagia during their lifetime (3,4). Moreover, this symptom accounts for 15% of referrals to gynecologists and 3% of all annual medical visits (5,6). As many as 20% of women with menorrhagia have an underlying bleeding disorder (7,8). (Other causes of menorrhagia include endometriosis, uterine cancer, polyp bleeding, hypothyroidism, and postpartum bleeding.) Menorrhagia is the most common presenting symptom and often the predominant clinical feature of women with a coagulopathy (9,10); it occurs four times more frequently in women with coagulopathy compared with normal women (7). No racial or ethnic group is spared (11). Menorrhagia occurs in over 90% of women with vWD, the most common inherited bleeding disorder (10). In fact, von Willebrand first recognized this mucosal bleeding disorder in a 13-year-old girl who died of menorrhagia (12). By contrast, little is known about the prevalence of menorrhagia among women with uncommon congenital coagulation disorders, for example, factor V or XI deficiency and factor VIII or factor IX (hemophilia A or B) carriers (13,14).

Unlike most anatomic causes of gynecologic bleeding (e.g., fibroids, endometrial cancer, infection), menorrhagia in women with a bleeding disorder commonly begins at menarche (9,10) and persists throughout life (6). Despite this, the diagnosis of a specific coagulopathy is often not considered (11), and, if so, it is only after invasive gynecologic examination is unrevealing (15). This results in delaying the diagnosis for a median of 4 years after the first bleeding symptoms (10). Moreover, invasive procedures performed prior to the diagnosis of an underlying bleeding disorder (e.g., dilatation and curettage, endometrial biopsy, transvaginal ultrasound, uterine imaging and sampling, and diagnostic hysteroscopy, laparoscopy, and hysterectomy) lead to excess morbidity and stress (1,16,17).

There are several reasons that the diagnosis of a bleeding disorder may not be appropriately pursued in women with menorrhagia: 1) some women may not seek medical attention unless there is a change in their normal menses, especially in those with a family history of heavy menstrual bleeding (9,18); 2) health care providers often associate bleeding disorders with male gender (e.g., hemophilia [11]); 3) menorrhagia symptoms are neither sensitive nor specific for the diagnosis of an underlying bleeding disorder (4); 4) the laboratory diagnosis of vWD and platelet-associated bleeding disorders can be difficult (e.g., blood group [19], estrogen [20], and stress [21] affect vWF levels and may obscure the diagnosis); and 5) routine diagnostic tests do not always detect variant bleeding disorders (e.g., a normal PTT may be seen in patients with vWD).

Therefore, any woman presenting with menorrhagia should have a complete personal and family history, thorough physical examination, and coagulation screening tests. It has been estimated that if a bleeding history were obtained in women with menorrhagia prior to undergoing diagnostic procedures or surgery, postoperative bleeding could be avoided in two thirds of these patients (10).

Etiology of Coagulation Disorders

Disorders of Vascular Endothelium

Disorders of the vasculature have similar symptoms to disorders of platelet plug formation (Table 9-1). Defects in the vessel wall may lead to telangiectasia, petechiae, or purpura, and menorrhagia may be present. Telangiectasias in the skin and along the gastrointestinal tract raise the suspicion of a primary vessel wall disorder (22). These may be sporadically acquired with aging or prolonged corticosteroid use, but their presence in large numbers or in unusual locations, for example, the lips, is suggestive of hereditary hemorrhagic telangiectasia (HHT), also known as Osler-Weber-Rendu disease. Individuals with HHT may have telangiectasias on the lips, nose, mouth, and the genitourinary and gastrointestinal tracts, but they often do not bleed until adulthood, when they manifest epistaxis, gastrointestinal bleeding, or menorrhagia, often associated with iron deficiency. Another vascular disorder is Ehlers-Danlos syndrome, in which bleeding results from abnormal collagen support of the blood vessel. Acquired vascular disorders can be associated with drugs, ascorbic acid deficit (scurvy), trauma, infection, and immunologic abnormalities. Immunologic disorders such as polyarteritis nodosa, rheumatoid vasculitis, Henoch-Schönlein purpura, drug reactions, cryoglobulinemia, or malignancies are often associated with palpable purpura and may lead to menorrhagia; bacterial, viral, or fungal infections cause both palpable and non-palpable purpura (22).

The diagnosis of bleeding disorders from vascular abnormalities is clear-cut. These occur in the setting of a normal platelet count, PT, and PTT. The bleeding time may be abnormal because of the vascular defect, but platelet closure times are normal. The specific abnormalities are diagnosed based on laboratory testing (e.g., low ascorbic acid levels in scurvy) or classic history and physical findings (e.g., multiple telangectasias in HHT). Treatment is aimed at the underlying disorder, and the specific therapy for bleeding and menorrhagia is mainly supportive, including iron supplementation and avoidance of platelet inhibitory drugs and anticoagulants.

Disorders of Platelet Plug Formation

Disorders of platelet plug formation, often termed *primary hemostasis*, present clinically as petechiae, purpura, bruising, or oozing from mucosal sites.

Table 9-1   Differential Diagnosis of Bleeding Disorders

Coagulation Disorders	Platelet Disorders	Vessel Wall Disorders
Congenital • Hemophilia A, B carrier • Factor XI deficiency • Other factor deficiencies	**Congenital** • von Willebrand disease • Bernard-Soulier syndrome • Glanzmann thromboasthenia • Storage pool disease	**Congenital** • Hereditary hemorrhagic telangiectasia • Ehlers-Danlos syndrome
Acquired • Acquired anti-VIII inhibitor • Vitamin K deficiency • Liver disease • DIC • Drug: warfarin, heparin, antibiotics	**Acquired** • ITP • TTP • Drug: ASA, NSAIDs, antibiotics, chemotherapy • Collagen diseases: SLE • Chronic renal disease • Leukemias • Myeloproliferative disorders	**Acquired** • Physical: valsalva, weight-lifting • Infection: bacterial, viral, rickettsial • Drug: heparin necrosis, warfarin necrosis • Dysproteinemias • Cutaneous vasculitis

◄──────────────── **Clinical Bleeding History** ────────────────►

General symptoms—Age at first bleeding; frequency, severity; requirement for transfusion; spontaneous vs. traumatic bleed; postoperative bleeding; family members affected, sex-linked; medication history

Type of bleeding • Fibrin clot defect: body cavity bleeding; hemarthroses; hematomas; postoperative, retroperitoneal, CNS bleeding	**Type of bleeding** • Platelet plug defect: mucosal bleeding; menorrhagia; epistaxis; bruising; post-operative, dental, GI, GU bleeding	**Type of bleeding** • Vessel wall defect: petechiae, ecchymoses, purpura, telangiectasia, gravity-dependent lesions, palpable vs. nonpalpable

◄──────────────── **Laboratory Screening Tests** ────────────────►

Tests of coagulation system • APTT • PT • Factor levels • Anti-VIII, APTT mix • Closure time	**Tests of platelet function** • Platelet count • Platelet adhesion, aggregation • Bleeding/closure time • von Willebrand factor • Platelet granule, secretion • Other diagnostic tests: creatinine, ANA, blood smear, CBC	**Tests of vascular integrity** • Inspection: nose, mouth, skin • Platelet count • CBC

Bleeding generally occurs at mucosal surfaces, in the oral, nasal, gastrointestinal, or genitourinary mucosa. Thus, epistaxis, dental bleeding, and menorrhagia are frequent; gastrointestinal bleeding is less common (see Table 9-1). Because platelet plug formation occurs early after vessel injury, bleeding in these disorders presents early after an insult, and adequate hemostasis is delayed. Post-surgical bleeding due to defective platelet plug formation may begin during or within minutes to hours following the procedure (23).

Platelet Disorders

Any of the causes of thrombocytopenia (e.g., hematologic malignancy, chemotherapy, immune thrombocytopenic purpura [ITP], HELLP syndrome, disseminated intravascular coagulation [DIC], thrombotic thrombocytic purpura [TTP]) may result in menorrhagia; management of the thrombocytopenia is best done by a consulting hematologist. Menorrhagia is more frequent when the platelet count is less than 50,000/μL, but genitourinary bleeding is most likely to be spontaneous when platelets fall below 10,000/μL (24). Platelet functional disorders may be congenital or acquired and may occur when the platelet count is normal. Congenital platelet function disorders include Bernard-Soulier syndrome (defective or absent GPIb/IX), Glanzmann thrombasthenia (GPIIb/IIIa defect), and abnormal platelet secretion, termed "platelet storage pool disease."

Acquired platelet function disorders are often drug-induced. Many platelet inhibitory drugs are now in common use to prevent vascular disease. Aspirin and NSAIDs, which inhibit the COX-1 enzyme, block the arachidonic acid pathway, preventing generation of thromboxane A_2. It is important to note that the highly selective COX-2 inhibitors (e.g., Celebrex) have little COX-1 effect and are not directly associated with increased bleeding risk. Other platelet inhibitors—for example, Plavix (ADP receptor blocker) and Abciximab (GPIIb/IIIa blocker)—interfere with platelet aggregation and are associated with clinical bleeding. Platelet dysfunction also occurs in chronic renal failure, especially before institution of hemodialysis; circulating platelets are, in effect, poisoned by some of the products of metabolism, which are renally cleared. Transfused platelets are also rapidly affected; thus, long-term platelet function may be optimized by frequent dialysis, correction of anemia (an adequate red cell mass enhances platelet-EC contact), and treatment with conjugated estrogens (25).

von Willebrand's Disease

The most common congenital disorder of platelet plug formation is von Willebrand's disease (vWD). vWD is an autosomal disorder characterized by deficient or defective vWF (19,26). Although platelet number and function are generally normal, platelet plug formation is defective because vWF is required for platelet adhesion at the site of vessel injury. Most individuals with vWD (65%-70%) have type 1 vWD, which is characterized by autosomal dominant inheritance and a quantitative decrease in normal vWF (26). Although bleeding is generally mild, over 90% of women with type 1 vWD have menorrhagia, which is usually their first bleeding symptom (10). Type 2 vWD is characterized by a qualitative defect in vWF, generally manifested by a reduction in the more hemostatically active high-molecular-weight vWF multimers (HMWM) (27). The different forms of type 2 vWD account for about 30% of vWD patients and usually cause more frequent clinical bleeding, including epistaxis, dental bleeding, and menorrhagia; unlike type 1 vWD, menorrhagia is usually not the initial symptom (10). Inheritance is autosomal dominant or, less frequently, recessive. Severe, or type 3, vWD, like type 2, rarely presents with menorrhagia, but this is still a common symptom. Type 3 disease accounts for 1%-5% of vWD; this generally results from the inheritance of two abnormal vWF genes and is manifested by absent vWF function and the most severe phenotype presenting in childhood.

There are also two variants of vWD: platelet-type and acquired. Platelet-type vWD is actually characterized by a platelet GPIb mutation that increases GPIb-GPIX binding to vWF, thereby causing increased clearance of HMWM and a "type 2 vWD-like" defect (28,29). Acquired vWD occurs in the setting of lymphoproliferative and myeloproliferative disorders, monoclonal gammopathies, hypothyroidism, some immunologic disorders and, occasionally, with drugs (30,31). Acquired vWD similarly presents mostly as a type 2 form, with decreased HMWM due to clearance; this variant is treated with vWF concentrate and/or IVIG, and generally resolves when the underlying disorder is cured.

It is important to note that individuals with vWD, especially mild type 1, may have normal screening tests, including PTT. Thus, in women with menorrhagia, it is absolutely necessary to screen for vWD. (Screening tests are described in the section on Laboratory Testing later in this chapter.)

Disorders of Fibrin Clot Formation

Disorders of fibrin clot formation, often called *secondary hemostasis*, are characterized by a defect or deficiency in one or more coagulation factors; these may be congenital or acquired. Congenital deficiencies typically affect a single clotting factor, whereas acquired deficiencies often affect multiple factors. With defective fibrin clot formation, primary platelet hemostasis is normal, but delayed thrombin generation and fibrin formation manifests as delayed bleeding after surgery or trauma. Bleeding in these disorders occurs in deep tissues, including muscle, resulting in hematomas, and in joints, hemarthroses. Menorrhagia has been described in several congenital disorders of fibrin clot formation, including factor XI and V deficiency, and in carriers of hemophilia A or B (factor VIII and IX, respectively). However, menorrhagia is very rare in female hemophilia carriers; fewer than 10% of female hemophilia carriers have factor VIII or IX levels low enough to induce abnormal bleeding under any circumstance (32). In rare subsets of female hemophilia carriers, for example, the Amish population, menorrhagia is actually much less common than postpartum bleeding, probably because normal platelet plug formation may prevent the former, while fibrin clot formation is more critical to hemostasis in the post-partum uterus (32). More commonly, acquired clotting disorders are associated with menorrhagia, including warfarin use, vitamin K deficiency, liver disease, and DIC (7,8,13,33-35).

Little is known about other coagulopathies causing menorrhagia, in part because of the rarity of most of these disorders. Fibrin clot formation is generally normal when factor levels are above 30%, and spontaneous bleeding is uncommon with factor levels greater than 5%. Although menorrhagia is a recognized symptom in women with congenital factor I, II, V, VII, X, or XI deficiency, such coagulopathies are rare, less than 1 in 500,000 incidence for each, and unlikely to be identified in small studies of women with menorrhagia (13,14). Moreover, as noted below, other mitigating factors may transiently increase factor levels and prevent excessive bleeding. Occasionally, multiple coagulation disorders may be inherited, for example, factor XI deficiency with hemophilia carrier status, or factor XI deficiency with vWD (35). As noted above, menorrhagia has not been reported in women with a prolonged PTT due to deficiency of factor XII, prekallikrein, or high-molecular-weight kininogen; these states are not associated with clinical bleeding (13). Similarly, menorrhagia is not associated with the prolonged PTT seen with lupus anticoagulants (LAC), which is actually a hypercoagulable disorder (36).

Evaluation and Diagnosis

The management of women with bleeding disorders is proactive and preventive. Evaluation for specific bleeding disorders must be considered in all women presenting with menorrhagia before any invasive tests, procedures, or surgeries are performed. The American College of Obstetricians and Gynecologists recommends testing specifically for vWD in all adolescents presenting with menorrhagia, women who are to undergo hysterectomy for menorrhagia, and adult women with menorrhagia without another cause (2). If the diagnosis of a bleeding disorder is confirmed, management is planned accordingly.

History and Physical Examination

The clinical evaluation of bleeding is aimed at determining which of the components of normal hemostasis (vascular endothelium, platelet plug formation, or fibrin clot) is defective. The recognition of bleeding disorders leading to menorrhagia depends on both the clinical presentation and an assessment of hemostatic function. The clinical evaluation should include a thorough physical examination, personal and family bleeding history, and a complete medication history. The physical examination should note the presence of mucosal hemorrhage, petechiae, and purpuric lesions, which tend to be associated with platelet-based hemostatic disorders versus hematomas and hemarthroses, which occur more often with coagulation factor deficiencies. Vascular abnormalities may manifest as skin laxity, thinning of dermal subcutaneous tissue, or telangiectasias on the lips and mucosal surfaces. The clinical bleeding history should include the site, severity, and frequency of bleeding; any incidence of bleeding with surgery or dental procedures; the presence of iron deficiency; the need for iron supplementation; or any requirement for transfusion, including the type of blood product received. It is very useful to know what has provoked bleeding in the past or whether bleeding occurs spontaneously. The timing of bleeding is also important, for example, bleeding that begins 24-48 hours after tooth extraction. Bleeding that persists for days after a procedure, leads to anemia, or requires the use of blood products is always considered abnormal.

The family history should include the type and severity of bleeding history in relatives, whether males or females are affected, and whether the severity is constant or variable among family members. The medication history should specifically include questions about aspirin, NSAIDs, platelet inhibitor drugs, sulfa- or quinine-based drugs, warfarin or heparin, and whether the patient has taken alternative medicines such as garlic, gingko, kava kava, or St. John's wort, which may cause platelet dysfunction, or herbs containing coumarin derivatives (37). In some women with mild bleeding disorders, menorrhagia may not come to clinical attention until there is a second coagulation defect. For example, a platelet inhibitory effect caused by ibuprofen superimposed on an underlying bleeding disorder such as mild vWD may result in newly appreciable menorrhagia; stopping the platelet inhibitory drug may reduce or resolve bleeding.

Laboratory Testing

Diagnostic screening tests to evaluate women with menorrhagia should always include a complete blood count, including hemoglobin, hematocrit, white blood count, differential, MCV, and platelet count, PT, and PTT (Tables 9-1 and 9-2). In addition, specific testing for vWD (a VW profile) should be done with a functional test, either RCoF or vWF:CBA, plus vWF:Ag, VIII:C, ristocetin platelet aggregation, and closure time with epinephrine and ADP. As mentioned earlier, because persons with vWD, especially mild type 1 vWD, may have normal screening tests, including the PTT, it is absolutely necessary to perform specific testing for vWD in women with menorrhagia. Screening

Table 9-2   Laboratory Diagnosis of Bleeding Disorders

Screening Laboratory Studies
- *Hematologic tests:* CBC, differential, platelet count
- *Endocrinologic tests:* Prolactin, FSH, progesterone (mid-cycle)
- *Liver function tests:* SGOT, SGPT, alkaline phosphatase, bilirubin
- *Kidney function tests:* BUN, creatinine, urinalysis
- *Gynecologic tests:* Pelvic ultrasound

◄──────────── **Screening Coagulation Laboratory Studies** ────────────►

Coagulation pathway	Coagulation abnormality	Congenital deficiency	Acquired coagulopathy
Intrinsic pathway	Prolonged APTT	FXI, XII, PK HMW-K FVIII, IX FVIII carrier FIX carrier vWD	Lupus anticoagulant (LAC) Specific anticoagulants: Anti-VIII Anti-V Heparin Acquired vWD
Extrinsic pathway	Prolonged PT	FVII	Vitamin K deficiency
Common pathway	Prolonged PT, APTT	FI, II, V, X	Vitamin K deficiency, liver disease, DIC

◄──────────── **Screening Platelet Function Studies** ────────────►

Platelet plug pathway	Platelet functional defect	Congenital platelet defect	Acquired platelet defect
Platelet adhesion	Platelet adhesion, ristocetin agglutination	Bernard-Soulier syndrome	ITP Myeloproliferative disorders
Platelet aggregation	Aggregation with epinephrine, ADP, collagen thrombin	Glanzmann thrombasthenia	Cardiopulmonary bypass Chronic renal disease Heparin
Platelet secretion	ATP:ADP ratio	Storage pool disease	
von Willebrand cofacter antigen	vWF:Ag: ELISA, Laurell immunoassay	von Willebrand disease	Acquired von Willebrand disease
vWF activity	FVIII:C, RCoF:VIII, Multimers (SDS PAGE) Collagen binding assay		
Vessel-platelet interaction	Closure time/ bleeding time	All above disorders	Aspirin, NSAIDs, antibiotics, platelet inhibitory drugs, ETOH

tests for vWD (38-50) include ristocetin cofactor activity (RCoF) (43), vWF antigen (vWF:Ag) (36), collagen binding activity (vWF:CBA) (47), and factor VIII clotting activity (FVIII:C). For screening, either RCoF or vWF:CBA, plus vWF:Ag, are required. Because vWF serves as a carrier molecule for VIII, if this level is low enough, then the PTT is prolonged. When screening tests for vWD are abnormal, vWF multimeric analysis is recommended to distinguish specific types of vWD, for example, type 2 vWD (48).

Several situations will increase vWF activity, including estrogen use, pregnancy, exercise, and inflammatory conditions (20). Therefore, if any of these circumstances are present in a woman with menorrhagia and the initial vWD screening tests are normal, it is critical to repeat those laboratory studies at least once or twice. It may also be optimal to obtain blood samples early in the morning, preferably during the first 3 days of the cycle (20,51). Another general rule is to delay vWD testing until 6-8 weeks postpartum or after estrogen cessation. One other difficulty in interpreting vWD testing is that vWF levels vary widely among individuals. If laboratory results for vWF are in the low-normal range in a patient with clear-cut evidence of a bleeding disorder (and no other laboratory diagnosis), one may consider vWD-specific treatment for excessive bleeding in that patient. One caveat is that vWF studies should be documented before and after treatment and correlated with clinical efficacy, especially because these treatments are not without complications.

Based on these results, other laboratory studies may be warranted: for example, SGOT, SGPT, alkaline phosphatase, and bilirubin to determine liver function; iron, ferritin, and TIBC for low MCV anemia; thyroid function tests; and creatinine tests. If the vW profile is normal, the tests should be repeated on the first 1-3 days of the cycle, on at least three occasions, to exclude vWD. Of course, if estrogen is used, it may mask a diagnosis: alternatively, if ASA or NSAIDs are used, these may prolong the closure (or bleeding times), thus medications should be carefully screened as part of the evaluation. Abnormal clotting tests require specific evaluation for congenital or acquired disorders (for example, specific factor levels, bleeding, closure-time) and are best conducted in association with the consultant hematologist.

The evaluation of platelet function always starts with a platelet count. A global measure of platelet function is the in vivo bleeding time; with platelet counts in the normal range and normal platelet function, the bleeding time is less than 8 minutes (45,46). The bleeding time does not usually become prolonged by thrombocytopenia alone until the platelet count is less than 100,000/μL. However, when the platelet count is less than 100,000/μL, the bleeding time does not distinguish between bleeding caused by thrombocytopenia and abnormal platelet function/vessel adhesion. The same caveat applies to the platelet closure time (e.g., the Dade PFA), an in vitro bleeding time, which is rapidly being adopted by laboratories (50). The closure time uses anticoagulated whole blood and determines the time required for platelet plug formation after stimulation with agonists such as collagen and ADP; closure time is prolonged by platelet dysfunction (e.g., aspirin) or by vWD. Other readily available laboratory testing for platelet function includes platelet aggregometry, which evaluates both primary platelet function and, with ristocetin-induced agglutination, vWf function; thromboxane B_2 synthesis, which evaluates COX-1 activity; and flow cytometry, which can evaluate for the presence or absence of platelet surface receptors (e.g., GPIb in Bernard-Soulier disease).

Treatment

Menorrhagia is the most common indication for hysterectomy in the United States, accounting for 300,000 such procedures per year (52,53). It is estimated that 20% or more of women with menorrhagia have an underlying bleeding disorder; thus, if noninvasive approaches to menorrhagia were implemented, the potential reduction in morbidity and health care costs would be dramatic. Treatment of menorrhagia in women with bleeding disorders requires 1) early diagnosis of the underlying bleeding disorder; 2) early intervention with hormonal therapy (e.g., OCPs) and/or DDAVP factor; 3) counseling regarding the disease and future expectations regarding pregnancy and future bleeding; and 4) establishing a physician-patient relationship to help with questions and future treatment and to serve as a resource when new issues arise.

The uterine bleeding itself may differ in association with other bleeding problems such as bruising, nosebleeds, and hematomas; bleeding with surgical procedures; worsened bleeding when gynecologic procedures are performed (e.g., hysterectomy, uterine ablation, D&C); potential for future postpartum bleeding or worsened bleeding during the menopause.

Oral contraceptives (OCP) generally reduce the severity of blood loss in most women with menorrhagia (54,55). vWD testing should be done prior to initiating estrogen therapy because estrogen may mask the diagnosis of vWD (20,56). These agents are obviously preferred in the management of menorrhagia over blood products, because the latter are costly, potentially infectious, and invasive. Estrogens not only increase the levels of clotting factors, including VIII, IX, and vWF (54,55), they also have direct beneficial effects on the endometrium (56,57). Estrogens are commonly prescribed as additional therapy for menorrhagia, which is not controlled with Stimate, IV DDAVP, amicar, or tranexamic acid alone (58,59).

When women with bleeding disorders discontinue estrogens (for example, in an attempt to become pregnant), the return of problematic menorrhagia may be lessened by reviewing with the patient the optimal timing for conception. During the postpartum fall in estrogen levels, women with vWD should be monitored for excessive or prolonged menstrual bleeding and treated symptomatically (60). In addition, the differential for excessive or prolonged postpartum bleeding should include the rare but life-threatening acquired inhibitor to factor VIII (see section on Congenital and Acquired Factor Deficiencies later in this chapter).

When surgery is required in the individual with an underlying bleeding disorder, there should be a discussion regarding the potential for bleeding during and after the procedure. For example, it is helpful to know the estimated blood loss expected in the normal patient undergoing the procedure, the length of the procedure, and the anticipated length of postoperative recovery. Women with menorrhagia must be evaluated for vWD or other abnormalities before undergoing any invasive diagnostic or therapeutic procedure such as dilatation and curettage (D&C), hysteroscopy, uterine ablation, or hysterectomy. Before the procedure, all potential interfering drugs should be stopped, including NSAIDs at least 3 days before surgery, aspirin 1 week before surgery, and warfarin 4-5 days before surgery (to reach an INR of less than 1.5).

If time permits, hepatitis vaccination can be administered before surgery per the current recommendations for individuals with bleeding disorders (61,62). In the patient with an established bleeding disorder, specific therapy is given immediately before the procedure; this therapy should accompany the patient to the procedure unit or operating room. One should also establish contact with the procedure unit and anesthesiologist to clarify the route, dose, and timing of therapy and to be available in the event of excessive bleeding. After the procedure, hemostasis is monitored and maintained with ongoing therapy as needed. Treatment is often continued for 1-2 days after minor procedures; when there is a major procedure or in those patients with severe platelet dysfunction or factor deficiency, treatment may be required for longer periods.

NSAIDs and COX inhibitors are generally avoided in individuals with bleeding disorders because they may contribute to bleeding by adding the additional defect of platelet dysfunction, which may greatly increase the bleeding symptoms.

Platelets are transfused in chemotherapy patients both prophylactically for platelet counts of less than 10-20K without bleeding and for counts of more than 20K when menorrhagia or other bleeding symptoms occur. There is no effective prophylaxis that prevents subsequent thrombocytopenic bleeding in menorrhagia patients who are about to undergo chemotherapy.

Medical treatment of bleeding disorders is summarized in Table 9-3. The following sections provide further discussion.

Platelet Disorders

The management of menorrhagia in patients with thrombocytopenia is straightforward; in addition to estrogens, platelet transfusion is the mainstay of therapy, with treatment, if possible, of the underlying condition. Thrombocytopenia due to ITP is usually treated with prednisone, 1 mg/kg/day, and tapering of the dosage once the platelet count is normal. When rapid platelet count correction is needed, for example, for surgery or massive hemorrhage, intravenous immunoglobulin (IVIG) may be given in a dose of 2 g/kg over 2-5 days (63,64), as well as platelet transfusions. In those individuals with drug-induced thrombocytopenia and bleeding, the offending drug should be stopped, and platelet transfusions can be given (24,65). For thrombocytopenia due to thrombotic thrombocytopenic purpura (TTP), the current treatment is plasma exchange, that is, plasmapheresis followed by infusion of FFP (66,67); platelet transfusion is contraindicated for TTP. The approach to management of thrombocytopenia and/or platelet dysfunction in individuals with myeloproliferative disorders is to treat the underlying disorder, use platelet transfusions sparingly (for bleeding and for counts less than 5-10,000/μL), and avoid drugs causing vitamin K deficiency or platelet dysfunction. The receptor disorders are not correctable, and any associated excessive bleeding must be treated with platelet transfusion.

Although storage pool disease in its most severe forms (Hermansky-Pudlak) is treated with platelet transfusion, bleeding in milder forms responds to DDAVP, the therapy for type 1 vWD (see below). As mentioned earlier, acquired platelet function disorders are often drug-induced. Like storage pool disease, bleeding with aspirin therapy can respond to DDAVP, but platelet transfusion is the definitive therapy for acquired platelet function disorders. For platelet dysfunction that occurs in chronic renal failure (particularly before the institution of hemodialysis), long-term platelet function may be optimized by frequent dialysis (25), correction of anemia, and treatment with conjugated estrogens. Acute bleeding in renal failure responds to DDAVP; anti-fibrinolytic therapy is also effective for oral, gastrointestinal, and genitourinary bleeding.

Von Willebrand's Disease

Menorrhagia associated with vWD can be managed with estrogen or progesterones such as Depo-Provera, with or without antifibrinolytic agents. Hormonal agents will increase the level of vWF (and also VIII) in type 1 vWD such that bleeding can be controlled; it should be emphasized that low-dose estrogens are often insufficient to reduce menorrhagia. If hormonal agents at a moderate dose are unsuccessful, hormones at a level that induces amenorrhea can be used to resolve bleeding and prevent the need for a hysterectomy; a gynecologist should be part of the management team in that circumstance.

DDAVP, 1-desamino-8-D-arginine vasopressin, is the treatment of choice for type 1 vWD (68). DDAVP triggers the release of vWF from endothelial cell Weibel-Palade bodies (69). DDAVP can be given intravenously in a dose of 0.3 micrograms per kilogram over 30 minutes. DDAVP is also administered as a highly concentrated nasal spray, Stimate, at a dose of 150 micrograms in one nostril for those weighing less than 50 kg; and 300 micrograms, one dose in each nostril, for those weighing more than 50 kg (70). A test dose of DDAVP should be given to establish laboratory-based effectiveness before the procedure. vWF levels achieved with intravenous DDAVP are generally higher, more rapidly achieved, and more durable than those with Stimate (68); thus, IV therapy is generally the first-line treatment for major surgery. Stimate is recommended for local procedures such as dental cleaning or tooth extraction, or for occurences of non-surgical bleeding such as epistaxis or menorrhagia (57,70). For the latter, Stimate is administered once daily on the first few days of the cycle (70). Among 307 menstrual cycles in 90 women with vWD, hemophilia A carriers, and congenital and acquired platelet defects, 88% of cycles were shortened or lightened by Stimate (70), similar to findings in smaller studies (71-73). Side effects include tachycardia, headache, and flushing due to vasodilatation, and hyponatremia and volume overload due to antidiuretic effects (70,71,74,75). The latter is more common in children (76) and can be prevented by avoiding excessive fluid intake (75). Tachyphylaxis occurs with repeated dosing of DDAVP as vWF stores are depleted. In most type 1 patients, only a few doses are required to control bleeding. However, if additional treatment is required beyond three doses, a vWF concentrate should be considered.

DDAVP is ineffective in individuals with type II vWD and is actually contraindicated in the type IIB variant because DDAVP increases platelet clearance through platelet-vWF binding and may lead to severe thrombocytopenia (77). For individuals with type 2 or 3 vWD, and the rare type 1 vWD unresponsive to DDAVP, effective therapy can be achieved with virally inactivated vWF-containing concentrate (57,74), for example, Humate-P. Plasma-derived products, unlike recombinant or highly purified factor VIII, contain significant amounts of vWF; Humate-P now lists the vWF activity on each unit, allowing for weight-dependent dosing. As mentioned earlier, acquired vWD is treated with vW concentrate and/or IVIG and generally resolves when the underlying disorder is cured. Based on several studies (78-80), about 75% of bleeding episodes are controlled with 1-2 doses of vWF concentrate, usually given initially at 40 U/kg and followed 12-24 hours later by 25 U/kg (79). Preclinical studies of a recombinant vWF concentrate have shown evidence of both safety and efficacy (81).

Table 9-3   Treatment of Bleeding Disorders

Agent	Dose	Disease Indication	Level of Evidence*	Mechanism	Side Effects
Desmopressin (DDAVP)	0.3 µg/kg IV	• Type 1 vWD • Hemophilia A carrier	(A)	• Releases vWF from endo-thelial cells by binding to ADH	• Flushing, headache, tachy-cardia, hyponatremia, volume overload, tachyphylaxis
Stimate (Intranasal) (1.5 mg/mL)	150 µg/nostril < 50 kg, one nostril > 50 kg, both nostrils	• Platelet dysfunction	(A)	• V2 receptor and activating CAMP	
von Willebrand factor concentrate	40 U/kg, then 25 U/kg q 12-24 h	• Type II, III vWD • Type 1 unresponsive to DDAVP	(A)	• Replaces vWF	• Allergic reaction, hepatitis, transmissible agent
Factor VIII concentrate (recombinant)	50 U/kg, then 25 U/kg q 8-12 h	• Factor VIII deficiency, severe or moderate • Acquired vWD	(A)	• Replaces FVIII	• Allergic reaction
Factor IX concentrate (recombinant)	75 U/kg, then 38 U/kg q 12-24 h	• Factor IX deficiency, • Hemophilia B carrier	(A)	• Replaces FIX	• Allergic reaction
Plasma, retested plasma	5 U = 20% level or 10 mL/kg	• Factor II, V, XI deficiency • Liver disease • Vitamin K deficiency • DIC, TTP • Marrow failure (malig-nancy, chemotherapy)	(A) (C)	• Replaces factors	• Fever, chills, hepatitis, transmissible agent, HIV
Cryoprecipitate	6 bags = 1200 mg fibrinogen	• Factor I deficiency • Dysfibrinogenemia • Factor XIII deficiency • Uremic bleeding, DIC	(C)	• Replaces fibrinogen factor XIII	• Fever, chills, transmissible agent, hepatitis, HIV

Agent	Dose	Indication	Level	Mechanism	Adverse effects
Factor VIIa (recombinant)	90 μg/kg q 2-3 h 20 μg/kg q 6-8 h	• Factor VIII inhibitor • Factor VII deficiency • Glanzmann thrombasthenia	(A) (A)	• Activates tissue factor, replaces FVII, FIX	• Thrombosis
Autoplex, FEIBA	75-100 U/kg, then 50 U/kg q 6-8 h	• Factor VIII inhibitor	(A)	• Replaces FIX, activates tissue factor	• Thrombosis, HIV, hepatitis, inhibitor transmissible agent
Platelet transfusion	1 U/10 kg (to 60 kg)	• Thrombocytopenia • Bernard-Soulier syndrome • Glanzmann thrombasthenia • ASA platelet defect • Platelet-type vWD • DIC	(A)	• Replaces platelets, restores platelet function	• Fever, allergic reactions
Amicar (epsilon-aminocaproic acid)	50 mg/kg q 6-8 h	• Congenital bleeding disorder	(A)	• Prevents lysis of clots by inhibiting plasminogen binding to fibrin	• Nausea, vomiting, kidney sludge, stone
Tranexamic acid	4 g/day (15 mg/kg)	• vWD • Hemophilia A, B carrier • Factor deficiencies	(C)	• Prevents lysis of clots by inhibiting plasminogen binding to fibrin	• Nausea, vomiting, diarrhea, hypotension
Estrogens	Mid-dose OCP	• vWD • Hemophilia A, B carrier • Factor deficiencies	(B,C)	• Increases factor levels • Endometrial changes	• Nausea, headache, thrombosis, cardiovascular risk
Hepatitis A vaccine, hepatitis B vaccine		• Congenital bleeding disorder	(A) (A)	• Protects from hepatitis A, B	• Soreness at site, nonspecific symptoms

* (A) = recommendation based on clinical trial data; (B) = recommendation based on laboratory data; (C) = recommendation based on opinion of experienced clinicians. The level of recommendation is based on general bleeding symptoms, not on menorrhagia.

Congenital and Acquired Factor Deficiencies

For menorrhagia occurring in any of the other congenital coagulation or platelet disorders, estrogens or OCPs, with or without DDAVP, are considered first-line treatment. If bleeding is difficult to control despite these measures, antifibrinolytic agents (Amicar, tranexamic acid) can be added. When coagulopathies are acquired due to a drug effect, eliminating the drug may be sufficient to stop menorrhagia. When the etiology cannot be eliminated, e.g., thrombocytopenia due to chemotherapy or transient anticoagulation, temporary transfusion support may be indicated.

The antifibrinolytic agents Amicar (epsilon-aminocaproic acid) and tranexamic acid can be used intravenously or topically for menorrhagia; these are commonly used for oropharyngeal and genitourinary bleeding in hemophilia A and B (82-84).

The specific treatment regimens for congenital bleeding disorders (see Table 9-3) have not been systematically evaluated for menorrhagia; guidelines are suggested, however, based on their general clinical use. When estrogens cannot be used because of contraindications, complications, or lack of efficacy, factor or blood products should be considered. In this context, it should be recognized that cryoprecipitate is not virally inactivated and thus is no longer recommended for mild hemophilia A (74). For symptomatic hemophilia A carriers, DDAVP at 30 μg/kg is the initial therapy of choice; for the very rare woman who is an extremely lionized hemophilia A carrier, recombinant or purified factor VIII is recommended (85). Similarly, menorrhagia in a severe hemophilia B carrier may require factor IX infusion (86). For such women who are pregnant, factor therapy is considered safer than DDAVP because of the latter's side effects. Factor therapy in pregnant women who are hemophilia carriers is used for symptomatic bleeding, and before and for 3-5 days after childbirth (32).

Cryoprecipitate is the product of choice for individuals with fibrinogen deficiency (87), dysfibrinogenemia, and factor XIII deficiency (59). Fresh-frozen plasma is the recommended treatment for coagulopathies for which purified factor is unavailable, including II, V, X, and XI (88). Before platelets contain factor V in their granules, platelet transfusion can also be used (in lieu of FFP) in factor V deficiency, especially when infrequent (e.g., outpatient) therapy is needed. Individuals with factor VII deficiency may be treated with recombinant factor VIIa (NovoSeven) (89).

For individuals with bleeding due to vitamin K deficiency, any offending drug (antibiotic, warfarin) should be stopped, and vitamin K replaced. This can be done on a non-emergency basis using oral vitamin K 2-10 mg daily. If bleeding is an emergency, or a procedure is needed, transfusion of FFP will achieve rapid correction, but vitamin K replacement may still be needed for chronic control of bleeding (90).

Genitourinary bleeding due to liver disease is generally treated with fresh frozen plasma to replace clotting factors and cryoprecipitate for hypo- and dysfibrinogenemia (14,60,91); platelets are rarely given for the mild thrombocytopenia associated with hypersplenism (92). Preliminary reports also suggest that recombinant VIIa (NovoSeven) may correct hepatic coagulopathy. It is important to realize that hepatic coagulation abnormalities without concomitant bleeding do not require treatment (unless an invasive procedure is anticipated); FFP causes significant volume overload, and recombinant VIIa has been associated with thrombosis. In contrast to liver failure, the bleeding patient with DIC should be vigorously treated to ameliorate the underlying disorder and supported simultaneously with platelets, cryoprecipitate, and FFP (87,93).

An extremely rare cause of postpartum bleeding is an acquired factor inhibitor or antibody, most often directed against factor VIII. Treatment of the underlying autoantibody is accomplished with prednisone and cytoxan (36,94). Bleeding symptoms are usually severe and have a hemophilia phenotype; effective therapy requires either a bypass factor complex (FEIBA, Autoplex) (95,96), or recombinant VIIa (NovoSeven) (89).

Chronic Medical Anticoagulation

Women who are chronically anticoagulated and develop menorrhagia require individualized management; several strategies can be evaluated. Induction of amenorrhea with hormonal treatment is one option. An IVC filter may be considered as a substitute for anticoagulation in the rare situations in which anticoagulation is not possible, with the recognition that the filter may be only temporarily helpful and may embolize. Different modes of anticoagulation can be considered, including low-intensity warfarin or low-molecular-weight heparin, to lessen the intensity of menorrhagia.

Summary

Menorrhagia is a significant health problem for women, particularly those with coagulation disorders. Menorrhagia should be considered to represent a bleeding disorder and should prompt a basic work-up for bleeding disorders. Through careful history and examination and judicious laboratory screening prior to invasive procedures, one can successfully treat these disorders, avoid unnecessary procedures, and improve the overall health care delivery for women with menorrhagia.

REFERENCES

1. Fraser IS. Menorrhagia: a pragmatic approach to the understanding of causes and the need for investigations. Br J Obstet Gynaecol. 1994;101(Suppl 11):3-7.

2. von Willebrand disease in gynecologic practice. ACOG Committee Opinion No. 263. American College of Obstetricians and Gynecologists. Obstet Gynecol. 2001;98:1185-6.

3. Foulkes J. Assessing blood flow in practice. Practitioner. 1996;240:235-41.

4. Hallberg L, Hogdahl AM, Nilsson L, Rybo G. Menstrual blood loss: a population study. Acta Obstet Gynecol Scand. 1966;45:320-51.

5. Smith SK. Hysterectomy: why and when? In: Smith SK, ed. Dysfunctional Uterine Bleeding. London: Royal Society of Medicine Press; 1994:107.

6. Shaw RW. Conference Proceedings: introduction. Br J Obstet Gynaecol. 1994;101:1-2.

7. Claessens EA, Cowell CA. Acute adolescent menorrhagia. Am J Obstet Gynecol. 1981; 139:277-80.

8. Edlund M, Blomback M, von Schoultz B, Andersson D. On the value of menorrhagia as a predictor for coagulation disorders. Am J Hematol. 1996;53:234-8.

9. Holmberg L, Nilsson IM. von Willebrand disease. Eur J Haematol. 1992;48:127-41.

10. Ragni MV, Bontempo FA, Cortese-Hassett AL. von Willebrand disease and bleeding in women. Haemophilia. 1999; 5:313-17.

11. Centers for Disease Control and Prevention. Report on the Universal Data Collection Program (UDC). Atlanta: U.S. Department of Health and Human Services; 2002;4:8.

12. von Willebrand EA. Hereditar pseudohemofili. Finska Lak Handl. 1926;67:7-12.

13. Roberts HR, Hoffman M. Other clotting factor deficiencies. In: Hematology: Basic Principles and Practice, 3rd ed. Hoffman R, Benz EJ, Shattil SJ, et al, eds. New York: Churchill Livingstone; 2000:1912-24.

14. Martinez J. Quantitative and qualitative disorders of fibrinogen. Basic Principles and Practice, 3rd ed. Hoffman R, Benz EJ, Shattil SJ, et al, eds. New York: Churchill Livingstone; 2000:1924-36.

15. Brenner PF. Differential diagnosis of abnormal uterine bleeding. Am J Obstet Gynecol. 1996;175:765-91.

16. Dodson MG. Use of transvaginal ultrasound in diagnosing the etiology of menometrorrhagia. J Reprod Med. 1994;39:362-72.

17. Foster PA. The reproductive health of women with von Willebrand disease unresponsive to DDAVP: results of an international survey. Thromb Haemostas. 1995;74:784-90.

18. La Fon J. Exploring von Willebrand Disease. New York: The National Hemophilia Foundation; 1992:1-21.

19. Gill JC, Endres-Brooks J, Bauer PJ, et al. The effect of ABO blood group on the diagnosis of von Willebrand disease. Blood. 1987;9:1691-5.

20. Mandalaki T, Louizou C, Dmitriadou C, Symeonides PH. Variations in factor VIII during the menstrual cycle in normal women. N Engl J Med. 1980;302:1093-4.

21. Rickles FR, Hoyer LW, Rick ME, Ahr DJ. The effects of epinephrine infusion in patients with von Willebrand's disease. J Clin Invest. 1976; 57:1618-25.

22. Coller BS, Schneiderman PI: Clinical evaluation of hemorrhagic disorders: the bleeding history and differential diagnosis of purpura. In: Hematology: Basic Principles and Practice, 3rd ed. Hoffman R, Benz EJ, Shattil SJ, et al, eds. New York: Churchill Livingstone; 2000:1824-40.

23. Wester J, Sixma JJ, Geuze JJ, Heynen H. Morphology of the haemostatic plug in human skin wounds: transformation of the plug. Lab Invest. 1979;41:182-92.

24. George JN, Woolf SH, Raskob GE, et al. Immune thrombocytopenic purpura: a practice guideline developed by explicit methods for the American Society of Hematology. Blood. 1996;88:3-40.

25. Daniak N. Hematologic complications of renal disease. In: Basic Principles and Practice, 3rd ed. Hoffman R, Benz EJ, Shattil SJ, et al, eds. New York: Churchill Livingstone; 2000:2357-73.

26. Sadler JE. A revised classification of von Willebrand disease. Thromb Haemost. 1994; 71:520-5.

27. Nichols WC, Ginsburg D. von Willebrand disease. Medicine. 1997;76:1-20.

28. Miller JL, Kupinski JM, Castella A, Ruggieri ZM. von Willebrand factor binds to platelets and induces aggregation in platelet-type but not type IIB von Willebrand disease. J Clin Invest. 1983;72:1532-42.

29. Weiss HJ, Meyer D, Rabinowitz R, et al. Pseudo-von-Willebrand disease: an intrinsic platelet defect with aggregation by unmodified human factor VIII/von Willebrand factor and enhanced absorption of its high-molecular weight multimers. N Engl J Med. 1982;306:326-3.

30. Joist JH, Cowan JF, Zimmerman TS. Acquired von Willebrand disease: evidence for a quantitative and qualitative factor VIII disorder. N Engl J Med. 1978;298:988-91.

31. Budde U, Bergmann F, Michiels JJ. Acquired von Willebrand syndrome: experience from 2 years in single laboratory compared with data from the literature and an international registry. Semin Thromb Hemostas. 2002;28:227-37.

32. Costa JM, Vidaud D, Laurendeau I, et al. Somatic mosaicism and compound heterozygosity in female hemophilia B. Blood. 2000;96:1585-7.

33. Bolton Maggs PHB. Bleeding problems in factor XI deficient women. Haemophilia. 1995;5:155-9.

34. Rodeghiro F, Castaman G, Dini E. Epidemiological investigation of the prevalence of von Willebrand disease. Blood. 1987;69:454-9.

35. Kadir RA, Economides EDL, Sabin CA, et al. Frequency of inherited bleeding disorders in women with menorrhagia. Lancet. 1999;36:21-7.

36. Feinstein DI. Inhibitors of blood coagulation. In: Basic Principles and Practice, 3rd ed. Hoffman R, Benz EJ, Shattil SJ, et al, eds. New York: Churchill Livingstone; 2000: 1963-82.

37. Norred CL. Complementary and alternative medicine use by surgical patients. AORN J. 2002;76:1013-21.

38. Zimmerman TS, Ratnoff OD, Powell AE. Immunologic differentiation of classic hemophilia (factor 8 deficiency) and von Willebrand disease, with observation on combined deficiencies of antihemophilic factor and proaccelerin (factor V) and an acquired circulating anticoagulant against antihemophilic factor. J Clin Invest. 1976; 50:244-54.

39. Sultan Y, Simeon J, Caen JP. Electrophoretic heterogeneity of normal factor VIII/von Willebrand protein, and abnormal electrophoretic mobility in patients with von Willebrand disease. J Lab Clin Med. 1976;87:185-97.

40. Lamme S, Wallmark A, Holmberg L, et al. The use of monoclonal antibodies in measuring factor VIII/von Willebrand factor. Scand J Clin Lab Invest. 1985;15:17-26.

41. Silveira AMV, Yamahoto T, Adamsson L, et al. Application of an enzyme-linked immuno-sorbent assay (ELISA) to von Willebrand factor and its derivatives. Thromb Res. 1986;43:91-102.

42. Ginsburg D, Handin RI, Bonthron DT, et al. Human von Willebrand factor (vWF): isolation of complementary DNA (cDNA) clones and chromosomal localization. Science. 1985;228:1401-6.

43. MacFarlane DE, Stibbe K, Kirby EP, et al. A method for assaying von Willebrand factor (ristocetin cofactor). Thromb Diath Haemorrh. 1975;34:306-8.

44. Ermens AAM, de Wild PJ, van der Graaf F. Four agglutination assays evaluated for measurement of von Willebrand factor (ristocetin cofactor) activity. Clin Chem. 1995;41: 510-14.

45. Mielke CH, Kaneshiro MM, Macher JA, et al. The standardized normal bleeding time and its prolongation by aspirin. Blood. 1969;34:204-15.

46. Kumar R, Ansell JE, Canoso RT, Deykin D. Clinical trials of a new bleeding time device. Am J Clin Pathol. 1978;70:642-5.

47. Favaloro EJ, Facey D, Grispo L. Laboratory assessment of von Willebrand factor: use of different assays can influence the diagnosis of von Willebrand disease, depending on differing sensitivity to sample preparation and differential recognition of high molecular weight von Willebrand factor forms. Am J Clin Pathol. 1995;104:264-71.

48. Raines G, Aumann H, Sykes S, Street A. Multimeric analysis of von Willebrand factor by molecular sieving electrophoresis in sodium dodecyl sulphate agarose gel. Thromb Res. 1990;60:201-12.

49. Howard M, Firkin BG. Ristocetin: a new tool in the investigation of platelet aggregation. Thromb Diath Haemorrh. 1971;26:362-9.

50. Carcao MD, Blanchette VS, Derek S, et al. Assessment of thrombocytopenic disorders using the platelet function analyzer (PFA 100). Br J Hematol. 2002;117:961-4.

51. Michhiels JJ, van de Velde A, van Vliet HHD, et al. Response of von Willebrand factor parameters to desmopressin in patients with type 1 and type 2 congenital von Willebrand disease: diagnostic and therapeutic implications. Semin Thromb Hemostas. 2002;28:111-31.

52. O'Connor H, Broadbent JAM, Magos AL, McPherson K. Medical Research Council randomized trial of endometrial resection versus hysterectomy in management of menorrhagia. Lancet. 1997;349:897-901.

53. Lalonde A. Evaluation of surgical options in menorrhagia. Br J Obstet Gynecol. 1994; 101:8-14.

54. Alperin JB. Estrogens and surgery in women with von Willebrand disease. Am J Med. 1982;73:36-71.

55. Mangal AK, Naiman SC. Oral contraceptives and von Willebrand disease. Can Med Assoc J. 1983;128:1274.

56. Harrison RL, McKee PA. Estrogen stimulates von Willebrand factor production by cultured endothelial cells. Blood. 1984;63:657-5.

57. Mannucci PM. How I treat patients with von Willebrand disease. Blood. 2001;97:1915-9.

58. Foster PA. The reproductive health of women with von Willebrand disease unresponsive to DDAVP: results of an international survey. Subcommittee on von Willebrand Factor of the Scientific and Standardization Committee of the ISTH. Thromb Haemost. 1995;74;784-90.

59. Amris CJ, Hilden M. Treatment of factor XIII deficiency with cryoprecipitate. Thromb Diath Haemorrh. 1968;20:528-33.

60. Kadir RA, Lee CA, Sabin CA, et al. Pregnancy in women with von Willebrand disease or factor XI deficiency. Br J Obstet Gynecol. 1998;105:314-21.

61. Ragni MV, Lusher JM, Koerper MA, et al. Safety and immunogenicity of subcutaneous hepatitis A vaccine in children with hemophilia. Haemophilia. 2000;6:98-103.

62. Health and Public Policy Committee, American College of Physicians. Hepatitis B vaccine. Ann Intern Med. 1984;100:149.

63. Bennett JS. Hereditary disorders of platelet function. In: Hematology: Basic Principles and Practice, 3rd ed. Hoffman R, Benz EJ, Shattil SJ, et al, eds. New York: Churchill Livingstone; 2000;2154-71.

64. Cines DB, Blanchette VS. Medical progress: immune thrombocytopenic purpura. N Engl J Med. 2002;346:995-1008.

65. Kelton JG. Heparin-induced thrombocytopenia: an overview. Blood Reviews. 2002;16:77-80.

66. Moake JL. Studies on the pathophysiology of thrombotic thrombocytopenic purpura. Semin Hematol. 1997;34:83.

67. George JN, Shattil SJ. Acquired disorders of platelet function. In: Hematology: Basic Principles and Practice , 3rd ed. Hoffman R, Benz EJ, Shattil SJ, et al, eds. New York: Churchill Livingstone; 2000:2172-86.

68. Mannucci PM, Ruggeri ZM, Pareti FI, et al. Deamino-8-D-arginine vasopressin: a new pharmacological approach to the management of hemophilia and von Willebrand disease. Lancet. 1977;1:869-72.

69. Kaufmann JE, Oksdhe A, Wollheim CB, et al. Vasopressin-induced von Willebrand factor secretion from endothelial cells involves V2 receptors and CAMP. J Clin Invest. 2000;106:107-16.

70. Leissinger C, Becton D, Cornell C, Gill JC. High-dose DDAVP intranasal spray (Stimate) for the prevention and treatment of bleeding in patients with mild hemophilia A, mild or moderate type 1 von Willebrand disease and symptomatic carriers of hemophilia A. Haemophilia. 2001;7:258-6

71. Rose EH, Aledort LM. Nasal spray desmopressin (DDAVP) for mild hemophilia A and von Willebrand. Ann Intern Med. 1991;114:563-8.

72. Vora AJ, Sampson BM, Farnsworth HJ, Preston FE. High dose intranasal desmopressin (DDAVP) in the management of women with menorrhagia and von Willebrand disease. Thromb Haemost. 1993;69:1184.

73. Lethagan S, Harris AS, Nilsson IM. Intransal desmopressin (DDAVP) by spray in mild hemophilia A and von Willebrand disease type 1. Blut. 1990;60:187-91.

74. Rodeghiero F, Castaman G, Meyer D, Mannucci PM. Replacement therapy with virus-inactivated plasma concentrates in von Willebrand disease. Vox Sang. 1992;62:193-9.

75. Dunn AL, Powers JR, Ribeiro MJ, et al. Adverse events during the use of intranasal desmopressin acetate for haemophilia A and von Willebrand disease: a case report and review of 40 patients. Haemophilia. 2002;6:11-4.

76. Smith TJ, Gill JC, Ambroso DR, Hathaway WE. Hyponatremia and seizures in young children given DDAVP. Am J Hematol. 1989;31:199-202.

77. Holmberg L, Nilsson IM, Borge L, et al. Platelet aggregation induced by 1-desamino-8-D-arginine vasopressin (DDAVP) in type IIB von Willebrand disease. N Engl J Med 1983;309:816-21.

78. Menache D, Aronson DL, Darr F, et al. Pharmaco-kinetics of von Willebrand factor and factor VIII:C in patients with severe von Willebrand disease (type 3 vWD): estimation of the rate of factor VIII:C synthesis. Br J Haematol. 1996;94:740-5.

79. Mannucci PM, Chediak J, Hanna W, et al. Treatment of von Willebrand disease with a high-purity factor VIII/ von Willebrand factor concentrate: a prospective, multicenter study. Blood. 2002;99:450-6.

80. Dobrokovska A, Krzensk U, Chediak JR. Pharmacokinetics, efficacy and safety of Humate-P in von Willebrand disease. Haemophilia. 1998;4:33-9.

81. Schwarz HP, Schlokat U, Mitterer A, et al. Recombinant von Willebrand factors: insight into structure and function through infusion studies in animals with severe von Willebrand disease. Sem Thromb Hemostas. 2002;28:215-25.

82. Walsh PM, Rizza CR, Matthews JM, et al. Epsilon aminocaproic acid therapy for dental extractions in haemophilia and Christmas disease: a double-blind controlled trial. BMJ. 1971;20:463-75.

83. Ong YL, Hull DR, Mayne EE. Case report: menorrhagia in von Willebrand disease successfully treated with single daily dose tranexamic acid. Haemophilia. 1998;4:63-5.

84. Bonnar J, Sheppard BL. Treatment of menorrhagia during menstruation: randomized controlled trial of ethamsylate, mefenamic acid, and tranexamic acid. BMJ. 1996;313: 579-82.

85. Lusher JM, Arkin S, Abildgaard CF, Schwartz RS. Recombinant factor VIII for the treatment of previously untreated patients with hemophilia A. N Engl J Med. 1993;328:453-9.

86. Roth DA, Kessler CM, Pasi KJ, et al. Human recombinant factor IX: safety and efficacy studies in patients with hemophilia B. Blood. 2001;98:3600-6.

87. Hattersley PG, Dimick ML. Cryoprecipitates in treatment of congenital fibrinogen deficiency. Transfusion. 1969;9:261-4.

88. National Institutes of Health Consensus Conference: Fresh-frozen plasma. Plasma. 1985;253:551.

89. Lusher J, Ingerslev J, Roberts H, Hedner U. Clinical experience with recombinant factor VIIa. Blood Coagul Fibrinolysis. 1998;9:119-28.

90. Furie BC, Furie B. Vitamin K metabolism and disorders. In: Basic Principles and Practice, 3rd ed. Hoffman R, Benz EJ, Shattil SJ, et al, eds. New York: Churchill Livingstone; 2000;1958-62.

91. Ragni MV. Liver disease, organ transplantation, and hemostasis. In: Consultative Thrombosis and Hemostasis. Kitchens CS, Alving B, Kessler C, eds. New York: Harcourt Brace; 2002:481-91.

92. Zalusky R, Furie B. Hematologic complications of liver disease and alcoholism. In: Basic Principles and Practice, 3rd ed. Hoffman R, Benz EJ, Shattil SJ, et al, eds. New York: Churchill Livingstone; 2000:2350-6.

93. Calverley DC, Liebman HA. Disseminated intravascular coagulation. In: Basic Principles and Practice, 3rd ed. Hoffman R, Benz EJ, Shattil SJ, et al. New York: Churchill Livingstone; 2000:1983-95.

94. Schaffer LG, Phillips MD. Successful treatment of acquired hemophilia with oral immunosuppressive therapy. Ann Intern Med. 1997;127:206-9.

95. Lusher JM, Shapiro SS, Palascak JE, et al. Efficacy of prothrombin-complex concentrates in hemophiliacs with antibodies to factor VIII: a multicenter therapeutic trial. N Engl J Med. 1980;303:421-5.

96. Sjamsoedin LJM, Heijnen L, Mauser-Bunschoten EP, et al. The effect of activated prothrombin-complex concentrate (FEIBA) on joint and muscle bleeding in patients with hemophilia A antibodies to factor VIII: a double-blind clinical trial. N Engl J Med. 1981;305:717-21.

10

Menstrual and Reproductive Issues in Women with Chronic Medical Problems

Deborah B. Ehrenthal, MD
Renee K. Kottenhahn, MD

There are a growing number of reproductive-age women who live with chronic medical problems. Chronic disease related to an unhealthy lifestyle is increasingly more common: one in three women in the United States are obese, almost 9% are diabetic, and 20% smoke tobacco. In addition, improved medical care has allowed women to enter their reproductive years with what were once life-threatening diseases. Women with underlying medical problems commonly develop changes in their menstrual cycles and fertility related to their underlying disease process or their medications. They also present complex clinical issues that may strongly affect their choices of contraception, preconception care, and pregnancy risk. This chapter provides the primary care provider with the tools needed to counsel these patients and guide them in important decision-making.

After an overview of contraceptive guidelines, the chapter is organized by disease state. The menstrual changes seen commonly with each medical problem are described briefly; further guidance on their evaluation and management is given in Chapters 2 to 6. Recommendations for contraceptive use are described in detail for each medical condition along with important clinical issues that need to be discussed as part of preconception counseling. For a complete discussion of pregnancy-related medical complications, the reader is referred to *Medical Care of the Pregnant Patient* (1).

Contraceptive Risk and Benefit

Contraceptive efficacy and risk are important issues for many female patients. The efficacy of the various methods of contraception are given in Table 10-1. Historically, clinicians have been reluctant to prescribe contraception, especially hormonal contraception, for women with medical disorders because of their concerns about safety and side effects. This resulted in the "withholding" of contraception from some of the women who most needed it: women with high pregnancy-related morbidity or mortality who should avoid pregnancy

Table 10-1   Contraceptive Efficacy (Percentage of Women Experiencing Unintended Pregnancy During the First Year of Typical and Perfect Use of Contraception)

Always very effective		
Method	Typical Use	Perfect Use
Norplant	0.05	0.05
Cu IUD	0.8	0.6
LNG-IUS	0.1	0.1
Male sterilization	0.15	0.1
Female sterilization	0.5	0.5

Effective as commonly used; very effective when used correctly and consistently		
Method	Typical Use	Perfect Use
COC /patch/ring	8	0.3
Depo-Provera	3	0.3

Only somewhat effective as commonly used; effective when used correctly and consistently		
Method	Typical Use	Perfect Use
Male condom	15	2
Female condom	21	5
Diaphragm	16	6
Cervical cap		
Parous	32	20
Nulliparous	16	9
Coitus interruptus	27	4
Spermicides	29	18
Periodic abstinence	25	—
No method: 85%		

Adapted from Hatcher RA. Contraceptive Technology, 18th ed. New York: Ardent Media; 2004:226.

and women in whom preconception stabilization would significantly improve pregnancy outcomes. In 1996 the World Health Organization (WHO) published evidence-based guidelines assembled by a panel of experts. Revised in 2004, the guidelines are updated periodically and can be found on the WHO Web site (2).

The expert consultants with WHO assessed each contraceptive method and posited a risk:benefit ratio for a large array of medical diagnoses and risk factors. The guidelines utilize a simple four-category classification system, which we will use in this chapter. According to the WHO classification system, a contraceptive method is considered to be *category 1* if it is always safe in any patient with a particular condition or risk factor. An example would be the use of the copper intrauterine device (IUD) in women with hypertension. A method falls into *category 2* if the advantages of the method generally outweigh the risks in the particular setting. This would be the case with the use of combined hormonal contraceptives by a woman with a history of pregnancy-induced hypertension. Use of the method would be recommended but would require clinical follow-up to ensure safety. Next, *Category 3* comprises methods for which the advantages generally outweigh the risks. Careful clinical judgement is needed in this category; consideration of other options for contraception and clinical follow-up is essential. An example of this category would be the use of combined hormonal contraceptives by a woman with controlled hypertension. Finally, a condition for which use of the contraceptive method represents an unacceptable health risk falls into *category 4*. Use of a combined hormonal contraceptive by a woman with hypertension and coexisting vascular disease would fall into this category.

Because the WHO document provides international guidance, and because the level of clinical knowledge and experience of clinicians who may practice in settings with variable resources may vary, the document lists two categories of classification within this framework. The classification varies depending on whether clinicians with expert knowledge, experience, and judgement are available or whether the clinicians and health care providers have more limited clinical experience (Table 10-2) (2).

For a woman with chronic medical problems, preconception counseling can have a major impact on reproductive outcome and should be addressed by her physician. The presence of a chronic disease may affect a woman's reproductive options. Some women will have diminished fertility; preconception medical optimization for women with some illnesses, such as diabetes mellitus, can significantly improve pregnancy outcome. Medications may need to be adjusted before conception to prevent potentially toxic effects of the medications on the developing fetus. Pregnancy may change the course of the underlying medical illness. All of these issues should be discussed with the patient prior to conception (1).

Table 10-2　WHO Classification System for Medical Eligibility of Contraceptive Methods

Classification	With Expert Clinical Judgment	With Limited Clinical Judgment
1	Use method in any circumstances	Yes (use the method)
2	Generally use the method	Yes (use the method)
3	Method not usually recommended unless other, more appropriate methods are not available or not acceptable	No (do not use the method)
4	Method not to be used	No (do not use the method)

From Medical Eligibility Criteria for Contraceptive Use, 3rd ed. Geneva: WHO; 2004; with permission.

Diabetes Mellitus

In the United States, a staggering 8.7% of all women over age 20 have diabetes (3). Diabetes is two to four times more common in African American, Hispanic/ Latino, American Indian, and Asian/Pacific Islander women than in white women. Each year 1.3 million new cases of diabetes are diagnosed (3). Women with diabetes have a high rate of unplanned pregnancy and a surprisingly low frequency of preconception care, given their frequent contact with the medical system for the management of their chronic disease (4). Contraceptive and preconception counseling are essential parts of routine care of diabetic women because pregnancy outcome is strongly correlated with the degree of glycemic control at the time of conception. For diabetic women, multiple issues need to be considered in order to fully assess the risks associated with pregnancy and to plan for the best possible pregnancy outcome.

Menstrual Disorders and Their Management

Several studies have confirmed an increased prevalence of menstrual disturbances among women with type 1 diabetes (5-9). Menarche is delayed on average approximately 1 year in girls who present with diabetes before they reach the age of 10 (9). Thereafter, 19%-32% of young women will have menstrual irregularity, including amenorrhea, oligomenorrhea, or polymenorrhea (6,9). In one study diabetic women were found to have about twice the frequency of menstrual disturbance than was seen in the control group (9). The incidence of menstrual disturbances appears to be higher in women with complications of diabetes: those with poor glycemic control and those with a higher body mass index (BMI). The cause of menstrual abnormalities has been attributed to disruption of the normal hypothalamic-pituitary-gonadal axis, but it is not well understood.

Menstrual cycle disturbances have not been well studied in women with type 2 diabetes. However, chronic anovulation with associated oligomenor-rhea or amenorrhea is associated with a substantial increase in risk for type 2 diabetes (10). Women with irregular menses have a higher BMI, larger waist circumference, and higher waist-to-hip ratio than women with regular menses. The risk factors for both are similar: hyperinsulinemia, obesity, and more central distribution of fat. This may be related to the polycystic ovary syndrome (PCOS), which is discussed in detail in Chapter 7.

Little is known about the menopausal transition in women with diabetes. In one large cohort of women with type 1 diabetes, this population was found to be twice as likely to reach menopause earlier than nondiabetic women, after adjusting for other factors (11). When diabetic women were compared with their non-diabetic sisters, they were found to have on average a 6-year reduction in child-bearing years caused by late menarche and early menopause. The menopausal transition with type 2 diabetes is probably earlier as well. One study of women in Mexico found that women with type 2 diabetes had an earlier mean age of menopause than the non-diabetic control group (12). The suggested mechanisms for this earlier menopause include the consequences of prolonged hyperglycemia, long-term consequences of diabetes, or consequences of autoimmune disease or genetic factors.

Optimization of medical therapy to treat diabetes is a cornerstone of managing menstrual disturbances associated with diabetes. Women with signs and symptoms of PCOS should undergo a diagnostic evaluation and be managed accordingly. It is important that women with chronic anovulation and bleeding undergo evaluation to rule out endometrial hyperplasia or cancer. For women with chronic anovulation and a benign endometrium, consideration should be given to using progestins or combined hormonal contraceptives to prevent the development of endometrial hyperplasia.

Contraceptive Options

Contraception is vitally important for women with diabetes because pregnancy outcome is strongly correlated with degree of glycemic control at the time of conception (1,4). The major contraceptive issue for women with diabetes is the risk associated with the use of hormonal contraceptives. Short-term use of combination hormonal contraceptives seems to have minimal metabolic consequences for diabetes. Small studies of women with type 1 diabetes have found that oral contraceptive pill (OCP) users have similar HbA1c values and no acceleration in the development of diabetic nephropathy or retinopathy, and no adverse changes in their lipids over short (1-7 years) duration of OCP use (13,14). For women with type 2 diabetes, there are no data on the use of combined hormonal contraceptives and their relationship to the development of the long-term complications of diabetes mellitus. However, because of theoretical concerns about the development of coronary artery disease and cerebrovascular disease, WHO currently recommends that combined hormonal contraceptive use should be limited to diabetic women who are not at increased risk for cardiovascular complications: non-smoking, otherwise healthy women under age 35 who have no evidence of hypertension, nephropathy, retinopathy, or other vascular disease and have had diabetes mellitus for less than 20 years (2). If combination hormonal contraception is used, blood pressure, weight, and lipids should be monitored periodically.

For the diabetic woman with vascular disease who desires hormonal contraception, progestin-only methods are often recommended (15). The 2004 WHO guidelines place progestin preparations in category 3 for diabetic women with nephropathy, retinopathy, neuropathy, and other vascular complications of diabetes (2). Thus, progestins are not contraindicated but are to be used with caution and closely followed up. There also remains controversy over the potential effects of the progestins on glycemic control because studies of long-acting injectable progestogens in non-diabetic women have shown some impairment in glucose metabolism (16,17). This has not been studied in diabetics, and the effect, if any, is probably small.

The IUD is an excellent contraceptive choice for women with diabetes because of its high efficacy, low risk, and rapid return to fertility once removed. The contraceptive diaphragm carries with it the theoretical risk of increasing the frequency of urinary tract infections, but no published data exist. At the completion of childbearing, surgical sterilization (for either partner) is an excellent choice; in a stable couple, male sterilization avoids the increased risks of surgical intervention for the diabetic woman.

Table 10-3 summarizes the WHO guidelines for medical eligibility for hormonal contraception for women with diabetes (2).

Preconception Counseling

Women with uncontrolled diabetes are at risk for significant maternal and fetal complications. Control of diabetes at the time of conception has a major impact on pregnancy outcome. The overall rate of fetal anomalies is at least five times higher in diabetics than the general population and is improved by tight glycemic control (18). The leading cause of fetal mortality and serious morbidity is major congenital malformations (4). Fetal macrosomia is more common, as are its associated risks. Risk of congenital anomalies is correlated with the HbA1c at the time of conception.

Table 10-3   WHO Guidelines for Medical Eligibility for Hormonal Contraception
for Women with Diabetes*

	COC/R/P	POP	DMPA/NE	Cu-IUD	LNG-IUD
History of gestational diabetes	1	1	1	1	1
Diabetes without vascular disease	2	2	2	1	2
Diabetes with nephropathy/retinopathy/neuropathy, diabetes with other vascular disease, or diabetes of >20 years' duration	3/4	2	3	1	2

*See Table 10-2 for explanation of WHO categories. COC/R/P = combination oral contraceptive, ring, patch; POP = progestin-only pill; DMPA/NE = depot medroxyprogesterone acetate/norethisterone enantate; Cu-IUD = copper-bearing IUD; LNG/IUD = levonorgestrel-releasing IUD (20 μg/24 hours).

Women with significant vascular complications of diabetes should understand the high risks associated with pregnancy, as should women with uncontrolled diabetes, end-stage renal disease, coronary heart disease, or untreated
proliferative retinopathy (1,4). Poor glycemic control, maternal nephropathy,
and hypertension increase the risk of fetal adverse outcomes. Pregnancy in
women with untreated coronary artery disease is associated with a high mortality rate, and women with significant risk factors for cardiac disease may benefit
from stress testing prior to conception. Pregnancy may accelerate the progression of diabetic nephropathy, but in most cases renal function will return to
baseline after delivery. Unfortunately, almost half of women with moderate-to-
severe renal disease will have a permanent decline in renal function. There can
be worsening of diabetic retinopathy during the pregnancy. These patients
should be seen by an ophthalmologist before conception and followed closely
during their pregnancy.

Fertility is generally preserved in women with diabetes until the development of renal insufficiency. For diabetic women, multiple issues need to be
considered in order to fully assess the risks associated with pregnancy and to
plan for the best possible pregnancy outcome. Preconception care of women
with diabetes has been shown to significantly improve outcome and is
strongly recommended by the American Diabetes Association (4). Adequate
contraception during the period of optimization is essential. Critical elements
of preconception counseling include an assessment of the complications of
diabetes, review and adjustment of medications, and optimization of glycemic
control. Ideally, angiotensin-converting enzyme (ACE) inhibitors or adrener-
gic receptor binders (ARBs) and statins are stopped during the time the patient is actively trying to conceive.

KEY POINTS FOR WOMEN WITH DIABETES

Menstrual changes	• Oligomenorrhea, amenorrhea, polymenorrhea, especially if poorly controlled.
Contraceptive options	• Combined hormonal contraceptives may be used by healthy non-smokers under age 35 who do not have hypertension, nephropathy, retinopathy, or vascular disease; otherwise, progestin-only preparations are a better choice.
	• Barriers, IUD, and sterilization are all good choices.
Fertility	• Generally preserved until renal insufficiency develops.
	• Menopause may be earlier.
Preconception counseling	• Determine the extent of end-organ damage.
	• Optimize glycemic control; stop ACE inhibitor/ARB (or follow closely and stop promptly upon confirmation of conception); stop oral hypoglycemics and lipid-lowering medications.
	• Refer for ophthalmologic evaluation.

Obesity

The prevalence of obesity continues to grow in the United States and other western countries. The 1999-2002 National Health and Nutrition Examination survey found that 30% of adults were obese (BMI ≥30) (19). These numbers are even higher among African American and Hispanic American women. Obesity and its co-morbidities (diabetes, hypertension, cardiovascular disease, PCOS) can affect a woman's menstrual and reproductive functions. Obese women are at increased risk of menstrual abnormalities, infertility, and endometrial cancer, as well as pregnancy-associated morbidity.

Menstrual Disorders and Their Management

Menarche occurs at a younger age in obese girls than in normal-weight girls (20). Obese women frequently experience menstrual irregularities such as amenorrhea, abnormal uterine bleeding, and premature menopause (21). This is usually the result of chronic anovulation and is attributed to the effects of higher levels of plasma androgens, insulin, and luteinizing hormone, as well as lower levels of sex-hormone binding globulin. There is significant overlap between women with "simple" obesity and women with hyperandrogenic obesity. Obese women with PCOS appear to be more likely to experience more menstrual irregularity than do thin women with PCOS (21).

Evidence suggests that sustained weight loss will lead to improvement in menstrual patterns (22). Exercise and weight loss have been shown to decrease androgen levels and to re-establish normal menstrual cycles. Clinical improvement is seen even with a modest degree (5%-10% of body weight) of weight loss. Evidence thus far does not support improved outcomes with the low-carbohydrate diets when compared with other types of low-calorie diets (23-25). Weight loss via bariatric surgery has been found to resolve the majority of menstrual irregularities and to improve fertility (26,27).

Obese women are at increased risk for the development of endometrial cancer. It is important in women with long-standing chronic anovulation to undergo evaluation of the endometrium if they are experiencing irregular bleeding to look for underlying endometrial hyperplasia and cancer. This is usually done by an endometrial biopsy in the office or by evaluating the endometrial strip by pelvic ultrasound.

In the absence of other contraindications, combination oral contraceptives manage irregular menses and lower the risk of endometrial cancer.

Contraceptive Options

There are no contraindications to the use of combined hormonal contraceptives in women who are overweight or obese, but weight may affect efficacy and side effects. Combined hormonal contraceptives may have a higher failure rate for women who are obese. This has been verified by studies using the contraceptive patch, leading to recommendations for use only in women under 199 lb (28,29). Women who are morbidly obese may be at a higher risk of venous thromboembolic disease, hypertension, and cardiac disease, and these risks should be taken into account when weighing contraceptive options. Injectable progestin methods may be associated with significant weight gain and bloating, although evidence for this remains mixed. There are theoretical risks of decreased efficacy of the diaphragm method if there are significant changes in weight. The IUD remains an excellent option for birth control.

Table 10-4 gives WHO guidelines for medical eligibility for hormonal contraception for obese women (2).

Table 10-4   WHO Guidelines for Medical Eligibility for Hormonal Contraception for Women with Obesity*

	COC/R/P	POP	DMPA/NE	Cu-IUD	LNG-IUD
BMI ≥ 30 kg/m²	2	1	1	1	1

*See Table 10-2 for explanation of WHO categories. COC/R/P = combination oral contraceptive, ring, patch; POP = progestin-only pill; DMPA/NE = depot medroxyprogesterone acetate/norethisterone enantate; Cu-IUD = copper-bearing IUD; LNG/IUD = levonorgestrel-releasing IUD (20 μg/24 hours).

Preconception Counseling

Obese women have significantly higher obstetric risks and should be encouraged to lose weight before conception. Obesity is associated with an increased risk of miscarriage, larger babies, longer hospital stays, and increased antepartum, intrapartum, and post-partum risks and complications (21,22,30,31). There is a clear association between increased BMI and a higher incidence of infertility. During pregnancy obese women are at increased risk for the development of chronic hypertension, gestational diabetes, preeclampsia, pregnancy-induced hypertension, obstructive sleep apnea, and urinary tract infections. At the time of delivery there is an increased risk of anesthesia-related difficulties, a higher caesarean section rate, macrosomia, preeclampsia/eclampsia, and shoulder dystocia. The postpartum period is more likely to be complicated by postpartum hemorrhage, endometritis, chronic hypertension, venous thromboembolic disease, preeclampsia/eclampsia, diabetes, wound dehiscence, and infection (22,30). Infants born to obese mothers have a two-fold increased risk of neural tube defects, suggesting that prenatal vitamin supplementation with folic acid is even more essential in this group (32).

Women who have undergone bariatric surgery and lost weight will see improved fertility (27). Although there have been some reports of poor pregnancy outcomes following bariatric surgery, larger reviews have found that if pregnancy occurs after the period of rapid weight loss (at least 1-2 years after surgery), it does not in general pose an increased risk for maternal or fetal complications (26,33,34). In fact, one study found that pregnancies carried by women after significant weight loss had fewer complications than during their pregnancies before bariatric surgery. It is generally recommended that women wait at least 1 year after surgery before attempting pregnancy, by which time the majority of weight loss has occurred.

KEY POINTS FOR OBESE WOMEN

Menstrual changes	• Amenorrhea, oligomenorrhea, and dysfunctional uterine bleeding due to chronic anovulation.
	• Increased risk of endometrial hyperplasia and endometrial cancer.
Contraceptive options	• Combination hormonal contraceptives may have a higher failure risk.
	• Risk of venous thromboembolism associated with estrogen use is higher.
	• Progestins may cause weight gain.

(cont'd.)

KEY POINTS FOR OBESE WOMEN *(continued)*	
Fertility	• Decreased; weight loss improves fertility.
Preconception counseling	• Higher obstetrical risks; weight loss prior to conception probably improves outcome.
	• Increased risk of neural tube defects makes folic acid supplementation more essential.
	• Pregnancy should be delayed 1-2 years following bariatric surgery.

Tobacco Use

The rate of smoking by women in the United States remains high (35). The well-known cardiovascular risks associated with smoking are further increased when women smokers use combined hormonal contraceptives. Smoking has some small effects on the menstrual cycle and fertility, but, more importantly, smoking among pregnant women is the major cause of low birth weight (36,37). Smoking cessation before conception and during pregnancy can significantly improve pregnancy outcome.

Menstrual Disorders and Their Management

A study of menstrual history in a group of women smokers found increased daily bleeding but a shortened duration of bleeding that was most pronounced in heavy smokers. There was no significant change in cycle length, but there was an increased duration of dysmenorrhea (38). Menopause occurs 1-2 years earlier in women who smoke (39).

Contraceptive Options

Cigarette smoking increases the cardiovascular risks associated with the use of combination hormonal contraception (40). The increased risk is significantly greater with increasing age and with increasing number of cigarettes smoked. Use of combined hormonal contraceptives by women who smoke should be strongly discouraged, especially in women 35 and older. Other methods are not associated with any significant risk and are the preferred methods of contraception in this group (2).

Table 10-5 gives WHO guidelines for medical eligibility for hormonal contraception for women who smoke (2).

Table 10-5   WHO Guidelines for Medical Eligibility for Hormonal Contraception for Women Who Smoke*

	COC/R/P	POP	DMPA/NE	Cu-IUD	LNG-IUD
Age < 35 years	2	1	1	1	1
Age ≥ 35 years					
<15 cigs/day	3	1	1	1	1
≥15 cigs/day	4	1	1	1	1

*See Table 10-2 for explanation of WHO categories. COC/R/P = combination oral contraceptive, ring, patch; POP = progestin-only pill; DMPA/NE = depot medroxyprogesterone acetate/norethisterone enantate; Cu-IUD = copper-bearing IUD; LNG/IUD = levonorgestrel-releasing IUD (20 µg/24 hours).

Preconception Counseling

Cigarette smoking is the most significant modifiable cause of adverse pregnancy outcomes (41). An extensive review by Hughes suggests that fertility is decreased in women who smoke, and a strong relationship was observed between the number of cigarettes smoked per day and decreased fertility (42). Smoking has long been known to have adverse effects on the developing fetus. Fetal effects are related to the effects of carbon monoxide from the smoke as well as the effects of nicotine, which crosses the placenta and is more concentrated in fetal circulation. Smoking is associated with an increased risk of preterm delivery, increased perinatal and neonatal mortality, and is the leading cause of low birth weight. Children of smokers have an increased risk of dying of sudden infant death syndrome and are more likely to have cognitive and behavioral problems (43).

Women who smoke should be urged to quit before conception. Smoking cessation during early pregnancy produces the most significant improvement in pregnancy outcome, but women who quit as late as the 30th gestational week will see benefits and reduction in low birth rate (44). Behavioral smoking cessation programs should be made available to all pregnant smokers and have been shown to have a significant impact.

Many experts believe that women who have been unable to quit smoking with behavioral therapy should consider pharmacologic therapy (45). All nicotine replacement products fall into pregnancy category D. Nicotine levels in the fetus, however, are lower when women use the nicotine patch or gum than when they smoke (46). This suggests that the risks associated with the use of nicotine replacement may be outweighed by the benefits for women who are heavy smokers (44,46). Bupropion, an antidepressant used to significantly improve quit rates, is a category B medication whose role in smoking cessation during pregnancy has not yet been evaluated (44).

Alcohol and Illicit Substance Abuse

Women who are chronic alcohol and illicit substance abusers have a high incidence of menstrual disturbances. Although there is a decreased fertility rate, the low rate of contraception use in this group leads to a high rate of unintended pregnancies (47). Alcohol and substance abuse strongly affect conscious choices about contraception and pregnancy.

Menstrual Disorders and Their Management

Women who are chronic alcohol abusers develop a variety of menstrual symptoms because of the effects of alcohol itself and the liver disease resulting from its use (48). Oligomenorrhea, amenorrhea, and menometrorrhagia are commonly seen due to ovulatory failure and histologic changes in the uterine epithelium caused by the alcohol (48). Alcohol also affects the pulsatile secretion of gonadotropin-releasing hormone, which affects dopamine levels, resulting in elevated prolactin levels. Alcohol can have direct toxic effects on the ovary, leading to decreased estrogen and progesterone production. Alcoholic women enter menopause earlier than control women (49).

A small number of studies of heroin users and women on methadone maintenance suggest that a majority of women using these substances experience abnormal menstrual patterns and infertility (50-52). Menstrual changes were found to be the result of hypothalamic dysfunction: an absence of cyclic gonadotropin release, resulting in amenorrhea (53). For women on a methadone maintenance program, tolerance appears to develop and ovulation can resume (53,54). For this reason, contraception is important for women on methadone maintenance who are at risk for future pregnancy even if they are initially amenorrheic. Women users of cocaine have been less well studied, but disruption in the menstrual cycle has been seen in small clinical studies as well as in animal models (55).

Amphetamine use was found in one study to be associated with increased duration of menstrual flow and increased cramping (51). Dysmenorrhea is also more common in this population, seemingly the result of the higher prevalence of pelvic inflammatory disease (50).

Contraceptive Options

The safety and efficacy of contraceptive options are affected by the presence of any medical complications of substance abuse, such as liver disease. In the absence of underlying medical problems, medication adherence is a major factor to be considered. A disorderly lifestyle makes it difficult to comply with oral contraceptives; long-acting methods such as the IUD may be the most appropriate choice (47). An IUD is contraindicated for a woman with pelvic inflammatory disease or purulent cervicitis but may be used in some settings even if she is currently at risk for sexually transmitted diseases (2). Women who are being closely monitored may be candidates for combination hormonal contraceptives or long-acting progestins. Contraception and protection from sexually transmitted diseases are both important goals, so condom use should be emphasized as well.

Preconception Counseling

Substance abuse during pregnancy carries with it substantial risk to the developing fetus and is a major public health problem. Alcohol use during pregnancy is the leading cause of mental retardation in the United States (56). The absolute risk associated with individual substances of abuse cannot be assigned due to difficulties in accurately evaluating dose and exposure (57). Some complications associated with substance abuse during pregnancy are listed in Table 10-6.

Withdrawal from opiates during pregnancy is not recommended. It is associated with significant fetal stress, and cases of fetal demise have been reported (58). The use of methadone maintenance with women who are opiate

Table 10-6 Complications Associated with Substance Abuse During Pregnancy

Alcohol	Fetal alcohol syndrome
Cocaine	Placental abruption
	Pregnancy-induced hypertension
	Uterine rupture
	Fetal growth retardation and low birth weight
	Congenital anomalies (e.g., urinary malformation, cardiac defects, ophthalmic anomalies, cerebral infarctions, hydrocephaly)
Narcotics	Fetal demise
	Low birth weight
	Premature delivery
	Symmetric growth retardation

dependent has been shown to improve perinatal outcomes (59,60). Women who use methadone as part of a comprehensive prenatal care and drug rehabilitation program have improved pregnancy outcomes (60).

KEY POINTS FOR FEMALE SUBSTANCE ABUSERS

Menstrual changes	• Narcotic users have a high frequency of amenorrhea and oligomenorrhea.
	• Alcohol users may have oligomenorrhea, amenorrhea, and menometrorrhagia as well as premature ovarian failure.
Contraceptive options	• Medical complications of abuse as well as issues of reliability direct contraceptive choice.
Fertility	• Variable.
Preconception counseling	• Address effects of addiction and recovery.
	• Improved outcome with methadone.

Eating Disorders

Anorexia nervosa and bulimia nervosa are complex disorders with psychological and medical attributes. *Anorexia* is characterized by a distorted body image and an overwhelming fear of being fat. Individuals with this disorder achieve and maintain unhealthy body weight through extreme dietary restriction, fasting, exercise, and other methods such as vomiting and purging. Anorectics tend to deny that their dieting behavior is a problem. *Bulimia* is defined by recurrent binge eating at least twice a week for at least 3 months. Patients often feel "out of control" of their behavior, compensating for these food binges by purging, vomiting, abusing laxatives or diuretics (which can lead to severe or lethal metabolic derangements), fasting, and excessive exercising. In contrast to anorexic patients, who are underweight, bulimic patients may be normal weight and even overweight and therefore often seem less visibly sick than patients with anorexia. A third category, Eating Disorder Not Otherwise Specified (assigned by the DSM IV), recognizes the nuances of disease manifestation. Menstrual disorders are extremely common in women with eating disorders and are associated with significant long-term health risks such as osteopenia and osteoporosis.

Menstrual Disorders and Their Management

Menstrual disorders are classic among girls and women with eating disorders. One of the diagnostic criteria for anorexia is, in fact, amenorrhea (for at least

3 consecutive menstrual cycles). Up to one fourth of patients with anorexia will experience loss of menses prior to weight loss (61). Patients with bulimia can have menstrual disturbances such as amenorrhea, bleeding related to anovulation, and luteal phase defects (62,63). The medical care provider should therefore be vigilant to detect eating disorders when evaluating patients with amenorrhea and other menstrual abnormalities. Questions that may be useful in eliciting a history of an eating disorder are detailed in Table 10-7.

Causes of eating disorders and the associated menstrual disturbances are multifactorial and remain poorly understood. Women with anorexia nervosa are demonstrably hypoestrogenic. Amenorrhea in patients with anorexia nervosa is attributed to impaired gonadotropin secretion, with follicle-stimulating hormone and luteinizing hormone levels measuring in the prepubertal range. Research has suggested that hypothalamic dysfunction may be attributed not just to weight loss but to nutritional insult. Hypoleptinemia has been implicated as a contributor to hormonal aberrations in both anorexic and normal weight bulimic patients (64-66).

Restoration of menstrual function can be achieved through weight recovery (for patients with anorexia) and improvement in behavior related to nutrition and eating disorders (for anorectic as well as bulimic patients). In one study of patients with anorexia, 86% had return of menses within 6 months when they reached, on average, 90% of standard body weight for their age and height (67). Thus, approximately 14% remained amenorrheic after regaining weight. The same research suggested two predictors of recovery of menstrual function: serum estradiol levels greater than 110.1 pmol/L or weight approximately 2.05

Table 10-7   Questions to Help Elicit a History of Eating Disorders

- What is the most you have ever weighed? When was that?
- What is the least you have ever weighed? When was that?
- What do you think you should weigh?
- Many women try different ways to control their weight. What have you tried?
- Have you ever had a binge, or a "pig out"? What makes up a binge? How much, how often? What ends the binge? Any triggers that you can identify that lead to a binge?
- Have you ever made yourself vomit? How many times per day? Any relation to meals? How long has this occurred?
- Have you ever used laxatives, diuretics, diet pills, or caffeine? How much, how often, and in what time frame?
- What do you do for exercise? How much, how often? How stressed do you feel if you miss a workout?
- Can you tell me what you ate in the past 24 hours? How many bites of ___?

Adapted from Gidwani GP, Rome ES. Eating Disorders. Clin Obstet Gynecol. 1997;40:601–15.

kg above the weight at which menses were lost (67). Resumption of menses is one of the primary goals of eating disorder management because amenorrhea and eating disorders of even relatively short duration may have great impact on bone density (68). Hormonal therapy with estrogen-progesterone pills, while a common practice, has not been proven to improve bone mineral density in patients with anorexia (69-71).

Contraceptive Options

Women with eating disorders should be counselled that it is possible to become pregnant despite amenorrhea, and appropriate precautions should be taken if they are sexually active. In one study, three quarters of the pregnancies were unplanned, resulting from mistaken beliefs about fertility in the presence of irregular menses (72). Combination hormonal contraceptives are a popular contraceptive choice, in part because of the unproven potential benefit for bone mineral density and the relative lack of significant medical risk in this young population. However, the use of combined hormonal contraceptives make it more difficult to use menses as a barometer for appropriate weight recovery in patients with anorexia. Depot medroxyprogesterone acetate (DMPA) should be used with extreme caution in women with eating disorders with known or potential osteopenia/osteoporosis because DMPA may further diminish bone density. IUDs do not pose any additional risk for women with eating disorders and are an excellent option. Barrier methods may be used as well.

Preconception Counseling

Limited research is available on fertility and pregnancy outcomes in women with eating disorders. Eating disorders exist on a continuum, and patients diagnosed with them require longitudinal care, whether they are overtly "sick" or in apparent recovery. Anorectic patients can be expected to have normal fertility if appropriate weight is restored, although some reports suggest an increase in pregnancy-related complications, low-birth weight, premature birth, postpartum depression, or neonatal feeding problems (73,74). In a limited study, researchers following patients over a 10-15 year period showed that current or previous history of bulimia nervosa appears to have little effect on ability to achieve pregnancy compared with the general population (75). Women whose eating disorders persist during pregnancy gain less weight, have more pregnancy-related complications, have smaller babies with lower 5-minute APGAR scores, and experience more difficulties in postpartum adjustment and breast feeding (72,76). Bulimic behaviors may progressively improve throughout pregnancy but may relapse postpartum, often with worse symptoms than before pregnancy (77). It is important for patients to understand that their ability to conceive is not a guarantee of a healthy pregnancy (or child), nor is it an indication that the eating disorder has resolved.

KEY POINTS FOR WOMEN WITH EATING DISORDERS

Menstrual changes	• Amenorrhea is part of the diagnostic criteria for anorexia.
	• Bulimics can have menstrual disturbances including amenorrhea and irregular bleeding.
Contraceptive options	• Combined hormonal contraceptives may be used but make it more difficult to use menses as a barometer for appropriate weight recovery.
	• DMPA should be used with caution due to its effect on bone mineral density.
Fertility	• Diminished in active eating disorder.
Preconception counseling	• Adverse pregnancy outcome is associated with active disease.
	• Longitudinal care of eating disorder is recommended to optimize health of mother and fetus and to prevent relapse.

The Female Athlete

Increased participation of women in sport activities has resulted in an appreciation of the effects of exercise on gynecologic health. In general, exercise is considered a beneficial activity and should be encouraged. Health risks of the highly trained female athlete, however, include psychological, reproductive, and skeletal disturbance. Among athletes, prevalence of amenorrhea ranges from 3.4% to 66%, significantly higher than the 2% to 5% prevalence of amenorrhea in the general population (78).

Menstrual Disorders and Their Management

The pathophysiology of menstrual disturbance in athletes is believed to involve disruption of the pulsatile secretion of gonadotropin-releasing hormone from the hypothalamus with resulting decreased secretion of follicle-stimulating hormone and luteinizing hormone. There is a higher incidence of delayed menarche and menstrual dysfunction in girls who started intensive athletic training before menarche (79). Decreased gonadotropin secretion results in estrogen deficiency, which, depending on severity, can delay puberty and cause oligomenorrhea, irregular menstruation, amenorrhea, osteopenia, and increased risk of fractures and osteoporosis. Young (adolescent) athletes with amenorrhea may enter adulthood with what could be an irreversible bone mass deficiency, putting them at risk for increased bone fractures throughout their lifetimes (71). Hormonal dysfunction in athletes has been attributed to alterations in estrogen metabolism, imbalance of caloric intake and energy expenditure, alterations in β-endorphin levels, and exercise changes in circulating growth factors, as well as hypoleptinemia (80,81). Hormonal profiles among amenorrheic athletes may vary depending upon the sport. Studies have shown that reproductive dysfunction in swimmers is caused by mild hyperandrogenism with a PCOS type of hormonal profile, which is distinct from the hypoestrogenic profile found in other athletes (82).

Intensity of training is another factor that can affect menstrual function in female athletes. However, research has shown that amenorrhea is seen more commonly in runners and ballet dancers (40%-50%) than in cyclists and swimmers (12%), suggesting that sports physique may be more important than sports intensity in affecting menstrual function (78,83). The "female athlete triad" diagnosis was coined to describe three synergistically detrimental disorders found in some female athletes: disordered eating, amenorrhea, and osteoporosis. It has been estimated that 15% to 62% of athletes and dancers have eating disorders, occurring more commonly among athletes participating in sports where low body weight is emphasized, such as ballet and ice skating (71).

Gynecologic evaluation of athletes is similar to non-athletes because "exercise-induced" menstrual disturbances are diagnoses of exclusion. Documentation of hypoestrogenism may be helpful in demonstrating a significant pathology in patients who are resistant to this diagnosis. Along with a comprehensive gynecologic history, patients should be questioned about their type of sport(s), intensity and quantity of training, and any history of any stress fractures. The nutritional part of the medical history should include body mass index (kg/m^2); current, desired, and maximal body weight; interest in losing weight; efforts to diet/control weight (including fasting, vomiting, laxative, diuretic and/or diet pill use, eating in isolation); and dietary restrictions (71).

For patients with the female athlete triad, the most effective treatment is modified or restricted exercise regimens and treatment of the eating disorder (84,85). Patients should be counseled that amenorrhea may take more than 6 months to reverse (67). Lifestyle changes will likely be difficult for the athlete to embrace, and consultation with an eating disorder or sports medicine specialist may be helpful. Athletes, coaches, trainers, families, and medical providers should be educated that weight is not an accurate estimate of fitness or fatness and that the consequences of the triad are significant and potentially irreversible (86).

It is not known to what extent osteopenia is reversible in women with the female athlete triad. Measurement of bone density should be part of the medical evaluation. Some experts recommend that bone densitometry scans should be performed on girls or women who have been amenorrheic for 6 months or longer and repeated yearly while they work on recovery (71). Utility of hormone replacement to improve skeletal health remains controversial because no randomized controlled studies of estrogen replacement in athletes have been published (87). To date, research has shown that estrogen therapy may be of limited or no benefit in the absence of weight gain (71). Furthermore, estrogen therapy may be contraindicated in the teenager with pubertal delay and incomplete growth. Bisphosphonates and calcitonin are also not sufficiently researched in young athletes (88). Physicians should recommend that athletes consume at least 1200 mg of calcium daily (by diet or dietary supplement).

Contraceptive Options

Combined hormonal contraceptives may be advantageous to athletes for reasons of lifestyle and convenience. Predictable, shorter, lighter periods are especially liked by athletes, who may also desire to use combined hormonal contraception to manipulate their menstrual cycles so that they not coincide with competitions (extended cycle contraception). Research has shown that OCP use has no significant effect on performance for most female endurance runners; furthermore, there is no evidence that the menstrual cycle phases significantly affect athletic (endurance running) performance (89).

As with other eating disorders, DMPA should be used with caution in women with female athlete triad because of its effect on bone mineral density. Barrier methods and IUDs are excellent contraceptive options for women athletes.

Preconception Counseling

For women who wish to conceive and for whom regular menstruation is not achieved with the primary interventions for exercise-related menstrual problems discussed previously, clomiphene citrate may be required to induce ovulation (80). Women should be advised that low weight and BMI at conception or delivery, as well as poor weight gain during pregnancy, are associated with low birth weight, premature birth, and maternal delivery complications (76).

Women athletes should be advised to discontinue any "sports enhancing" drugs or supplements before conception. They should be encouraged to have an evidence-based discussion of any complementary medicine use with their medical provider so that risks can be assessed. For the healthy pregnant woman, daily, moderate exercise (30 minutes or more) is considered beneficial. The American College of Obstetricians and Gynecologists (ACOG) advises that pregnant women avoid sports using supine positioning and sports that put them at risk for abdominal trauma or falling. Scuba diving is contraindicated in pregnancy. Warning signs to terminate exercise include vaginal bleeding, dyspnea before exertion, dizziness, headache, chest pain, muscle weakness, calf pain or swelling, preterm labor, decreased fetal movement, and amniotic fluid leakage. Women with health conditions that complicate their pregnancies should avoid physical activity until consultation with their obstetrician (90).

KEY POINTS FOR FEMALE ATHLETES

Menstrual changes	• There is a higher incidence of delayed menarche and menstrual dysfunction in girls who started intensive athletic training before menarche.
	• High-intensity training and low-percent body weight are also factors that can affect menstrual function, depending on the sport.
	• Medical providers should be vigilant to diagnose early or fully manifest female athlete triad.
	• Hormonal (estrogen) therapy for underweight and/or osteopenic athletes remains controversial.
Contraceptive options	• No restriction of contraceptive options based on athletics alone.
	• DMPA should be used with caution in patients with female athlete triad due to its effect on bone mineral density.
Fertility	• Diminished if female eating disorder/female athlete triad is present.
Preconception counseling	• Encourage patient to optimize weight, stop sport-enhancing drugs and supplements, and modify exercise.

Acute and Chronic Liver Disease

The spectrum of liver disease encompasses a wide range of processes such as infectious, toxin-induced, autoimmune, inherited, thrombotic, and pregnancy-related. Both acute and chronic liver disease can have a broad range of effects on the reproductive system and on drug metabolism.

Menstrual Disorders and Their Management

Menstrual disorders are common in women with liver disease. Changes in the menstrual cycle often precede the usual clinical manifestations of overt liver disease and may in fact be the presenting symptom (91). Women with acute and chronic liver disease often experience amenorrhea, oligomenorrhea, and metrorrhagia.

The mechanism of endocrine effects of liver disease in women is not as well understood as it is in men but is presumably similar. The physiologic changes eventually lead to amenorrhea in as many as 50% of women with chronic liver disease (91). Women with menstrual abnormalities in the setting of liver disease fall into two groups. The first group has normal gonadotropin levels but elevated levels of estrogen and testosterone. This may be due to decreased sex-hormone binding globulin produced by the liver or to decreased metabolism of estrogens due to portosystemic shunting of weak androgens, which are then converted to estrogens. The second group of women are hypogonadotropic: they are thin and underweight, and their menstrual changes may be related to malnutrition (92).

Alcoholic liver disease is more severe in women than in men. Women whose liver disease is due to alcohol will develop menstrual symptoms caused by the liver disease and by the effects of alcohol itself.

Women with primary biliary cirrhosis are more likely to develop menorrhagia. In Wilson's disease, copper deposition in the pituitary and hypothalamus may result in secondary hypogonadism (93). Treatment with penicillamine can ameliorate the menstrual irregularities in these patients. Contraceptive counseling is critical because fertility in these women is frequently preserved even with advanced liver disease (94).

Contraceptive Options

Contraceptive counseling is critical in this population because pregnancy should be deferred until the liver disease is stable or in remission. Half of all women with severe liver disease or cirrhosis will develop complications during pregnancy.

The use of hormonal contraception in women with liver disease has not been well studied, and recommendations are made on the basis of small clinical studies and expert opinion, as discussed below. In general, estrogen-containing contraceptives are contraindicated in women with active liver disease or with decompensated cirrhosis (95,96). Progestin-only contraceptives are recommended as safe, based on a study of their use in six patients with chronic active hepatitis or primary biliary cirrhosis (97). Contraceptive recommendations will depend upon the etiology, acuity, and severity of the liver disease.

Acute Hepatitis

Hormonal contraceptives are contraindicated in patients with acute hepatitis (98,99). IUD or barrier methods are the best choices. Use of barrier methods by women with viral hepatitis is encouraged to prevent transmission of infection. Once liver function tests return to normal, combination hormonal contraceptives are considered safe.

Chronic Hepatitis

The use of estrogen-containing contraceptives is controversial due to concern about the increased risk of the development of hepatocellular carcinoma (98). Some experts believe that estrogen-containing contraception may be used if the liver disease is stable and liver function tests are followed and remain unaffected (100). For women with mild liver dysfunction, the clinician is advised to weigh the risks and benefits with each individual patient (96). Use of estrogens is said to be safe for women who are asymptomatic carriers of viral hepatitis infections. There are no data on the use of hormonal contraceptives in women with hepatitis C. Barrier methods are especially important in reducing transmission rates for patients with viral hepatitis. The IUD is a safe alternative, as well, in women without cirrhosis and ascites; the levonorgestrel-containing IUD may be helpful in decreasing menorrhagia. Women with ascites are at risk for spontaneous bacterial peritonitis, and, theoretically, the increased risk of pelvic inflammatory disease associated with an IUD can further increase this risk. IUD use is not recommended for women taking immunosuppressive medications because of the increased risk of infection. Tubal ligation for women who have completed childbearing is an excellent choice but can be difficult to perform if a patient has ascites or extensive vascular collateralization.

Cholelithiasis, Cholestatic Liver Disease, and Cholestasis of Pregnancy

Women with a history of cholestasis related to OCP use are at an increased risk of cholestasis with subsequent use, so oral contraception should be reintroduced with caution, only if there are no other acceptable options, and only if the risks and benefits are carefully weighed. Women who have experienced pregnancy-related cholestasis may use combined hormonal contraceptives, but there may be a small increase in the risk of recurrence. Combined hormonal contraceptive use may cause a small increase in the risk of gallbladder disease or may worsen pre-existing gallbladder disease in women who are susceptible.

Wilson's Disease

Estrogen use is controversial in patients with Wilson's disease. Some believe that estrogens will increase plasma ceruloplasmin, leading to increased absorption of copper, although there are no clinical data to support this (94). If an estrogen-containing contraceptive is used, close follow-up is needed to watch for evidence of exacerbation (98). The use of the copper IUD is not recommended because of the theoretical possibility that it may increase copper absorption, thus exacerbating this copper storage disease. There is, however, little evidence that the amount of copper absorbed is significant. Progesterone-only hormonal methods and barrier methods are considered to be the contraceptives of choice (94).

Primary Biliary Cirrhosis
There is very little clinical evidence on the effect of hormones on the course of primary biliary cirrhosis. Current expert consensus favors the use of progestins but is against the use of estrogens in this group (98).

Budd-Chiari Syndrome
Estrogen-containing contraceptives are contraindicated in women with Budd-Chiari syndrome because of the increased risk of thrombosis associated with their use (98).

Alcoholic Liver Disease
Use of estrogens is not recommended in women with alcoholic liver disease. Both acute alcohol ingestion and alcoholic hepatitis have been shown to elevate serum estrogen levels. Diminished contraceptive efficacy is related to poor compliance; alcoholic hepatitis may affect metabolism of the contraceptive as well.

Post-Transplantation
Use of combination hormonal contraceptives is acceptable in many cases. They are not recommended for patients with a history of thrombosis and must be used cautiously in women with hypertension or active liver disease. Cyclosporin levels must be monitored when using combined hormonal contraceptives. The steroid hormones can decrease cyclosporin metabolism, leading to hepatotoxicity due to elevated cyclosporin levels. Progestin-only methods of contraception have not been well studied but may be a good choice in women with contraindications to estrogens. Immunosuppressant levels should be followed with use of progestins (101). The use of the IUD by women on immunosuppressive therapy may be associated with an increased risk of ascending infection (101,102).

Table 10-8 summarizes WHO guidelines for medical eligibility for hormonal contraception for women with liver disease (2).

Preconception Counseling

Fertility is diminished by hepatic dysfunction, and rates of pregnancy are low in women with cirrhosis and decompensated liver disease. Because half of women

Table 10-8   WHO Guidelines for Medical Eligibility for Hormonal Contraception for Women with Liver Disease*

	COC/R/P	POP	DMPA/NE	Cu-IUD	LNG-IUD
Viral hepatitis					
Active	4	3	3	1	3
Carrier	1	1	1	1	1
Cirrhosis					
Mild (compensated)	3	2	2	1	2
Severe (decompensated)	4	3	3	1	3
Liver tumors					
Benign (adenoma)	4	3	3	1	3
Malignant (hepatoma)	4	3	3	1	3
History of cholestasis					
Pregnancy-related	2	1	1	1	1
Past COC-related	3	2	2	1	2
Gall bladder disease					
Symptomatic					
Post-cholecystectomy	2	2	2	1	2
Medically treated	3	2	2	1	2
Current	3	2	2	1	2
Asymptomatic	2	2	2	1	2

*See Table 10-2 for explanation of WHO categories. COC/R/P = combination oral contraceptive, ring, patch; POP = progestin-only pill; DMPA/NE = depot medroxyprogesterone acetate/norethisterone enantate; Cu-IUD = copper-bearing IUD; LNG/IUD = levonorgestrel-releasing IUD (20 μg/24 hours).

with severe liver disease will develop maternal complications during pregnancy, it is crucial that the high risks of pregnancy are understood by the patient. Women with portal hypertension are at increased risk for variceal hemorrhage, and the fetus is at increased risk for premature birth and intrauterine fetal demise. As a general rule, pregnancy should be deferred until the hepatic disease is stable or in remission in order to optimize outcome. Medications should be reviewed before conception to minimize risk to the fetus. Use of beta-blockers to decrease the risk of variceal bleeding is readily justified during pregnancy.

KEY POINTS FOR WOMEN WITH LIVER DISEASE

Menstrual changes	• Amenorrhea, oligomenorrhea, metrorrhagia early in course; eventually, amenorrhea with chronic liver disease.
Contraceptive options	• Advisability of hormonal method depends upon the etiology, acuity, and severity of the disease.

(cont'd.)

KEY POINTS FOR WOMEN WITH LIVER DISEASE *(continued)*	
Contraceptive options *(cont'd.)*	• Barrier methods are safe for all; IUD carries risks for some.
Fertility	• Diminished.
Preconception counseling	• Women with severe liver disease are at very high risk for maternal complications. Medications should be reviewed.

Renal Disease

Compared with some other chronic organ system diseases, women with kidney disease can be relatively optimistic about their reproductive function.

Menstrual Disorders and Their Management

Impaired renal function can affect the timing of both menarche and menopause. Girls who develop renal insufficiency or renal failure before menarche may show delayed puberty and delayed menarche. The average age of menopause in women on dialysis is 47 years, about 5 years earlier than the average woman not receiving dialysis (103). As renal function diminishes, women of reproductive age who have renal disease will generally experience irregular menstrual bleeding. Women with renal insufficiency who develop amenorrhea tend to have higher prolactin levels than women with renal insufficiency who continue to have normal menstrual cycles. The effect of the hyperprolactinemia frequently seen in this group is not understood, although complete amenorrhea is more common in women with symptoms of galactorrhea and hyperprolactinemia (104). Premature ovarian failure appears to be more common in this population (105). Women with renal disease who are post-menopausal will have appropriately elevated follicle-stimulating hormone and luteinizing hormone levels (104). The majority of women with chronic renal failure will eventually become anovulatory due to a hypothalamic defect in gonadotropin secretion. They may become amenorrheic or develop irregular menstrual bleeding.

Dialysis will lead to the re-establishment of the menstrual cycle in most women. Improvements in dialysis techniques and the addition of erythropoietin have led to significant improvement in menstrual function and fertility, and recent studies found that 42% to 67% of women on dialysis were menstruating (106). Those women who do reestablish menses with initiation of dialysis often develop menorrhagia, with 64% of women in one study reporting heavier flow than before dialysis (107). Menorrhagia is important to recognize and control because it may affect the management of anemia.

Contraceptive Options

If the underlying renal disease is caused by diabetic nephropathy or lupus nephritis, or if the woman has poorly controlled hypertension, combination hormonal contraception is contraindicated (2). Progestin-only contraceptives are a good choice, as long as endogenous estrogen levels are adequate to protect the bones and to prevent breakthrough bleeding. If blood pressure is well controlled, combination hormonal contraception is safe if used with careful monitoring (2). Barrier methods are safe in women with renal failure. The advisability of IUD in this population is questionable because of general concern about the use of IUDs in women who are immunosuppressed. The copper IUD may also worsen menorrhagia. Conversely, the levonorgestrel-IUD may decrease bleeding.

Preconception Counseling

Women with renal disease generally have a decreased level of fertility, the cause of which is usually multifactorial. It may be related to cyclophosphamide used to treat renal disease, premature ovarian failure, and chronic anovulation (105). Women with chronic renal failure on dialysis have diminished fertility, but pregnancy is possible (103).

Women with renal disease should be carefully counseled about pregnancy and its complications. Pregnancy outcomes can be greatly affected by renal disease, and the long-term effect of pregnancy on the prognosis of the underlying renal disease likewise depends upon the degree of renal dysfunction (Table 10-9). A team approach to perinatal management during pregnancy in women with renal disease is recommended and should include a nephrologist and a perinatologist (108,109).

Table 10-9   Outcomes During Pregnancy in Women with Renal Disease

	Pregnancy Outcomes
• Mild renal insufficiency	Good pregnancy outcome (85% successful outcome)
• Cr > 1.5	Preterm delivery, IUGR problems
• Cr > 2.5	Poor pregnancy outcome
	Prognosis of Renal Disease During Pregnancy
• Cr < 1.5	Little effect on long-term prognosis
• Cr > 1.5	Worsening of renal function
• Proteinuria with preserved renal function	Worsening of proteinuria (will return to baseline after delivery); increased risk of preeclampsia

---

KEY POINTS FOR WOMEN WITH RENAL DISEASE

Menstrual changes	• Irregular bleeding or amenorrhea due to chronic anovulation.
Contraceptive options	• Combination hormonal contraception contraindicated in women with diabetic nephropathy or lupus nephritis and in women with uncontrolled hypertension. IUD should not be used by women on immunosuppressants.
Fertility	• Diminished.
Preconception counseling	• Pregnancy outcome depends upon the degree of renal insufficiency. Pregnancy may lead to irreversible worsening of renal function in some women.

Systemic Lupus Erythematosus and the Antiphospholipid Syndrome

Menstrual disorders are common and varied in women with rheumatologic diseases. It is crucial that the physician understand the contraception and fertility issues for these women because many rheumatologic diseases have their highest prevalence during the childbearing years. Timing of childbearing is particularly important for women with rheumatologic diseases. Of all the rheumatic diseases, systemic lupus erythematosus (SLE) most commonly affects pregnancy because it often presents in younger women and there tends not to be a remission of the disease during pregnancy.

Menstrual Disorders and Their Management

Menstrual disturbances are common in women with SLE and are related to multiple medical issues in this group of women. The menstrual changes experienced are quite varied and include menorrhagia, oligomenorrhea, and amenorrhea. They tend to occur more often during the initial stage of the illness or during periods of increased disease activity (110). It is speculated that the effect may be an SLE-induced oophoritis or possibly an effect at the level of the endometrium. The use of alkylating agents in treating SLE is known to cause amenorrhea and gonadal dysfunction as well. Sixty percent of SLE patients treated with intravenous cyclophosphamide will develop premature ovarian failure.

Contraceptive Options

In women with SLE, safety of combination hormonal contraceptives is controversial because of risks associated with the estrogen component of these agents (111). There is increased risk of side effects such as hypertension, thromboembolism, myocardial infarction, and stroke. Study results are controversial; however, women with lupus nephritis seem to be at particular risk of flare when taking combination hormonal contraceptives. Women with antiphospholipid antibody syndrome are prone to thromboses during pregnancy, in the postpartum period, and while on combination hormonal contraceptives. They are also at increased risk of recurrent miscarriages.

It is recommended that combination hormonal contraceptives not be prescribed for women with active lupus nephritis, antiphospholipid antibodies, or active SLE. If combination hormonal contraceptives are used by patients with inactive SLE, the patient should be monitored for signs of a flare and for the development of antiphospholipid antibodies (111).

For women with SLE or antiphospholipid antibodies, progestin-only contraceptives can be recommended. Small series have shown no increase in the risk of thrombosis with the use of progestin-only methods (111,112). Barrier methods are safe in women with SLE but as a single method do not provide the required degree of reliability needed by women who have medical contraindications to pregnancy. IUDs are considered safe in this population, but they are not recommended for use by women who are on immunosuppressive medications because of the possible increased risk of infection (111).

Preconception Counseling

Medications used to treat rheumatologic disorders can significantly affect a woman's fertility (113). Alkylating agents decrease fertility, most extensively in women who are older or have had a longer duration of therapy. Studies are underway to assess the efficacy of gonadotropin-releasing hormone agonists in preserving ovarian function and fertility.

Pregnancy is contraindicated for women receiving cyclophosphamide, so a reliable contraceptive should be used. Women with antiphospholipid antibody syndrome who are on chronic warfarin should be converted to heparin or low-molecular-weight heparin immediately upon diagnosis of pregnancy at the time of the first missed period. For women with irregular menses, a monthly pregnancy test is recommended in order to detect pregnancy as early as possible. For women with SLE, pregnancy outcome is best if conception occurs when the disease is inactive and if there is no nephropathy. SLE increases the risk of perinatal morbidity and mortality, and a team approach to management with a rheumatologist and a perinatologist is recommended. Maternal morbidity is also increased in women with SLE.

KEY POINTS FOR WOMEN WITH SYSTEMIC LUPUS ERYTHEMATOSUS

Menstrual changes	• Varied, including menorrhagia, oligomenorrhea, and amenorrhea. More often in early stages of disease and at times of increased disease activity.
Contraceptive options	• Use of combination hormonal contraceptives (CHCs) containing estrogen is controversial due to increased risk of HTN, VTE, MI, and stroke. CHCs are contraindicated in women with lupus nephritis, antiphospholipid antibodies, or active SLE. • IUD should not be used by women who are on immunosuppressant medications.
Fertility	• Medications may decrease fertility and can cause premature ovarian failure.
Preconception counseling	• Pregnancy is contraindicated for women on cyclophosphamide, and other medications need to be reviewed before contraception. • Perinatal morbidity and mortality are increased. • Pregnancy may increase flare rate in SLE. • The best time for conception is during remission.

KEY POINTS FOR WOMEN WITH OTHER RHEUMATIC DISEASES

Rheumatoid arthritis	• Combination hormonal contraceptives are safe in this population. • Disease tends to improve during pregnancy: 75% of patients generally undergo a remission. More than 90% will relapse post-partum. There is no increased risk for the fetus.
Scleroderma	• Raynaud's symptoms tend to improve, GERD and arthralgias tend to worsen, but there is no increase in preeclampsia or renal crisis. • Women with cardiopulmonary involvement have higher risks during pregnancy. Fetus is at increased risk of premature delivery and IUGR.
Dermatomyositis/ polymyositis	• Combination hormonal contraceptives are safe in this population. (In fact, they may improve symptoms.) • There is a risk of flare during pregnancy and an increased risk of prematurity. Fetal outcome is worse if disease is active, and there is a high rate of fetal loss. • Pregnancy should be planned during remission.

Hypertension, Hyperlipidemia, and Heart Disease

Menstrual abnormalities are not a common problem for women with cardiovascular diseases, but contraceptive and reproductive issues are an essential part of primary care for women with congenital heart disease, valvular heart disease, hypertension, hyperlipidemia, and vascular disease. With evolving medical technology, more women with congenital heart diseases are living until reproductive age. Patients with complex lesions pose unique clinical challenges, and their reproductive care, especially during pregnancy, should be managed by specialists. Drug management and end organ disease will affect contraceptive choice and pregnancy care; these should routinely be reevaluated in women of childbearing age.

Menstrual Disorders and Their Management

There are limited data on menstrual patterns in women with congenital heart disease. In general, women with cyanotic disease report later onset of menarche, a higher frequency of menstrual cycle irregularities, and increased incidence of longer or shorter menstrual cycles when compared with women with acyanotic disease and healthy controls (114). The presence of hypertension or hyperlipidemia does not affect the menstrual cycle. Women on anticoagulants for management of their cardiac disease may experience problems with menorrhagia.

Contraceptive Options

Contraceptive recommendations vary depending on the specific cardiovascular disease (hypertension, hyperlipidemia, and structural and atherosclerotic heart disease) and are discussed accordingly in the following sections.

Hypertension

Onset of hypertension during contraceptive use and return to pretreatment levels within 1 year of cessation is diagnostic of oral contraceptive–induced hypertension (OCIH) (115). The mechanism for OCIH is not well understood. Research has been limited by the small number of participants and inadequate controls and confounded by the lower dose (30 µg or less of estrogen) and different combinations of estrogen/progestin preparations currently in use. Estimated prevalence of OCIH is 15.5% to 18%, but these data are limited by the same factors that limit research (116,117). Women who are at risk for OCIH include those with a family history of hypertension, personal history of renal disease, obesity, age over 35, or a history of pregnancy-induced hypertension.

Women who develop hypertension after starting a combined hormonal contraceptive should stop the medication and have their blood pressure monitored to see if it returns to normal. If hypertension persists, more intensive treatment may be warranted for blood pressure control.

Women with chronic hypertension are at an increased risk for myocardial infarction and stroke when using combined hormonal contraceptives (118). Women with well-controlled and monitored hypertension who are under age 35 are candidates for a trial of estrogen-containing contraceptives as long as there is no evidence of end-organ vascular disease and they do not smoke cigarettes (119). The hormonal contraceptive can be continued if blood pressure remains well controlled after several months of careful monitoring. Women with chronic hypertension who do not meet these criteria, however, should be advised against the use of combined hormonal methods (2). Progestin-only methods are an alternative as long as the blood pressure remains under 160/100. Barrier methods and IUDs are good alternatives. Effective contraception is especially important if the patient is on ACE inhibitors or ARBs to control hypertension because these drugs are teratogenic. If the patient is not using a highly effective method of contraception, ACE inhibitors and ARBs should be avoided.

Hyperlipidemia

Estrogens and progestins can affect lipid levels, but the levels generally stay within the normal range and the changes may not be clinically relevant in women without significant risk factors for cardiovascular disease (96,120). ACOG recommendations state that most women with controlled dyslipidemia can use low-dose formulations (35 µg or less of estrogen) safely (119). Periodic monitoring of lipid levels, especially during the first few months after initiating therapy, is recommended. In patients with an LDL cholesterol level above 160 or with multiple risk factors for coronary artery disease (smoking, diabetes, obesity, hypertension, family history of premature heart disease and/or lipid disorders, HDL below 35 mg/dL), alternative contraceptive measures should be considered. Progesterone-only contraception or an IUD would be an acceptable choice for these patients (121).

Progestin-only contraception or an IUD is probably preferable in the presence of overt hypertriglyceridemia. Women with hypertriglyceridemia (fasting serum triglyceride above 250) should avoid the use of combined hormonal contraception because the estrogen component can cause elevation in triglyceride levels, which can lead to pancreatitis (122).

Structural and Atherosclerotic Heart Disease

Combination hormonal contraceptives, with their inherent pro-thrombotic effects, are not advisable for women who have structural, functional, or hematologic abnormalities that increase their risk of thromboembolism. Combined hormonal contraceptives are contraindicated for use by patients with prosthetics, cyanosis, pulmonary hypertension, low cardiac output, dilated cardiac chambers, atrial dysrhythmia, sluggish venous conduit flow (e.g., a Fontan circuit), ischemic heart disease, history of subacute bacterial endocarditis, and certain shunts (2,123). Estrogen-containing contraception is acceptable in women with uncomplicated valvular heart disease, such as asymptomatic, non-regurgitating mitral valve prolapse (2,124).

Progestin-only methods may be used with caution by women with an increased risk of thromboembolism, coronary disease, or valvular heart disease. Progestin-only methods are recommended contraceptive choices for patients with complex cyanotic heart disease (tricuspid atresia, transposition of the great arteries, tetralogy of Fallot) (112). Although highly effective, long-acting progestin-only methods have the disadvantage of causing menstrual irregularity, which may be especially troublesome for patients using anticoagulants. In patients with impaired systemic or pulmonary ventricular function, fluid retention while using this method may also be problematic (112,124). Progestogen-only pill preparations are of limited use in young women because of their high failure rate and requirement for strict compliance with daily use (125).

IUDs are good options for women with coronary artery disease. They should be used with caution in patients on anticoagulants due to potential uterine bleeding, although this may not be an issue for the levonorgestrel IUD. Vasodepressor reflexes occurring at the time of IUD insertion may be poorly tolerated. Some experts recommend against the use of IUDs in women with complex cyanotic heart disease, prosthetic valves, valvular heart disease, a history of endocarditis, or congenital heart disease such as pulmonary disease anemia, ventricular septal defect, and coarctation of the aorta because of concerns about the increased risk of pelvic inflammatory disease associated with the IUD, which could lead to endocarditis (112). The WHO, however, does not consider this to be a contraindication (2).

Sterilization is the method of choice for patients with Eisenmenger's syndrome or New York Heart Association class IV symptoms (123). Barrier methods have many advantages but used alone do not provide sufficient protection against pregnancy in the face of congenital heart disease.

Table 10-10 summarizes WHO guidelines for medical eligibility for hormonal contraception for women with cardiovascular disease (2).

Preconception Counseling

Hypertension

Most women with chronic hypertension will have an uneventful pregnancy. Women who are most likely to have difficulties during pregnancy are those with end-organ damage due to hypertension (118). Although there is a deficiency in research data to guide clinicians caring for chronically hypertensive

Table 10-10   WHO Guidelines for Medical Eligibility for Hormonal Contraception for Women with Cardiovascular Disease*

	COC/R/P	POP	DMPA/NE	Cu-IUD	LNG-IUD
History of hypertension where BP cannot be evaluated	3	2	2	1	2
Adequately controlled hypertension	3	1	2	1	1

Elevated blood pressure
  Systolic 140-159 or
  Diastolic 90-99
	3	1	2	1	1

Systolic ≥ 160 or Diastolic ≥ 100	4	2	3	1	2
Vascular disease	4	2	3	1	2
History of hypertension during pregnancy but current blood pressure normal	2	1	1	1	1
Known hyperlipidemias	2/3	2	2	1	2
Valvular heart disease Uncomplicated	2	1	1	1	1
Complicated (pulmonary hypertension, atrial fibrillation, history of SBE)	4	1	1	2	2
Multiple risk factors for CVD (older age, smoking, diabetes, hypertension)	3/4	2	3	1	2
History of and current ischemic heart disease	4	2(I)/3(C)	3	1	2(I)/3(C)
Stroke (history of cerebrovascular accident)	4	2(I)/3(C)	3	1	2
Known thrombotic mutation (e.g., factor V Leiden, prothrombin mutation, protein S, protein C and antithrombin deficiencies)	4	2	2	1	2

*See Table 10-2 for explanation of WHO categories. COC/R/P = combination oral contraceptive, ring, patch; POP = progestin-only pill; DMPA/NE = depot medroxyprogesterone acetate/norethisterone enantate; Cu-IUD = copper-bearing IUD; LNG/IUD = levonorgestrel-releasing IUD (20 µg/24 hours); I = guideline for initiation of this method; C = guideline for continuation of this method.

women who desire pregnancy, it is important to note that there is no evidence that pharmacologic treatment of hypertension in women whose blood pressure is below 160/100 improves outcome for either the mother or fetus (109,118). Choice of antihypertensive during the preconception period and during pregnancy is important. Methyldopa and labetalol are considered first-line therapy.

ACE inhibitors and ARBs are not a good choice of anti-hypertensive in women of childbearing age unless there is a compelling clinical indication such as diabetes. When women who are on ACE inhibitors or ARBs plan to become pregnant, the ACE inhibitor or ARB should be stopped because of a high risk of teratogenicity when taken during the second trimester. Some experts advocate continuing these medications during the preconception period in order to maintain the reno-protective effects and stopping them as soon as pregnancy is confirmed.

Hyperlipidemias

Lipid-lowering medications such as the statins and niacin are contraindicated during pregnancy and lactation and should be discontinued. Appropriate diet, activity, and lifestyle modifications should be reinforced during preconception counseling and pregnancy-related care. Although LDL cholesterol levels rise during pregnancy, there is little evidence that pregnancy aggravates coronary heart disease (121).

Structural and Atherosclerotic Heart Disease

Preconception counseling should address maternal morbidity and mortality as well as risk of congenital heart defect in offspring. Poor outcome is anticipated with certain cardiac lesions. Women with pulmonary hypertension have a maternal mortality rate approaching 50%. Consultation with the patient's cardiologist is strongly recommended before conception (126).

KEY POINTS FOR WOMEN WITH CARDIOVASCULAR DISEASE	
Menstrual changes	• Presence of hypertension or hyperlipidemia does not affect the menstrual cycle.
	• Amenorrhea, menorrhagia, and metrorrhagia are concerns for women with cyanotic heart disease.
Contraceptive options	• Combination hormonal contraception is contraindicated in women with uncontrolled hypertension, hypertriglyceridemia, ischemic and complicated valvular disease, vascular disease, and some shunts.
	• Hemodynamic status and anticoagulation may pose challenges in IUD and progestin-only methods use.
	• Sterilization is recommended for women with Eisenmenger's syndrome or NYHA IV symptoms.
Fertility	• Variable; diminished in women with cyanotic heart disease.

(cont'd.)

Seizure Disorders

Seizures affect approximately 1% of the population and are common neurological disorders seen in the reproductive years (127). Menstrual and fertility problems in women with epilepsy are common and may be attributed to the seizure disorder itself or to antiepileptic medications. The comprehensive care of women with epilepsy should balance seizure management with drug side effects and reproductive function.

Menstrual Disorders and Their Management

Amenorrhea, menorrhagia, and metrorrhagia are common concerns for women with epilepsy. It is difficult to determine whether the etiology of menstrual aberrations is related to the seizures, their treatment, or sometimes a related pathology, especially PCOS. Seizures can disrupt the hypothalamic pituitary ovary axis, altering pulsatile release of pituitary luteinizing hormone and elevating prolactin (128). Anti-epileptic drugs (AEDs) that induce the cytochrome P450 system alter the metabolism of steroid hormones and consequently reduce their concentration. Concomitant use of combination hormonal contraceptives with these AEDs can lead to an increased frequency of break-through bleeding and contraceptive failure. Weight gain associated with AEDs (including but not limited to valproate, carbamazepine, vigabatrin, and gabapentin) can promote PCOS (and subsequent menstrual disturbance) in predisposed women who have no previous hormonal abnormality (129). Women taking Depakote have been found to have androgen abnormalities with a PCOS-like picture.

Catamenial seizures, whereby there is a more than two-fold increase in seizure frequency perimenstrually or before ovulation, have an incidence of 12.5% (130). Hormonal triggers are not entirely understood, but they may be related to levels of estrogen (midcycle seizures triggered by estrogen surges), progesterone (seizures triggered by a relative deficit in progesterone), or possibly hormone ratios (high estrogen-to-progesterone before ovulation and menstruation, which would trigger seizures). Another potential trigger is AED level fluctuations related to the menstrual cycle (the premenstrual decline in hormones could allow for an increased number of hepatic enzymes available to degrade AEDs) (130).

Evaluation for PCOS is often indicated in epileptic women with menstrual disorders, particularly if they are obese, hirsute, or have experienced significant weight gain during treatment with AEDs. Prolactin levels should be included in the evaluation of a reproductive endocrine disorder. The clinician should be sure to have the patient's prolactin levels drawn at 8 a.m., *not* during a post-ictal period. AEDs may affect prolactin levels, but it is important to rule out hypothyroidism or a pituitary tumor as causative.

If a diagnosis of PCOS is established, a decision must be made about whether weight gain is related to seizure therapy medications and whether it is prudent to switch to another AED regimen. Treatment of PCOS, or non-PCOS–related anovulatory cycles, otherwise is similar to that of non-epileptic women.

Preliminary evaluation of catamenial epilepsy includes appropriate documentation of seizure frequency and investigation into total and free serum drug levels throughout the menstrual cycle. Supplemental AED dosages may be necessary to optimize drug levels, and the choice of anti-seizure drug may need to be re-evaluated. There are limited data on the benefits of specific hormonal treatments, and none have yet been approved by the FDA for treating catamenial seizures. Hormonal treatments have included low-estrogen/high-progesterone oral contraceptives, supplemental oral or vaginal progesterone during the second half of the menstrual cycle, extended hormone regimens, and DMPA (130).

Contraceptive Options

The failure rate of oral contraceptives is high among women taking AEDs that induce the cytochrome P450 system (Table 10-11). The American Academy of Neurology recommends that women taking these AEDs may benefit from combination-type oral contraceptives at higher doses (127). Many experts recommend using the 50-μg pill in this setting, but there are no clinical data to support this. It may be prudent to advise women to also use a barrier method

Table 10-11   Anti-Epileptic Drugs and the Cytochrome P450 System

Inducers of the cytochrome P450 system	Phenobarbital, primidone, phenytoin, felbamate, carbamazepine, oxcarbazepine, ethosuximide, topiramate (weakly)
Non-inducers of the cytochrome P450 system	Valproic acid, benzodiazepines, gabapentin, lamotrigine, vigabatrin, tiagabine

of contraception for several cycles until suppression of ovulation is confirmed (with ovulation kits). Levonorgestrel implants are contraindicated in women receiving AEDs that induce the cytochrome P450 system because of cases of contraceptive failure. It is recommended that medroxyprogesterone injections be given every 10, rather than 12, weeks to women who are receiving AEDs that induce hepatic microsomal enzymes (131).

Women on AEDs that do not induce the cytochrome P450 system can use combined hormonal contraceptives at standard doses. DMPA, barrier methods, and IUDs are also options. Oral contraceptives have been shown to significantly decrease serum levels of lamotrigine, and this AED may need to be adjusted after starting or stopping hormonal contraception (as directed by the manufacturer's prescribing information) (132).

Table 10-12 summarizes WHO guidelines for medical eligibility for hormonal contraception for women with seizure disorders (2).

Preconception Counseling

Women with seizures have a lower fertility rate and a higher rate of spontaneous abortion and other complications of pregnancy than the general population. Over 90% of women with epilepsy, however, can expect good pregnancy outcomes (127). During pregnancy women should be aware that poorly controlled generalized seizures present health risks for the mother as well as the fetus as a result of hypoxia and acidosis. Anti-epileptic therapy, apart from the seizure disorder, also poses significant problems during pregnancy because most anticonvulsants are teratogenic (133). AEDs assigned Pregnancy Risk Category D (evidence of human fetal risk, although the benefits may outweigh the risks) include phenytoin, phenobarbital, primidone, and valproic acid. Carbamazepine, ethosuximide, and the newer AEDs (felbamate, gabapentin, lamotrigine) have been assigned to Category C (documented adverse effects in animal studies without controlled studies in women, or studies in women and

Table 10-12 WHO Guidelines for Medical Eligibility for Hormonal Contraception for Women with Seizure Disorder*

	COC/R/P	POP	DMPA/NE	Cu-IUD	LNG-IUD
Seizure disorder	1	1	1	1	1
Certain anticonvulsants (phenytoin, carbamazepine, barbiturates, primidone, topiramate, oxcarbazepine)	3	3	2	1	1

*See Table 10-2 for explanation of WHO categories. COC/R/P = combination oral contraceptive, ring, patch; POP = progestin-only pill; DMPA/NE = depot medroxyprogesterone acetate/norethisterone enantate; Cu-IUD = copper-bearing IUD; LNG/IUD = levonorgestrel-releasing IUD (20 μg/24 hours).

animals are not available). Malformations are more common in infants exposed to polytherapy and high-serum AED concentrations.

Seizure control on the fewest number of medications is the therapeutic goal during pregnancy (134). Changing AED therapy during the course of pregnancy, however, can potentially cause added risk to mother and fetus.

Pre-conceptual care is critical; at least 6 months before conception and in conjunction with a neurologist, drug therapy should be re-evaluated. AED dosage may need to be adjusted throughout pregnancy because increased estrogen levels may reduce the seizure threshold, expansion of plasma volume may cause drug levels to fall, and high-dose folic acid supplementation may increase the metabolism of AEDs. Non–protein-bound AED levels should be monitored during pregnancy. In the patient who is clinically stable, levels should be ascertained prior to conception, at the beginning of each trimester, and in the last month of pregnancy. Additional levels should be done with each seizure occurrence and as otherwise clinically indicated. If AED doses have been increased during pregnancy, physicians must be careful to readjust AED dosage post-partum in order to avoid toxicity.

Some AEDs, including phenytoin, carbamazepine, and phenobarbital, cause folate malabsorption, and valproate reduces serum folate levels; these drugs may therefore be associated with fetal malformations. Women should begin folic supplementation (4 mg daily) at least 3 months prior to conception and throughout pregnancy. Vitamin K supplements (10 mg daily) are necessary during the last month of pregnancy in women taking enzyme-inducing AEDs.

KEY POINTS FOR WOMEN WITH SEIZURE DISORDER

Menstrual changes	• Amenorrhea, menorrhagia, and metrorrhagia are common concerns.
Contraceptive options	• Anti-epileptic drugs (AEDs) that induce cytochrome P450 can lead to contraceptive failure and an increased frequency of spotting and break-through bleeding.
Fertility	• Diminished.
Preconception counseling	• Seizure control on the fewest number of medications is the therapeutic goal. AED therapy should be optimized at least 6 months prior to conception.
	• Folate supplementation of 4 mg daily at least 3 months prior to conception.
	• Medication compliance and AED level monitoring are important.
	• Vitamin K supplementation in the last month of pregnancy may be required.

REFERENCES

1. Lee RV, Rosene-Montella K, Barbour LA, et al. Medical Care of the Pregnant Patient. Philadelphia: American College of Physicians; 2000.

2. Medical Eligibility Criteria for Contraceptive Use, 3rd ed. Geneva: World Health Organization; 2004.

3. National Diabetes Fact Sheet: General Information and National Estimates on Diabetes in the United States, 2003. Atlanta: U.S. Department of Health and Human Services, Centers for Disease Control and Prevention; 2003. Accessed at www.cdc.gov/diabetes/pubs/factsheet.htm on August 30, 2003.

4. American Diabetes Association. Preconception care of women with diabetes. Diabetes Care. 2002;25(Suppl):S82-4.

5. Schroeder B, Hertweck SP, Sanfilippo JS, Foster MB. Correlation between glycemic control and menstruation in diabetic adolescents. J Reprod Med. 2000;45:1-5.

6. Yeshaya A, Orvieto R, Dicker D, et al. Menstrual characteristics of women suffering from insulin-dependent diabetes mellitus. Int J Fertil Menopause Stud. 1995;40:269-73.

7. Griffin ML, South SA, Yankov VI, et al. Insulin-dependent diabetes mellitus and menstrual dysfunction. Ann Med. 1994;26:331-40.

8. Adcock CJ, Perry LA, Lindsell DR, et al. Menstrual irregularities are more common in adolescents with type 1 diabetes: association with poor glycemic control and weight gain. Diabetic Med. 1994;11:465-70.

9. Kjaer K, Hagen C, Sando SH, Esho JO. Epidemiology of menarche and menstrual disturbances in an unselected group of women with insulin-dependent diabetes mellitus compared to controls. J Clin Endocrinol Metab. 1992;75:524-9.

10. Roumain J, Charles MA, de Courten MP, et al. The relationship of menstrual irregularity to type 2 diabetes in Pima Indian women. Diabetes Care. 1998;21:346-9.

11. Dorman JS, Steenkiste AR, Foley TP, et al. Menopause in type 1 diabetic women: is it premature? Diabetes. 2001;50:1857-62.

12. Malacara JM, Huerta R, Rivera B, et al. Menopause in normal and uncomplicated NIDDM women: physical and emotional symptoms and hormone profile. Maturitas. 1997;28:35-45.

13. Garg SK, Chase HP, Marshall G, et al. Oral contraceptives and renal and retinal complications in young women with insulin-dependent diabetes mellitus. JAMA. 1994;271:1099-1102.

14. Petersen KR, Skouby SO, Vedel P, Haarber AB. Hormonal contraception in women with IDDM: influence on glycometabolic control and lipoprotein metabolism. Diabetes Care. 1995;18:800-6.

15. Jones KP, Wild RA. The role of hormonal contraceptives: contraception for patients with psychiatric or medical disorders. Am J Obst Gynecol. 1994;170:1575-80.

16. Kjos SL, Peters RK, Xiang A, et al. Contraception and the risk of type 2 diabetes mellitus in Latina women with prior gestational diabetes mellitus. JAMA. 1998;280:533-8.

17. Fahmy K, Abdel-Razik M, Sharaway M, et al. Effect of long-acting progestagen-only injectable contraceptives on carbohydrate metabolism and its hormonal profile. Contraception. 1991;44:419-30.

18. Kitzmiller JL, Buchanan TA, Kjos S, et al. Pre-conception care of diabetes, congenital malformations, and spontaneous abortions. Diabetes Care. 1996;19:514-41.

19. Hedley AA, Ogden CL, Johnson CL, et al. Prevalence of overweight and obesity among US children, adolescents, and adults, 1999-2002. JAMA. 2004;291:2847-50.

20. Bray GA. Complications of obesity. Ann Intern Med. 1985;103:1052-62.

21. Norman RJ, Clark AM. Obesity and reproductive disorders: a review. Reprod Fertil Dev. 1998;10:55-63.

22. Dickerson VM. Evaluation, management, and treatment of obesity in women. Obst Gynecol Survey. 2001;56:650-63.

23. Kiddy DS, Hamilton-Fairley D, Bush A, et al. Improvement in endocrine and ovarian function during dietary treatment of obese women with polycystic ovary syndrome. Clin Endocrinol. 1992;36:105-11.

24. Moran LJ, Noakes M, Clifton PM, et al. Dietary composition in restoring reproductive and metabolic physiology in overweight women with polycystic ovary syndrome. J Clin Endocrinol Metab. 2003;88:812-9.

25. Stamets K, Taylor DS, Kunselman A, et al. A randomized trial of the effect of two types of short-term hypocaloric diets on weight loss in women with polycystic ovary syndrome. Fertil Steril. 2004;81:630-7.

26. Deitel M, Stone E, Kassam HA, et al. Gynecologic-obstetric changes after loss of massive excess weight following bariatric surgery. J Am Coll Nutr. 1988;7:147-53.

27. Brolin RE. Bariatric surgery and long-term control of morbid obesity. JAMA. 2002;288: 2793-6.

28. Zieman M, Guillebaud J, Weisberg E, et al. Contraceptive efficacy and cycle control with the Ortho Evra/Evra transdermal system: the analysis of pooled data. Fertil Steril. 2002;77(Suppl2):S13-8.

29. Holt VL, Cushing-Haugen KL, Daling JR. Body weight and risk of oral contraceptive failure. Obstet Gynecol. 2002;99:820-7.

30. Weiss JL, Malone FD. Caring for obese obstetric patients. Contemp Obstet Gynecol. 2001:13-26.

31. Castro LC, Avina RL. Maternal obesity and pregnancy outcomes. Curr Opin Obstet Gynecol. 2002;14:601-6.

32. Shaw GM, Velie EM, Schaffer D. Risk of neural tube defect-affected pregnancies among obese women. JAMA. 1996;275:1093-6.

33. Moore KA, Ouyand DW, Whang EE. Maternal and fetal deaths after gastric bypass surgery for morbid obesity. N Engl J Med. 2004;351:721-2.

34. Sheiner E, Levy A, Silverberg D, et al. Pregnancy after bariatric surgery is not associated with adverse perinatal outcome. Am J Obstet Gynecol. 2004;190:1335-40.

35. Cigarette smoking among adults: United States, 2001. MMWR. 2003;52:953-6.

36. Latts LM. Tobacco and alcohol use. In: Medical Care of the Pregnant Patient. Philadelphia: American College of Physicians; 2000:160-73.

37. Howe G, Westhoff C, Vessey M, Yeates D. Effects of age, cigarette smoking, and other factors on fertility: findings in a large prospective study. BMJ. 1985;8:1697-700.

38. Hornsby PP, Wilcox AJ, Weinberg CR. Cigarette smoking and disturbance of menstrual function. Epidemiology. 1998;9:193-8.

39. Gold EB, Bromberger J, Craford S, et al. Factors associated with age at natural menopause in a multiethnic sample of midlife women. Am J Epidemiol. 2001;153:865-74.

40. Chasan-Taber L, Stampfer MJ. Epidemiology of oral contraceptives and cardiovascular disease. Ann Intern Med. 1998;128:467-77.

41. Cnattingius S, Lambe M. Trends in smoking and overweight during pregnancy: prevalence, risks of pregnancy complications, and adverse pregnancy outcomes. Semin Perinatol. 2002;26:286-95.

42. Hughes EG, Brennan BG. Does cigarette smoking impair natural or assisted fecundity? Fertil Steril. 1996;66:679-89.

43. Perkins KA. Smoking cessation in women: special considerations. CNS Drugs. 2001;15: 391-411.

44. Okuyemi KS, Ahluwalia JS, Harris KJ. Pharmacotherapy of smoking cessation. Arch Fam Med. 2000;9:270-81.

45. Klesges LM, Johnson KC, Ward KD, Barnard M. Smoking cessation in pregnant women. Obstet Gynecol Clin. 2001;28.

46. Wright LN, Thorp JM, Kuller JA, et al. Transdermal nicotine replacement in pregnancy: maternal pharmacokinetics and fetal effects. Am J Obest Gynecol. 1997;176:1090-4.

47. Hankoff LD, Darney PD. Contraceptive choices for behaviorally disordered women. Am J Obstet Gynecol. 1993;168:1986-9.

48. Marks JB, Sklyer, JS. The liver and the endocrine system. In: Schiff's Diseases of the Liver, 8th ed. Philadelphia: JB Lippincott; 1999.

49. Teoh SK, Lex BW, Mendelson JH, et al. Hyperprolactinemia and macrocytosis in women with alcohol and polysubstance abuse. J Studies Alcohol. 1992;53:176-82.

50. Bai J, Greenwald E, Caternini H, Kaminetzky HA. Drug-related menstrual aberrations. Obstet Gynecol. 1974;44:713-9.

51. Stoffer SS. A gynecologic study of drug addicts. Am J Obstet Gynecol. 1968;101:779-83.

52. Wallach RC, Jerez E, Blinick G. Pregnancy and menstrual function in narcotics addicts treated with methadone. Am J Obstet Gynecol. 1969;105:1226-9.

53. Santen RJ, Sofsky J, Bilic N, Lippert R. Mechanism of action of narcotics in the production of menstrual dysfunction in women. Fertil Steril. 1975;26:538-48.

54. Cushman P. The major medical sequelae of opioid addiction. Drug Alcohol Depend. 1980;5:239-54.

55. Mello NK, Mendelson JH. Cocaine's effects on neuroendocrine systems: clinical and preclinical studies. Pharmacol Biochem Behavior. 1997;57:571-99.

56. Cook, PS. Fetal alcohol syndrome (FAS), the leading known cause of mental retardation. In: Alcohol, Tobacco and Other Drugs May Harm the Unborn. US Department of Health and Human Services; 1990. Publication Number 90-1711, page 17.

57. Bolnick JM, Rayburn WF. Substance use disorders in women: special considerations during pregnancy. Obstet Gynecol Clin. 2003;30:545-58.

58. Mason E. Illicit drug use. In: Medical Care of the Pregnant Patient. Philadelphia: American College of Physicians; 2000.

59. Curet LB, Hsi AC. Drug abuse during pregnancy. Clin Obstet Gynecol. 2002;5:73-88.

60. Archie C. Methadone in the management of narcotic addiction in pregnancy. Curr Opin Obstet Gynecol. 1998;10:435-40.

61. Katz J, Weiner J. The aberrant reproductive endocrinology of anorexia nervosa. In: Behavior and Bodily Disease. Weiner H, Stunkard AJ, eds. New York: Raven Press; 1981:165.

62. Pirke KM, Fichter MM, Chlond C, et al. Disturbances of the menstrual cycle in bulimia nervosa. Clin Endocrinol. 1987;27:245-51.

63. Gidwani GP, Rome ES. Eating disorders. Clin Obstet Gynecol. 1997;40:601-15.

64. Mehler PS, Eckel RH, Donahoo WT. Leptin levels in restricting and purging anorectics. Int J Eat Disord. 1999;26:189-94.

65. Grinspoon S, Gulick T, Askari H, et al. Serum leptin levels in women with anorexia nervosa. J Clin Endocrinol Metab. 1996;81:3861-3.

66. Warren MP, Voussoughian F, Geer EB, et al. Functional hypothalamic amenorrhea: hypolepinemia and disordered eating. J Clin Endocrinol Metab. 1999;84:873-7.

67. Golden NH, Jacobson MS, Schebendach J, et al. Resumption of menses in anorexia nervosa. Arch Pediatr Adolesc Med. 1997;151:16-21.

68. Bachrach LK, Guido D, Katzman D, et al. Decreased bone density in adolescent girls with anorexia nervosa. Pediatrics. 1990:86:440-7.

69. Golden NH, Lanzkowsky L, Schebendach MA, et al. The effect of estrogen-progestin treatment on bone mineral density in anorexia nervosa. J Pediatr Adolesc Gynecol. 2002;15:135-43.

70. Klibanski A, Biller BM, Schoenfeld DA, et al. The effects of estrogen administration on trabecular bone loss in young women with anorexia nervosa. J Clin Endocrinol Metab. 1995;80:898-904.

71. Rome ES. Eating disorders. Obstet Gynecol Clin N Am. 2003;30:353-77.

72. Stewart DE, Raskin J, Garfinkel PE, et al. Anorexia nervosa, bulimia, and pregnancy. Am J Obstet Gynecol. 1987;157:1194-8.

73. Franko DL, Blais MA, Becker AE, et al. Pregnancy complications and neonatal outcomes in women with eating disorders. Am J Psychiatry. 2002;159:1249-50.

74. Bulik CM, Sullivan PF, Fear JL, et al. Fertility and reproduction in women with anorexia nervosa: a controlled study. J Clin Psychiatry. 1999;60:130-5.

75. Crow SJ, Thuras P, Keel PK, Mitchell JE. Long-term menstrual and reproductive function in patients with bulimia nervosa. Am J Psychiatry. 2002;159:1048-50.

76. Ehrenberg HM. Low maternal weight, failure to thrive in pregnancy, and adverse pregnancy outcomes. Am J Obstet Gynecol. 2003;189:1726-30.

77. Morgan JF, Lacey JH, Sedgwick PM. Impact of pregnancy on bulimia nervosa. Br J Psychiatry. 1999;174:135-40.

78. West RV. The female athlete: the triad of disordered eating, amenorrhea and osteoporosis. Sports Med. 1998;26:63-71.

79. Warren WP. The effect of exercise on pubertal progression and reproductive function in girls. J Clin Endocrinol Metab. 1980;51:1150-7.

80. Pfeifer SP, Patrizio P. The female athlete: some gynecologic considerations. Sports Med Arthroscopy Rev. 2002;10:2-9.

81. Warren MP. Health issues for women athletes: exercise-induced amenorrhea. J Clin Endocrinol Metab. 1999;84:1892-6.

82. Constantini NW, Warren MP. Menstrual dysfunction in swimmers: a distinct entity. J Clin Endocrinol Metab. 1995;80:2740-4.

83. Sanborn CF, Martin BJ, Wagner WW Jr. Is athletic amenorrhea specific to runners? Am J Obstet Gynecol. 1982;143:859-61.

84. ACSM position stand on the female athlete triad. Sports Exerc. 1997;29:1-9.

85. Sanborn CF, Horea M, Siemer BJ, Dieringer KI. Disordered eating and the female athlete triad: the athletic woman. Clin Sports Med. 2000;19:199-213.

86. American Academy of Pediatrics, Committee on Sports Medicine and Fitness. Medical concerns in the female patient. Pediatrics. 2000;106:610-3.

87. Cummings DC, Cummings CE. Estrogen replacement therapy and female athletes. Sports Med. 2001:31:1025-31.

88. Lebrun CM, Rumball JS. Female athlete triad. Sports Med Arthroscopy Rev. 2002;10:23-32.

89. Burrows M, Bird S. The physiology of the highly trained female endurance runner. Sports Med. 2000;4:281-300.

90. ACOG Committee on Obstetric Practice. Exercise during pregnancy and the postpartum period. Obstet Gynecol. 2002;99:171-3.

91. Brenner PF. Differential diagnosis of abnormal uterine bleeding. Am J Obstet Gynecol. 1996;175:766-9.

92. Cundy TF, Butler J, Pope RM, et al. Amenorrhea in women with non-alcoholic chronic liver disease. Gut. 1991;32:202-6.

93. Marks JB. The liver and the endocrine system. In: Schiff's Diseases of the Liver, 8th ed. Philadelphia: JB Lippincott. 1999;477-88.

94. Haimov-Kochman R, Ackerman Z, Anteby EY. The contraceptive choice for a Wilson's disease patient with chronic liver disease. Contraception. 1997;56:241-4.

95. World Health Organization. Medical eligibility criteria for contraceptive use. In: Improving Access to Quality Care in Family Planning, 2nd ed.

96. Wallach M, Grimes DA. Modern Oral Contraception: Updates from the Contraceptive Report. Totowa, NJ: Emron; 2000.

97. Sotaniemi EA, Hynnynen T, Ahlqvist J, et al. Effects of medroxyprogesterone on the liver function and drug metabolism of patients with primary biliary cirrhosis and chronic active hepatitis. J Med. 1978;9:117-28.

98. Connolly TJ, Zuckerman AL. Contraception in the patient with liver disease. Semin Perinatol. 1998;22:178-82.

99. ACOG Technical Bulletin 198, Hormonal Contraception; October 1994.

100. Decherney AH. The use of birth control pills in women with medical disorders. Clin Obstet Gynecol. 1981;24:965-75.

101. Laifer SA, Guido RS. Reproductive function and outcome of pregnancy after liver transplantation in women. Mayo Clin Proc. 1995;70:388-94.

102. George ED, Schluger LK. Special women's health issues in hepatobiliary diseases. Clin Fam Pract. 2000;2:155-69.

103. Holley JL, Schmidt RJ, Bender FH, et al. Gynecologic and reproductive issues in women on dialysis. Am J Kidney Dis. 1997;29:685-90.

104. Lim VS. Reproductive function in patients with renal insufficiency. Am J Kidney Dis. 1987;9:363-7.

105. Cochrane R, Regan L. Undetected gynaecological disorders in women with renal disease. Hum Reprod. 1997;12:667-70.

106. Rush H, Neugarten J, Coco M. Women's health issues in a dialysis population. Clin Nephrol. 2000;54:455-62.

107. Chao AS, Huang JY, Lien R, et al. Pregnancy in women who undergo long-term hemodialysis. Am J Obstet Gynecol. 2002;187:1.

108. Samuels P, Colombo DF. Renal disease. In: Obstetrics: Normal and Problem Pregnancies, 4th ed. New York: Churchill Livingstone; 2002:1065-79.

109. Powrie RO, Rosene-Montella K, Davidson JM, Hayslett JP. Hypertension and renal disease. In: Medical Care of the Pregnant Patient. Philadelphia: American College of Physicians; 2000:185-233.

110. Pasoto SG, Mendonca BB, Bonfa E. Menstrual disturbances in patients with systemic lupus erythematosus without alkylating therapy: clinical, hormonal and therapeutic associations. Lupus. 2002;11:175-80.

111. Lautenbach GL, Petri M. General medical care of the patient with rheumatic disease. Rheum Dis Clin N Am. 1999;25:539-65.

112. Frederiksen MC. Depot medroxyprogesterone acetate contraception in women with medical problems. J Reprod Med. 1996;41(5S):414-8.

113. Rosene-Montella K. Rheumatologic disorders and the antiphospholipid antibody syndrome. In: Medical Care of the Pregnant Patient. Philadelphia: American College of Physicians; 2000.

114. Canobbio MM, Rapkin JK, Perloff JK, et al. Menstrual patterns in women with congenital heart disease. Pediatr Cardiol. 1995;16:12-5.

115. Weir RJ. Oral contraceptives and hypertension. In: Textbook of Hypertension. Swales JD, ed. New York: Blackwell Scientific Publications; 1994:153-68.

116. Tyson JE. Oral contraception and elevated blood pressure. Am J Obstet Gynecol. 1968;100:875-6.

117. Saruta T. A possible mechanism for hypertension induced by oral contraceptives. Arch Intern Med. 1970;26:621-6.

118. ACOG Committee on Practice Bulletin. Chronic hypertension in pregnancy. Obstet Gynecol. 2001;98:177-85.

119. ACOG Committee on Practice Bulletin. The use of hormonal contraception in women with co-existing medical conditions. Int J Gynaecol Obstet. 2001;75:93-106.

120. Chasen-Taber L, Stampfer MJ. Epidemiology of oral contraceptives and cardiovascular disease. Ann Intern Med. 1998;128:467-77.

121. Knopp RH, LaRosa JC, Burkman, RT. Contraception and dyslipidemia. Am J Obstet Gynecol. 1993;168:1994-2005.

122. Davidoff F, Tishler S, Rosoff C. Hyperlipidemia and pancreatitis associated with oral contraceptive therapy. N Engl J Med. 1973;289:552.

123. Swan L, Hillis WS, Cameron A. Family planning requirements of adults with congenital heart disease. Heart. 1997;78:9-11.

124. Sullivan JM, Lobo RA. Considerations for contraception in women with cardiovascular disorders. Am J Obstet Gynecol. 1993;168(6S):2006-11.

125. Mendelson MA. Gynecologic and obstetric issues in the adolescent with heart disease. Adolesc Med State Art Rev. 2001;12:163-74.

126. Poppas A. Congenital and acquired heart disease. In Medical Care of the Pregnant Patient. Philadelphia: American College of Physicians; 2000:355-70.

127. Practice parameter: management issues for women with epilepsy (summary statement). Report of the Quality Standards Subcommittee of the American Academy of Neurology. Epilepsia. 1998;51:944-8.

128. Morell MJ. Effects of epilepsy on women's reproductive health. Epilepsia. 1998;39 (Suppl 8):S32-S37.

129. Bauer J, Isojarvi JIT, Herzog AG, et al. Reproductive dysfunction in women with epilepsy: recommendations for evaluation and treatment. J Neurol Neurosurg Psychiatr. 2002;73:121-5.

130. Logsdon-Pokorny VK. Mini-review. Epilepsy in adolescents: hormonal considerations. J Pediatr Adolesc Gynecol. 2000;13:9-13.

131. Crawford P. Interactions between antiepileptic drugs and hormonal contraception. CNS Drugs. 2002;16:263-72.

132. GlaxoSmithKline. Lamictal (lamotrigine tablets) Prescribing Information, August 2004.

133. Holmes LB, Harvey EA, Coull BA, et al. The teratogenicity of anticonvulsant drugs. N Engl J Med. 2001;344:1132-8.

134. Borbour L, Pickard J. Epilepsy. In: Medical Care of the Pregnant Patient. Philadelphia: American College of Physicians; 2000:669-81.

Management Details

11

Procedural Management of Abnormal Uterine Bleeding

D. Paul Shackelford, MD
Matthew K. Hoffman, MD, MPH

Procedural management of abnormal uterine bleeding continues to be re-served for patients who fail medical management. Before procedural management of menstrual abnormalities is initiated, a thorough diagnostic evaluation that includes an assessment of the endometrium must be performed to exclude underlying endometrial carcinoma and hyperplasia.

Historically, hysterectomy has been the mainstay of procedural treatment of menstrual irregularities, and it remains the most commonly performed nonpregnancy-related surgical procedure performed in the United States (1). However, recent advances in technology have provided women with other options. These include endometrial ablation (using a variety of techniques), uterine artery embolization, hysteroscopic resection of endometrial polyps and myomas, and radiation. It is important that providers caring for women understand the indications, success rates, limitations, and complications of these various procedures. Unfortunately, the paucity of comparative trials that examine the long-term success and complications of the different techniques makes direct comparisons and directed counseling more difficult.

Before any procedure is considered, two separate issues need to be addressed. First, does the patient desire future pregnancy? As women choose alternatives to hysterectomy, those who want to become pregnant in the future must be offered procedures with an established pregnancy safety record (e.g., myomectomy). Second, the patient must be assessed for individual medical risks. Risks associated with surgery depend on the choice of procedure and the patient's underlying medical conditions; hysterectomy, for example, confers more risk than the minimally invasive procedures.

Hysterectomy

Hysterectomy remains the most definitive and effective surgical therapy for abnormal uterine bleeding. Because of the many advances that have been made in surgical technique, hysterectomy has become a safe choice for the majority of patients. Currently, the overall death rate is 0.6/1000 (2). The rate is lower for nonemergent cases, noncancer cases, and cases not related to obstetric complications. Irregular uterine bleeding and symptomatic uterine leiomyomas are the two most common indications for hysterectomy. Vaginal hysterectomy remains the safest of the techniques, with an overall lower rate of surgical morbidity and lesser direct and indirect costs (Table 12-1) (1-3). Despite these benefits, vaginal hysterectomy continues to be underutilized, representing only 25% of the hysterectomies performed in the United States (4). Abdominal hysterectomy is believed to confer higher rates of morbidity, in part due to the added surgical trauma of the abdominal incision and use of this technique in more difficult cases.

With the development of advanced laparoscopic surgical techniques, the laparoscopic-assisted vaginal hysterectomy and the laparoscopic hysterectomy have gained acceptance among gynecologic surgeons. Advantages include a shorter overall hospital stay and a more rapid return to work compared with abdominal hysterectomy. Surgical morbidity rates lie between those of vaginal and abdominal hysterectomy. Steep learning curves, the high cost of the instruments, and the longer operative time are issues that have impeded universal acceptance of laparoscopic-assisted procedures (4). A promising development is the introduction of surgical robotics. The improved visualization and removal of natural hand tremor may improve the safety and the speed of the procedure (5).

Patient satisfaction studies have suggested that patients are generally satisfied with the long-term results of hysterectomy. This is particularly true of patients who received treatment for abnormal uterine bleeding and symptomatic uterine myomas. This may be less true of patients with other surgical indications such as pelvic pain (6,7).

Table 12-1   Complication Rates by Type of Hysterectomy

	Abdominal Hysterectomy	Vaginal Hysterectomy	Laparoscopically Assisted Vaginal Hysterectomy
Transfusion	15%	8%	?
Infection	7-9%	3-5%	6%
Bowel and bladder injury	2%	2%	3%

Myomectomy

An increasingly accepted alternative to hysterectomy for women with leiomyomas (fibroids) is myomectomy. Leiomyomas are endemic among women in their 40s and remain one of the most common reasons for gynecologic surgery. They are detected in 25% of women undergoing clinical examination, approximately 50% of asymptomatic women who undergo transvaginal sonography, and 80% of women at the time of necropsy (8-10).

Given that leiomyomas are nearly universal in women aged 40 years and older, it is generally accepted that it is necessary to treat them only when they are symptomatic (causing pressure and bleeding) and/or raise concern for leiomyosarcoma. Historically, rapidly expanding leiomyomas have been viewed as a high-risk factor for leiomyosarcoma. Interestingly, the only study that has examined this found that the risk of leiomyosarcoma in patients with rapidly expanding leiomyomas (2-3/1000 hysterectomies performed for fibroids) was no greater than in women without such leiomyomas (11).

The location and size of the leiomyoma dictate the patient's symptoms as well as the surgical approach. Myomectomy may be performed abdominally, hysteroscopically, or laparoscopically. Leiomyomas that are submucous (below the endometrium) tend to manifest as irregular bleeding and can be approached hysteroscopically. Those that are subserosa (below the serosal layer) or intramural (within the uterine wall) are more likely to result in pelvic pressure and require a transabdominal approach. The decision to perform a myomectomy (selective removal of the leiomyoma) is appropriate in women who choose to retain their pregnancy potential or who choose not to undergo hysterectomy. It is important that patients considering myomectomy understand the risk of recurrent fibroids that will require subsequent surgery. In one large series, the risk for subsequent surgery was 11% in women with a solitary fibroid and 26% in women with multiple fibroids (12).

Abdominal Myomectomy

Historically, abdominal myomectomy has been the surgical approach of choice. Although there has been a perceived higher rate of complications with this procedure, recent studies have suggested that the risks are in keeping with those of hysterectomy (13,14). Moreover, this procedure has a proven history of safety in subsequent pregnancy. The rate of uterine rupture of the endometrial cavity appears to be quite low at 0.1% or less; however, the exact incidence is unknown (15).

Laparoscopic Myomectomy

Laparoscopic myomectomy is an option for women with a solitary leiomyoma in the range of 5-8 cm. Currently, the safety of pregnancy after laparoscopic myomectomy has not been validated. Cases of uterine rupture and uterine peritoneal fistula after laparoscopic myomectomy have been clearly documented, although large series have not been reported (16).

Hysteroscopic Myomectomy

This approach offers shorter patient recovery compared with the other forms of myomectomy. Despite the ease of this procedure, hysteroscopic myomectomy appears to be a very effective method of resolving menorrhagia, with no more than approximately 15% of patients requiring subsequent surgery (17). Fertility remains acceptable after this procedure, with as many as 59% of women achieving pregnancy (18).

Uterine Artery Embolization

Uterine artery embolization has increasingly been viewed as an alternative to myomectomy. This procedure involves catheterizing the fine branches of the uterine arteries and selectively embolizing the vessels supplying the leiomyomas. Normal myometrium quickly develops collateral blood supply after the embolization, whereas leiomyomas do not. Short-term studies have demonstrated that uterine artery embolization results in both shrinkage of the leiomyomas and improvement in menstrual and volume-related symptoms (19,20). Long-term studies and studies identifying patients at greater risk for failure are lacking. Immediate complications include febrile morbidity (2%), hemorrhage (0.75%), performance of unintended procedure (2.5%), life-threatening event (0.05%), and need for readmission (3.5%) (21). Although pregnancy after embolization has been reported, longitudinal safety data are lacking.

Endometrial Ablation

Endometrial ablation attempts to resolve abnormal bleeding by destroying the endometrium while leaving the underlying myometrium intact. The ability to destroy all of the endometrium is inhibited by the anatomy of the uterus. Specifically, the cornu and the lower uterine segment are difficult to reach with the majority of techniques.

This anatomic limitation is thought to be the major reason for the varied success rates among different procedures. Anatomic distortion associated with uterine myomas precludes the use of most endometrial ablation techniques in many patients. In general, endometrial ablation, irrespective of technique, is associated with amenorrhea in 20% to 60% of patients and a subjective improvement in 80% of patients up to 1 year after ablation (22). Some long-term studies of endometrial ablation note a 40% success rate at 5 years, with a significant portion of patients requiring a second procedure (23,24).

Hysteroscopic techniques include endomyometrial resection and contact electrosurgical ablation (commonly referred to as rollerball ablation). Both techniques have a significant learning curve and operator-dependant success rates. Surgical morbidity is uncommon, occurring in 2.5% of cases (25). Surgical morbidity is increased to 9.3% in patients treated with a second hysteroscopic ablation (26). Surgical morbidity, specifically fluid overload and resulting electrolyte imbalance, is a significant concern with hysteroscopic techniques. Other complications associated with hysteroscopic ablation include uterine perforation and associated bowel or bladder injury.

Nonhysteroscopic ablative techniques have become popular due to their simplicity of use, similar success rates, and lower surgical morbidity compared with hysteroscopic modalities. Several techniques are available, including thermal balloon, cryosurgical technique, and radiofrequency. Long-term randomized studies are available for the thermal balloon technique only. Success rates of the thermal balloon technique are similar to those of the hysteroscopic techniques (22). Fertility after endometrial ablation has been reported. Nevertheless, endometrial ablation should not be used in patients who desire future pregnancy, because a higher rate of pregnancy complications, particularly malplacentation, has been reported (27). It is thus generally recommended that surgical sterilization be performed concurrently with any form of endometrial ablation. Uterine perforation remains the most common complication with nonhysteroscopic techniques.

Hysteroscopic Resection of Endometrial Polyps

Endometrial polyps remain a common cause of abnormal bleeding, being found in approximately 20% to 25% of reproductive-age women, with a peak incidence in women in their 40s (28). Although natural history studies have suggested that more than 50% of polyps may resolve spontaneously, hysteroscopic resection remains the mainstay of treatment for most women (29). The goal of resection is to restore normal menstrual cycles and rule out the possibility of underlying hyperplasia and/or carcinoma. The risk of endometrial hyperplasia arising in a polyp is approximately 11%; the risk of endometrial hyperplasia with atypia is 3.3%; and the risk of endometrial carcinoma is 3% (30). These risks appear to be higher in women who are postmenopausal. Hysteroscopic resection can be achieved by various instruments, such as grasping forceps, microscissors, and electrosurgery. With successful resection, eumenorrhea can be achieved in more than 90% of women without other underlying pathology (31).

Radiation Therapy

The use of ionizing radiation to manage abnormal uterine bleeding dates back to the early use of radiation in medicine. Initially the technique was believed to be safe and was highly effective. The technique was abandoned due to the high occurrence of uterine sarcomas and leukemia 10 to 20 years after the initial treatment (32-34). With the development of modern equipment and a better understanding of radiation biology, the technique may be considered in patients for whom medical therapy has failed and surgical therapy is not an option.

Summary

Abnormal uterine bleeding is a common gynecologic problem encountered by primary care physicians and gynecologists alike. Various procedural options are available for patients who fail medical management. Hysterectomy offers safe and definitive treatment. Less invasive alternatives, such as endometrial ablation, uterine artery embolization, myomectomy, and resection of endometrial polyps, are gaining in popularity and offer new options for many women. Thus, surgical treatment can now be individualized based upon the patient's desires, medical condition, and anatomy. It is crucial that providers understand the complications and limitations of these various procedures.

REFERENCES

1. Lepine LA, et al. Hysterectomy Surveillance: United States, 1980-1993. Vol. 46. No. SS-4 MMWR 1.
2. Dicker RC, Greenspan JR, Stauss LT, et al. Complications of abdominal and vaginal hysterectomy among women of reproductive age in the United States. Am J Obstet Gynecol. 1982;144:841-8.
3. Harris WJ. Early complications of abdominal and vaginal hysterectomy. Obstet Gynecol Survey. 1995;50:795-804.
4. Farquhar CM, Steiner CA. Hysterectomy rates in the United States, 1990-1997. Obstet Gynecol. 2002;99:229-34.

5. Margossian H, Falcone T. Robotically assisted laparoscopic hysterectomy and adnexal surgery. J Laparoendosc Adv Surg Tech. 2001;11:161-5.

6. Kjerulff KH, Rhodes JC, Langenberg PW, Harvey LA. Patient satisfaction with results of hysterectomy. Am J Obstet Gynecol. 2000;183:1440-7.

7. Weber AM, Walters MD, Schover LR, et al. Functional outcomes and satisfaction after abdominal hysterectomy. Am J Obstet Gynecol. 1999;181:530-5.

8. Buttram VC, Reiter RC. Uterine leiomyomata: etiology, symptomatology and management. Fertil Steril. 1981;36:443-5.

9. Baird DD, Dunson DB, Hill MC, et al. High cumulative incidence of uterine leiomyoma in black and white women: ultrasound evidence. Am J Obstet Gynecol. 2003;188:100-7.

10. Cramer SF, Patel A. The frequency of uterine leiomyomas. Am J Clin Pathol. 1990;94:433-8.

11. Parker WH, Fu YS, Berek JS. Uterine sarcoma in patients operated on for presumed leiomyoma and rapidly growing leiomyoma. Obstet Gynecol. 1994;83:414-8.

12. Malone LJ. Myomectomy: recurrence after removal of solitary and multiple myomas. Obstet Gynecol. 1969;34:200-3.

13. Hillis SD, Marchbanks PA, Peterson HB. Uterine size and risk of complications among women undergoing abdominal hysterectomy for leiomyomas. Obstet Gynecol. 1996;87:539-43.

14. Iverson RE Jr, Chelmow D, Strohbehn K, et al. Relative morbidity of abdominal hysterectomy and myomectomy for management of uterine leiomyomas. Obstet Gynecol. 1996;88:415-9.

15. Garnet JD. Uterine rupture during pregnancy: an analysis of 133 patients. Obstet Gynecol. 1964;23:898-905.

16. Harris WJ. Uterine dehiscence following laparoscopic myomectomy. Obstet Gynecol. 1992;80:545-6.

17. Derman SG, Rehnstrom J, Neuwirth RS. The long-term effectiveness of hysteroscopic treatment of menorrhagia and leiomyomas. Obstet Gynecol. 1991;77:591-4.

18. Ubaldi F, Tournaye H, Camus M, et al. Fertility after hysteroscopic myomectomy. Hum Reprod Update. 1995;1:81-90.

19. Pron G, Bennett J, Common A, et al. The Ontario Uterine Fibroid Embolization Trial. Part 2. Uterine fibroid reduction and symptom relief after uterine artery embolization for fibroids. Fertil Steril. 2003;79:120-7.

20. Broder MS, Goodwin S, Chen G, et al. Comparison of long-term outcomes of myomectomy and uterine artery embolization. Obstet Gynecol. 2002;100:864-8.

21. Uterine Artery Embolization. ACOG Committee Opinion Number 293, February 2004.

22. Meyer WE, Walsh BW, Grainger DA, et al. Thermal balloon and rollerball ablation to treat menorrhagia multicenter comparison. Obstet Gynecol. 1998;92:98-103.

23. A randomized trial of endometrial ablation versus hysterectomy for the treatment of dysfunctional uterine bleeding: outcome at four years. Aberdeen Endometrial Ablation Trials Group. Br J Obstet Gynaecol. 1999;106:360-6.

24. Boujida VH, Philipsen T, Pelle J, Joergensen JC. Five-year follow-up of endometrial ablation: endometrial coagulation versus endometrial resection. Obstet Gynecol. 2002;99:988-92.

25. Propst AM, Liberman RF, Harlow BL, Ginsburg ES. Complications of hysteroscopic surgery: predicting patients at risk. Obstet Gynecol. 2000;96:517-20.

26. MacLean-Fraser E, Penava D, Vilos GA. Perioperative complication rates of primary and repeat hysteroscopic endometrial ablations. J Am Assoc Gynecol Laparosc. 2002;9:175-7.

27. Hoffman MK, Sciscione AC. Placenta accreta and intrauterine fetal death in a woman with prior endometrial ablation: a case report. J Reprod Med. 2004;49:384-6.

28. Woodruff ENJ. Novak's Gynecologic and Obstetic Pathology with Clinical and Endocrine Relations, 8th ed. Philadelphia: WB Saunders; 1979.

29. DeWaay DJ, Syrop CH, Nygaard IE, et al. Natural history of uterine polyps and leiomyomata. Obstet Gynecol. 2002;100:3-7.

30. Ben-Arie A, Goldschmit C, Laviv Y, et al. The malignant potential of endometrial polyps. Eur J Obstet Gynecol Reprod Biol. 2004;115:206-10.

31. Preutthipan S, Herabutya Y. Hysteroscopic polypectomy in 240 premenopausal and postmenopausal women. Fertil Steril. 2005;83:705-9.

32. Nikolic B, Spies JB, Lundsten MJ, Abbara S. Patient radiation dose associated with uterine artery embolization. Radiology. 2000;214:121-5.

33. Nikkanen V, Salmi T, Gronroos M. Uterine malignant degeneration after low-dose endometrial irradiation. Int J Gynaecol Obstet. 1980;18:240-2.

34. Inskip PD, Monson RR, Wagoner JK, et al. Leukemia following radiotherapy for uterine bleeding. Radiation Res. 1990;122:107-19.

Index

A

Abdominal examination in dysmenorrhea, 103
Abdominal myomectomy, 247
Abdominal wall pain, 118
Ablation
    endometrial, 248-249
        post-ablation syndrome after, 116
    laparoscopic uterosacral nerve, 111
Abnormal uterine bleeding. *See* Bleeding,
    abnormal uterine
Abuse
    of mentally disabled patient, 164
    substance, 209-211
Acanthosis nigricans, 59-60, 146-147
Acetaminophen, 107
Acne, 153
Acupuncture, 112
Acute liver disease, 217-222
Adenoma, prolactin-secreting, 60-61, 144
Adenomyosis, 114-115
Adolescent
    abnormal bleeding in, 16-18
    cycle length in, 12
    pelvic examination in, 104
    perimenarchal, bleeding in, 31-32
    primary amenorrhea in, 52-54
Adrenal disorder, 63-64
Adrenal hyperplasia, congenital, 144, 147, 149
Adrenarche, 7
African American
    menarche in, 7
    precocious puberty in, 10
Age
    abnormal bleeding and, 29-30
    at menarche, 6-7
    premature ovarian failure and, 58
Agenesis, müllerian, 56
Alcohol abuse, 209-211
Alcoholic liver disease, 218, 220
Algorithm
    for dysmenorrhea, 102
    for menorrhagia, 181
    for secondary amenorrhea, 68
Alopecia, 152-153
Alternative therapy for dysmenorrhea, 111-112
Amenorrhea, 51-76
    alcohol abuse and, 209
    characteristics of, 30
    chronic anovulation in, 59-64
    in developmentally disabled patient, 163-164
    in diabetes mellitus, 200-201
    differential diagnosis of, 85
    drug-related, 64-65
    eating disorder and, 211-213
    in female athlete, 215
    hypergonadotropic hypogonadism with, 57-58
    hypothalamic, 62-63

Amenorrhea *(cont'd.)*
    hypothyroidism and, 42
    in liver disease, 218
    outflow tract abnormality as, 54-57
    overview of, 51-52
    primary
        in adolescent, 19, 52-54
        defined, 51
        diagnosis of, 65-66
        in hypergonadotropic hypogonadism, 57-58
        puberty and, 7
        treatment of, 70-71
        in renal disease, 222
    secondary, 19, 51
        diagnosis of, 66-70
        in hypergonadotropic hypogonadism, 57-58
        structural abnormality in, 56-57
        treatment of, 71-73
American Academy of Neurology, 233
Amicar
    for bleeding disorder, 187
    for factor deficiency, 188
Amphetamine, 209-210
Anatomic lesion
    bleeding due to, 33
    dysmenorrhea with, 116
Androgen-insensitivity hormone, 56
Androgen-receptor antagonist, 152
Angiotensin-converting enzyme inhibitor, 228
Anorexia nervosa, 72-73, 211-213
    amenorrhea and, 32
Anovulation
    chronic, 59-64
        Cushing's disease and, 63-64
        hyperandrogenism causing, 59-60
        hyperprolactinemia in, 60-62
        hypogonadotropic hypogonadism and, 62-
            63
        in pituitary insufficiency, 63
        in thyroid disease, 63
        treatment of, 72-73
    in diabetes mellitus, 201
    in mentally disabled patient, 164
    in polycystic ovarian syndrome, 153
    in renal disease, 222
    in young girl, 4
Anovulatory bleeding, 32-33
    in developmentally disabled patient, 161-163
    in early gynecologic years, 10-11
Antagonist, androgen-receptor, 152-153
Anti-epileptic drug, 232-235
Anti-inflammatory drug
    in bleeding disorder, 176, 184
    for developmentally disabled patient, 162
    for dysmenorrhea, 104-105, 105, 106
    for perimenopausal bleeding, 89-90
    for premenstrual syndrome, 135

Antiandrogen, 152-153
Anticoagulant therapy, 189
Anticonvulsant, 158
    oral contraceptives and, 166
Antifibrinolytic agent, 188
Antihypertensive therapy, 230-231
    prolactin and, 61
Antiphospholipid syndrome, 224-226
Antispasmodic, 110
Artery embolization, uterine, 248
Arthritis, rheumatoid, 226
Asherman's syndrome, 56-57
    treatment of, 71-72
Aspirin, 106
Atherosclerotic heart disease, 228-229, 231
Athlete
    contraception for, 216
    menstrual disorders in, 214-216
    preconception counseling for, 216-217
Atrophy, endometrial, 45
Atypical endometrial hyperplasia, 45
Atypical glandular cell, 38
Autoantibody, 189
Autoimmune disease, 58
Autoplex, 189

B
Bariatric surgery, 206
Barrier contraception for mentally disabled
        patient, 165, 166
Behavior disorder, 162
Bernard-Soulier syndrome, 180
Beta-adrenergic antagonist, 109
Beta-human chorionic gonadotropin, 36
Biliary cirrhosis, 218, 220
Bipolar disorder, 129
Birth control pill. *See* Hormonal contraceptive
Bleeding
    abnormal uterine, 29-49
        in adolescent, 16-18
        anatomic lesions causing, 33-34
        anovulatory, 32-33, 33, 43-44
        coagulation studies in, 42
        complete blood count in, 42
        in developmentally disabled patient, 161-163
        endometrial, 38-42
        endometrial ablation for, 248-249
        endometrial cells on Pap smear in, 37-38
        etiology of, 30-35
        evaluation of, 35-42
        fibroids and, 44-45
        history in, 35-36
        hysterectomy for, 246
        in infant, 30-31
        menorrhagia and, 43
        myomectomy for, 247-248
        overview of, 245
        Pap smear in, 37-38
        in perimenarchal adolescent, 31-32
        perimenopausal, 34, 77-96. *See also*
                Perimenopause
        physical examination in, 36-37
        polyps and, 44, 249-250

Bleeding *(cont'd.)*
    abnormal uterine *(cont'd.)*
        postmenopausal, 23, 34-35, 37-38, 44-46
        pregnancy testing in, 36
        procedural management of, 245-252
        radiation therapy for, 250
        recurrent, 46
        terminology about, 30
        of thyroid function, 36
        treatment of, 42-46
        uterine artery embolization for, 248
    break-through, 4
    in early gynecologic years, 10-11
Bleeding diasthesis, in adolescent, 17
Bleeding disorder, 171-195
    etiology of
        of fibrin clot formation, 177-178
        of platelet plug formation, 174-177
        vascular, 174
    evaluation of, 178-182
    overview of, 172-173
    in perimenopausal patient, 83
    treatment of, 182-189
        in chronic medical anticoagulation, 189
        drugs for, 186-187
        for factor deficiency, 188-189
        of platelet disorder, 184-185
        of von Willebrand disease, 184-187
Bleeding time, 181-182
Blood count, 42
Blood pressure, 227-232
    contraception and, 227-228, 231
    fertility and, 231
    menstrual disorder and, 227, 231
    in polycystic ovarian syndrome, 145
    preconception counseling and, 229-232
Body mass index, 80
Bone density in female athlete, 216
Bone loss, 162-163
Bowel disease, inflammatory, 116-117
Break-through bleeding, 4
Breast development, 9
Budd-Chiari syndrome, 220
Bulimia, 211-213
Butylbromide, 110

C
Calcium antagonist, 109
Calendar, menstrual
    for normal cycle, 14, 15
Cancer
    in adolescent, 18
    endometrial
        Pap smear in, 37
        postmenopausal bleeding in, 45-46
    in obesity, 205
    in perimenopause, 81-82
    postmenopausal bleeding and, 34
Carbamazepine, 235
Catamenial seizure, 232, 233
Celecoxib, 105
Cell
    atypical glandular, 38

Cell (cont'd.)
  endometrial, on Pap smear, 37-38
Cervical stenosis, 115-116
Chasteberry fruit, 133
Child, uterine bleeding in, 31
Cholelithiasis, 219
Cholestasis of pregnancy, 219
Cholestatic liver disease, 219
Cholesterol, 228
Chorionic gonadotropin, human, 6
Chromosomal abnormality, 57-58
Chronic anovulation, 59-64
  causes of, 59-64
  treatment of, 72-73
Chronic illness, 197-242. See also Medical
  condition
Chronic medical coagulation, 189
Chronic pelvic infection, 115
Cirrhosis, 218, 220
Citalopram, 133
Climacteric, 21-22
Clomiphene, 154-155
Clotting disorder. See Coagulation disorder
Coagulation disorder. See also Bleeding disorder
  abnormal bleeding in, 42
  in adolescent, 32
  diagnosis of, 85
  differential diagnosis of, 175
  etiology of, 173-178
    platelet plug formation as, 173-177
    vascular endothelium defect as, 173
  in perimenopausal patient, 83
  undiagnosed, 35
Coagulation factor deficiency, 177-178
  diagnosis of, 180
  treatment of, 188-189
Complete blood count, 42
Complications
  of hysterectomy, 246
  of pregnancy, 210
Conception. See also Preconceptionn counseling
  diabetes and, 202
  smoking and, 208
Congenital disorder
  adrenal hyperplasia as, 144, 147, 149
  cardiac, 229
  of coagulation, 180
  diabetes and, 202
  factor deficiency as, 188-189
  of platelet function, 180
Congestion, pelvic, 115
Contraception. See also Contraceptive, hormonal
  in atherosclerotic heart disease, 228-229
  in cardiovascular disease, 231
  for developmentally disabled patient, 164-167
  in eating disorder, 213
  efficacy of, 198
  for female athlete, 216, 217
  liver disease and, 218-219, 221, 222
  in obesity, 205, 206
  in renal disease, 223, 224
  smoking and, 207-208
  substance abuse and, 210, 211

Contraception (cont'd.)
  in systemic lupus erythematosus, 224-225, 226
Contraceptive, hormonal
  for abnormal perimenopausal bleeding, 90,
    91-92
  amenorrhea and, 64-65
  in atherosclerotic heart disease, 228-229
  as cause of amenorrhea, 52
  in diabetes, 201-202
  for dysmenorrhea, 107-108
  hypertension induced by, 227-228
  in liver disease, 218-220
  for menorrhagia, 182-183
  for mentally disabled patient, 165-166
  in polycystic ovarian syndrome, 148, 150-151
  for premenstrual syndrome, 135
  progestin-only
    in atherosclerotic heart disease, 229
    in diabetes, 202
    for dysmenorrhea, 108-109
    in hyperlipidemia, 228
    in liver disease, 218, 220
    in renal disease, 223
  in renal disease, 223
  in systemic lupus erythematosus, 225
Copper deposition, 218, 219-220
Coronary artery disease, 228-229
  in diabetes, 203
Corpus luteum, 5, 6
Cortisol test for Cushing syndrome, 67-68, 150
Counseling. See Preconception counseling
COX-2 inhibitor
  in bleeding disorder, 184
  bleeding disorder and, 176
  for dysmenorrhea, 107
Cramping, 20-21. See also Dysmenorrhea
Cryoprecipitate
  for bleeding disorder, 186
  for factor deficiency, 189
Cultural factors, 78
Cushing's syndrome, 63-64
  diagnosis of, 67-70
Cyclooxygenase inhibitor
  for dysmenorrhea, 104-105
  for perimenopausal bleeding, 90
Cyclosporine, 220
Cyst, functional, 20
Cystic acne, 153
Cystic follicle, 20
Cytochrome P450 system, 233, 232
Cytotoxic drug, 65

D
Danazol, 135
DDAVP
  for factor deficiency, 188
  for platelet disorder, 184-185
  in von Willebrand disease, 184-187
Dehydroepiandrosterone sulfate, 149
Dermatomyositis, 226
Depression, 129
1-Desamino-8-D-arginine vasopressin, 185, 186, 188
Desmopressin, 185, 186, 188

Developmentally disabled patient, 157-169
   abnormal uterine bleeding in, 161-163
   amenorrhea in, 163-164
   contraception for, 164-167
   epidemiology of menstrual cycles in, 157-158
   gynecological examination of, 159-161
   health history of, 158-159
   menarche in, 158
Dexamethasone suppression test, 64, 68-69
DHEA-S, 149
Diabetes mellitus
   contraceptive options in, 201-202
   menstrual disorders with, 200-201
   preconception counseling in, 202-204
   premature ovarian failure in, 58
Dialysis, 222
Diaphragm in diabetes, 202
Diclofenac, 105
Diet, 132
Diflunisal, 105
Disseminated intravascular coagulation, 176
DMPA. *See* Medroxyprogesterone acetate, depot
Down syndrome, 158
Drug therapy
   for abnormal perimenopausal bleeding, 89-90
   amenorrhea caused by, 64-65, 73
   anti-epileptic, 232-234
   anticoagulant, 189
   prolactin excess caused by, 61
   for smoking cessation, 208
Dysfunctional uterine bleeding, 32
Dysmenorrhea, 19-20, 97-123
   amphetamine abuse and, 209-210
   in developmentally disabled patient, 162
   overview of, 97-98
   primary, 98-112
      alternative therapy for, 111-112
      antispasmodics for, 110
      beta-adrenergic antagonist for, 109
      calcium antagonists for, 109
      COX-2 inhibitors for, 107
      epidemiology of, 98
      etiology of, 99
      evaluation of, 101-104
      narcotics for, 110
      oral contraceptives for, 107-108
      pathophysiology of, 99-101
      progestational drugs for, 108-109
      prostaglandin synthetase inhibitors for, 104-107
      risk factors for, 98-99
      surgery for, 110-111
      treatment of, 104-112
   secondary, 97, 112-118
      adenomyosis causing, 114-115
      endometriosis causing, 113-114
      gastrointestinal pain and, 116-117
      infection causing, 115
      musculoskeletal disorders in, 117-118
      pelvic congestion syndrome in, 115
      referral for, 113
      signs and symptoms of, 113
      urologic conditions in, 117

Dysmenorrhea *(cont'd.)*
   secondary *(cont'd.)*
      uterine anomalies causing, 115-116
Dyspareunia, 102
Dysphoric disorder, 129

E
Early perimenopause, 77
Eating disorder, 72-73, 211-214
   amenorrhea and, 32
   menstrual disorder in, 211-213
Eflornithine, 152-153
Eisenmenger's syndrome, 229
Electrical nerve stimulation, transcutaneous, 111-112
Embolization, uterine artery, 248
Embryology/American Society for Reproductive Medicine, 141-142
Endocervical polyps, 33-34
Endometrial ablation, 248-249
   dysmenorrhea after, 116
Endometrial bleeding, 3-4
Endometrial cancer
   in obesity, 205
   Pap smear in, 37
   postmenopausal bleeding in, 45-46
Endometrial cell on Pap smear, 37-38
Endometrial hyperplasia, 45
Endometrial polyp, 33
   hysteroscopic resection of, 249-250
Endometriosis, 113-114
Endometrium
   in anovulatory cycle, 11
   atrophy of, 45
   evaluation of, 38-42
      D&C in, 41-42
      piston suction device for, 39-40
      sonohysterography in, 41
      ultrasonography in, 41
   in perimenopause, 86-89
      biopsy of, 87
      dilation and curettage and, 88-89
      hysteroscopy of, 88
      magnetic resonance imaging of, 89
      sonohysterography of, 88
      ultrasonography of, 87
   progesterone stimulation of, 6
   in secondary amenorrhea, 56-57
Epilepsy, 158, 232-235
Epsilon-aminocaproic acid, 187, 188
Estrogen
   anovulatory bleeding and, 11, 33
   for bleeding disorder, 187
   in female athlete, 215
   in hyperandrogenism, 60
   in liver disease, 218, 219-220
   for menorrhagia, 183
   for mentally disabled patient, 166
   prolactin and, 61
Estrogen-containing contraceptive. *See also* Hormonal contraceptive
   in hepatitis, 219
   in hypertension, 228

Estrogen replacement therapy
  for abnormal perimenopausal bleeding, 90-92
  for mentally disabled patient, 164
Ethical issue, sterilization as, 167
Ethinyl estradiol, 166
Ethnic differences in menarche, 6-7
Etodolac, 105
European Society of Human Reproduction, 141-142
Exercise, 132

F
Factor deficiency, 177-178
  diagnosis of, 180
  treatment of, 188-189
Factor VIIA, 187-189
Factor VIII, 186, 189
  evaluation of, 179
Factor IX, 186
Female athlete, 214-217
Fertility
  in cardiovascular disease, 231
  in diabetes, 203, 204
  in liver disease, 220-221
  in polycystic ovarian syndrome, 145
  in seizure disorder, 234
  in systemic lupus erythematosus, 226
Fetal anomaly, in diabetes, 202
Fibrin clot formation disorder, 177-178
Fibroid
  bleeding due to, 33-34
  in perimenopausal patient, 80
Fibromyalgia, 118
Fluoxetine, 133-134
Flurbiprofen, 105
Flutamide, 152
Folic supplementation, 235
Follicle, cystic, 20
Follicle-stimulating hormone
  anovulatory cycle and, 10, 53
  in developmentally disabled patient, 157
  in normal menstrual cycle, 4-5
  in perimenopause, 86
  in polycystic ovarian syndrome, 148
  in secondary amenorrhea, 69
Follicular phase of menstrual cycle, 4-5
46,XY karyotype, 57
Fragile X syndrome, 58
Fresh frozen plasma, 189
Functional cyst, 19

G
Galactorrhea, 144
Genetic factors in polycystic ovarian syndrome, 145
Genital tract abnormality
  amenorrhea caused by, 54-57
  dysmenorrhea with, 116
Glandular cell, atypical, 38
Glanzmann thrombasthenia, 180
Gonadal dysgenesis, 57-58
Gonadotropin
  in female athlete, 214-215
  human chorionic, 6

Gonadotropin-releasing hormone
  anovulatory cycle and, 10, 53
  in developmentally disabled patient, 157
  dysmenorrhea and, 109
  in female athlete, 214
Gynecological examination. See Pelvic examination

H
Hair
  in polycystic ovarian syndrome, 145, 146-147
  pubic, 8
Heart disease, 228-232, 231
  atherosclerotic, 228-229
Heat treatment for dysmenorrhea, 112
HELLP syndrome, 175-176
Hemorrhagic telangectasia, hereditary, 173
Hemostasis
  normal, 171
  primary, 172
    disorders of, 173-174
  secondary, 172
    disorders of, 177-178
Hepatic coagulopathy, 189
Hepatitis, 219
Hepatitis vaccination, 183, 187
Herbal remedy, 133
Hereditary hemorrhagic telangectasia, 173
Hermansky-Pudlak disease, 184
Heroin abuse, 209
High-density lipoprotein, 228
Hirsutism, 146, 152
Histiocyte, 38
History, patient
  in amenorrhea, 66
  of dysmenorrhea, 100-101
  menstrual, 35
Hormonal contraceptive. See Contraceptive, hormonal
Hormone
  abnormal bleeding in adolescent and, 16
  age-related changes in, 79
  amenorrhea and, 64-65
  in female athlete, 215
  in hyperandrogenism, 60
  in hypogonadotropic hypogonadism, 62-63
  in liver disease, 218
  in menopause, 23
  menstrual cycle and, 4-6
  in perimenopause, 86
  in polycystic ovarian syndrome, 148
  seizures and, 232-233
  uterine bleeding and, 3-4
Hormone replacement therapy
  for abnormal perimenopausal bleeding, 90-92
  for mentally disabled patient, 164
Human chorionic gonadotropin, 6
  in pregnancy testing, 36
Humate-P, 185
17-α-Hydroxyprogesterone, 149
Hygiene, menstrual, 160
Hymen, imperforate, 55, 71
Hyoscine, 110

Hyperandrogenism, 59-60
Hypergonadotropic hypogonadism, 57-58
Hyperinsulinemia, 143
    in polycystic ovarian syndrome, 146-147
Hyperlipidemia, 231
Hypermenorrhea, 19
Hyperplasia
    congenital adrenal, 144, 147, 149
    endometrial, 45
Hyperprolactinemia, 60-62
Hypertension, 227-232
    contraception in, 227-228, 231
    fertility in, 231
    menstrual disorder in, 227, 231
    preconception counseling in, 229-232
Hypoestrogenism, 215
Hypogonadism
    hypergonadotropic, 57-58
    hypogonadotropic, 62-63
Hypoleptinemia, 212
Hypomenorrhea, 19
Hypothalamic disease, 62-63
    diagnosis of, 70
    prolactin excess and, 61
    treatment of, 72-73
Hypothalamic-pituitary axis, 12-13, 53
Hypothyroidism, 42
Hysterectomy
    for abnormal bleeding, 246
    for menorrhagia, 182
    in mentally disabled patient, 163
Hysteroscopic myomectomy, 248
Hysteroscopic resection of endometrial polyp,
    249-250

I
Ibuprofen for dysmenorrhea, 105
Imaging
    in amenorrhea diagnosis, 65
    in dysmenorrhea, 104
Immune thrombocytopenic purpura, 175-176
Immunoglobulin in platelet disorder, 184
Immunologic disorder, 173
Imperforate hymen, 55, 71
Index, body mass, 80
Indomethacin, 106
Infant, uterine bleeding in, 30-31
Infertility. See Fertility
Inflammatory bowel disease, 116-117
Insulin resistance
    in hyperandrogenism, 59-60
    in polycystic ovarian syndrome, 142-143,
        153
Intrauterine device
    in atherosclerotic heart disease, 229
    in diabetes, 202
    for dysmenorrhea, 109
    in hyperlipidemia, 228
    for mentally disabled patient, 165, 166-167
    in renal disease, 223
Intravenous immunoglobulin, 184
Irregular bleeding in developmentally disabled
    patient, 161-163

K
Karyotype in gonadal dysgenesis, 57
Ketoprofen, 105
Ketorolac, 105
Kidney disease, 222-224

L
Laboratory evaluation
    of amenorrhea, 67-70
    of bleeding disorder, 179-182
    of dysmenorrhea, 104
    of polycystic ovarian syndrome, 148-150
Laparoscopic hysterectomy, 246
Laparoscopic myomectomy, 248
Laparoscopic uterosacral nerve ablation, 111
Laparoscopy for dysmenorrhea, 110-111
Leiomyoma
    bleeding due to, 33-34
    in perimenopausal patient, 80
Leukotriene, 100
Lipoprotein, 228
Liver disease, 217-222
    alcoholic, 220
    bleeding with, 189
    Budd-Chiari syndrome as, 220
    cholestatic, 219
    cirrhosis as, 220
    contraception in, 218-219, 221, 222
    hepatitis as, 219
    menstrual disorders in, 218, 221
    post-transplantation, 220
    preconception counseling in, 220-222
    spectrum of, 217
    Wilson's, 219-220
Low-density lipoprotein, 228
LUNA, 111
Lupus erythematosus, systemic, 224-226
Luteal phase symptoms, 127-128
Luteinizing hormone
    anovulatory cycle and, 53
    anovulatory cycles and, 11
    in developmentally disabled patient, 157
    in perimenopause, 86
    in polycystic ovarian syndrome, 148

M
Malignancy
    in adolescent, 17
    endometrial
        Pap smear in, 37
        postmenopausal bleeding in, 45-46
    in obesity, 205
    in perimenopause, 81-82
    postmenopausal bleeding and, 34
Medical coagulation, chronic, 189
Medical condition, 197-242
    antiphospholipid syndrome as, 224-226
    athletic participation and, 214-217
    cardiovascular, 227-232
    contraception in, 198-200
    diabetes as, 200-204
    eating disorder as, 211-214
    liver disease as, 217-222

Medical condition *(cont'd.)*
  obesity as, 204-207
  renal disease as, 222-224
  seizure disorder as, 232-235
  substance abuse and, 209-211
  systemic lupus erythematosus as, 224-226
  tobacco use and, 207-209
Medroxyprogesterone acetate, depot
  amenorrhea and, 64-65
  for developmentally disabled patient, 162
  for mentally disabled patient, 165, 166
  weight gain with, 162, 163
Mefenamic acid, 105
Menarche, 4
  in developmentally disabled patient, 158
  in diabetes mellitus, 200
  in female athlete, 214
  in obesity, 204
  pubertal development and, 6-10
Menometrorrhagia, 19, 30
  alcohol abuse and, 209
Menopause, 21-22
  abnormal bleeding in, 77-96. *See also*
    Perimenopause
  bleeding after, 34-35
    endometrial cells on Pap smear in,
      37-38
    etiology of, 34-35
    recurrent, 46
    treatment of, 45-46
  in diabetes mellitus, 201
  transition to, 77
Menorrhagia, 19
  bleeding disorder with, 171-195. *See also*
    Bleeding disorder
  characteristics of, 30
  coagulopathy and, 32, 42
  in developmentally disabled patient,
    162
  polyps causing, 33
  von Willebrand disease causing, treatment of,
    185-188
Menstrual calendar
  for normal cycle, 14, 15
Menstrual cycle, normal, 3-25, 30
  in adult, 18-21
    abnormal bleeding patterns in, 18-19
    ovulation in, 19-20
  in early gynecologic years, 10-16
    abnormal bleeding patterns in, 16-18
    transition to ovulatory, 12-16
  hormonal patterns in, 4-6
  in menopause, 21-22
  pubertal development and, 6-10
  types of uterine bleeding and, 3-4
Menstrual disorder
  in cardiovascular disease, 231
  in female athlete, 217
  in liver disease, 218, 221
  in obesity, 206
  in renal disease, 222, 224
  substance abuse and, 211
  in systemic lupus erythematosus, 224, 226

Mentally disabled patient, 157-169. *See also*
    Developmentally disabled patient
Metabolic disease, 61
Metformin, 151-152, 154-155
Methadone maintenance, 209
Metoclopramide, 158
Metrorrhagia, 19, 30
Mineral supplement, 132-133
Mirena intrauterine system, 109
Mittelschmerz, 20
Moliminal symptoms, 4, 20-21
  in anovulatory cycle, 11
Mood disorder, 128-129
Mucous, in normal cycle, 20
Müllerian agenesis, 56
Myomectomy, 247-248

N
Nabumetone, 105
Naproxen, 105
Narcotic for dysmenorrhea, 110
Nerve ablation, uterosacral, 111
Nerve stimulation, transcutaneous electrical, 111-
    112
Neurogenic disease, 61
Neuroleptic drug, 158
Neuropsychiatric drug, 61
Newborn, uterine bleeding in, 30
Nicotine replacement, 208
Nonsteroidal anti-inflammatory drug
  in bleeding disorder, 176, 184
  for developmentally disabled patient, 162
  for dysmenorrhea, 104-105, 105, 106
  for premenstrual syndrome, 135
Nutrition, 132-133

O
Obesity
  contraception and, 205, 206
  menstrual disorders and, 204-205
  preconception counseling in, 206, 207
Oligomenorrhea, 19
  alcohol abuse and, 209
  characteristics of, 30
  in diabetes mellitus, 200
  in mentally disabled patient, 164
Oophorectomy, 135
Oral contraceptive. *See* Contraceptive, hormonal
Osler-Weber-Rendu disease, 173
Osteopenia, 216
Outflow tract abnormality, 54-57
  treatment of, 71-72
Ovarian failure
  amenorrhea with, 52, 55
  premature
    causes of, 57-58
    in mentally disabled patient, 164
    treatment of, 72
Ovarian syndrome, polycystic. *See* Polycystic
    ovarian syndrome
Ovulation
  in polycystic ovarian syndrome, 153-155
  signs and symptoms of, 19-20

Ovulatory cycle
  in adolescent, 54
  hormones in, 4-6
  transition to, 12-16
Oxaprozin, 105

P
Pain. See also Dysmenorrhea
  abdominal wall, 118
  gastrointestinal, 116-117
  musculoskeletal, 117-118
  urologic, 117
Pap smear
  in abnormal bleeding, 37-40
  atypical glandular cells on, 38
  in developmentally disabled patient, 161
  endometrial cells on, 37-38
  histiocytes on, 38
Paroxetine, 133
Partial thromboplastin time, 179
Patch, contraceptive, 165
PCOS. See Polycystic ovarian syndrome
Pelvic congestion syndrome, 115
Pelvic examination
  for abnormal bleeding, 36-37
  of developmentally disabled patient, 159-161
  in dysmenorrhea, 103-104
  in polycystic ovarian syndrome, 147-148
Pelvic infection, 115
Perimenarchal adolescent, 31-32
Perimenopause, 22
  abnormal bleeding in, 34
    diagnosis of, 81-89
    differential diagnosis of, 85
    etiology of, 80
    recognition of, 81
    treatment of, 89-92
  epidemiology of, 78-79
  normal hormonal changes in, 79
  risk factors in, 79-80
  transition to menopause and, 77
Phenobarbital, 235
Phenytoin, 235
Phospholipase A2, 99-100
Physical examination
  for abnormal bleeding, 36-37
  in amenorrhea diagnosis, 67
  in bleeding disorder, 178-179
  in dysmenorrhea, primary, 103-104
  of perimenopausal patient, 83
Piroxicam, 105
Pituitary disorder
  amenorrhea with, 63
  prolactin excess and, 61
Plasma exchange, 184
Plasma for bleeding disorder, 186, 189
Platelet disorder
  differential diagnosis of, 175
  laboratory evaluation of, 182
  of plug formation, 173-177
    thrombocytopenia and, 175-176
    von Willebrand disease as, 176-177
  Platelet inhibitor, 176

Platelet transfusion
  for bleeding disorder, 187
  in bleeding disorder, 184
Polycystic ovarian syndrome, 141-156
  in adolescent, 32
  anovulation in, 59-60
  criteria for, 142
  definition of, 141
  in diabetes mellitus, 201
  diagnosis of, 143-150
    history in, 144-145
    laboratory evaluation of, 148-150
    physical examination for, 145-148
  pathophysiology of, 142-143
  seizure disorder and, 232-233
  treatment of, 150-155
    of acne, 153
    of hirsutism and alopecia, 152-153
    hormonal contraceptive in, 150-151
    metformin for, 151-152
    ovulation and, 153-155
Polymenorrhea, 19, 30
  in diabetes mellitus, 200
Polymyositis, 226
Polyp
  bleeding due to, 33-34
  endometrial, 249-250
  in perimenopause, 80
Positioning for pelvic examination, 160
Post-coital bleeding, 33-34, 36
Post-coital contraception, 167
Post-transplantation contraception, 220
Postmenopausal bleeding
  endometrial cells on Pap smear in, 37-38
  etiology of, 34-35
  recurrent, 46
  treatment of, 45-46
Precocious puberty, 10
Preconception counseling
  in cardiovascular disease, 229-232
  in chronic illness, 198
  in diabetes, 202-204
  in eating disorder, 213-214
  for female athlete, 216-217
  in obesity, 206, 207
  in renal disease, 223, 224
  smoking and, 208
  substance abuse and, 210-211
  in systemic lupus erythematosus, 225, 226
Prednisone, 184
Pregnancy
  abnormal bleeding in, 36
  in adolescent, 17
  amenorrhea and, 52
  bariatric surgery and, 206
  cholestasis of, 219
  diabetes and, 202-203
  eating disorder and, 213-214
  in mentally disabled patient, 164
  in renal disease, 223
  substance abuse and, 210
  in systemic lupus erythematosus, 225
  testing for, 36

Premature ovarian failure, 57-58
   in mentally disabled patient, 164
   treatment of, 72
Premenstrual dysphoric disorder, 136
Premenstrual syndrome, 125-138
   clinical criteria for, 126
   diagnosis of, 129-130
   differential diagnosis of, 128-129
   epidemiology of, 127-128
   terminology about, 125-126
   treatment of, 130-135
      exercise as, 132
      hierarchical approach to, 131
      of isolated symptoms, 134-135
      nutrition in, 132-133
      ovulation suppression in, 135
      selective serotonin reuptake inhibitors for,
         133-134
Prepubertal child, bleeding in, 31
Primary amenorrhea
   in adolescent, 52-54
   in hypergonadotropic hypogonadism, 57-58
Primary dysmenorrhea, 98-112. See also
   Dysmenorrhea, primary
Primary hemostasis, 173-174
Progestational drugs for dysmenorrhea, 108-109
Progesterone
   in anovulatory cycle, 11
   break-through bleeding and, 33
   in menstrual cycle, 5-6
Progestin
   for abnormal perimenopausal bleeding, 90
   for mentally disabled patient, 166
Progestin challenge test, 69-70
Progestin-only contraceptive
   in atherosclerotic heart disease, 229
   in diabetes, 202
   for dysmenorrhea, 108-109
   in hyperlipidemia, 228
   in liver disease, 218, 220
   in renal disease, 223
Prolactin
   hyperprolactinemia and, 60-62
   in seizure disorder, 233
Prolactin-secreting adenoma, 60-61, 144
Prostaglandin, 99-100
Prostaglandin synthetase inhibitor, 104-107
Puberty, precocious, 10
Pubic hair
   menarche and, 31
   Tanner staging of, 8
Purpura, thrombocytopenic, 175-176
   treatment of, 184

R
Racial differences in menarche, 7
Radiation therapy for abnormal bleeding, 250
Rectal examination
   of developmentally disabled patient, 161
   in dysmenorrhea, 103
Recurrent postmenopausal bleeding, 46
Renal disease, 222-224
Reproductive health evaluation, 158-161

Resection of endometrial polyp, 249-250
Rheumatic disease, 224-226
Risk factors
   age-related, 79-80
   for dysmenorrhea, 98-99
   for premenstrual syndrome, 127-128
Risk:benefit ratio for contraceptive, 198-200

S
St. John's wort, 133
Scleroderma, 226
Secondary amenorrhea, 57-58
Secondary dysmenorrhea, 112-118
Secondary hemostasis, 177-178
Sedation, 161
Seizure disorder, 232-235
   contraception in, 233-234
   menstrual disorders in, 232-233
   preconception counseling in, 234-235
Selective serotonin reuptake inhibitor, 133-134
Septum, transverse vaginal, 55, 56
   surgery for, 71
Sertraline, 133
Sexual maturity, 6-10
Sexuality of developmentally disabled patient,
   159
Sheehan's syndrome, 63
Simmond's syndrome, 63
Skin in polycystic ovarian syndrome, 145, 146-
   147
Smoking, 207-209
   contraception and, 207-208
   menstrual disorders and, 207
   preconception counseling and, 208
Sonography, transvaginal, 150
Spironolactone
   for polycystic ovarian syndrome, 152
   for premenstrual syndrome, 134-135
Stenosis, cervical, 115-116
Sterilization
   in atherosclerotic heart disease, 229
   for mentally disabled patient, 165, 167
Stimate, 185
Stimulation, transcutaneous electrical nerve,
   111-112
Storage pool disease
   treatment of, 184
Stress-related amenorrhea, 62-63
Structural heart disease, 231
Substance abuse, 209-211
   contraception and, 210
   menstrual disorders in, 209-210
   preconception counseling and, 210-211
Sulindac, 105
Supplement, nutritional, 132-133
Surgery
   for abnormal uterine bleeding, 245-252
      endometrial ablation, 248-249
      hysterectomy, 246
      myomectomy, 247-248
      overview of, 245
      perimenopausal, 90
      uterine artery embolization, 248

Surgery *(cont'd.)*
  for anatomic abnormality, 71
  in bleeding disorder, 182, 183
  for dysmenorrhea, 110-111
  for menorrhagia, 182
Swyer's syndrome, 57-58
Systemic lupus erythematosus, 224-226

T
Tanner staging, 8
Telangiectasia, hereditary hemorrhagic, 173
Temperature in normal cycle, 20
Terbutaline, 109
Terminology
  menstrual, 30
  of premenstrual syndrome, 135-136
Testosterone in polycystic ovarian syndrome, 143,
    148-149
Thelarche, 7
  menarche and, 31
Thrombasthenia, Glanzmann, 180
Thrombocytopenia
  bleeding disorder with, 175-176
  bleeding time in, 181-182
  treatment of, 184
Thrombocytopenic purpura, 175-176
Thromboembolism, 165-166
Thrombotic thrombocytopenic purpura, 176, 184
Thyroid disorder
  amenorrhea in, 63
  differential diagnosis of, 85
  premature ovarian failure in, 58
Thyroid testing, 42
Tobacco use, 207-209
Transcutaneous electrical nerve stimulation,
    111-112
Transfusion, platelet, 184
Transition, menopausal, 20
Transplantation, liver, 220
Transvaginal sonography, 150
Transverse vaginal septum, 55
  surgery for, 71
Turner's syndrome, 57

U
Ultrasonography, 104
Urine testing for pregnancy, 36

Uterine anomaly, 115
Uterine artery embolization, 248
Uterine bleeding
  types of, 3
Uterine bleeding, abnormal. *See* Bleeding,
    abnormal uterine
Uterosacral nerve ablation, 111

V
Vaginal hysterectomy, 246
Vaginal septum, transverse, 55, 71
Vanishing testes syndrome, 58
Vascular disorder
  in diabetes, 203
  differential diagnosis of, 175
Vascular endothelium, 173
Vasopressin
  dysmenorrhea and, 100
  for von Willebrand disease, 185, 186, 188
Vicoprofen, 110
Virginal adolescent, 104
Vital signs in polycystic ovarian syndrome,
    145
Vitamin K deficiency, 188
von Willebrand disease
  abnormal bleeding in, 35-36
  forms of, 176-177
  laboratory testing for, 179-182
  screening for, 171
  treatment of, 184-185
von Willebrand factor concentrate, 186

W
Weight gain, 162, 163
Weight loss
  eating disorder and, 211-213
  in obesity, 205
Wilson's disease, 218, 219-220
World Health Organization contraception
    guidelines
  for diabetes, 203
  in obesity, 205
World Health Organization contraceptive
    guidelines
  for cardiovascular disease, 230
  in liver disease, 221
  for seizure disorder, 234

Lasers

THE PERIOPERATIVE CHALLENGE

SECOND EDITION

KAY A. BALL

Director of Education
United Medical Network
Lewis Center, Ohio

with 250 illustrations and 20 color plates

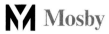 Mosby

St. Louis Baltimore Boston Carlsbad Chicago Naples New York Philadelphia Portland
London Madrid Mexico City Singapore Sydney Tokyo Toronto Wiesbaden

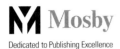

Dedicated to Publishing Excellence

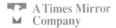

A Times Mirror
Company

PUBLISHER: NANCY L. COON
EDITOR: MICHAEL S. LEDBETTER
ASSOCIATE DEVELOPMENTAL EDITOR: CECILY S. BAROLAK
PROJECT MANAGER: CAROL SULLIVAN WEIS
PRODUCTION EDITOR: RICK DUDLEY
DESIGNER: ELIZABETH FETT
MANUFACTURING SUPERVISOR: TIM STRINGHAM
ORIGINAL ART: JACK REUTER

A NOTE TO THE READER:
The author and publisher have made every attempt to check dosages and nursing content for accuracy. Because the science of pharmacology is continually advancing, our knowledge base continues to expand. Therefore we recommend that the reader always check product information for changes in dosages or administration before administering any medication. This is particularly important with new or rarely used drugs.

SECOND EDITION
Copyright © 1995 by Mosby–Year Book, Inc.

Previous editions copyrighted 1990

Printed in the United States of America

Composition by Top Graphics
Color separation by Color Dot Graphics, Inc.
Printing/binding by R.R. Donnelley & Sons Company

Mosby–Year Book, Inc.
11830 Westline Industrial Drive
St. Louis, Missouri 63146

International Standard Book Number ISBN 0-8151-0524-X

95 96 97 98 99 / 9 8 7 6 5 4 3 2 1

CLINICAL CONSULTANTS

Wanda Lou Dunkel, RN, BAN, CNOR
Clinical Nurse III–Lasers & Microscope
 Coordinator
Memorial Medical Center
Springfield, Illinois

Kevin C. Kauffman, RN, ASN
Director of Endoscopy Training
Nevada OB/GYN Educational Foundation
Las Vegas, Nevada

To Mom and Dad (Betty and Don),

who continue to give me life.

PREFACE

During the past thirty years, health care has witnessed the birth, maturation, and expansion of laser technology. For many specialties today, the laser is a valuable and accepted tool. But recently, with health care reform activities focused on cost containment, all high technology has been forced to prove its worth. Sometimes lasers have been replaced by alternate tools based only on perceived cost savings and not on total patient outcomes. Laser technology faces the challenge of surviving in this type of demanding environment today. Therefore, a thorough understanding of lasers is needed to enhance the evolution and survival of this amazing tool.

The tissue interaction, safety, applications, and benefits of the laser are still not totally understood and may even become overwhelming to the health care professional. Becoming more familiar with lasers will replace insecurity with excitement. This book will clarify laser technology and highlight the advancements that continue to expand its uses.

The many illustrations throughout the book will enhance the reader's understanding of laser technology. An extensive glossary is also included to provide a quick reference of laser terminology. The purpose of this book is to provide an easy-to-understand educational guide that simplifies the many complex aspects of laser technology.

Part I, "Laser Biophysics, Systems, and Safety," simplifies the basics of this technology to provide a strong foundation for the complete understanding of its applications and potential uses. Simple, understandable language takes this sophisticated technology and makes it less confusing and very user-friendly. Sample safety guidelines are presented as models for developing policies and procedures needed to provide a safe laser environment.

Part II, "Clinical Laser Applications," describes various laser procedures and perioperative considerations. Each chapter deals specifically with one specialty area and/or related applications. The surgical team must understand the complete operative plan and implementation techniques before participating in any laser procedure. Applications are described in detail and new investigational procedures are introduced.

Part III, "Administrative Aspects of a Laser Program," describes specifically how to develop a comprehensive laser program and, more importantly, how to maintain it. Tips on increasing laser volume are discussed and economic considerations are emphasized.

In preparing this book, I relied on research and my clinical experiences that I gained managing two comprehensive laser programs. I also tried to address questions that I often hear from nurses, physicians, and other laser team members while I teach laser courses throughout the world. I appreciate the support of my nursing colleagues and physicians who have edited these chapters or offered their advice and comments.

Special recognition must be given to my husband, Dan Flynn, who reads every word I write and critiques my works. My two sons, Christopher and Trevor, also give me strength. But mostly I would like to recognize my parents, Betty Atkinson and Donald Atkinson, for always being there for me. They gave me a life that I hope will have a lasting impact on my professional colleagues.

Contents

PART I

LASER BIOPHYSICS, SYSTEMS, AND SAFETY

1 LASER BIOPHYSICS   3
   Principles of light   4
   Basic atomic physics   7
   Laser light characteristics   8
   Laser power   10
   Laser-tissue interaction   14
   Laser vs. electrosurgery   19
   Laser benefits   25

2 LASER SYSTEMS   28
   Laser wavelengths and colors   29
   Laser system parts   29
   CO_2 laser   32
   Neodymium: yttrium-aluminum-
      garnet (Nd:YAG) laser   39
   Frequency doubled YAG laser   50
   Holmium:YAG laser   51
   Argon laser   52
   Krypton laser   53
   Tunable dye laser   54

   Q-switched ruby laser   54
   Copper vapor laser   55
   Diode laser   55
   Excimer laser   55
   Free electron laser   56

3 LASER SAFETY   58
   Laser safety references and regulatory
      bodies   58
   Laser classifications   61
   Laser committee   61
   Laser safety officer and laser team
      members   62
   Eye safety   64
   Controlled treatment area   76
   Fire safety   78
   Other safety measures   88
   Laser plume   91
   Laser safety policies   103

PART II

CLINICAL LASER APPLICATIONS

4 OPHTHALMOLOGY LASER
  APPLICATIONS 109
  Anatomy 110
  Retinal photocoagulation for
    retinopathies 111
  Laser repair of retinal tears and
    detachments 118
  Laser procedures for glaucoma 118
  Posterior capsulotomy 124
  Recent ophthalmological laser
    applications 126

5 EAR, NOSE, AND THROAT AND
  RELATED LASER APPLICATIONS
  131
  Laser procedures for the ear 131
  Laser procedures for the nose and
    sinus 135
  Laser microlaryngoscopy 138
  Laser bronchoscopy 147
  Laser tonsillectomy 150
  Laser procedure of the
    temporomandibular joint 151
  Laser treatment for snoring 151
  Laser procedures in the oral cavity
    153
  Soft-tissue laser procedures 154
  Laser applications in dentistry 154

6 DERMATOLOGY AND PLASTIC
  SURGERY LASER APPLICATIONS
  157
  Laser surgery for vascular lesions 161
  Laser surgery for cutaneous lesions,
    172
  Laser surgery for tattoo removal 178
  Laser blepharoplasty and other plastic
    repair procedures 182

7 GASTROENTEROLOGY AND
  COLORECTAL LASER
  APPLICATIONS 186
  Laser endoscopy 186
  Laser surgery for rectal and perianal
    conditions 195

8 GYNECOLOGY LASER
  APPLICATIONS 200
  Lower tract laser applications 200
  Laparoscopic laser applications
    206
  Hysteroscopic laser applications
    214
  Intraabdominal laser applications for
    infertility 220

9 UROLOGY LASER APPLICATIONS
  224
  Endoscopic laser applications 224
  External and open laser procedures
    235

10 GENERAL SURGERY AND
  ONCOLOGY LASER
  APPLICATIONS 239
  Laser procedures of the breast 240
  Laser procedures of the neck 244
  Laser procedures of the chest 246
  Laser procedures involving
    abdominal organs 248
  Photodynamic therapy 255

11 CARDIOVASCULAR LASER
  APPLICATIONS 261
  Atherosclerosis 261
  Peripheral laser angioplasty 262
  Coronary artery procedures 270

Vascular welding and intravascular sealing 272
Future cardiovascular laser applications 273

12 PODIATRY, ORTHOPEDIC, AND NEUROSURGERY LASER APPLICATIONS 275
Podiatric laser applications 275

Orthopedic laser applications 286
Neurosurgical laser applications 296

13 LASER TECHNOLOGY AND ANIMALS 300
Animal use in laser research 300
Laser applications in veterinary medicine 302

PART III

ADMINISTRATIVE ASPECTS OF A LASER PROGRAM

14 FORMING THE INFRASTRUCTURE OF A LASER PROGRAM 317
Laser committee 317
Business plan development 321
Physician credentialing 323
Staffing: The laser team 325
Ethics 333
Expanding laser services 334

15 FINANCES OF A LASER PROGRAM 342
Procurement of laser systems 342
Laser economics 350
Cost containment 353
Maintaining adequate laser utilization 356

16 LEGAL ASPECTS OF LASER SURGERY 359
Laser program administration 359
Patient consent and education 363
Physician liability 365

17 MARKETING A LASER PROGRAM 367
Developing a marketing plan 367
Implementing a marketing plan 370
Evaluating a marketing plan 380

18 LASER EDUCATION 383
Perioperative patient education 383
Community education 393
Health care professional education 397

APPENDIX STANDARDS OF PERIOPERATIVE CLINICAL PRACTICE IN LASER MEDICINE AND SURGERY 409

GLOSSARY 415

INDEX 418

COLOR PLATES 18-19

PART ONE

LASER BIOPHYSICS, SYSTEMS, AND SAFETY

Laser technology has evolved quickly since the first practical system was built in 1960. Advances continue to refine laser applications while the true potential of this amazing tool is still being realized. It is essential to understand laser biophysics before trying to comprehend the variety of laser systems available today and the safety concerns associated with them. Part I introduces laser energy and tissue interaction concepts. The basics of electrosurgery are reviewed and compared with laser technology. Various laser systems are described, including their specific characteristics and delivery systems. Safety practices are detailed that protect the patient, personnel, and environment from potential laser hazards. Sample safety guidelines are highlighted for easy reference for the development of policies and procedures. This foundation of laser knowledge is imperative before participating in clinical laser applications.

1

LASER BIOPHYSICS

ight has been used for medicinal purposes since early times. Over 6000 years ago, the Egyptians realized the therapeutic power of natural sunlight and used it for medical treatments. In Europe, during the Industrial Revolution, factory smoke filtered out most of the beneficial ultraviolet radiation components, and many workers developed a calcium deficiency that led to rickets and pulmonary tuberculosis. It was found that unblocked sunlight helped alleviate the symptoms of these conditions. During the late nineteenth century, Nils Finsen, a Danish scientist, used ultraviolet radiation from a fabricated arc-lamp to treat vitiligo and psoriasis. This was the first time an artificial light source was used for therapeutic light treatments (Laserscope, 1990).

Light technology expanded greatly during the last three decades as the health care industry witnessed the creation and evolution of an amazing tool called the laser. The roots of laser technology began in 1917, when Albert Einstein formulated the theory of stimulated emission that was to be the foundation of laser technology (Einstein, 1917). Einstein stated that the ability of molecules to absorb radiation was dependent upon the number of molecules present and whether the molecules were in their upper or lower energy states. When more molecules are in the upper states than lower states, the molecules are stimulated to emit rather than absorb radiation.

In 1958, A.L. Schawlow and C.H. Townes investigated this concept and developed the principle of LASER, which stands for *L*ight *A*mplification by the *S*timulated *E*mission of *R*adiation (Schawlow and Townes, 1958). They suggested that mirrors could be used to amplify this stimulated emission of radiation.

In 1960, Dr. Theodore H. Maiman of the Hughes Aircraft Co. built the first true laser based on earlier concepts (Figure 1-1). The lasing material was a ruby crystal equipped with mirrors to amplify the lasing action. This introductory laser, which produced an intense, deep red beam, was the first of many lasers to be developed.

The laser field continues to expand as the popularity of this technology increases with new advances. Laser use, like computerization, has blossomed from theoretical concepts to actual application. The laser has grown from a complex to an uncomplicated piece of equipment over a short time.

3

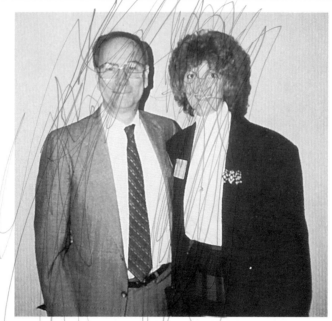

Fig. 1-1   Dr. Theodore Maiman and author, Kay Ball.

Nurses working in this field must understand the foundation of laser technology so as to promote safety and ensure appropriate operation. Laser light must be distinguished from ordinary light. To accomplish this, the nurse must understand basic laser biophysics.

PRINCIPLES OF LIGHT

The acronym LASER defines the process by which a form of energy is converted into light energy. The term also can refer to the device that produces the light, and to the light itself.

Although the exact nature of light is not fully understood, it has been determined that light (or electromagnetic energy) is released as a photon and travels in waves. A photon is the basic component of all light, including laser light. A wave can be characterized by four properties: wavelength, amplitude, velocity, and frequency.

Wavelength

Wavelength is the distance between two successive peaks of a wave, as illustrated in Figure 1-3. This length is measured in nanometers (nm); 1 nm is equal to 10^{-9} m, an extremely short measurement. Wavelengths have also been measured in micrometers (μm) and angstroms (Å). The relationships of these measurements are provided on page 5.

Radiant energy comes in all forms, from sunlight to radios, and is considered "wave energy." If this wave energy were to be graphed, a continuum from very long waves to extremely short waves would be drawn. This continuum is known as the electromagnetic spectrum and illustrates the relationship between all waves traveling in space. This spectrum can be compared with the row of strings in a piano. At one end of the spectrum are the longer waves in the infrared region, just as the lower sounding notes come from the end of the piano with the longer strings. The shorter waves are in the ultraviolet region at

Wavelength Measurement Comparisons

Millimeters (mm) > Micrometers (μm) > Nanometers (nm) > Angstroms (Å)

$$1 \text{ μm} = 0.0001 \text{ mm}$$
$$= 1000 \text{ nm}$$
$$= 10{,}000 \text{ Å}$$
$$1 \text{ nm} = 0.000001 \text{ mm}$$
$$= 0.001 \text{ μm}$$
$$= 10 \text{ Å}$$
$$1 \text{ Å} = 0.0000001 \text{ mm}$$
$$= 0.0001 \text{ μm}$$
$$= 0.1 \text{ nm}$$

the other end of the spectrum, just as the higher notes are produced by the shorter strings at the other end of the piano. Visible light occupies only a small portion of the electromagnetic spectrum, just as only a few strings are used to play the popular tunes we hear on the piano. Lasers deliver light energy within a small portion of the electromagnetic spectrum; some waves are visible and some are invisible. Laser energy extends from the near ultraviolet portion, through the visible waves, to the far infrared region, as illustrated in Figure 1-2.

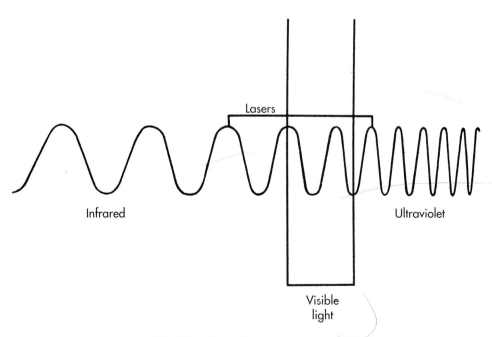

FIG. 1-2   The electromagnetic spectrum.

The length of the wave determines the color of the light. Visible light has a wavelength range of approximately 400 to 750 nm. Red light is about 630 nm, whereas blue light is around 488 nm. The carbon dioxide (CO_2) laser has a very long wavelength (10,600 nm) in the invisible, mid-infrared region of the electromagnetic spectrum. The Nd:YAG laser wavelength (1064 nm) is 10 times shorter than the CO_2 laser wavelength in the invisible, near-infrared area. The following chart describes these basic segments (Fuller, 1993):

Type of light	Wavelength
Ultraviolet (uV)	100-400 nm
Visible	400-750 nm
Near-infrared (NIR)	750-3000 nm
Mid-infrared (MIR)	3000-30,000 nm
Far-infrared (FIR)	30,000 nm-1 mm

Amplitude

Amplitude is half of the height of the wave from the top of one peak to the bottom of the next. Amplitude measures the magnitude or power of the wave. The taller the wave, the more power or amplitude it contains (Figure 1-3).

Velocity

Velocity is the rate of speed at which the wave travels. All wavelengths travel at the same speed within a vacuum. The speed of light is constant at approximately 186,300 miles per second, or about 300,000 km per second in a vacuum.

Frequency

Frequency is expressed in cycles per second or hertz (Hz) and is the number of wave peaks that pass a given point per second. Frequency is inversely related to wavelength. It is expressed in the following equation:

$$\text{Frequency} = \frac{\text{Speed of light (constant)}}{\text{Wavelength}}$$

A shorter wavelength has a higher frequency since more wave peaks pass a given point each second. Conversely, longer wavelengths have a lower frequency since fewer wave peaks are able to pass a given point in a second.

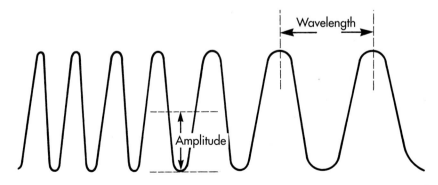

FIG. 1-3   Light properties of wavelength and amplitude.

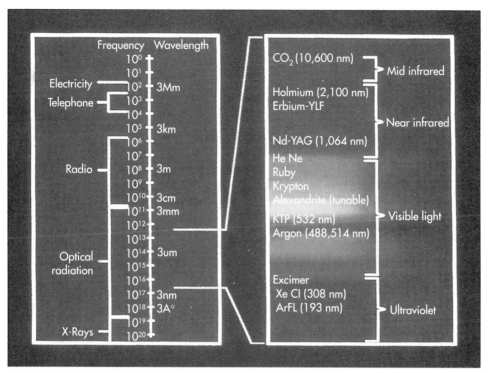

FIG. 1-4   The relationship between frequency and wavelength. (Courtesy Surgical Laser Technologies, Inc., Oaks, PA.)

At any point along the electromagnetic spectrum, a wave can be described by its wavelength or frequency. Convenience and preference have determined how a wave is portrayed. For example, radio waves are specified in terms of frequency, whereas laser light is described by its wavelength. The relationship between frequency and wavelength is described in Figure 1-4.

X-rays, cosmic rays, and gamma rays have the shortest wavelengths and highest frequencies and are known as ionizing radiation. These waves possess great energy, have great penetrative ability, and can disrupt molecular structure by effecting DNA activity. Special precautions, such as the use of lead shields, are taken when x-rays are emitted to decrease their penetration into areas not intended for irradiation.

Longer wavelengths (such as lasers or microwaves) characterize nonionizing radiation, since the penetration of these waves basically does not effect DNA . The lasers used clinically today are listed as producing nonionizing radiation; therefore, special penetration precautions are not necessary. Nonionizing radiation is not a hazard to pregnant women.

BASIC ATOMIC PHYSICS

Laser light differs from ordinary light, such as light from a lamp, in that it is organized light. Laser is to light as music is to noise, that is, while music is organized noise, laser light is finely tuned energy that exists in an organized and pure form. Because of this pre-

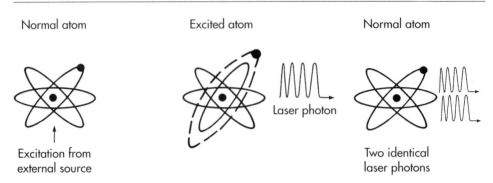

FIG. 1-5   Photon generation. An external energy source excites the atom to spontaneously emit a photon. This photon can stimulate the emission of two identical photons.

cision, laser light can be used to perform astounding feats. An understanding of basic atom activity is required to comprehend how laser light is produced.

In simple terms, an atom consists of negatively charged electrons orbiting a positively charged nucleus. The electrons circle at discrete energy levels at various distances from the nucleus. These electrons are able to move from one orbital shell to another and can produce energy as a result of this activity.

Briefly, laser energy is generated in the following way. When a negatively charged electron orbits close to its positively charged nucleus, the atom is in its ground or resting state, which is known to be at its lowest possible level of energy. When the atom is excited by an outside source, energy is absorbed, and the electron jumps to a higher, less stable orbital shell. Since the atom is unstable in this excited state, it will return almost immediately to its resting state once again. As this process occurs, a tiny bundle of surplus energy called a *photon* is spontaneously released or emitted.

If the photon is close to another atom still in the excited state, it will then interact with this atom. The photon will trigger the excited second atom to return to its resting state, and in this process another photon of laser light will be emitted. Thus, the process of stimulated emission has occurred, and laser energy has been initially formed. These two photons of identical energy and frequency will then travel together in perfect harmony (Figure 1-5).

This excitation process can continue until more atoms are in the excited state than the resting state. This condition is known as population inversion of the lasing medium, and laser energy can then be discharged.

LASER LIGHT CHARACTERISTICS

Laser light differs from ordinary light in three characteristic ways: Laser light is monochromatic, collimated, and coherent.

Monochromatic

Monochromatic refers to the highly purified color produced by the laser. Laser energy is composed of photons that are all the same color or wavelength. For example, pure red light consists of wavelengths that are all 630 nm. In contrast, ordinary light from a lamp produces white light that consists of many wavelengths or colors.

The color of the laser beam sometimes determines how it interacts with various tissues. For example, an argon beam of 488/514 nm is absorbed readily by red-pigmented tissue.

Collimated

Laser light is collimated, that is, its waves are parallel to each other and do not diverge significantly as they travel outward. In contrast, the beam of ordinary light from a flashlight diverges and spreads out as it travels away from its source (Figure 1-6).

Laser light maintains a collimated pattern so well that if a certain kind of laser were pointed toward the moon, which is 240,000 miles away, the beam would only spread out to approximately ½ mile. For all practical purposes, this deviation is insignificant (Absten and Joffe, 1985).

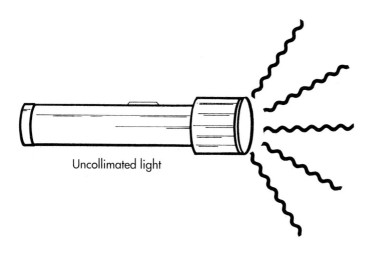

Uncollimated light

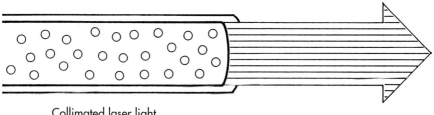

Collimated laser light

FIG. 1-6   Collimated laser beam compared with the uncollimated beam from a flashlight.

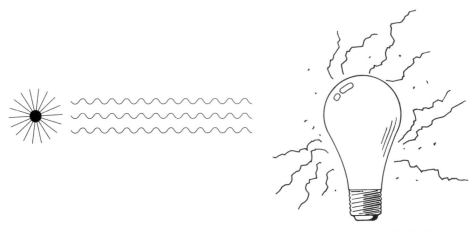

FIG. 1-7   Coherent laser beam compared with the incoherent waves from a light bulb.

The collimated property of a laser beam is extremely important in surgical applications because it minimizes any loss of power. When this collimated laser energy passes through a lens, the beam can be focused into a tiny spot that concentrates the energy to allow for ultimate precision.

Coherent

Laser light is coherent in that the waves travel in phase and in the same direction. Waves are in phase with each other when all of the peaks and troughs move in synchrony with each other in time and space. When all of the waves are in phase, this coherence has an additive effect on the amplitude or power (Figure 1-7).

Ordinary light from a light bulb travels randomly from its source in all directions and is known as incoherent. This pattern is analogous to the pattern of small choppy waves flowing in every direction that are produced by water skiers on a crowded lake. The pattern of ocean waves breaking in a neat and organized manner on the beach is analogous to the coherent pattern.

LASER POWER

Power Density

The rate of laser energy delivery is called power and is measured in watts. The wattage is equal to the amount of energy, measured in joules, divided by the duration of exposure, measured in seconds.

$$\text{Watts (W)} = \frac{\text{Joules (J)}}{\text{Seconds (s)}}$$

An important factor in the effective application of the laser is a concept of power density, or irradiance. Power density is defined as the amount of power that is concentrated into a spot, or watts/cm^2.

$$\text{Power density} = \frac{\text{Watts}}{\text{Spot size (cm}^2)}$$

Power density is the amount of power distributed within the area of the spot. This relationship can be compared with the relative ease of walking in deep snow with or without snowshoes. When wide snowshoes are worn, it is easy to walk over the snow because the body weight is spread over a larger area. When regular shoes are worn, the weight of the body on the smaller surface area causes the person to sink into the snow. With a given amount of power, a larger spot size will spread the laser power over a greater area, thus decreasing the impact of the beam. A smaller spot size will concentrate the power, thus making the beam more intense.

The *focal length of the lens* determines the size of the beam spot, as a general rule (Figure 1-8). A lens with a short focal length can provide a smaller spot size, thus increasing the intensity of the beam. A CO_2 laser with a 50-mm lens can produce a spot size of 0.1 mm, whereas a 400-mm lens can produce a spot size of 0.8 mm. Thus the shorter 50-mm lens can concentrate the power in a smaller spot area. Lenses can be modified to achieve spot sizes in the range of 0.025 to 0.05 mm for very precise surgeries, such as in laser welding or ophthalmological applications.

When the laser is used as a cutting tool, the spot size must be small to concentrate the power into a tiny area. When coagulation is desired, the laser beam is defocused to allow for an increased spot size that will spread the beam over a larger area. A surgeon can easily manipulate the beam to achieve the desired tissue effects.

The *wavelength of the laser* also limits the spot size and beam focusing. When all other factors are equal, shorter wavelengths can generate smaller spots. Thus, an argon laser at 488/514 nm can produce a much smaller spot than the CO_2 laser can at 10,600 nm. The choice of laser should be based on the specific effects of the laser on the tissue rather than based on its spot-size capabilities.

The *transverse electromagnetic mode* (TEM) determines the precision of the spot by the power distribution over the spot area. A TEM_{01} mode is an example of a common multimode distribution, meaning that the spot has a cool area in the center of the beam. This doughnutlike effect is analogous to cutting with a dull knife. The most common and fundamental mode is the TEM_{00}, which produces an even power distribution over the

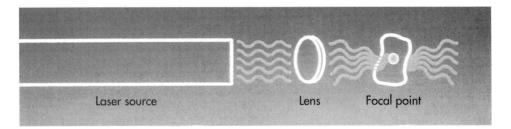

Laser source   Lens   Focal point

FIG. 1-8   The focusing lens focuses the laser beam on the target. (Courtesy Surgical Laser Technologies, Inc., Oaks, PA.)

spot, with most of the power concentrated in the center and the rest decreasing in intensity towards the periphery of the beam. The spot size of a TEM_{00} beam is the region that has approximately 86% of the total beam power. This mode, with a gaussian (bell-shaped) distribution, produces the smallest precise spots (Figure 1-9).

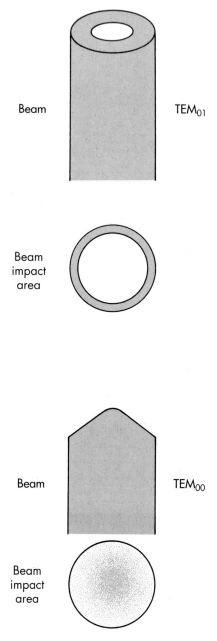

FIG. 1-9   Transverse electromagnetic modes.

Fluence

Fluence is one of the most important and critical concepts that affects precision during laser surgery. It involves three properties: watts, time, and spot size (or area). The tissue effect will vary if any of these parameters are changed.

$$\text{Fluence} = \frac{\text{Watts} \times \text{Time}}{\text{Spot size (cm}^2)}$$

A laser beam can impact tissue at 100 W for 1 second, thereby delivering 100 J to tissue. Another beam can impact tissue at 1 W for 100 seconds, thereby also delivering 100 J to tissue. The difference in tissue effect is that more adjacent tissue damage will occur with the longer duration of impact because of the laser's tissue-heating effects. Using the highest appropriate wattage for the shortest time minimizes any damage to adjacent healthy tissue.

Many of the surgical lasers produce a thermal tissue effect. Light energy is converted into thermal energy within the tissue, and a surgical effect occurs. The amount of time that the laser beam is in contact with the tissue determines the amount of thermal tissue effect. The control panel on the surgical laser unit often includes a switch or button to determine the length of exposure of the beam to the tissue. The continuous wave (CW) option allows the laser beam to be emitted for whatever duration the operator selects as long as the laser is being activated. A gated CW mode allows the continuous wave to be turned on and off in a predetermined manner. A time pulsed mode can deliver higher powers in shorter times than can the CW mode, whereas the Q-switched lasers create even higher power pulses in yet shorter durations (Figure 1-10).

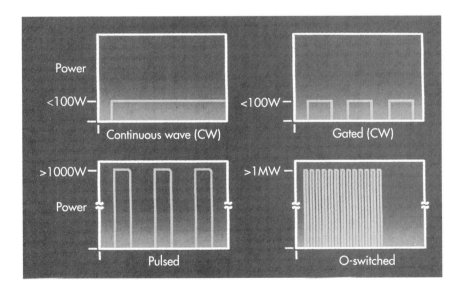

FIG. 1-10   Temporal characteristics of lasers. (Courtesy Surgical Laser Technologies, Inc., Oaks, PA.)

LASER-TISSUE INTERACTION

When laser energy is delivered to tissue, four specific interactions can occur: reflection, scattering, transmission, or absorption. The extent of the interaction depends on the wavelength of the laser, fluence, and tissue types.

Reflection

The laser beam has no effect on the target when it is reflected off the impact site (Figure 1-11), but it can cause harm where the beam eventually hits. The laser beam can be reflected by specular reflection or diffuse reflection.

Specular reflection occurs when the angle of the reflection is equal to the angle of the oncoming light; therefore, the quality of the beam is kept intact. This reflection can be used to treat hard-to-reach areas, such as the undersurface of an ovary, by causing the beam to be specularly reflected off a laser mirror. Specular reflection also can cause safety hazards because the laser beam can be inadvertently reflected off a shiny instrument, causing the laser to hit elsewhere. An anecdotal report noted that a nurse's mask caught on fire when a CO_2 beam was reflected off the surface of a shiny instrument and impacted the mask during a laparotomy procedure.

Diffuse reflection occurs when the light has been reflected, but the beam has been scattered. If a laser beam strikes the curved surface of an instrument, the beam will be diffused and spread out. This scattering decreases the potential for damage caused by the laser beam impact.

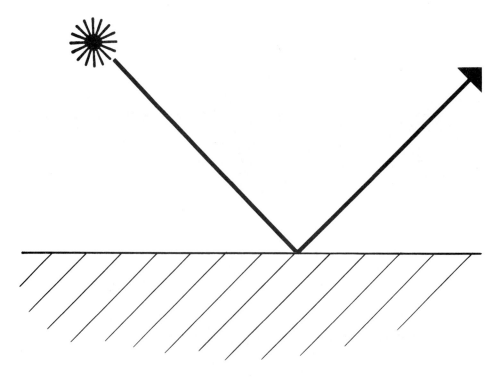

FIG. 1-11   Reflection.

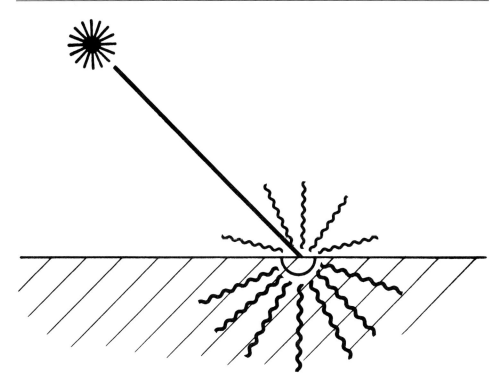

FIG. 1-12   Scattering.

Scattering

The distribution of the laser light energy within the tissue can be altered when the beam is scattered through the tissue (Figure 1-12). If the scattered energy is ultimately absorbed, then it will be converted to heat. The laser beam can also backscatter, causing a potential hazard. For example, when an endoscope is used, an Nd:YAG laser beam can backscatter up the endoscope and cause damage to the optics and the distal end of the scope.

Transmission

Some laser wavelengths can be transmitted through certain tissue but have little or no thermal effect (Figure 1-13). For example, the argon laser beam is transmitted through the clear portions of the anterior chamber of the eye to coagulate a blood vessel on the retina. Nd:YAG energy can be transmitted through the distending media in the bladder to vaporize a tumor on the bladder wall.

Absorption

Thermal damage caused by the laser energy being absorbed by the tissue depends on the wavelength and fluence of the beam and the tissue color, consistency, and water content (Figure 1-14). As the tissue absorbs the laser energy, heat energy is produced and tissue damage occurs. Heat dissipation depends on the tissue consistency and the blood flow

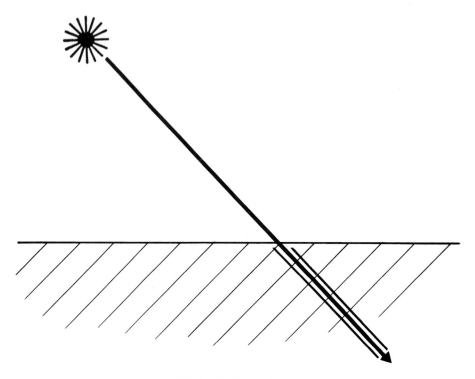

FIG. 1-13   Transmission.

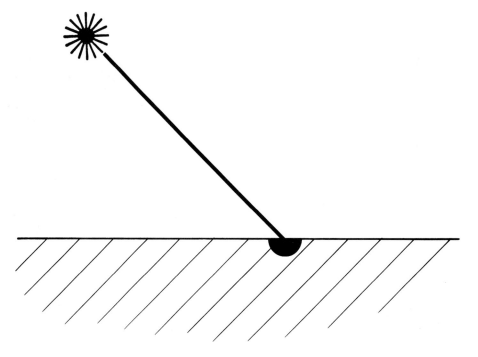

FIG. 1-14   Absorption.

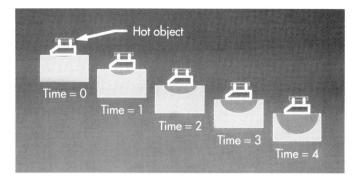

FIG. 1-15   Heat can be conducted through the target as long as the hot object remains in contact with the target. (Courtesy Coherent, Inc., Palo Alto, CA.)

in the surrounding tissue that helps cool the impact site. The conduction of heat through tissue is similar to touching a hot object. The longer the hot object is in contact, more conduction of the heat occurs (Figure 1-15).

When laser light strikes tissue and absorption takes place, the cellular water is super-heated to over 100° C. Intracellular protein is destroyed as the heat continues to build. The water inside the cell then turns to steam. Since 1 g of steam occupies more space than does 1 g of water, the cellular membrane bursts under this extreme pressure. Debris and smoke (laser plume) is spewed from the tissue. Adjacent tissue is warmed by the intense heat produced at the point of incidence. Short pulses of laser energy will decrease the radiation of heat and, therefore, will decrease the region of thermal necrosis.

The degree of thermal damage depends upon the temperature to which the laser energy heats the tissue. Table 1-1 notes the changes that occur as the laser beam is absorbed. The mechanism of thermal laser surgery is illustrated in Figure 1-16. At the immediate laser-tissue impact site there is a zone of vaporization. Immediately adjacent to this site is a zone of necrosis caused by the thermal spread. Farther from the impact site is a zone of coagulation as thermal injury decreases (Figure 1-17).

The *depth of penetration* of the laser beam depends upon the laser wavelength, color and consistency of the tissue, power of the beam, duration of beam exposure, and beam spot size.

TABLE 1-1

Tissue Changes with Temperature Increases

Temperature	Visual change	Biological change
37-60° C	No visual change	Warming, welding
60-65° C	Blanching	Coagulation
65-90° C	White/grey	Protein denaturization
90-100° C	Puckering	Drying
100° C	Smoke plume	Vaporization, carbonization

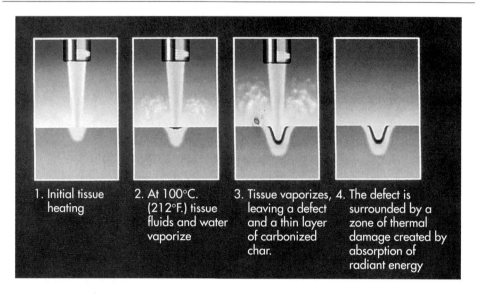

1. Initial tissue heating
2. At 100°C. (212°F.) tissue fluids and water vaporize
3. Tissue vaporizes, leaving a defect and a thin layer of carbonized char.
4. The defect is surrounded by a zone of thermal damage created by absorption of radiant energy

FIG. 1-16   Absorption of laser energy in tissue. (Courtesy Surgical Laser Technologies, Inc., Oaks, PA.)

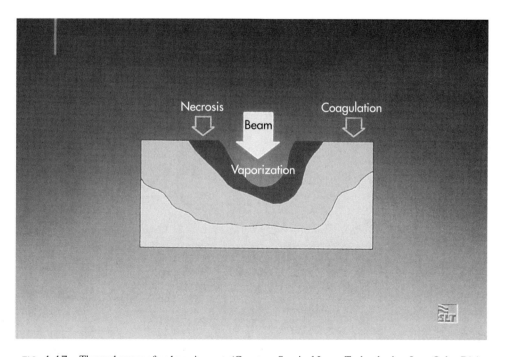

FIG. 1-17   Thermal zones after laser impact. (Courtesy Surgical Laser Technologies, Inc., Oaks, PA.)

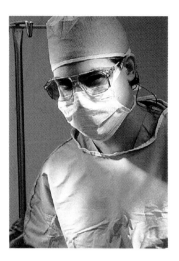

PLATE 1   Laser eyewear should have side shields to provide complete protection against specific laser wavelengths. (Courtesy Titmus Optical, Inc., Petersburg, VA.)

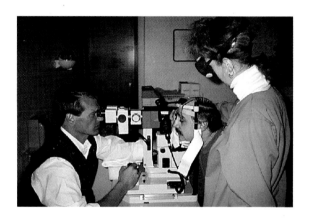

PLATE 2   During a panretinal photocoagulation, the surgeon's eyes are protected by an internal slit lamp filter while the attending nurse wears protective goggles.

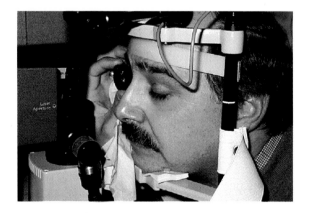

PLATE 3   For ophthalmic laser surgery, the patient's position at the slit lamp is stabilized by a chin rest and forehead bar.

PLATE 4   A tattoo is assessed for treatment with a Q-switched ruby laser. (Courtesy Derma-Lase, Hopkinton, MA.)

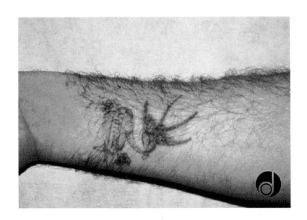

PLATE 5   Postoperative results of treating the tattoo with a Q-switched ruby laser. (Courtesy Derma-Lase, Hopkinton, MA.)

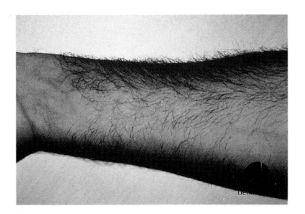

PLATE 6   19-year-old patient with a hemangioma on the neck (top). After 5 treatments (bottom).

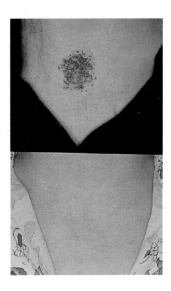

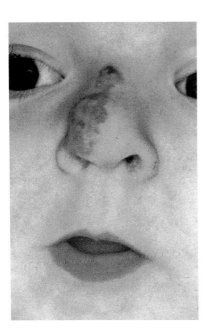

PLATE 7   Infant with a disfiguring and rapidly growing hemangioma of the nose. (Courtesy Dr. Dennis Duddley and Candela Laser Corporation, Wayland, MA.)

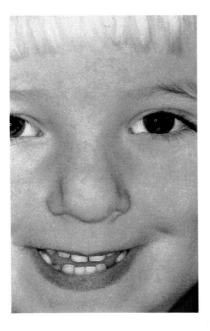

PLATE 8   The hemangioma is no longer visible after three treatments with a vascular lesion laser. (Courtesy Dr. Dennis Duddley and Candela Laser Corporation, Wayland, MA.)

PLATE 9   A contact Nd:YAG
delivery device is used to
hemostatically excise soft tissue.
(Courtesy Surgical Laser
Technologies, Inc., Oaks, PA.)

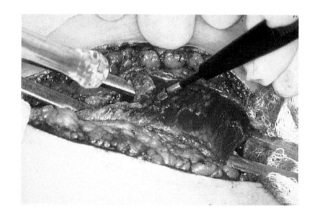

PLATE 10   A right angled Nd:YAG
fiber is used to treat a benign
hypertrophied prostate. (Courtesy
Myriadlase, Inc., Forest Hill, TX.)

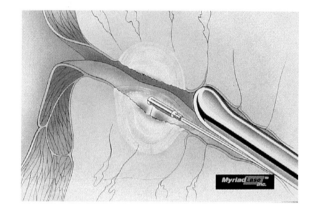

PLATE 11   The CO_2 laser beam is
directly reflected off the surface of a
laser mirror to impact a hard-to-reach
area.

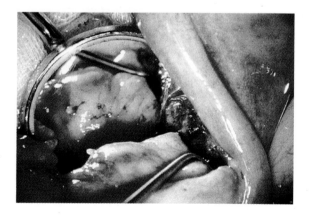

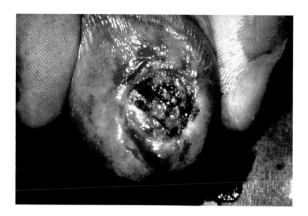

PLATE 12　Penile carcinoma is excised and the treatment area ablated with a CO_2 laser. (Courtesy Dr. Frank Aledia.)

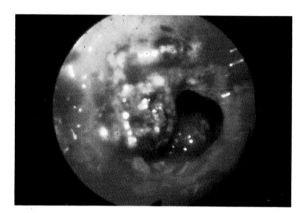

PLATE 13　A gastrointestinal lesion is identified and assessed for laser treatment. (Courtesy Surgical Laser Technologies, Inc., Oaks, PA.)

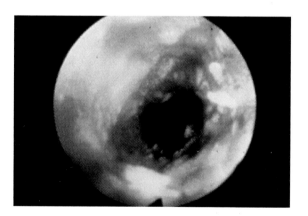

PLATE 14　A gastrointestinal lesion is vaporized using Nd:YAG laser energy to open the lumen. (Courtesy Surgical Laser Technologies, Inc., Oaks, PA.)

PLATE 15 An inguinal hernia is hemostatically repaired with contact Nd:YAG laser energy using local anesthesia. (Courtesy Surgical Laser Technologies, Inc., Oaks, PA.)

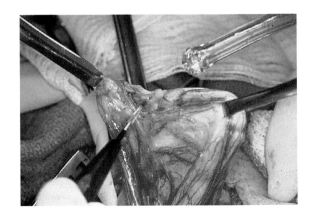

PLATE 16 The tunable dye laser light is delivered to a malignancy during photodynamic therapy.

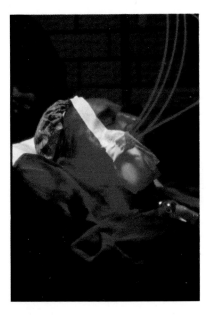

PLATE 17 The "cold laser" (helium-neon laser) for biostimulation is used experimentally to treat an area on the ear lobe that controls hunger.

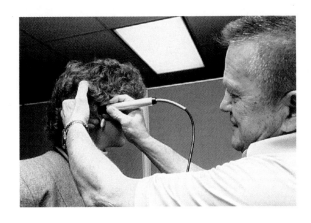

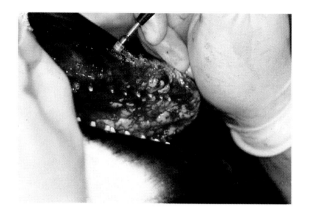

PLATE 18   An abnormal and expanding lesion on the mouth of a dolphin is hemostatically and precisely vaporized with laser energy to control its spread. (Courtesy SeaWorld, Inc., Aurora, OH.)

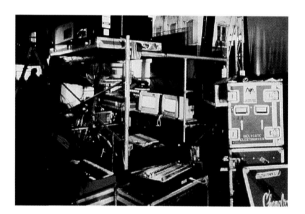

PLATE 19   Equipment setup for lasers being used for an entertaining laser light show. (Courtesy of Chameleon Productions, Orlando, FL.)

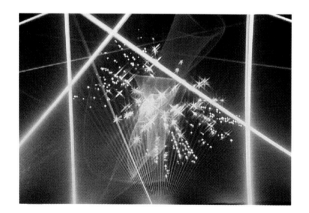

PLATE 20   A laser light show is produced by many of the same wavelengths used in surgery. (Courtesy of Chameleon Productions, Orlando, FL.)

As the laser beam cuts through tissue, it will continue to heat and destroy deeper tissues. If there is concern about accidental damage to adjacent tissues, a backstop may be used. Materials such as wet sponges, quartz rods, or titanium rods can be used as backstops.

The absorption of some lasers, such as argon and Nd:YAG lasers, depends upon the chromophore content of the tissue. Examples of tissue chromophores are hemoglobin and melanin. The color or wavelength of some beams are greatly absorbed by these chromophores, causing heating of selective tissues. The argon laser will be selectively absorbed by red or dark tissue to a depth of 0.5 to 2 mm, whereas the Nd:YAG laser beam exhibits color selectivity for darker tissues, with absorption to a depth of 2 to 6 mm.

CO_2 laser energy absorption is independent of tissue color. This beam is almost completely absorbed by cellular water to a shallow depth of 0.1 to 0.2 mm. There is little scattering because nearly all of the CO_2 energy is used to heat the cellular water.

Laser surgery can be divided into three broad categories regarding tissue response: thermal, mechanical, and chemical effects. Approximately 85% of lasers used today produce a thermal effect at the tissue level. These lasers cut, coagulate, vaporize, and ablate tissue from the interaction site where the thermal response originates. The mechanical effect on tissue is produced by some lasers as the laser beam generates sonic energy that mechanically disrupts tissue. Breaking apart kidney stones in the ureter or disrupting the posterior capsule within the eye are examples of this type of mechanical effect. The chemical effect of some lasers is produced as the laser energy activates light-sensitive drugs to disrupt and change tissue. This process is used in photodynamic therapy to selectively destroy malignant cells.

LASER VS. ELECTROSURGERY

In today's surgical arena, the question of whether to use the electrosurgery unit (ESU) or the laser during surgery continues to be debated. To judge the merits of each technology, the perioperative nurse must also understand the basic concepts and physics of electrosurgery.

It has often been stated that the ESU is the most widely used tool in surgery and the least understood. Electrosurgical technology was first used in the 1920s and has evolved into a sophisticated and useful tool in the operating room. Physicians often prefer to use the ESU because it is usually readily available, its costs are low, and no specific specialized training or credential is required. These benefits sometimes outweigh those of laser technology, thus ESU utilization may be greater than laser utilization in different surgical arenas.

To fully comprehend some of the disadvantages of ESU technology, one must understand the basic concepts of electrosurgery. ESU energy can cut, coagulate, or vaporize tissue by generating an electrical current that causes very intense localized heating at the tissue site. Electrical current requires a complete circuit to function properly. The current flowing out of the generator must be returned to complete the electrical cycle (Figure 1-18).

A monopolar ESU delivers highly concentrated current through an active electrode, such as an electrocautery pencil, to the target surgical site. This concentrated electrical energy heats the immediate tissue, and a response to this current occurs. The energy then travels on through the body and is collected by the dispersive electrode (ESU pad) and is then returned to the generator. A complete circuit has therefore been achieved (Figures

1-19 and 1-20). The dispersive pad receives the scattered current over a larger area, thus keeping the concentration of the energy low. Therefore, no tissue heating occurs at the pad site unless the pad is not adhered well or is only partially contacting tissue; then a secondary burn will occur.

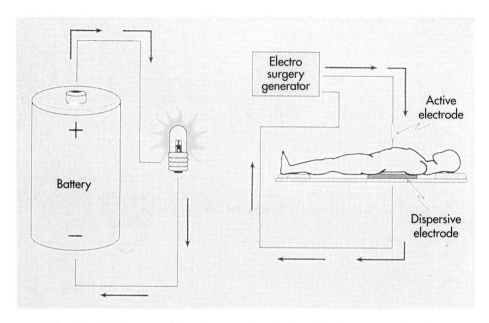

FIG. 1-18   Electrical current must make a complete circuit to function, even during electrosurgery. (Courtesy Ethicon Endo-surgery, Inc., Cincinnati.)

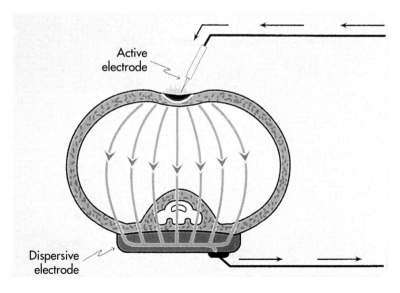

FIG. 1-19   The active electrode delivers the electrosurgery energy and the dispersive electrode collects the energy. (Courtesy Ethicon Endo-surgery, Inc., Cincinnati.)

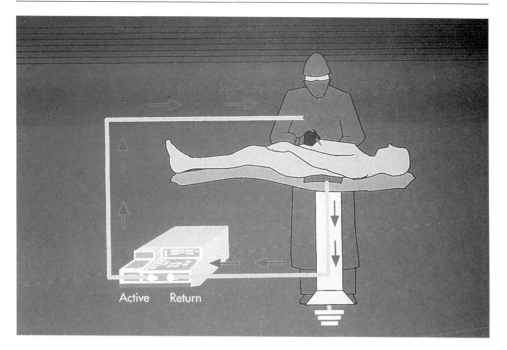

FIG. 1-20   Monopolar electrosurgery. (Courtesy Ethicon Endo-surgery, Inc., Cincinnati.)

Bipolar ESUs work similarly to monopolar ESUs in that a complete circuit takes place. The energy is delivered through the active electrode, which is usually one prong of a bipolar forceps, while the energy is returned through the other prong of the forceps. Since the energy is delivered and received through the prongs of the bipolar forceps, a dispersive pad is not needed (Figure 1-21). Other instruments, such as bipolar scissors, are being developed that use this bipolar effect.

The merits of using the laser or the ESU during laparoscopy are also argued in today's surgery suite. Laparoscopy poses different concerns, as these energies must be directed into the body cavity via a long tube. New laser delivery devices are being perfected, but ESU energy must be delivered through an insulated instrument that is passed through a trocar sheath or the biopsy port of the laparoscope. Electrosurgical energy can be passed through many different types of instruments, such as scissors, probes, hooks, and needles. This energy is then delivered through the instrument and is returned to the generator to complete the electrical circuit.

Safety concerns have arisen regarding electrosurgery instruments. If the insulation of the long shaft of the active electrode has a crack or a defect, then the electrical energy could escape from the instrument wherever it comes in contact with tissue and could cause a burn at that site (Figure 1-22). For example, if the insulation of a probe has a crack or break, then the electrical energy could escape at this site and cause a bowel burn that could lead to major postoperative complications.

Another concern regarding the use of an ESU during laparoscopy is a concept known as capacitive coupling. This condition has caused patient injury because it is still not completely understood. For capacitive coupling to occur, a unique set of circumstances

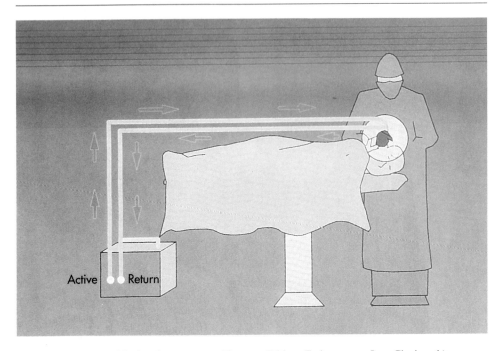

FIG. 1-21   Bipolar electrosurgery. (Courtesy Ethicon Endo-surgery, Inc., Cincinnati.)

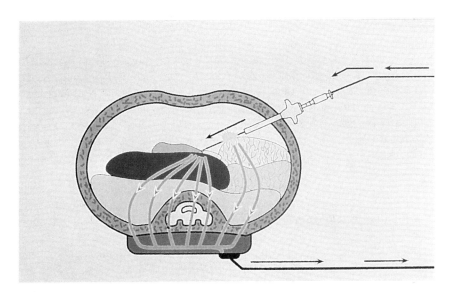

FIG. 1-22   Injury resulting from electrical current escaping from a break in the probe's insulation. (Courtesy Ethicon Endo-surgery, Inc., Cincinnati.)

must be present. As the electrical energy is emitted from the end of a well-insulated active laparoscopic electrode, this energy can flow through air like radio frequency current to a nearby metal surface, such as the trocar sheath or the laparoscope. This current can then cause the metal surface to be charged with electrical energy (Figure 1-23). This occurs as a result of the high-frequency current produced by the ESU. If the metal surface of the charged trocar sheath or laparoscope then touches other tissue while charged, the electrical current will be emitted and cause a thermal tissue response or a burn (Figures 1-24 and 1-25). This situation could go undetected if it is out of the operator's view, and then problems are noted when untoward symptoms arise postoperatively.

When capacitive coupling occurs, the charged metal usually has nowhere to be discharged. For example, if a plastic stability thread is used with a metal trocar sheath placed through the abdominal wall and fat, then the electrical charge cannot be discharged safely. The plastic stability thread must be eliminated so that the metal can be discharged directly through contact with the abdominal wall and fat layer. This surface is large enough to continually discharge the metal sheath (Figure 1-26).

Hazards associated with ESU utilization, especially during laparoscopic procedures, can be minimized easily. Well-insulated electrosurgical instruments should be used that have been routinely inspected for defects or nicks. To minimize the dangers of capacitive coupling, plastic and metal should not be mixed. When an ESU device is used through a metal trocar sheath, plastic stability threads should not be employed. Nonconductive (nonmetal) radiolucent trocar sheaths can also be used. Also available today are devices that can be connected via a cable or wire to the metal trocar sheath or laparoscope so that constant electrical discharging can occur to eliminate the problem of capacitive coupling.

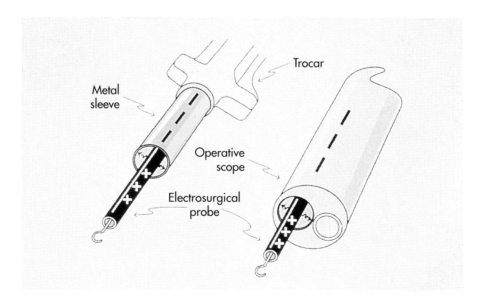

FIG. 1-23   Capacitive coupling occurs when electrical energy flowing from an instrument charges a nearby metal trocar sheath or laparoscope. (Courtesy Ethicon Endo-surgery, Inc., Cincinnati.)

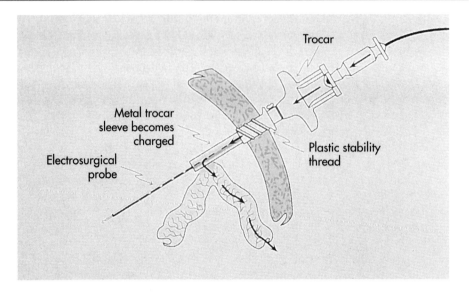

FIG. 1-24   Capacitive coupling to the metal trocar sheath and a bowel injury. (Courtesy Ethicon Endo-surgery, Inc., Cincinnati.)

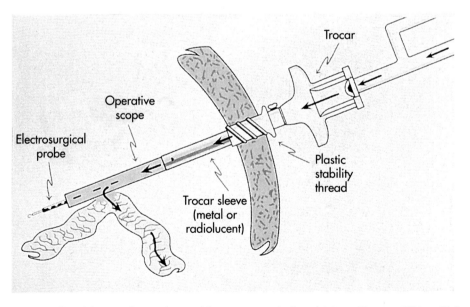

FIG. 1-25   Capacitive coupling to the metal laparoscope and a bowel injury. (Courtesy Ethicon Endo-surgery, Inc., Cincinnati.)

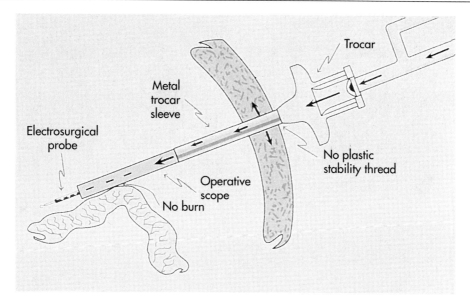

FIG. 1-26 Discharging the laparoscope charge within the abdominal wall and fat layer. (Courtesy Ethicon Endo-surgery, Inc., Cincinnati.)

When comparing the laser with the ESU, laser energy tends to cause a uniform zone of thermal buildup (Figure 1-27), unlike electrocautery, which causes an irregular zone of tissue damage because the electrical current it uses flows along the path of least resistance, such as a blood vessel (Figure 1-28). The laser beam does not flow toward the path of least resistance, thus it creates a more uniform zone of damage in the tissue. Therefore, the laser offers more precision than the ESU.

Whether to use a laser or an ESU will continue to be a controversial issue in the surgical environment. One must weigh the pros and cons of each technology before deciding which would be most appropriate for each specific procedure. Physician preference, skill level, availability of the technology, potential hazards, and cost seem to be the most important deciding factors today. When deciding which tool to use, one should place the emphasis on what is best for the patient, including benefits during the surgical intervention, patient safety, and the patient's recovery phase.

LASER BENEFITS

Many beneficial effects have been reported as a result of the laser beam interacting with the tissue to cut, coagulate, ablate, or vaporize, including the following:

- Sealing smaller blood vessels (dryer field of surgery)
- Sealing lymphatics (decreasing postoperative edema and the spread of malignant cells)
- Sealing nerve endings (on selective tissue, decreasing postoperative pain)
- Sterilizing tissue (from the heat buildup at the laser-tissue interaction site)
- Decreasing postoperative stenosis (by decreasing the amount of scarring)

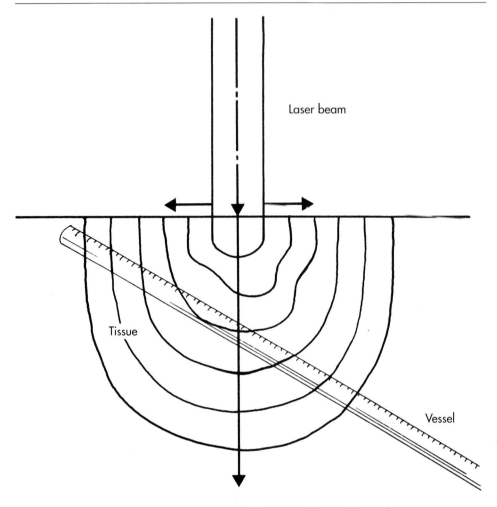

FIG. 1-27   The laser causes a uniform zone of thermal destruction.

Finally, because of these laser-tissue effects, laser application leads to:

- Quicker recovery and return to daily living
- Shorter surgery time
- A shift to more outpatient and local anesthesia applications

REFERENCES

Absten GT and Joffe SN: *Lasers in medicine: an introductory guide,* London, 1985, Chapman Hall, Ltd.

Einstein A: On the quantum theory of radiation, *Physio Z* 18:121, 1917.

Fuller TA: *Thermal surgical lasers, a technical monograph,* Oaks, PA, 1993, Surgical Laser Technologies, Inc.

Laserscope: Monograph: *Tissue interaction and safety considerations of lasers,* San Jose, CA, 1990.

Schawlow AL and Townes CH: Infrared and optical lasers, *Phys Rev* 112:1940, 1958.

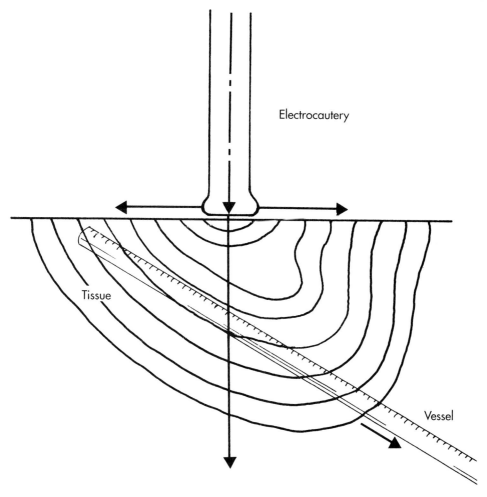

Electrocautery

Tissue

Vessel

FIG. 1-28 Electrosurgery causes an irregular zone of tissue damage.

SUGGESTED READINGS

Achauer BM, Vander Kam VM, and Berns MW: *Lasers in plastic surgery and dermatology,* New York, 1992, Thieme.

Ball KA: *Lasers in the O.R.,* Thorofare, NJ, 1988, Slack.

Fuller TA, editor: *Surgical lasers, a clinical guide,* New York, 1987, Macmillan.

Fuller TA: *Thermal surgical lasers,* a technical monograph, Oaks, PA, 1993, Surgical Laser Technologies, Inc.

Joffe SN, editor: *Lasers in general surgery,* Baltimore, 1989, Williams & Wilkins.

Meeker MH and Rothrock JC: *Alexander's care of the patient in surgery,* St. Louis, 1995, Mosby.

Sliney DA and Trokel SL: *Medical lasers and their safe use,* New York, 1993, Springer-Verlag, Inc.

Wright VC and Fisher JC: *Laser surgery in gynecology, a clinical guide,* Philadelphia, 1993, WB Saunders Co.

2

LASER SYSTEMS

Laser technology has developed from the constant efforts of researchers and physicians dedicated to advancing laser applications. Every day new wavelengths are being explored for use in medicine and surgery. The beginning developments of laser systems and the first laser applications are noted in Table 2-1.

TABLE 2-1

Developments in Laser Technology

Year	Contributor	Contribution
1917	Einstein	Principle of "stimulated emission"
1958	Schawlow & Townes	"LASER" principle
1960	Javan	Helium-neon
1960	Maiman	Developed ruby laser
1961	Goldman	First ruby laser clinical application
1961	Schnitze	Developed Nd:Glass laser
1964	Bridges	Argon
1964	Patel	Developed CO_2 laser
1964	Gordon	Developed argon laser
1964	Geusic, Marcos, Van Uitert	Developed Nd:YAG laser
1965	Polanyi	First CO_2 laser clinical application
1968	L'Esperance	First argon laser clinical application
1977	Kiefhaber	First Nd:YAG laser clinical application
1980	Dougherty	Described Photodynamic Therapy
1981	Bierlein	KTP
1984	Daikuzono, Joffe	Developed Nd:YAG contact technology

LASER WAVELENGTHS AND COLORS

Lasers are identified by their wavelength, which also indicates their color. Table 2-2 describes some of the most common lasers that are being used or investigated for use in clinical applications. The appropriate wavelength is determined for a particular surgery or laser treatment depending upon the desired tissue effects and delivery system of the laser.

TABLE 2-2

Description of Laser Color and Wavelength

Laser	Color	Wavelength (nm)
Excimer	Ultraviolet	
ArF		193
KrCl		222
KrF		248
XeCl		308
XeF		351
Helium-cadmium		325
Dye	Variable	400-1000
Argon	Blue	488
	Green	514
Copper vapor	Green	511
	Yellow	578
Frequency doubled YAG (KTP)	Green	532
Krypton	Green	531
	Yellow	568
	Red	647
Gold vapor	Red	627
Helium-neon	Red	632
Dye laser	Variable with dyes	400-1000
	Red	632
	Yellow-green	577
Diode	Near-infrared	670-1550
Ruby	Deep red	694
Alexandrite	Near-infrared	760
Nd:YAG	Near-infrared	1064
		1318
Thulium:YAG	Near-infrared	2010
Holmium:YAG	Near-infrared	2100
Erbium:YAG	Near-infrared	2900
CO_2	Mid-infrared	10,600

LASER SYSTEM PARTS

There are five parts to any laser system: excitation source, laser head, ancillary components, control panel, and delivery system. Figure 2-1 illustrates the various parts of a laser system.

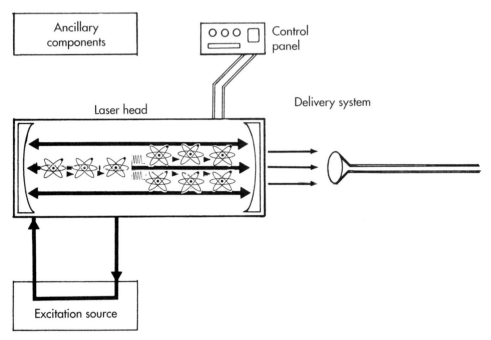

FIG. 2-1   Laser system parts.

Whenever a laser malfunctions, a systematic review of these different parts will help determine the source of the trouble. Laser preventive maintenance and service must be documented as required by the Joint Commission on Accreditation of Healthcare Organizations because the laser is a piece of electrical equipment. Computerizing this information makes it much easier to retrieve and store. Any trends noted involving increased laser repairs helps justify the procurement of a replacement laser.

Excitation Source

The excitation source provides energy to the laser head for the production of the laser light. This source can be electrical, chemical, flash lamps, or other laser systems. Basically, gas lasers are excited electrically, whereas solid or liquid lasers are optically pumped with flash lamps. Some CO_2 lasers are excited by a radio frequency. A small, handheld, helium neon laser pointer uses battery energy for the excitation mechanism.

A CO_2 laser usually requires 110 V, adding to its versatility and mobility, since it can be operated by merely plugging it into a regular electrical outlet. The earlier Nd:YAG and KTP lasers have special electrical requirements to activate the excitation mechanism. This necessitates an additional electrical line with the specified electrical power. Today many of these units can use 110-V electrical current. Most of the nonmobile tunable dye or argon systems today still require either 208- or 220-V current. Appropriate planning for special electrical needs is essential when determining where the lasers will be used.

Laser Head

The *active medium* is located in the laser head or optical resonator and is the substance energized to produce the photons or laser energy. Lasers are usually named after their active medium. For example, argon laser energy is produced from the active medium argon (a gas). Active mediums can be grouped into four major classifications:

1. Gas: The molecules in a gas-active-medium environment become excited when an electric current is passed through the gas. The current may be pulsed or continuous, thus the laser energy generated will be either pulsed or continuous. Gas lasers are available with wavelengths from the ultraviolet range (excimer) to the infrared region (CO_2). Other examples of gas lasers are argon, krypton, and helium-neon lasers.

2. Solid: Solid lasers are crystal lasers. The active medium is normally an optically clear type of material that is composed of a host crystal and is laced with an impurity called a dopant. Examples of host crystals are yttrium-aluminum-garnet (YAG), yttrium-lithium-fluoride (YLF), yttrium-aluminum-oxide (YALO), and glass. The type of host crystal is chosen for its thermal conductivity, brittleness, and mechanical and optical stability (Sliney and Trokel, 1993). The dopant actually produces the lasing energy. An arc or flash lamp is used to activate the dopant, causing the stimulated emission of radiation to generate the laser beam. Examples of solid crystal lasers are neodymium, holmium, ruby, and erbium.

3. Liquid: The active medium in a liquid laser is a flowing organic dye that, when activated by another laser beam, produces a wide range of wavelengths. Since this type of laser is more complex and involves a specific dye, more maintenance is required, and sometimes these lasers can be less reliable. An example of a liquid laser is a tunable dye laser.

4. Semiconductor diode: Semiconductor diode lasers have been used extensively in consumer products and in optical fiber communication systems. In recent years, this technology has been developed for use in clinical applications. This small and efficient laser consists of layers of semiconductor crystal material that are used as the active medium. Since semiconductor lasers are new to the medical arena, their potential is still being investigated. An example of a semiconductor laser is a diode laser endolaser and photocoagulator for ophthalmic applications.

The *feedback mechanism* of laser light production is a critical factor in amplifying the light produced by stimulated emission. A system of mirrors is positioned at each end of the laser head. The laser energy is propagated and reflected between these two mirrors. As the photons are fed back into the active medium, more photons are produced, building the intensity of the power and producing an excited state called population inversion. At this stage the laser energy can be emitted from the laser head and delivered to the target site.

The mirror at one end of the laser head is fully reflective, and at the other end a partially reflective mirror permits the escape of some of the laser energy. This semitransparent mirror allows the laser light to leave the cavity. The narrow, concentrated beam of light can then be focused by a lens or passed into an appropriate delivery system.

Ancillary Components

Ancillary components are the additional laser system parts that are needed to help with the production of the laser energy. Depending on the laser system, different laser components are required.

The *console* of the laser provides protective housing for the various components within the laser. The console's framework helps protect the laser during transportation and discourages easy access by unqualified personnel.

The *cooling system* of the laser keeps the laser head from overheating. Some laser systems are air-cooled, meaning that the laser head is cooled by a constant stream of air produced by an internal fan. Other laser systems are cooled by a continual flow of water that is either recycled from within the unit or obtained from an external plumbing source.

A *vacuum pump* is needed in the free-flowing CO_2 laser systems. The vacuum pump provides the force to pull the special CO_2 laser mixture from the gas tank and deliver it to the laser head.

Other laser components may be needed, depending upon the type of laser and its design. These components are described in detail in the service manual for each individual laser.

Control Panel

The control panel is the source of laser operation. Various laser modes, wattages, durations, and other parameters are relayed through the control panel. Computerization has allowed complex laser operational panels to become more user-friendly over recent years. The laser team member and the physician should be acutely familiar with the control panel of the laser.

Some lasers are controlled by a dial system that scrolls the laser to the desired wattage, duration, and mode. Trends have led to the development of a microprocessor system that responds immediately to the push of a button to indicate the desired settings.

For safety purposes, lasers are equipped with a standby mode that will not permit the beam to be emitted even if the foot pedal is activated. Lasers also have a master key that must be inserted into the control panel to make the laser operational. Also, feedback security measures have been added to the control panel to help ensure laser safety. For example, many Nd:YAG and argon lasers cannot be activated unless the fiber delivery system is properly in place.

Delivery System

The delivery system is the device or attachment that transmits the laser energy to the tissue from the laser head. A typical delivery system includes a fiber, an articulated arm, or a fixed optical array. The CO_2 laser light is delivered to the tissue via an articulated arm, which is a hollow tube that has special mirrors to transmit the laser beam. The Nd:YAG and argon laser light can be delivered to the tissue through laser fibers. Other attachments to the various delivery systems are available that refine the method of laser delivery to the tissue. For example, computerized scanning devices can be attached to the delivery system. Automatically controlled pulsations of laser energy can then be delivered to the target within a preselected desired pattern, providing a high level of precision and accuracy.

CO_2 LASER

CO_2 Laser Characteristics

The CO_2 laser has been one of the primary instruments for laser surgery. The invisible CO_2 beam of 10,600 nm is located in the middle-infrared region of the electromagnetic spectrum. Since the beam is invisible, a helium-neon laser light is transmitted coaxially with the CO_2 laser light and serves as the aiming beam.

The active medium in the CO_2 laser is really a combination of specific concentrations of CO_2, nitrogen, and helium gases designed to increase the efficiency of the output. This active medium is excited by electrical currents to generate the production of laser photons.

The hallmark of the CO_2 beam is its precision qualities resulting from the absorption characteristics of the energy. The CO_2 beam is strongly absorbed by water in the tissue. Since biological tissue contains 75% to 90% water, the CO_2 beam is readily absorbed and heats the cellular contents. Adjacent tissue is affected only by thermal transmission from the target cells. If the tissue is heated to lower temperatures, coagulation or protein denaturization can occur (Table 1-1). If the cell is heated to above the boiling point, the cellular membrane will explode and a laser plume will be produced. The amount of thermal buildup determines whether the tissue will be cut, vaporized, or coagulated.

When the CO_2 laser beam hits tissue, its absorption is independent of tissue color, unlike the argon laser. Therefore, lighter tissue can absorb the beam as readily as darker tissue can. Also, the CO_2 beam does not scatter like the noncontact Nd:YAG beam.

The CO_2 laser produces a very superficial tissue effect. "What you see is what you get" is often said of the CO_2 laser because the actual tissue damage can be observed. The lateral zone of damage or the depth of penetration of the CO_2 laser beam is limited 0.1 to 0.2 mm. This depth can be compared with the zone of damage of the argon laser at 0.5 to 2 mm, the Nd:YAG laser at 2 to 6 mm, and the holmium laser at 0.4 to 0.6 mm (Figure 2-2). The zone of thermal damage is expanded by increasing the exposure time of the beam to the tissue.

The depth of penetration of the CO_2 beam is controlled by the power density and the duration of exposure (fluence). Therefore, when cutting is desired, higher power with a small focused beam, coupled with a short exposure, is used to decrease the thermal spread

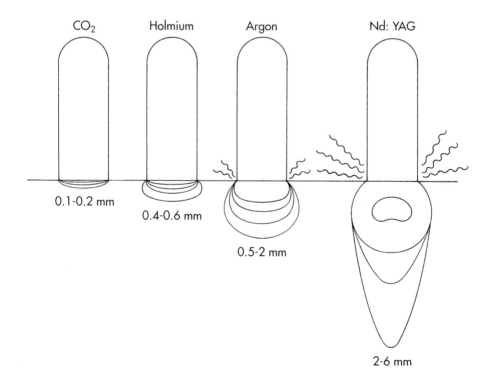

FIG. 2-2 The CO_2 laser depth of penetration is less than that of the argon, Nd:YAG, and holmium lasers.

to adjacent tissues. Debulking (removal of a large portion of tissue) or coagulation requires defocusing of the beam to enlarge the spot size and spread the energy over a larger area. Vessels up to 0.5 mm in diameter can be coagulated while the beam is in focus, but a defocused beam is needed to coagulate vessels of up to 2 mm (Absten and Joffe, 1985).

After the CO_2 laser cuts or coagulates tissue, the beam will continue to travel, hitting the tissue behind the target site. Therefore, backstops are required to decrease damage to surrounding tissues. Wet sponges or rods made out of quartz or titanium have been used as backstops.

The CO_2 beam can be used to make skin incisions. When compared with the healing that occurs after a conventional scalpel incision, the healing pattern of the laser-induced wound is clinically similar even though the healing processes are different. Of greatest concern is the wound strength of a CO_2 laser incision vs. a steel scalpel cut. Studies have shown that a wound produced by a CO_2 laser achieves the same tensile strength as a scalpel incision 21 days after the operation. Therefore, the relative weakness of the laser incision is only temporary (Absten and Joffe, 1985).

CO_2 Laser Types

Two types of CO_2 lasers are available today: the free flowing CO_2 laser and the sealed tube CO_2 laser.

The *free flowing* CO_2 laser requires a gas cylinder containing a special mixture of CO_2, nitrogen, and helium. The concentration of these gases must be exact for the mixture to be activated and create the laser beam. Since subatmospheric pressure must be maintained within the laser tube, a vacuum pump within the system is used to pull the gas through the laser head during the lasing period. This is necessary because the energy discharged breaks down the CO_2 into carbon monoxide and ozone. The broken down or disassociated gas is discarded from the laser system into the environment and is not hazardous. The gas cylinder must be replaced when empty. All of the different components within this laser add to the maintenance, noise, and expense of operating the laser.

The *sealed tube* laser system contains a special mixture of CO_2, nitrogen, helium, and several other gases sealed within the laser tube. When the gas mixture is activated to produce a laser beam, very little of the CO_2 breaks down. The CO_2 that is split apart is then catalyzed to regenerate the mixture necessary for the lasing action to continue. The gas mixtures and catalysts are continually being refined by laser companies that successfully make sealed tubes. The companies that originally made these lasers were spinoffs from U.S. aerospace or military companies.

Sealed lasers have two types of life: operating life and shelf life. Operating life is the anticipated life of the laser unit itself, whereas the shelf life is the expected life of the laser tube before it needs recharging. The shelf life affects the budget because the system needs to be maintained; thus shelf life is usually the more important factor to consider. The normal shelf life of a sealed tube laser ranges from 1 to 4 years depending upon the technology used by the manufacturer. At the end of that life, the tube can be recharged for costs that range from nominal to quite expensive. When evaluating a sealed CO_2 laser system, questions should be asked and answered about this type of laser system. What is the cost of recharging the sealed tube at the end of its shelf life? Can the tube be recharged onsite, or does the laser have to be returned to the manufacturer for this service? When the tube needs recharging, will the power slowly drop over time, or will the laser shut down all at once?

Sealed tube technology uses either direct electrical current (DC) or radio frequency (RF) to excite the CO_2 gas. A vacuum pump and replacement gas cylinder is not necessary in these CO_2 laser units since the tube is sealed. As a result, these systems are often mechanically and electronically simpler and produce less noise than the free flowing lasers.

CO_2 Laser Delivery Systems

Because of the long wavelength of the CO_2 laser at 10,600 nm, the beam must be delivered to the tissue through a hollow tube called an articulated arm (Figure 2-3). The arm contains special mirrors, positioned at joints, that sequentially reflect the invisible CO_2 and visible helium-neon beams forward. Care must be taken not to accidentally hit the articulated arm against a wall or another object that would cause these two laser beams to become misaligned. If misalignment did occur, the aiming beam would appear on the tissue at a different point than where the actual CO_2 laser energy would impact. This could cause major problems, especially in very delicate surgeries such as vocal cord polyp removals. Also, if the CO_2 and helium-neon beams are not aligned, then conducting the laser energy through a laparoscope to the target site is extremely difficult.

The long wavelength of the CO_2 laser beam cannot be effectively conducted through solid flexible fibers. Advances in technology are furthering the development of CO_2 laser fibers today. Several companies have developed flexible hollow core fibers that reflect the beam within the internal lumen. This process causes much of the power to be lost along the transmission length of the hollow fiber. For example, 100 W of CO_2 laser energy may enter the hollow core delivery device but probably only 50 W would be emitted from the end, thus indicating a 50% transmission loss.

A variety of lensed devices can be attached to the end of an articulated arm to deliver the CO_2 beam to tissue. The lens causes the raw CO_2 beam to be concentrated into a small spot. The point at which the beam is most intense or at its smallest size is called the focal point of the beam, and the distance from one lens to this focal spot is called the focal length of the beam (Figure 2-4). If a lens is not positioned in front of the raw CO_2 beam, the parallel beam can travel great distances, potentially causing tremendous safety problems.

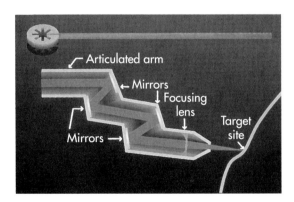

FIG. 2-3   The CO_2 laser beam is delivered to the tissue via an articulated arm. (Courtesy Coherent, Inc., Palo Alto, CA.)

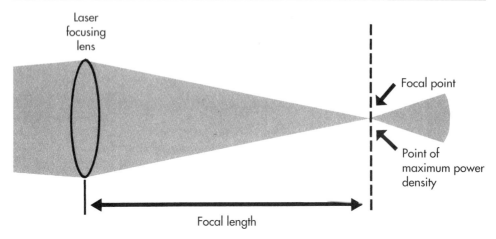

FIG. 2-4   The CO_2 laser focusing lens determines the focal length of the beam.

A handpiece can be attached to the end of the articulated arm to allow the surgeon to use the laser in the freehand style, much like a scalpel. A lens is contained in the handpiece that causes the beam to focus at a certain distance from the lens. For example, a 125-mm lens focuses the beam 125 mm from the lens. An indicator tip is often placed on the end of the handpiece barrel to designate the true focal point or, in this example, exactly 125 mm from the lens. The spot size of the beam can be adjusted by moving the indicator tip closer or farther from the target. The handpiece lens action is similar to focusing sunlight through a magnifying glass to increase the light's intensity on the target.

The CO_2 beam can cut or coagulate, depending upon the spot size that is made by passing the beam through a lens. If cutting is desired, the tissue would be positioned at the focal point of the lens. The spot size would be smallest with all the laser energy concentrated within the tiny spot. If coagulation is desired, the lens is held farther from the target or in the defocused mode, thus spreading the beam intensity over a larger area (Figure 2-5).

The CO_2 laser focusing lenses must be handled with care. Usually the barrel of the handpiece can be autoclaved, whereas the lens must never be soaked or autoclaved. These lenses are coated with a special substance, such as zinc selenide or gallium arsenide, that provides antireflection and ensures that the helium-neon and CO_2 beams are approximately the same size. Because of the precision these expensive lenses provide, they must be properly handled, cared for, and protected.

When dust accumulates on the lens surface, pressurized air can be blown onto the lens to remove the dust. If the lens surface is smudged, soap and water must not be used because the lens coating can easily be destroyed. Manufacturer's recommendations must be followed for specific lens care. Some guidelines suggest that if aggressive care is needed, a drop of absolute alcohol, acetone, or special lens cleaner can be placed on the lens surface. The drop is then rotated on the lens and gently shaken off, and the lens is allowed to dry. If the lens must be mechanically cleaned, soft optical lens paper can be used if specified by the manufacturer.

Many CO_2 handpieces are designed with tubing connected to the handpiece barrel. This tubing allows compressed air, CO_2, or nitrogen to purge the barrel to prevent smoke or splatter from coating the focusing lens (Figure 2-6). Some CO_2 laser systems have been built with an internal air compressor to provide a constant flow of purge air whenever the laser is activated. This eliminates the need for cylinders of medical-grade purge gas.

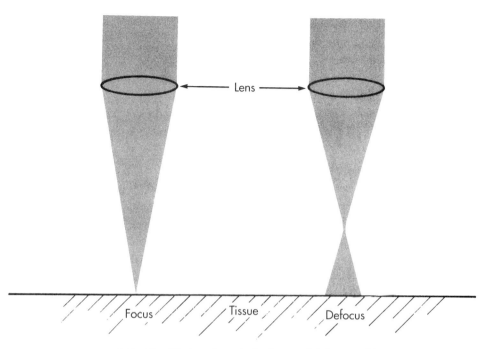

FIG. 2-5   The CO_2 laser beam in the focus and defocus positions.

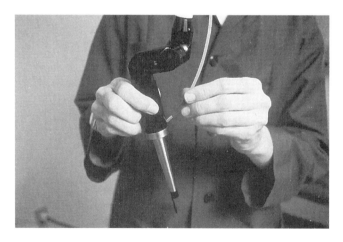

FIG. 2-6   A small tube connected to the handpiece conducts the purge gas.

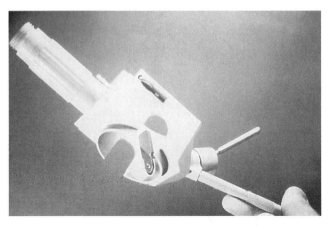

FIG. 2-7   The microscope adapter connects the articulated arm of the CO_2 laser to the microscope.

The articulated arm of the CO_2 laser system can also be adapted to a microscope to deliver the laser energy. A special micromanipulator allows the laser to be connected to a microscope or colposcope (Figure 2-7). The focal length of the microscope lens must be coordinated with the focal length of the laser lens. Most micromanipulators today have an adjustable lens so that the laser lens power can coincide easily with the microscope lens. For example, if a microlaryngoscopy is being performed with a 400-mm microscope lens, the laser micromanipulator is adjusted to provide a 400-mm laser lens focal length. The CO_2 beam is moved within a small area by rotating a joystick that turns a mirror to reflect the beam to the tissue (Figure 2-8).

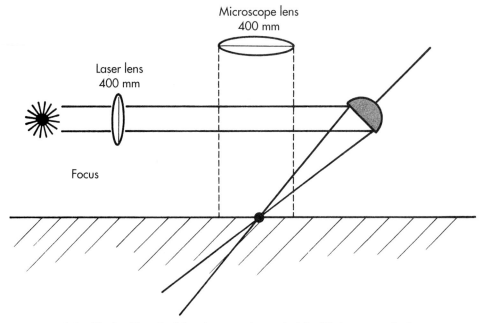

FIG. 2-8   The focal length of the microscope lens and of the CO_2 beam must be the same.

The CO_2 beam can also be delivered to the tissue by connecting the articulated arm to a coupling device that is attached to a rigid endoscope (e.g., laparoscope, bronchoscope). Rigid endoscopic/laparoscopic waveguides have been developed that are small enough to fit through the biopsy port of the endoscope. The waveguide then conducts the CO_2 laser energy directly to the tissue while producing a very small spot, thus offering more precision by decreasing the problems of alignment and focusing.

CO_2 Operational Modalities

The CO_2 laser system usually has a variety of operational modality options, including continuous wave (CW), pulsed, repeat pulse, and superpulse (Figure 2-9).

The CW modality allows the CO_2 beam to be emitted continually while the foot pedal is depressed. The pulsed modality delivers a single pulse for a specified duration (e.g., 0.1 or 0.5 second). This short burst of laser energy reduces heat spread and provides more control for the surgeon. A single pulse is generated by a timer on the CW mode. A repeat pulse or timed pulse allows the beam to be emitted in an automatic repeat sequence as long as the foot pedal is depressed.

The superpulse modality appears to be a continuous beam, but actually the laser is cycling on and off several hundred times per second. The peak power of each spiked pulse may go to 5 to 10 times the maximum output of the laser. For example, an 80-W CO_2 laser may produce a superpulse of 500 W at peak power. The average wattage is much more significant than the peak power. The superpulse action allows the tissue to cool, thus decreasing adjacent tissue damage. This mode is often used when precision is critical because it reduces the amount of charring. Depending on the target tissue and the skill of the physician, the appropriate operational modality will be chosen for the desired tissue effect.

Some CO_2 lasers can now be equipped with a special microprocessor-controlled scanner. With this unique scanner, the physician can program the area to be lased and then activate the laser to deliver the laser energy automatically and uniformly to the tissue at specified pulse durations.

NEODYMIUM: YTTRIUM-ALUMINUM-GARNET (ND:YAG) LASER

Nd:YAG Laser Characteristics

The Nd:YAG laser wavelength is located in the near-infrared region of the electromagnetic spectrum with a usual wavelength of 1064 nm. The Nd:YAG laser consists of a solid crystal of yttrium-aluminum-garnet. It is doped (laced) with a rare earth element called neodymium that actually produces the laser light energy when exposed to bright flash lamps.

Since the Nd:YAG wave is invisible, an aiming beam is required. Often a milliwatt helium-neon laser light is used as the pilot to mark the target for the Nd:YAG therapeutic beam.

When the noncontact Nd:YAG laser energy impacts tissue, there is a high degree of scattering. Thermal damage can occur to a depth of 2 to 6 mm, producing a homogenous coagulative effect. Therefore, the noncontact Nd:YAG laser is appreciated for its controlled coagulative properties without vaporization. During noncontact Nd:YAG laser-tissue interaction, slow heating of large tissue volumes occurs at the point of impact, followed by deep, slowly progressive coagulation. The Nd:YAG laser can coagulate arteries of less than 2 mm in diameter and veins of less than 3 mm because of the combined effects of the coagulation process and tissue shrinkage from vaporization of the cellular protoplasm (Joffe and Oguro, 1988).

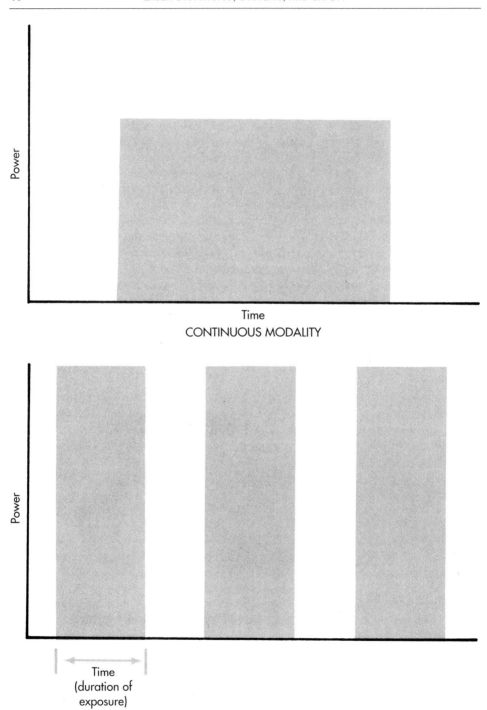

CONTINUOUS MODALITY

TIMED PULSE MODALITY

FIG. 2-9 Different operational modalities determine the duration of exposure of the CO_2 laser energy to the tissue.

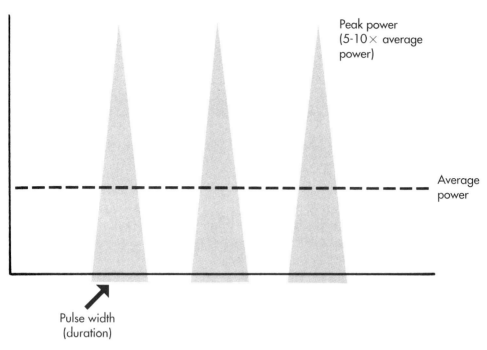

Peak power
(5-10× average
power)

Average
power

Pulse width
(duration)

SUPERPULSE MODALITY

FIG. 2-9, CONT'D.   For legend see opposite page.

As the Nd:YAG laser continues to coagulate, vaporization will result, causing carbonization. Since the Nd:YAG beam is more readily absorbed by darker pigments, the carbonized tissue will absorb the beam more rapidly, causing greater tissue absorption and reaction.

The Nd:YAG laser light is transmitted through clear fluids or structures, unlike the CO_2 laser beam, which is strongly absorbed by fluids. Therefore, the Nd:YAG laser energy can be used to effectively coagulate and vaporize a bladder tumor through the fluid medium of the bladder.

Another Nd:YAG wavelength being introduced is in the 1318-nm range. This wavelength is being investigated and utilized for its ability to provide a more efficient conversion of laser energy into heat in the tissue. The absorption by water and saline of the 1318-nm beam is greater than that of the 1064-nm Nd:YAG wavelength, causing less heat dissipation and greater cutting precision.

Besides the CW mode, a special type of Nd:YAG laser was developed to provide a pulsed mode, delivering the Nd:YAG beam to the tissue in nanoseconds. This laser is used in ophthalmology and is known as a photodisruptor. The Q-switched Nd:YAG laser provides quality switching of the optical resonator to create high peak powers delivered at 50,000 to 200,000 W in tens of nanoseconds (10^{-9} seconds) to disrupt a membrane or strand within the eye. This pulsing is extremely short in duration and does not have a thermal effect on the tissue. Mode-locked Nd:YAG lasers also produce pulses of tens of millions of watts in tens of picoseconds (10^{-12} seconds), referred to as ultrashort pulses. This pulsing is achieved by fixing the way the photons bounce back and forth in the laser head. The Q-switched and mode-locked pulsed lasers create photomechanical effects on tissue and are completely different Nd:YAG laser systems than the CW unit (Fuller, 1993).

Other Q-switched Nd:YAG lasers have been developed to deliver high peak powers (i.e., 35 mW) within very short wavelengths (i.e., 10 ns). This type of pulsed Nd:YAG laser, because of the color selectivity of the beam, is being used to remove dark ink tattoos. The laser beam destroys the dark chromophores while leaving the surrounding tissue unharmed.

The continuous wave Nd:YAG laser system may have special electrical requirements. For example, some of the Nd:YAG lasers available today require 220-V, single-phase electricity, or 208-V, three-phase electrical connections or a dedicated 110-V line. Some of the older Nd:YAG lasers require external plumbing connections to provide a constant flow of water to cool the laser tube. These are called water-cooled systems. Adequate water flow must be available to provide proper cooling. The water is usually tapped from a water line close by and then returned to a drain. Quick-release plumbing helps facilitate the set-up process for this type of system. The newer Nd:YAG laser systems are air-cooled with an internal closed water supply cooled by a fan system, not unlike the setup in an automobile radiator. As the fan air-cools the water, the closed water system circulates to cool the laser tube. The Q-switched Nd:YAG laser has no special electrical or water requirements.

Noncontact Fiber Delivery System

The wavelength of the Nd:YAG laser can be delivered to the tissue via a quartz fiber. The laser light is introduced into the proximal fiber end by a lens system and is transmitted through the fiber length by a process known as total internal reflection (Fuller, 1993) (Figure 2-10).

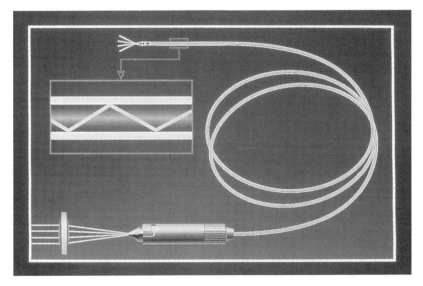

FIG. 2-10   Transmission of light through a fiber optic system. (Courtesy Surgical Laser Technologies, Inc., Oaks, PA.)

Nd:YAG Laser Fiber Design

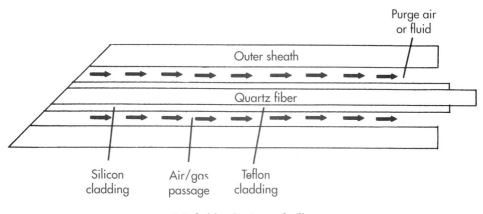

FIG. 2-11   Anatomy of a fiber.

Fiberoptics are composed of two parts: the core and the cladding. The quartz core of the fiber is surrounded by a silicon and Teflon cladding that provides high flexibility and mechanical stability. The fiber can be easily bent and still conduct the laser energy. Fiber units made this way are known by various names, such as bare fiber or straight fiber. If this fiber unit is surrounded by a catheter sheath, the fiber is often called a catheter fiber. The catheter fiber allows purge air/gas or fluid to flow along the length of the fiber to cool the distal tip. Fiber sizes vary widely today because researchers have been developing increasingly smaller fiber diameters. The sizes used in most clinical applications range from 0.2 to 0.6 mm in diameter. Figure 2-11 illustrates the anatomy of a fiber.

The exit divergence of the distal fiber end usually is between 6 and 24 degrees (Joffe and Oguro, 1988). As the Nd:YAG beam exits the fiber and hits the tissue, the beam tends to spread out as the distance increases (Figure 2-12). This leads to a decrease in power density as the fiber is held farther from the tissue and spreads the beam over a larger area. Approximately 30% to 40% of the Nd:YAG beam intensity is lost to backscatter (Joffe and Oguro, 1988). To achieve fullest efficiency in the Nd:YAG beam, the fiber should be held perpendicular to the tissue when the laser is activated. If the fiber is at another angle from the tissue, then the spot configuration will be altered (Figure 2-13).

Focusing handpieces have been developed that place a lens in front of the exiting Nd:YAG beam. This reusable fiber system allows the beam to be focused by adjusting the distance of the lens from the target area.

A reusable laser fiber should be calibrated before each use according to the manufacturer's instructions. The calibration process notes the power of the beam as it enters the fiber compared with the power of the beam as it exits the fiber (Figure 2-14). Manufacturers usually recommend repolishing or discarding a fiber showing over 25% loss of power transmission.

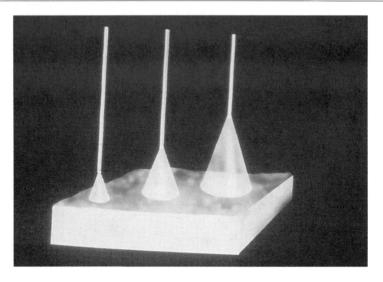

FIG. 2-12   Divergence of laser energy from a noncontact fiber.

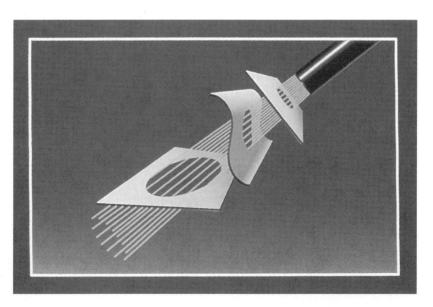

FIG. 2-13   The noncontact fiber should be held at right angles to the tissue. Positioning at any other angle will change the optimal beam configuration. (Courtesy Surgical Laser Technologies, Inc., Oaks, PA.)

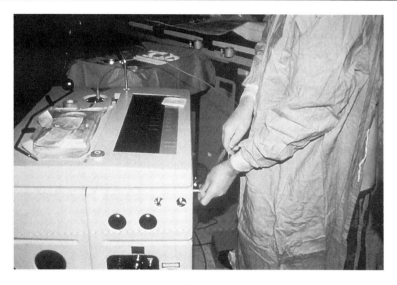

FIG. 2-14   Calibrating the laser fiber.

Reusable fibers were originally used when Nd:YAG laser technology first became popular. These fibers were soon replaced by disposable fibers. Now surgical personnel are relooking at the merits and potential cost savings of reusing bare fibers. Repolishing a fiber should be performed according to the manufacturer's instructions. A sample fiber-polishing procedure is provided below.

Fiber Repair Procedure for Bare Fibers

If a physician touches a noncontact fiber to the tissue, or fires too closely to the tissue, the end of the fiber may burn. When this happens, the light will no longer emerge from the tip within a small concentric spot, and the fiber will need to be repaired. To do this, follow the steps below.

1. Scrape off the Teflon and silicon cladding over about ½ inch.
2. Cleave or break the distal end of the fiber by scoring it with a diamond cutter or a No. 15 blade and then snapping off the damaged end.
3. Polish the fiber end by securing the bare fiber in a polishing tool (to stabilize the fiber) and gently rotating the fiber end on the special fiber-polishing paper. Circular or figure-eight movements will help ensure adequate polishing of the tip.
4. Examine the polished end of the fiber by viewing the tip through a magnifying glass or other type of optical enhancement system.
5. Recalibrate every polished fiber immediately before use to note the power transmissibility. If there is more than 25% loss of power, then the length of the fiber should be checked for damage, the tip should be repolished, or the fiber should be discarded.
6. Store the fibers with a dust cover on the proximal end that attaches to the laser, and protect the distal end of the fiber.
7. Sterilize or disinfect the fiber as needed.

Technology has perfected disposable fibers for single use. Since these fibers can be costly, some health care facilities have written protocols for reprocessing them. Sterilization cases are available from instrument companies to contain and protect the fibers for gas sterilization. If disposable fibers are reprocessed, the health care facility assumes liability for the processing and subsequent uses. Therefore, a written protocol must be developed by the institution to ensure that appropriate procedures are being followed and that the fiber's sterilization/decontamination and integrity are ensured. A sample protocol for justifying the need to reprocess disposable laser fibers is provided below.

Noncontact fibers must not come in contact with the tissue. If tissue is present on the end of the fiber, the tissue will bake on it, leading to fiber destruction. Therefore, preventing the fiber from coming in direct contact with tissue is extremely important.

The air/gas or fluid that flows through to purge a catheter fiber helps keep the tip of the fiber free from debris and cools the end to decrease fiber destruction.

Protocol to Justify the Reuse of Single-Use Laser Fibers

1. Obtain approval for this protocol by the hospital risk manager and the Laser Committee.
2. Conduct a survey of 10 major hospitals to determine whether they reprocess disposable fibers and what method they use for reprocessing.
3. Develop criteria to determine which fibers to reprocess. Examples may include the following:
   a. The fiber can be cleaned adequately.
   b. The fiber's physical characteristics or quality will not be adversely affected by the reprocessing.
   c. The product will remain safe and effective for its intended use.
4. Determine which fibers could be reprocessed. Examples may include the following:
   a. Bare fibers—used for urology (i.e., bladder tumor procedures).
   b. Right-angle fibers—used for prostatic procedures.
   c. Handpiece fibers—used for open or laparoscopic procedures with air or gas purge.
   d. Sculpted fibers.
   e. No fluid-cooled fibers.
   f. No fibers that have been grossly contaminated with blood, pus, or fecal material.
5. Communicate with fiber manufacturers for written recommendations for reprocessing single-use fibers.
6. Conduct a cost analysis of the cost of the fiber vs. reusing the fiber (e.g., cost of the sterilization container, staff time, and supplies to reprocess the fiber).
7. Develop a draft procedure policy including the steps to be followed when reprocessing single-use fibers.
8. Obtain permission from the appropriate sources within the hospital to conduct a pilot study that involves reprocessing disposable fibers after they have been used on inanimate tissue models.
9. Conduct the study noting the sterility/decontamination and integrity of the fiber.
10. Evaluate the results of the study and report to the Laser Committee to determine whether reprocessing disposable fibers is justified.

Contact Fiber Delivery System

Manufacturers have developed special tips to deliver laser energy while the laser tip is in contact with the tissue. Since these tips are held directly in contact with the tissue, tactile sensation is restored for the physician.

Most contact tips are made of a physiologically neutral synthetic sapphire crystal. The special properties of the tip make it very useful in delivering laser energy directly to the tissue. These tips have been shown to have high melting temperatures (2030 to 2050° F), low thermal conductivity, and mechanical strength.

Contact tips are attached to a catheter endoscopic fiber or a handpiece fiber by a universal connector that has threads so that various tips can be screwed on and off as needed. The laser energy is then conducted through the probe body and exits at the probe-tissue interface. A wavelength conversion occurs as the tip transforms the predetermined amount of laser power into heat at the probe-tissue connection (Fuller, 1993) (Figure 2-15). The tip is coated with a special material to optimize the optical distribution of the energy for increased precision and performance.

Fluid or air/gas can flow through the length of the fiber and exit at the point of the contact tip. This purge is essential for cooling the tip during the procedure. Care must be taken not to clog the purge side holes so that the flow will continue and the tip will remain cool.

Laser tips of different geometric configurations are available to shape the laser energy distribution. Depending on the tissue type and desired tissue effects, individual tips are chosen to cut, coagulate, or vaporize tissue. Figure 2-16 illustrates the laser energy distribution with various contact tips. Some tips may be frosted with a special coating to allow the light to be dispersed from the lateral walls instead of being channeled down only

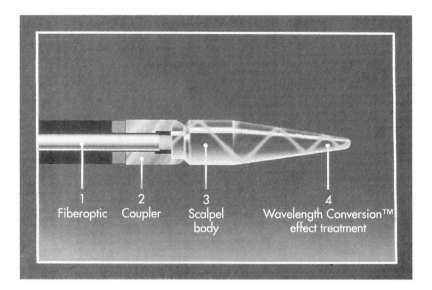

FIG. 2-15   Contact tip and fiber combination conducts the laser energy to the tissue. (Courtesy Surgical Laser Technologies, Inc., Oaks, PA.)

through the distal tip. Approximately 15% to 20% of the energy is then permitted to exit through the frosting on the sides while 80% to 85% of the energy still exits at the distal tip.

Various tip shapes cause the laser power to be dispersed so that optimal light intensity is delivered to the tissue. This beam-distribution capability helps control the thermal effect of the beam, thus providing tremendous control to vaporize, ablate, or coagulate (Figure 2-17).

The diameter of the distal tip of the probe determines the spot size of the beam. Smaller tip ends cause increased power density by concentrating all of the energy within a smaller area, thus requiring less wattage. The depth of penetration of the contact tip depends on the laser power (wattage), tip diameter, and duration of exposure.

There is no need to focus the beam because the tip is in contact with the tissue, and therefore the spot size and power density are accurately controlled. The tissue provides a

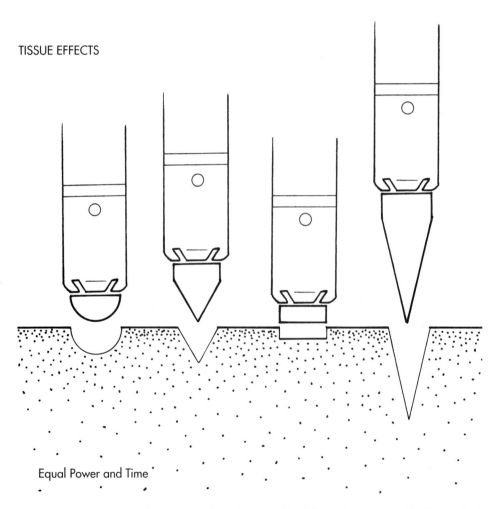

TISSUE EFFECTS

Equal Power and Time

FIG. 2-16   Contact tips of various configurations provide different laser energy distribution in the tissue.

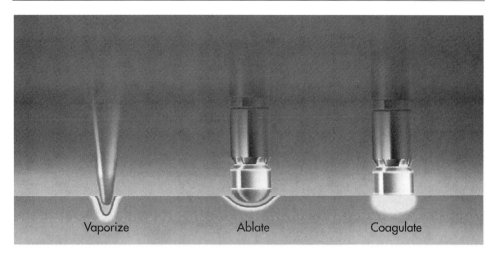

FIG. 2-17 Contact tips provide precise cutting, coagulation, and ablation. (Courtesy Surgical Laser Technologies, Inc., Oaks, PA.)

heat sink, or a dispersal of heat, from the tip. If the tip is not in contact with the tissue during continued laser activation, then the tip may overheat and fracture.

Since the tip is in direct contact with the tissue, less laser energy is required. Less than 25 W of power is usually needed to deliver the Nd:YAG energy to the tissue. If the contact tip is larger, then greater powers can be used. For example, 40 to 50 W of energy can safely be used through a 10-mm rounded contact probe. Since the energy is concentrated within the tip, less adjacent tissue heating and damage occur with the contact system. The contact tip delivery system decreases the backscatter of the beam to only 5% (Joffe and Oguro, 1988). The contact tip provides excellent thermal coagulation and penetration with minimal laser smoke or plume production.

A study comparing noncontact with contact technology illustrated that to provide comparable tissue coagulation, the noncontact technology caused 3 mm of adjacent tissue necrosis, whereas the contact technology caused only 0.5 mm of adjacent tissue damage. Therefore, adjacent tissue damage can be decreased by 75% when contact tips are used. This in turn leads to decreased sloughing of necrotic tissue postoperatively, possibly decreasing subsequent infection. There is also less chance of perforation of a structure as a result of the greater precision offered by the contact delivery system (Joffe and Oguro, 1988).

The contact tip often causes slower cutting, but the tip also coagulates as it cuts. Hemostasis results from the tissue edema and protein coagulation.

If lateral stress is exerted on the contact laser scalpel during cutting, fracture of the tip can occur. The physician must allow the laser energy to cause the cutting, not the actual mechanical movement of the scalpel through the tissue.

Contact tips should be stored, cleaned, and handled according to the manufacturer's recommendations. Contact tips can be soaked in hydrogen peroxide to help loosen tissue debris before the cleaning process begins. Most contact tips can be steam-sterilized and stored in special contact tip cases. Extreme care must be taken not to misplace or lose these small contact tips during cleanup. Operating room personnel and physicians should be cognizant of the expense of each tip and fiber to encourage proper handling and care.

Other contact technology has been developed to provide tactile feedback for the surgeon. Contact fibers have been designed by a process in which the distal end is sculpted into a geometrical configuration, such as a conical or rounded shape. Individual contact tips are not needed since the sculpted fiber itself can actually touch the tissue. Tissue reaction is similar to that of the contact tips, however. Because the energy is concentrated at the end of the sculpted fiber when it exits, decreased power is necessary. The physician determines which contact system to use.

A limitation of sculpted fibers is the inability to change the geometrical configuration of the fiber end during the procedure (another fiber must be used). Also, the fiber's heat tolerance is less than that of a contact tip. Research continues on other materials, such as a ceramic jacket around a quartz fiber, to provide contact capabilities.

The benefits derived from Nd:YAG laser contact technology are as follows:

- Less power needed to deliver the Nd:YAG laser energy
- Less blood loss because of direct coagulation
- Less smoke production
- Less adjacent tissue damage
- Less backscatter and reflection of the beam
- Tactile feedback provided
- Uniform performance in all soft tissue

FREQUENCY DOUBLED YAG LASER
Frequency Doubled YAG Laser Characteristics

In current technology a solid state laser has been developed that is designed to pass an Nd:YAG primary beam of 1064 nm through a potassium titanyl phosphate crystal to produce an intense green laser light of 532 nm. This process of delivering the primary beam through the KTP crystal causes the wavelength of 1064 nm to be shortened to half—532 nm—while doubling the beam's frequency. The emergent beam is therefore visible. Figure 2-18 illustrates the frequency doubling process.

TWIN CRYSTAL ARRANGEMENT

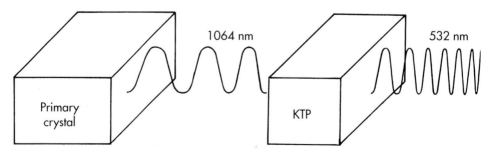

FIG. 2-18   Frequency doubled YAG laser principle. A primary beam passes through a special crystal to double the frequency and halve the wavelength.

This monochromatic green beam is similar in wavelength to that of the argon beam as it is strongly absorbed by hemoglobin, melanin, and other similar pigments. This beam also can be transmitted through clear fluids or structures.

Older KTP lasers have special electrical and water requirements for operation. Normal water flow and pressure is adequate to cool the laser. A special safety feature shuts down the laser if the water pressure or flow is not sufficient. The newer KTP lasers have internal water-cooling systems, so external hookups are not needed. Many of the newer models also can be connected to 110-V outlets for operation.

Advances have produced a modified laser unit that allows either the primary Nd:YAG beam or the 532-nm emergent beam to be delivered to the tissue. When one selects a certain button on the control panel, the primary beam or the emergent beam can be activated by controlling the positioning of the KTP crystal.

Frequency Doubled YAG Laser Delivery Systems

The 532-nm wavelength is delivered to the tissue through a fiber that can be connected to a microscope or handpiece. A computerized eye safety filter is available to attach to the microscope or an endoscope. This shutter, activated only when the laser is fired, allows an eye safety filter to fall in place to protect the surgeon's eyes. By filtering the light only during the laser activation, the surgeon is afforded a clear view of the field with no discoloration from an optical filter.

The KTP laser fiber is made of a quartz core surrounded by silicon cladding and a nylon coating to prevent breakage or other damage. The same fiber can be used to deliver the 1064- or 532-nm wavelength to the tissue. Fibers are available that normally range from 0.2 to 0.6 mm in diameter. Fiber repair is quickly and easily performed by following the manufacturer's instructions.

The reusable fibers should be calibrated before each use to determine the amount of transmission loss from the entry of the laser energy into the fiber to its emergence from the fiber end. If the transmission loss is significant (over 25%), the fiber should be repaired or replaced. The disposable fibers do not need calibration before use because the laser usually assumes an 85% calibration factor (transmission) with a 2% variation.

Fiber handpieces of various configurations are available today to offer the physician greater ease of operation and the ability to deliver the energy to less accessible areas (such as the middle ear). These handpieces provide the physician with tactile sensation because the fiber can be held directly in contact with the tissue or can be used in the noncontact manner.

Many KTP lasers, like the argon lasers, can also be attached to a computerized scanning system, such as the Hexascanner (see section on argon laser delivery systems later in this chapter). This system allows for precision delivery of the energy within a specific pattern.

HOLMIUM:YAG LASER

Another type of YAG solid state laser is the holmium:YAG, which emits a pulsed beam of 2100 nm. This laser energy is conducted to the tissue via a flexible fiber. When the laser energy is being delivered through a fluid medium, a vapor bubble is produced that allows the beam to be transmitted to the tissue. The tip of the fiber must be held close to the target site. If cutting is desired, then the fiber must be touching or almost touching the tissue. If tissue sculpting or ablating is needed, then the fiber must be within 2 mm of the tissue. If the tissue is more than 5 mm away from the fiber tip, no significant tissue response will occur. This beam is not color-selective and produces a depth of thermal damage limited from 0.4 to 0.6 mm, similar to the CO_2 laser's thermal damage. The holmium:YAG laser is being used widely by orthopedists during arthroscopic procedures because it can be used in fluid environments and causes tissue response similar to the CO_2 laser. Other specialists are realizing the unique properties of this laser wavelength and are beginning to use it during different surgical applications. The holmium:YAG laser is portable and does not need water hookups; however, it usually requires special electrical powers (e.g., 208-volt, 30-amp, single phase power).

ARGON LASER
Argon Laser Characteristics

The argon laser produces an intense visible blue light and green light of approximately 488 and 514.5 nm, respectively. In clinical use, the combination of the blue and the green light allows for more complete tissue absorption. Some systems are designed to offer a green-only argon light option for delicate surgery in which specific absorption is critical (e.g., ophthalmology retinal procedures).

The core of the argon laser is the plasma tube that contains the argon. High electrical current is passed down the barrel of the tube through the gas to excite the argon atoms to produce the laser energy. Over the years, through sophisticated engineering, the argon laser has become more reliable. The disadvantage of the argon laser is that the plasma tubes must be replaced periodically. These tubes sometimes cost about one fourth the original price of the laser itself.

Hemoglobin, melanin, or other similar pigmentation selectively and readily absorb the argon wavelength. The laser energy is then converted into heat upon absorption, and this thermal effect produces coagulation or vaporization. Because of this selective absorption, the localized heat generation controls the spread of the thermal energy and decreases laser damage to adjacent tissue.

Argon laser energy is transmitted through clear fluids and structures, as is the Nd:YAG wavelength. Therefore, the argon laser can be successfully directed through the clear structures of the eye to coagulate a bleeding vessel on the retina without having to enter the eye surgically. The argon laser can also be used through a cystoscope to effectively vaporize a tumor in the fluid-filled environment of the bladder.

The aiming beam for the argon laser is usually low-power argon laser energy. Since this light is in the visible range, the low-power argon beam appropriately and safely indicates where the high-power therapeutic beam will strike. This type of aiming system and fiber delivery system do not cause alignment problems like those encountered with the CO_2 laser mirror and articulated arm system.

The low-power argon laser systems, powered by 5 W or less, usually require a 208-V, three-phase or 220-V, single-phase electrical line for operation. Some of these lasers have internal fans that air-cool the argon tube. The high-power argon laser systems need higher electrical voltage connections plus external plumbing to provide water flow for adequate tube cooling. Some of these lasers require that the external water supply continue to circulate for a period of time even after the system has been turned off. This ensures that the tube is properly cooled to prolong its life. Special attention is needed to determine the flow (gallons per minute) and the pressure (pounds per square inch) of water needed to appropriately cool the laser. Often the upper floors of older buildings do not have adequate water flow and pressure to maintain proper cooling of the system. In such situations, a booster pump will help increase the water flow and pressure to the laser.

Argon laser technology is being challenged by tubeless laser technology that uses a solid-state type of system. These smaller compact units require less maintenance and are usually less expensive to operate. Advances in these systems continue to provide cost-effective, reliable, and convenient lasers that will replace the older argon units.

Argon Laser Delivery Systems

Argon laser energy can be delivered to the tissue through a slit lamp, microscope, or fiber. The slit lamp and microscope delivery systems usually are equipped with an internal optical filter that protects the surgeon's eyes when the foot switch or hand-control button is depressed to activate the laser. This shutter unit should be checked routinely for proper operation.

An argon fiber can be directed through the biopsy port of a rigid or flexible endoscope to perform surgery from within an organ or structure. At the end of the fiber, the beam diverges approximately 10 to 14 degrees. Therefore, the spot size can be altered by changing the distance of the fiber tip from the tissue. The fiber is usually used in the noncontact manner, but some fibers can also be used in contact with the tissue. A fiber that is used inside the eye or ear may be designed with the fiber encapsulated in a cannula for maximum handling control.

A handpiece can also be affixed to the fiber to deliver the energy to the tissue. Often these handpieces come in different shapes with the fiber permanently attached. There are two basic types of handpieces that alter the argon beam. One type is the focused device, which ensures the spot size is a specific diameter when the handpiece is held a certain distance from the tissue. For example, a 100-μm, focused device handpiece is in focus when the tip is held 2 inches from the tissue. To vary the spot size, the handpiece end is moved closer to or farther from the tissue. The other type of handpiece contains an internal lens that can be moved to change the focal length and spot size of the beam.

Today many argon fibers are being produced as disposable or single-use fibers. Some surgical facilities have chosen to reprocess these fibers and are assuming the liability for doing so (see Fiber Repair Procedure for Bare Fibers on page 45). If a fiber is reusable, the manufacturer's recommendations for fiber repair should be followed.

Many argon and other types of lasers can be connected to a computerized scanning delivery device, such as the Hexascanner. This type of automatic scanner will deliver small bursts of laser energy to the tissue in preselected patterns. The microprocessor-controlled scanner delivers the laser energy in a certain sequence, allowing tissue to cool between exposures and thus reduce the risk of thermal tissue damage. This type of delivery system provides precision and successful results for dermatology procedures, such as lightening port-wine stains. Because maximum power and minimum exposure tissue are provided, tissue heating and intraoperative pain are minimized. The total treatment time can be decreased and reproducible results obtained with each sequential treatment.

KRYPTON LASER

The krypton laser is a gas laser similar to the argon laser. An electrical current activates the krypton active medium to produce laser energy. The krypton laser usually has special water and electrical requirements.

The krypton laser has various wavelengths from green (531 nm) and yellow (568 nm) to red (647 nm). Red laser light is the type most frequently used and produces more power in the red spectrum than does the ruby laser or the helium-neon laser.

Since the krypton laser beam is absorbed less by hemoglobin than the argon laser beam is, ophthalmologists are using this wavelength to more selectively destroy tissue on the retina.

TUNABLE DYE LASER

The ultimate dream of the physicist involved in laser technology development is to create a laser whose beam wavelength or color could be controlled by the mere turn of a dial. The tunable dye laser is the closest realization of this dream. In the tunable dye laser, a liquid organic dye dissolved in water or an alcohol solvent of a specific molar concentration is exposed to an intense light source, usually an argon laser beam. The dye absorbs the laser light of one wavelength and then fluoresces and emits light over a broad spectrum of visible colors. A special tuning element can be inserted into the cavity to cause a specific wavelength to lase. The operator can turn the element, usually a birefringent crystal, through various angles to dial in the desired wavelength within a certain range. Usually the tunable dye laser can be tuned from 400 to 1000 nm by changing the dye and certain other parameters. The dye in the laser is subjected to photo-induced dye disintegration, thus requiring frequent changes of dye after a certain number of pulses. Tunable dye lasers can be used in either the continuous or the pulsed modes. Today the tunable dye laser is being used for spectroscopy, cell sorting, laboratory counting devices, dermatology procedures, and selective destruction of malignancies.

Tuning the dye laser to yellow light at approximately 577 to 585 nm causes highly selective vascular damage in clinical applications. Since hemoglobin has a local absorption peak of these yellow light wavelengths, a vascular lesion will readily absorb this laser energy, while the nonvascularized tissue will cause the beam to diffuse. Thus, lightening a port-wine stain can be successfully achieved by using this wavelength.

A flashlamp-pumped pulsed dye (FLPPD) laser consists of a tube filled with a dye solution that is excited by a flashlamp within the laser head. The wavelength may be tuned from 400 to 1000 nm by changing the dye. Precisely tuning in a particular wavelength can be achieved through the use of prisms to control the dye's fluorescence spectra. This FLPPD laser produces high peak powers with short single pulses and is ideal for treating dermatology conditions involving specific pigmentations.

The tunable dye laser is also used for photodynamic therapy with the wavelength tuned to red light at 630 nm. When a special light-sensitive drug whose absorption peak is also at 630 nm is injected or used topically, the tunable dye laser energy is absorbed, causing a reaction that can selectively destroy a malignancy. The key to the success of this treatment is the type of fiber used and the accurate measurement of the output.

Pulsed dye lasers have gained popularity in recent years. A 504-nm pulsed system is being used for laser lithotripsy to fragment stones. A tiny 0.2-mm fiber can be delivered through an endoscope to reach the stone. The fiber is held very close to the stone, or in contact with the stone, and a photoacoustical effect causes the fragmentation.

Q-SWITCHED RUBY LASER

The Q-switched ruby laser emits a red beam of 694 nm. The Q-switching causes the laser to concentrate the energy into a single, intense pulse with energy of approximately 10 J and a duration of 25 ns. This is achieved through a fast electromagnetic switch, usually known as a Pockel's cell, located in the laser cavity, that causes the active medium to build up excited energy in excess of what it would normally. A shutter prevents the actual lasing. When the excitation is at its greatest, the shutter is opened so that lasing occurs, and a great burst of energy is emitted from the cavity. The outcome is a brief nanosecond pulse or a series of powerful pulses.

High-powered flashlamps are used to excite the ruby crystal, which consists of aluminum trioxide that is doped with chromium ions. The extremely short pulses have high peak powers of greater than 106 W/cm^2. This energy is transmitted to the target through an articulated arm that contains a focusing lens that concentrates the energy in a uniform pattern.

This 694-nm energy penetrates several millimeters into the skin or the target. Dark blue and black pigmentation readily absorbs the beam, making this laser highly appropriate for tattoo removals of this color pigmentation.

COPPER VAPOR LASER

The copper vapor laser emits a green light of 510 nm and a yellow light of 578 nm. The heart of this laser consists of a neon gas-filled ceramic tube containing copper pellets. A high-voltage electrical current is passed through the gas pellet mixture, causing the metal to emit the laser energy. A prism positioned between the end mirrors is then used to select the specific wavelength desired.

The copper vapor laser energy is directed to the tissue via quartz optical fibers in a flexible tube with a handpiece on the end. The laser can emit a series of very short pulses (10 to 40 ns) at a very quick repetition rate. Each pulsation has a few millijoules of energy at very high peak powers (>10 kW).

The main use of the copper vapor laser has been for dermatology and plastic surgery. The choice of this laser is based on physician preference since more research is needed to determine convincing data to support the use of this laser over another.

DIODE LASER

Diode lasers are compact and efficient lasers used today mainly in computers, fiberoptic communication, video disc players, and a range of other electronic instruments and equipment. Low-output diode lasers today emit red and orange wavelengths and are used for ophthalmology applications. Researchers are developing diode laser systems for other surgical applications. The advancement of this technology will continually threaten other laser systems because these units are more compact and cost-effective.

EXCIMER LASER

The excimer laser alludes to an excited dimer, which refers to a molecule that is relatively stable when excited. This molecule breaks up into its component parts when it loses its energy and emits a photon. Excimer laser systems today use compounds of rare gases and halogens that are excited complexes rather than excited dimers, but the name has remained the same.

Depending upon the exact chemical composition of the active medium, a variety of ultraviolet (UV) wavelengths can be produced. The four most popular gases used in the excimer lasers are argon fluoride (ArF), producing a wavelength of 193 nm; krypton fluoride (KrF), 248 nm; xenon chloride (XeCl), 308 nm; and xenon fluoride (XeF), 351 nm.

When the pulsed, high-intensity UV laser energy is absorbed on the surface of tissue, photoablation occurs. Because of the rapid surface absorption of the laser beam, penetration depths are less than 1 μm. The bonds of the absorbing molecules are disassociated without the production of thermal energy. Therefore, no significant damage occurs to the other surrounding molecules, and a sharp, clean cut is produced. In comparison, other lasers break apart molecular bonds with thermal energy (Achauer, Vander Kam, and Berns, 1992).

The hazard associated with the excimer laser system is that most of the gases used in the unit are extremely toxic or even fatal. The challenge has been for the physicist to develop a laser design to encapsulate these toxic gases and provide protection from high-voltage discharges. Appropriate system housing, engineering designs, and exhaust systems have been critical in the expansion of the clinical use of this type of laser. The large size of the excimer laser helps accommodate the number of vital parts needed to produce the lasing energy. As technology advances, excimer laser units are becoming more compact.

Another concern about excimer laser technology is the possible undesired side effects of its high-intensity UV radiation. Studies are being conducted to determine whether it has a mutagenic and carcinogenic effect on cells.

Excimer lasers are being investigated for tissue ablation of the cornea and within occluded arteries. The ultraviolet excimer laser energy is strongly absorbed by protein. Therefore, research is being conducted to note the results of correcting the shape of the cornea in radial keratoplasty and opening occluded arteries in laser angioplasty. The excimer laser's popularity arises from its tremendous precision in cutting or coagulating with no notable thermal spread to adjacent tissue.

FREE ELECTRON LASER

Researchers are currently investigating the development and use of the free electron laser. This large laser system consists of a magnetic field that has a series of magnets whose poles alternate along the pathway of flowing electrons. As these free electrons pass through the magnetic field close to the speed of light, their polarity is altered. The electrons travel in a wiggling motion through the magnetic field, which is called the wiggler. As the electrons pass through this field, they give up a certain amount of energy in the form of photons. One can tune the laser to a broad range of wavelengths rather than to only a narrow range by varying the electron energy and the force of the magnetic field (Achauer, Vander Kam, and Berns, 1992). The versatility of this laser in emitting a variety of wavelengths, coupled with its precision capabilities, will make it extremely useful in medicine.

REFERENCES

Absten GT and Joffe SN: *Lasers in medicine: an introductory guide,* London, 1985, Chapman & Hall.

Achauer BM, Vander Kam VM, and Berns MW: *Lasers in plastic surgery and dermatology,* New York, 1992, Thieme.

Fuller TA: *Thermal surgical lasers,* Oaks, PA, 1993, Surgical Laser Technologies, Inc.

Joffe SN and Oguro Y, editors: *Advances in Nd:YAG laser surgery,* New York, 1988, Springer-Verlag.

Sliney DH and Trokel SL: *Medical lasers and their safe use,* New York, 1993, Springer-Verlag.

SUGGESTED READINGS

Apfelberg DB, editor: *Evaluation and installation of surgical laser systems,* New York, 1987, Springer-Verlag.

Ball KA: The evolution of surgical lasers, *Today's OR Nurse,* 8:9, June 1986.

Fuller TA: *Thermal surgical lasers, a technical monograph,* Oaks, PA, 1993, Surgical Laser Technologies, Inc.

Joffe SN, editor: *Lasers in general surgery,* Baltimore, 1989, Williams & Wilkins.

Meeker MH and Rothrock JC: *Alexander's care of the patient in surgery,* ed 10, St. Louis, 1995, Mosby.

Pfister JI, Kneedler JA, and Purcell SK: *The nursing spectrum of lasers,* Denver, 1988, Education Design, Inc.

Ratz JL: *Lasers in cutaneous medicine and surgery,* Chicago, 1986, Year Book.

3

LASER SAFETY

A s laser programs develop and expand, one question becomes critical: How hazardous is the laser? With the constant evolution of laser technology, potential hazards and safety measures are also continually changing. The laser team member must become acutely aware of the many controls needed to ensure the safe and appropriate use of the laser.

LASER SAFETY REFERENCES AND REGULATORY BODIES

There are many laser safety references and regulatory bodies that have developed guidelines or standards for the safe use of lasers in health care. The following paragraphs describe some of these expert resources for laser safety.

American National Standards Institute (ANSI)

ANSI, a nongovernmental organization, comprises experts from trade associations, technical societies, professional groups, and consumer organizations that have developed appropriate standards for the safe use of lasers. In 1973, the ANSI Z136.1 standards were formulated, addressing laser safety in warfare, industry, and health care. In 1988, ANSI Z136.3 standards were published that address laser safety in health care specifically. The appendix of these standards establishes a consensus on laser safety in each specialty area of medicine and surgery. The Z136.3 standards will be updated in the mid 1990s and will continue to be revised in the future as needed. When a revision is needed, teams of experts are convened to assist with any changes in wording.

Center for Devices and Radiological Health (CDRH)

The CDRH is the combination of two previous groups called the Center for Medical Devices and the Bureau of Radiological Health. This agency is the regulatory section of the Food and Drug Administration (FDA) in the Department of Human Services. Congress has given the CDRH the responsibility of standardizing the manufacture of laser units. This organization also issues the Investigational Device Exemption to allow the investigation of new laser applications. If the laser's effectiveness in an application is proven, the laser can then be marketed for that clinical application or use.

The CDRH requires specific labeling on the laser head of Class IV lasers informing the operator of the type of laser radiation as well as the peak power that can be produced. The exit port of the laser beam must be clearly identified.

The Safe Medical Device Act that was signed into law on November 28, 1990, requires that user facilities and manufacturers of medical devices, including lasers, report certain device-related problems to the FDA. Reports must be filed if the device has caused death or serious illness or injury. The FDA identifies serious illness or injury as "life threatening, that which results in permanent impairment of a body function or permanent damage to a body structure or necessitates immediate medical or surgical intervention to preclude permanent impairment of a body function or permanent damage to a body structure" (U. S. Department of Health and Human Services, Medical Device Reporting for User Facilities, 1991). The FDA also encourages the reporting of any device malfunction, no matter what the damages may be. User facilities also must submit a semiannual report to the FDA summarizing any incidents with medical devices (U.S. Department of Health and Human Services, Highlight of the Safe Medical Device Act of 1990, 1991).

The FDA is measuring compliance with this ruling. Between November 28, 1991, and December 10, 1992, the FDA received reports from manufacturers that there were 1,444 deaths associated with the use of medical devices. During that same time, though, only 268 deaths were reported by user facilities. This confirms that user facilities are probably reporting deaths caused by medical devices to the manufacturer instead of reporting them directly to the FDA (*Clinical Laser Monthly,* February 1993). The FDA is continuing to address the issue of noncompliance with this regulation.

Occupational Safety and Health Administration (OSHA)

OSHA is within the U.S. Department of Labor and is primarily responsible for ensuring worker safety during laser intervention. This agency depends on the ANSI standards and addresses physical environment problems, such as the safe placement of power cords and whether surgical smoke is being evacuated properly. OSHA also reviews the results of research conducted by NIOSH (see below), a federal agency that conducts studies involving safety hazards in the workplace.

National Institute for Occupational Safety and Health (NIOSH)

NIOSH, a federally funded institute, conducts research to prove or disprove hazards within the workplace. For example, NIOSH has conducted studies that prove laser plume contents are potentially hazardous. OSHA often uses the results of NIOSH research to mandate compliance to minimize hazards in the work environment.

Joint Commission on Accreditation of Healthcare Organizations (JCAHO)

The JCAHO examines facilities to determine whether they comply with specific standards and guidelines that JCAHO has published. The JCAHO does not specifically reference laser safety issues because they consider lasers to be like any other equipment that is covered by the broad general standards. The JCAHO surveyors are being educated about the use of lasers and about the details of the ANSI Z136.3 standards. Therefore, they may ask some general questions of the surgical team regarding lasers such as these: How is the competency of a laser team member assessed? What kind of orientation program is in place to prepare staff members to operate a laser during a procedure? What policies are in the surgery manual that specifically address laser safety? The JCAHO appears to be very interested in education and documentation and examines these aspects closely.

Association of Operating Room Nurses (AORN)

The AORN, the professional organization of perioperative nurses, has developed recommended practices that serve as guidelines for the safe use of lasers. Originally, the recommended laser practices were listed as part of the "recommended practices for radiation safety in the OR (including lasers)" (AORN, 1989). In 1989, the revised version of the original laser section, "recommended practices for laser safety in the operating room," was published, and then it was revised again in 1993. It will continue to be reviewed for possible revision at least every 3 to 5 years. These recommended practices are intended to represent what is believed to be the optimal level of practice for nurses who work with lasers.

American Society for Laser Medicine and Surgery (ASLMS)

The ASLMS was founded in 1980 through the pioneering efforts of Dr. Leon Goldman. His endeavors were financially supported by a generous grant from the A. Ward Ford Memorial Institute in Wausau, Wisconsin. Others instrumental in the formation of this organization were Drs. Ellet Drake and William B. Mark. The goal of this organization is to unite health care professionals in clinical laser application, laser education, and laser research to benefit humanity. This body of experts has developed standards and guidelines for the use of the laser in the health care environment.

The ASLMS was patterned after the International Laser Surgery Society, which was organized through the efforts of Dr. Isaac Kaplan of Tel Aviv, Israel, in 1975. The ASLMS has been vital in helping to expand laser technology in health care worldwide.

State and Local Regulations

State and local regulations vary from area to area. Restrictions range from no regulations to yearly inspection or certification. Those involved in procuring a laser system must become familiar with state and local regulations.

Many states are adopting some type of regulatory process for the control of lasers. Some states that have laser safety regulations include but are not limited to Texas, Florida, Arizona, Alaska, Georgia, New York, California, Illinois, Massachusetts, Oregon, Virginia, and Vermont. In 1983, a guide for state legislation was published, called *Suggested State Regulations for the Control of Radiation, Volume II, Nonionizing Radiation, Lasers* (U.S. Department of Health and Human Services). These suggestions include a state agency registration system for lasers, the responsibilities and qualifications of the laser safety officer, training program requirements, and various safety requirements.

Hospital Policies and Procedures

Safety policies and procedures vary with each health care institution. Guidelines for safety rules must be specific enough for users to be able to follow, but must be general enough to truly address the situation. The health care facility is held liable for following its own safety policies and procedures. The standard of care for laser use in the health care arena must be realized and acknowledged so that appropriate guidelines can be instituted that are attainable and realistic for the facility.

LASER CLASSIFICATIONS

A laser is classified as a medical device and falls under the jurisdiction of medical device regulations as published in the *Federal Register,* Volume 40, Part II, July 30, 1975. During 1976, the FDA mandated a definition of medical devices and their development processes. This law further classified medical devices into three groups, according to the difficulty in guaranteeing their safety. The laser has been designated as a Class III medical device. Further subclassifications by federal regulations and ANSI divide lasers into four more classifications (U. S. Department of Health and Human Services, 1988).

Class I Lasers

Class I lasers include the self-contained (enclosed) systems (such as those used in laboratories for diagnostic work) that do not inflict harm under normal circumstances. These lasers do not require hazard-warning labeling because the laser output is at or below the acceptable emission limits.

Class II Lasers

Class II lasers are low-powered devices that emit visible laser light (for example, the helium-neon laser). The normal aversion reflex, such as blinking or turning the head, provides adequate protection against Class II lasers. These lasers are safe for momentary viewing, but constant, deliberate viewing without eye protection could cause degenerative eye changes, especially if the aversion reflex is absent. A sedated patient may have a compromised aversion response and should be protected against a laser port that may emit a helium-neon aiming beam.

Class III Lasers

Class III lasers require special training to operate and have the potential to cause injury if viewed directly or if specularly reflected. Some ophthalmology Nd:YAG lasers are listed as Class III lasers.

Class IV Lasers

Most lasers used in medicine and surgery are Class IV lasers (CO_2, argon, continuous wave, Nd:YAG). These lasers are potentially hazardous and could cause fire, skin burns, and optical damage from either direct or scattered radiation. Specific safety measures must be employed to prevent injury from Class IV lasers.

LASER COMMITTEE

The first action of a health care facility becoming involved with laser technology should be to develop a laser committee. This group is essential, basic, and absolutely vital in monitoring and ensuring laser safety. The laser committee can begin as an adhoc committee of the surgical committee, but as more laser units are procured, a separate laser committee should be formed. The laser committee consists of individuals dedicated to the growth of the laser program. Such members could include but are not limited to the following:

Hospital administration representative
Laser safety officer
Laser team members

Operating room director

Hospital risk manager

Physician representative from each specialty area (neurosurgery, ophthalmology, otorhinolaryngology, general surgery, urology, gynecology, internal medicine, cardiology and peripheral vascular, pulmonary, colorectal, oncology, orthopedics, podiatry, etc)

Physician representatives from each ancillary area (radiology, pathology, etc)

Other areas that may send a representative to the laser committee meeting could include the following:

Library services (to develop a laser resource center)

Accounting (to coordinate patient charges, reimbursement, and equipment/supply costs)

Computer information services department (to access computer programs to help with tracking statistics and credentialing)

Training and education department (to help develop laser training programs)

Development foundation department (to help generate donation funds to benefit the laser program)

Marketing and public relations (to develop marketing plans for the laser program)

Many other health care professionals could be added to the list of laser committee members because this technology affects many areas within the hospital's complex environment. The laser committee meetings should be open because a laser program affects many of the other hospital departments. Usually a laser committee meets at least once per quarter or, ideally, once per month.

The laser committee usually is chaired by a physician if it is an official medical staff committee. Other chairpersons may be the laser safety officer or the laser program director. The chairperson is responsible for presiding over meetings, developing the agenda, and making sure that pertinent issues are addressed in a timely manner.

The laser committee is responsible for ensuring that the laser is used appropriately and safely. The committee develops policies and procedures for safe laser use and functions as the ultimate advisor for enforcement. For example, physician-credentialing protocols must be developed and monitored by the laser committee. ANSI standard Z136.3 offers basic guidelines for physician credentialing. The structure and responsibilities of the laser committee are discussed in detail in Chapter 13.

LASER SAFETY OFFICER AND LASER TEAM MEMBERS

ANSI Z136.3 guideline recommends that health care facilities designate a laser safety officer (LSO) to direct laser safety practices. The LSO has the tremendous responsibility and authority of ensuring that up-to-date safety parameters are being followed and are in compliance with policies, standards, and regulations. The LSO investigates laser accidents immediately and prepares necessary reports to notify the laser committee. The LSO oversees and coordinates laser safety through laser team members. This individual has the ultimate authority and responsibility to enforce safety within the laser program.

The LSO monitors the safety practices employed by the laser team members and communicates any changes needed. Since the laser team is usually the ultimate resource in providing a safe laser environment, most facilities give the laser team the authority to shut down a laser if the institution's written safety standards are not being followed. To provide continuity in the execution of laser safety measures, the laser committee then stands behind this action of the laser team.

Some of the expanded responsibilities that the LSO may authorize the laser team member to fulfill are listed:

- Set up and test-fire the laser system
- Operate the laser control panel
- Place the laser on standby when it is not actually being used to prevent accidental and uncontrolled laser firing
- Perform preventive maintenance and minor troubleshooting on the laser
- Monitor and enforce laser safety according to written policies and procedures
- Participate in quality management activities
- Report to the LSO any infractions of the written policies
- Document the laser procedure, laser charges, and laser service
- Inventory and maintain laser supplies and accessories
- Attend laser committee meetings when requested
- Assist with patient education
- Help monitor physician credentialing
- Stay abreast of laser technology by attending continuing education conferences or reading laser publications
- Actively assist with laser system evaluations when a new laser is needed
- Act as the laser resource person for the surgical team
- Make suggestions to enhance the laser program
- Assist with a laser marketing program to increase visibility and utilization

All laser team members should participate in a hands-on training program and must completely understand the operation of each laser they are expected to operate. ANSI standard Z136.3 offers suggestions on credentialing and education of the LSO and laser team members. Training and education are discussed in more detail in Part III.

The laser team members must also remain current in laser technology so that advances in new procedures and laser systems can be addressed and handled appropriately. The team members also become the resource persons for laser information for the rest of the surgical and nursing staff. A well-educated and skilled team helps decrease the fear of laser technology and fosters a positive attitude toward the laser program.

Open verbal communication is imperative between the physician and the laser team members during the laser procedure. Each should be acutely aware at all times of the laser power, mode, and status (i.e., standby or ready). Miscommunication can easily result in misunderstanding and laser accidents that could compromise patient and surgical team safety.

Laser safety is each laser team member's responsibility when assisting with laser procedures. Learning about laser safety should begin with a comprehensive review of the ANSI guidelines. The laser team can visit different facilities to learn how others promote laser safety. Manufacturer's safety recommendations should also be reviewed for detailed information pertinent to a specific laser. The policies and recommended practices of recognized groups and professional organizations, such as ANSI, AORN, and ASLMS, should be referenced when safety policies are drafted for a facility. As all of these external resources are analyzed, specific needs must be determined so that a safety policy can

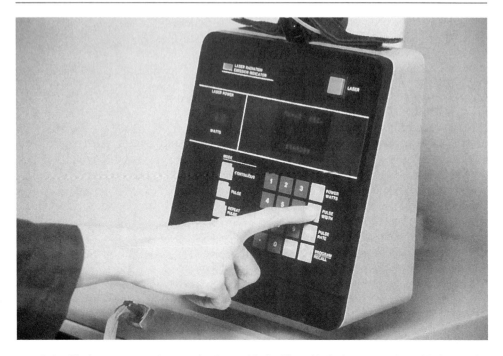

FIG. 3-1   The laser team member must be thoroughly familiar with the laser control panel before participating in the laser procedure.

be formed that will adequately address these needs. After safety policies are in place, then
they must be reviewed frequently for needed revision.

The laser team members should thoroughly understand the control panel of the laser
and must perform a safety check on the laser before each use to ensure proper functioning
(Figure 3-1). Some facilities include a laser safety checklist as a permanent part of the patient record. Other facilities merely note that a safety check was performed on the laser as
listed in the facility policy and procedure manual.

Different safety checks may be performed on different laser systems. A CO_2 laser
should be evaluated for proper alignment to ensure that the aiming beam coincides with
the site the CO_2 laser beam strikes. Reusable argon and Nd:YAG fibers must be calibrated
to note the amount of energy entering the fiber compared with the amount exiting. The
ready and standby features must be tested for proper operation. During the testing
process, the laser team member must make sure that everyone in the room wears the
proper eye protection. The physician is responsible for being aware of the status of the
laser before it is used clinically. A sample laser safety checklist for the CO_2 laser is provided on page 65.

EYE SAFETY

Enforcing eye safety measures is critically important during laser procedures. Since
the eye is extremely sensitive to laser radiation, maximum care must be taken to provide
optimum protection. Relatively low levels of laser radiation can cause permanent eye

---

Sample Laser Safety Checklist for CO_2 Laser

1. Move laser into the room, making sure to protect the articulated arm from bumping into walls or overhead lights. Make sure the appropriate smoke evacuation system is available for use.
2. Hang laser warning signs at all entrances to the room.
3. Place CO_2 glasses or goggles at each entrance to the room.
4. Plug laser into wall outlet.
5. If free-flowing CO_2 laser:
   Open valves on the laser gas tank and the purge tank. Note how much gas is in each tank. Replace tank if gas contents are low.
   If sealed CO_2 tube:
   Open valve on purge tank unless laser is equipped with air compressor. (Some lasers may not have a purge tank or compressor.)
6. Attach articulated arm to appropriate lens or coupler that will be connected to a handpiece, waveguide, CO_2 laparoscope, or microscope.
7. Put key in slot and turn key to "on" position. Dial in access code if needed.
8. Test control panel by adjusting knobs or pushing buttons to desired settings.
9. Make sure everyone in the room is wearing the appropriate eye protection. Test-fire the laser on a wet tongue blade to note alignment and proper operation using approximately 10 W of power.
10. Place laser in the standby mode.
11. Drape the articulated arm or microscope if needed.
12. Position laser near the patient after draping is complete.
13. Position laser foot pedal in a convenient location for the operating physician.
14. Ensure that everyone, including the patient, has appropriate eye safety.
15. Constantly monitor that all laser safety policies and procedures are being followed.
16. Activate laser at the physician's verbal request. Make sure that the laser plume is being evacuated properly. Place laser in the standby mode when the physician is not actively using the laser.
17. When the physician is finished with the laser, turn the laser off. The laser may be removed when the procedure is complete.
18. The laser team member must document the laser use on the patient's permanent record. A laser log or the surgical intraoperative notes may be used for this documentation.
19. The laser and laser parts must be cleaned, disinfected, or sterilized according to the manufacturer's instructions and stored appropriately.
20. The laser warning signs are removed and stored.
21. The CO_2 glasses and goggles are cleaned in a germicidal solution, dried, and stored.

---

damage. The ophthalmological hazards to the eye depend on the wavelength of the laser and the tissue absorption of this energy.

Eye protection requires the understanding of two terms: *maximum permissible exposure* (MPE) and *nominal hazard zone* (NHZ). ANSI Z136.3 standard (ANSI, 1988) defines these terms as follows:

The MPE is the level of laser radiation to which a person may be exposed without hazardous effects or adverse biological changes in the eye or skin. MPE levels are determined as a function of laser wavelength, exposure time, and pulse repetition.

The NHZ is the space in which the level of the direct, reflected, or scattered radiation during normal laser operation exceeds the maximum permissible exposure. Exposure levels beyond the boundary of the NHZ are below the appropriate MPE level. The NHZ is the boundary line for the maximum permissible exposure of laser energy.

The principal use of the NHZ criterion is to define the region near the laser operation within which control measures are required. Anyone inside the NHZ must wear appropriate eye protection because the MPE level is exceeded. The NHZ outlines the perimeter of the MPE area of laser energy. Persons outside the NHZ would be exposed to laser energy below the MPE level and are considered in the safe territory.

The NHZ can be calculated using a laser range equation that considers such factors as the laser wavelength, beam divergence, laser power, beam size at the aperture and/or lens, lens focal length, and range from the laser to the target. Diffuse reflection and scattering are also taken into account when determining the NHZ of the beam. Charts have been developed that list the calculated NHZ for specific lasers. ANSI Z136.3 standard has NHZ reference tables for selected surgical lasers.

The NHZs vary for laser wavelengths that are delivered through fibers. Figure 3-2 describes these differences.

Since the laser power, spot size, and other parameters may be changed during a procedure, continual calculations to determine the NHZ would have to be done throughout the surgery. To simplify this situation for surgical environments, the NHZ is considered to be within the surgery room. Therefore, NHZ calculations are not needed because appropriate eye protection is required for entering any surgery room in which the laser is being used. This concept is being challenged by those who feel that determining the NHZ eliminates unnecessary use of protective eyewear.

Biomedical technicians may want to calculate the NHZ when providing laser service since the protective housing of the laser is removed, and thus optical hazards are in-

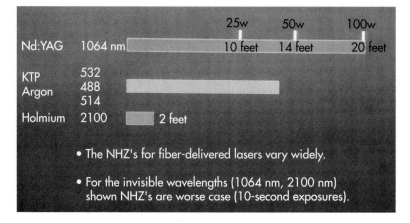

FIG. 3-2   Nominal hazard zones of lasers delivered via fibers. (Courtesy Coherent, Inc., Palo Alto, CA.)

creased. Eye protection should always be used when one is servicing a laser or providing preventive maintenance if the laser is to be activated.

Eye Injuries

At 10,600 nm, CO_2 laser light is readily absorbed by the surface tissue of the eye and can easily result in corneal or scleral damage (Figure 3-3). The holmium laser beam at 2100 nm also can cause this type of eye injury. Eye protection with lenses that filter these specific wavelengths is needed. Side shields are highly recommended for the persons near the laser-tissue impact area to guard against corneal injury from the side (Figure 3-4). Persons who are farther away from these beams are usually out of the CO_2 NHZ and are not required to wear side shields. Prescription glasses are usually not recommended as appropriate protection because the glass or plastic lens material may not absorb the beam adequately, and transmission to the eye could occur. Contact lenses are not sufficient eye protection because the sclera is left unprotected.

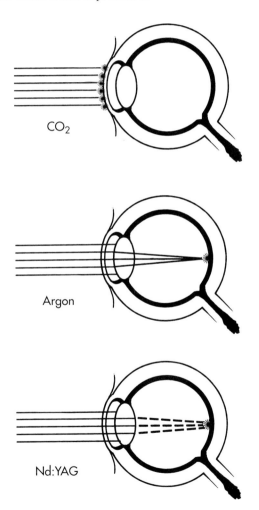

FIG. 3-3 The CO_2 laser can cause corneal damage; the argon and Nd:YAG lasers can cause retinal damage.

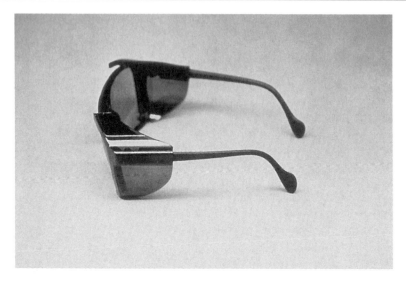

FIG. 3-4   Side shields prevent the laser beam from impacting the eye from the side.

Because argon (488 and 515 nm) and Nd:YAG (1064 nm) laser light is transmitted through clear fluids or structures, the beams can easily pass through the cornea and be focused by the lens onto the retina. This focusing action increases the beam's power density tremendously and thus can easily injure retinal tissue. Therefore, protective eyewear must be in place before one enters a room in which these lasers are being activated (Figure 3-3).

Retinal damage can result from an acute incident or from slow degeneration caused by chronic low-power exposures to the beam. Both types of damage may go unnoticed. A direct accident (exposure) can damage a small area of the retina and can result in a scotoma (blind spot in the field of vision). Continual low-power exposure can promote cataract formation in the lens of the eye and can also damage the retina. Retinal cones, the structures that detect color, are usually the first to be affected. Difficulty in distinguishing between blue and green can indicate early retinal cone damage.

Eye Protection

Providing eye protection requires an understanding of laser wavelengths and laser-tissue interaction. Every laser facility must formulate policies and procedures that appropriately address the eye protection needed when using the lasers. A sample of eye protection policy is provided on page 69.

Recommendations suggest that protective goggles, glasses, and lens covers should have the appropriate filtering capabilities, and optical density should be specifically noted on the eyewear (Figure 3-5). For example, a pair of Nd:YAG glasses may be inscribed with, "for use with 1064 nm, 5 OD." The optical density of the lens is the ability of the material to absorb a specific wavelength; it is expressed in mathematical terms. A higher optical density does not necessarily mean better eye protection. Some lenses with higher optical densities are darker and can decrease visibility, making it difficult to see the laser

Sample Safety Policy and Procedure:
Eye Protection During Laser Procedures

Purpose:

To provide eye safety and protection for laser team members and patients during laser procedures.

General Statement:

By definition, a Class IV laser can cause eye injury either by direct contact with the beam or by reflection of the beam off a reflective surface.

Procedure:

1. During laser procedures performed under general anesthesia or regional anesthesia, the patient's eyes will be protected with moistened gauze pads or appropriate laser protective eyewear (glasses or goggles).
2. During local anesthesia procedures, the patient's eyes will be protected by moistened pads, towels, special laser eye shields, or appropriate protective eyewear (glasses or goggles).
3. ALL persons (including visitors) within the laser treatment area must wear appropriate eye protection during the laser procedure.
4. Different laser wavelengths require different eyewear. Nd:YAG or argon protective eyewear should have an optical density of at least 4.0.
5. For CO_2 procedures:
   a. Side shields are recommended for anyone near the laser-tissue interaction site.
   b. Prescription glasses are NOT considered appropriate eye protection because the lens material may not stop the transmission of the laser beam.
   c. Half-glasses and contact lenses are NOT considered appropriate eye protection because the sclera is left exposed.
6. Protective eyewear (glasses or goggles) must be regularly inspected by the laser team members. Any scratched surface will allow the laser beam to be transmitted, and the wearer's eye could be harmed.
7. When using the laser through a microscope or endoscope, ALL persons in the laser treatment room or operating room must use appropriate eye protection.
8. Warning signs stating that eye protection is needed must be placed on all access doors to the laser treatment room or surgical room where a laser procedure is in progress. Appropriate protective eyewear should be available at the entry door(s).
9. Windows must be covered appropriately, depending upon the wavelength of the laser used.
10. To prevent reflection of the laser beam, special precautions must be followed. Instruments that are not dulled or ebonized should be covered with wet towels or sponges to decrease reflection.

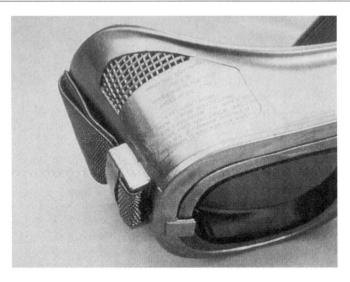

FIG. 3-5   The wavelength and optical density should be inscribed on the lens or elsewhere on the protective eyewear.

control panel readings or observe the patient's color. Lighter shades of protective lenses with adequate optical densities are being developed as technology advances.

Choosing the appropriate lens material involves issues of comfort and efficiency. Plastic lenses tend to be lighter weight, but glass lenses are more likely to withstand a direct laser beam impact (*Clinical Laser Monthly,* July 1992).

One would think that the ideal laser protective eyewear would protect the wearer from all wavelengths since more than one laser may be used during a procedure. In reality, this type of eyewear would be extremely difficult to see through because the lenses would be filtering a range of different wavelengths. Therefore, eyewear that filters out only one or two wavelengths is needed so that other colors and wavelengths can be seen.

Protective eyewear can be expensive, so proper care and handling is mandatory (Figure 3-6). Protocols should be developed to designate responsibility for distributing, collecting, and maintaining the laser eyewear. Glasses and goggles should be inspected periodically to detect scratching, cracking, or other damage. Protective eyewear can be stored in lengths of stockinette or in their original packing containers for protection (Figure 3-7).

Some lasers used in microscopic surgery have an automatic shutter with a filter that connects to the microscope head. When the laser is activated, the shutter allows a protective eye filter to be positioned in the line of sight to shield the physician's eyes from any scattering of the beam. Some microscope configurations allow the filter to be placed above the observer optics. This setup allows protection for the main viewer but possible eye injury to the observer. Persons viewing the surgery through unprotected optics must use protective eyewear. Care must be taken to set the filter below all sets of optics on the microscope for proper protection for everyone viewing through the equipment.

Lens eye filters are available that can be placed over the top of a rigid or flexible endoscope viewing port to protect the physician's eye from laser backscatter (Figure 3-8). The eye filter must be appropriate for the wavelength of laser being used. The physician must

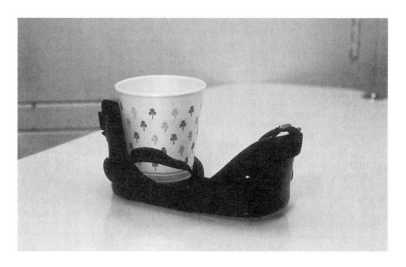

FIG. 3-6   A pair of argon goggles is being damaged from misuse.

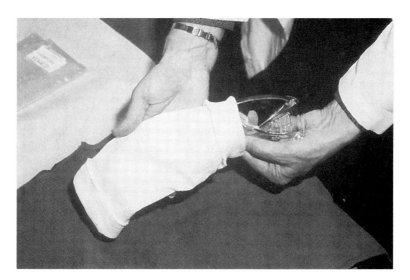

FIG. 3-7   Protective glasses can be stored in lengths of stockinette to keep the lenses from getting scratched.

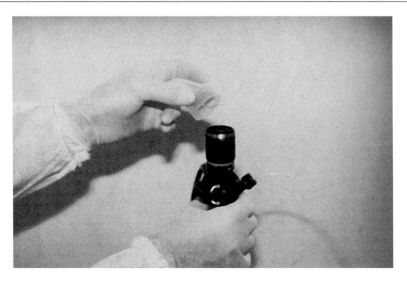

FIG. 3-8   A special laser lens can be placed over the eyepiece of a laparoscope.

understand that the other eye is not protected and that neither eye will be protected if the energy escapes from the fiber at any area other than the tip.

The use of an eye filter does not preclude the need for protective eyewear for the rest of the operating room team. Some have asked if the team really needs eye protection if the laser energy is being released inside an organ, such as during laparoscopic or other endoscopic procedures. A break in the fiberoptic cable, sudden accidental dislodging of the fiber, or inadvertent disconnection of the CO_2 coupler during laser activation can easily cause ocular damage to unprotected eyes. The Laser Committee must decide on the risks involved and determine whether eye protection should be required during these procedures. Many Laser Committees prefer to have consistency within the program and require protective eyewear for all laser procedures.

Whether physicians should be required to wear eye protection during laser procedures, especially during laparoscopies, continues to be debated in the surgical arena. Some hospitals require noncompliant physicians to sign eyewear refusal waiver forms releasing the hospital from liability if they incur an eye injury. Some attorneys disagree with this practice, stating that the waiver forms are not the appropriate response to this issue of noncompliant physicians and that the waiver form could be used against the hospital in court.

Opponents of using waiver forms state that a signed waiver is evidence that the hospital realizes a problem exists and that nothing is being done to prevent potential injury to the physician. Hospitals should make sure that physicians follow all hospital rules and regulations as a condition of maintaining hospital privileges. If an accident occurred and the physician sustained eye damage, he or she could sue the facility, claiming that safety practices were inadequate (*Clinical Laser Monthly,* February 1993).

Other attorneys state that a signed waiver form indicates that a physician is well-informed of the laser hazard and chooses to not wear eye protection. Some physicians state that their vision is compromised by eyewear and that this in turn leads to safety concerns for the patient. Physicians choose the risk of possibly sustaining an eye injury over making a wrong cut or vaporizing the wrong tissue when the surgical site cannot be easily seen.

Often the laser team members are caught in the middle of this argument between the hospital and the nonhospital employees (the physicians). Hospitals must address this dilemma directly and develop policies accordingly. Laser safety should always be the top priority rather than something considered for the sake of convenience. When one takes a stance on this issue, the best resource is the hospital risk manager, who can assist the Laser Committee in making a final decision.

Patient Eye Protection

The patient's eyes must always be protected from laser energy. If the patient is awake, appropriate goggles or glasses must be worn (Figure 3-9). Complete preoperative education provides the patient with the rationale for eye protection during the laser intervention. If the patient is under general anesthesia, eye pads can be gently taped over the patient's closed eyes (Figure 3-10). A wet towel or a laser-retardant drape should cover the eye pads if the laser is to be used in the immediate vicinity of the face. Manufacturers have developed special eye protection pads that are covered by a reflective surface that deflects stray laser beams. This eye protection adheres to the patient's face and is easily removed after the procedure is completed.

Whenever laser energy is used in the immediate vicinity of the eye, such as to lighten a port-wine stain on the eyelid, a metal eye shield can be positioned to protect the eye. A drop of an ophthalmological local anesthetic is instilled before the eye shield is carefully placed on the surface of the eye. If these metal shields are sterilized in the autoclave, they must be completely cooled before being placed on the surface of the eye.

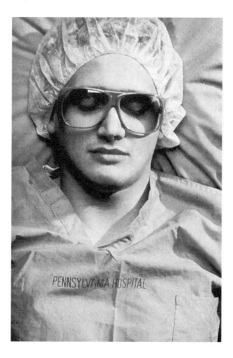

FIG. 3-9   Protective glasses are worn by a patient during a local anesthesia laser procedure.

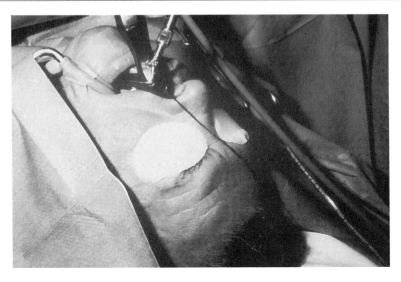

FIG. 3-10   The patient's eyes are protected with moistened gauze pads during a laser procedure.

Baseline Eye Examination

To document the laser team's ocular health, a baseline eye examination can be performed on those health care professionals who routinely work with laser systems. Another eye examination should be performed after any ophthalmological accident and also upon termination of employment. Noting and documenting the health of an employee's retina decreases the chance of future litigation that would hold the facility responsible for ocular injury during employment. Performing routine eye examinations has nothing to do with guaranteeing safety but can be used for medical/legal purposes if an employee decides to sue a hospital for not supplying appropriate eye protection.

Baseline eye examinations usually include documentation of the employee's ocular history, visual acuity, macular function, contrast sensitivity, and retinal condition. The reason for conducting this eye screen is to provide baseline information on visual performance and condition, for making comparisons that will indicate whether any ophthalmological injury occurred and to document ocular health upon termination. Each health care facility must formulate its own protocol regarding ophthalmological medical surveillance. Samples of a medical surveillance eye examination policy and form are provided on pages 75 and 76.

Many laser team members and physicians are challenging this need for eye examinations, and many issues are involved. Who should have eye examinations—only the laser team members or everyone who participates in the laser procedure? What is the cost of performing these examinations? Does this cost justify the reason for conducting the eye examinations? Who monitors the system to ensure that everyone has had a baseline eye examination and anyone terminating has had another eye examination? How extensive should the examination be? Should annual examinations also be performed? How are employees handled who refuse the eye examination? These are just a few of the questions that have been posed concerning required eye examinations. The main point is that these examinations are performed to ensure that no eye damage (especially retinal damage) has occurred during laser procedures. This protects the facility from potential litigation at a

Sample Safety Policy and Procedure:
Eye Examinations for Medical Surveillance

Purpose:
1. To establish a baseline against which ocular damage can be measured in the event of an injury.
2. To provide documentation of ocular health for legal purposes.

Procedure:
1. Laser team members will have the following ocular examination upon hiring and upon termination:
   a. Ocular history
   b. Visual acuity test
   c. Central vision field examination
   d. Contrast sensitivity test
   e. Fundoscopic examination
   Laser team members include the clinical laser nurse, laser safety technicians, and biomedical laser technician.
2. Other personnel actively involved in the laser procedure will have the following ocular examination upon hiring and upon termination:
   a. Ocular history
   b. Visual acuity test
   c. Central vision field examination
   d. Contrast sensitivity test
   If any abnormalities are noted, then further fundoscopic examination is necessary. Other personnel include the secretary, operating room director, OR staff nurses, OR technicians, and orderlies.
3. Any person involved in a laser ocular accident will have a complete ophthalmological examination, including a fundoscopic examination.
4. All reports of the ocular examinations will be kept in the employee's health file.
5. All physicians or student physicians will assume their own responsibility for ocular health.

future date. This policy does not ensure eye safety during laser procedures. A facility must explore the rationale of incorporating eye examinations into the laser program to provide sound and logical justification for this expense.

Some facilities perform eye examinations only after potential eye damage has occurred. Other facilities perform baseline eye examinations only on the biomedical engineers or technicians who are at increased risk for eye damage when they remove the protective housing from the laser for servicing. Some facilities continue to involve all surgical employees in the eye examination policy, while others do not conduct examinations at all. Each facility should determine the rationale for performing eye examinations before developing a policy. If a policy is then formed to conduct eye examinations, it must be followed as written and not only as convenience and scheduling permits.

Sample Eye Examination Form for Medical Surveillance

Baseline_____   Incident _____   Termination _____

Name _____ Clock Number_____

Department_____ Position _____

Date _____

  I. Ocular history

  II. Visual acuity

  III. Physical examination (including central vision field & contrast sensitivity examination)

  IV. Fundoscopic examination (if required or recommended)

  V. Comments

Physician signature_____

CONTROLLED TREATMENT AREA

The area where the laser is to be used must be controlled by the laser team members. Access to the room should be granted only to those individuals who have been appropriately educated in laser safety.

Laser warning signs must be placed at all entrances to the laser treatment area. ANSI standard Z136.3 recommends that the laser warning sign be consistent with suggested regulations (Figure 3-11). For example, a Class IV laser sign should illustrate the laser hazard symbol, which is a sunburst pattern consisting of two sets of radial spokes of different lengths and one long spoke radiating from a common center. "Danger" should be written at the top of the sign with "Laser Radiation—Avoid eye or skin exposure to direct or scattered radiation." Often the appropriate glasses or goggles are located near the sign for persons who need to enter the secured area while the laser is being activated.

Laser signs should always be removed when the laser procedure is completed. Laser signs may also be removed when the laser segment of the procedure is completed and the rest of the surgery continues. Some laser signs have been designed to be turned around

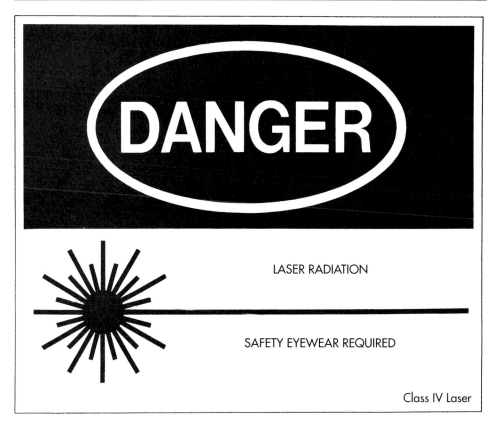

DANGER

LASER RADIATION

SAFETY EYEWEAR REQUIRED

Class IV Laser

FIG. 3-11   Warning signs notify personnel that a laser is being used and appropriate eye protection is needed before entering the room.

when the laser is not being used so that those entering the room realize that the laser is not being used and eye protection is not needed.

Windows or ports into the laser treatment area should be covered from the inside of the room with a blocking barrier that stops transmission of the beam. Blockage is needed only to protect from those laser wavelengths that can penetrate the window (i.e., argon, Nd:YAG). Many times, easy-to-clean, pull-down window blinds are installed (Figure 3-12). Windows that are positioned extremely high in the surgery room may not need to be covered since no one would be directly on the other side who could be harmed.

ANSI standards note that door interlocks may be used during laser procedures. A door interlock does not allow the laser to be activated or shuts down the laser when the surgical or treatment room door is opened. Door interlocks may provide safety for the surgical team but can compromise patient safety. For example, a physician may be coagulating a bleeding vessel when the door is opened. With a door interlock system, the laser would be automatically discontinued, thus compromising patient care. Therefore, during laser surgery door interlocks are not needed because the laser team member makes certain that only authorized persons are in the room, that protective eye wear is immediately available upon entry, and that safety precautions are being followed.

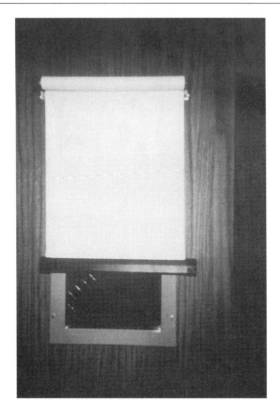

FIG. 3-12   Windows can be covered with a light-blocking shade inside the laser treatment room.

The laser key should be available only to authorized personnel and must not be left in the laser during storage. Some facilities store the key in the narcotics box; others may have a secured box designated especially for laser keys. A sample key storage policy is provided on page 79.

FIRE SAFETY

Fire prevention is critical during laser surgery. Awareness of laser biophysics is valuable in understanding the laser-tissue interaction and the problems that could occur. A fire can be started by a reflected beam as readily as by a direct beam impact. An inadvertent impact from a stray laser beam can ignite flammable material. Control of the laser beam results from the constant efforts of the physician and laser team members. Even though a fire during a laser procedure is an uncommon occurrence, health care professionals must be prepared to react quickly to contain a fire should one start. Immediate action will minimize injury to the patient and the surgical team. A sample fire safety policy is provided on page 80.

Portable fire extinguishers should be mounted in convenient locations for emergency use on the laser if it catches on fire. Personnel should be properly trained to respond to a fire by disconnecting the electrical equipment from the power source and by using a fire extinguisher to put out the fire.

Sample Safety Policy and Procedure:
Key Storage for Laser Units

Purpose:

To provide controlled access to laser keys.

General Statement:

The laser key will not be left in the laser unit when the laser is not in use.

Procedure:

1. Laser keys will be stored in a special security key box in the laser center for the lasers in the outpatient, local anesthesia facility.
2. Laser keys will be stored in the narcotics box for lasers in the operating room areas.
3. Laser keys will not be given to or used by any unqualified personnel.
4. Lasers will NOT be operated unless a qualified laser safety officer is present to operate the laser.

Halon Fire Extinguisher

A halon fire extinguisher consisting of hydrogenated halocarbons is recommended for laser unit fires because it does not produce a residue and has low toxicity. This extinguisher disrupts combustion by interrupting the flaming process (*Clinical Laser Monthly,* February 1993). Halon fire extinguishers are known to be an environmental concern because the halon disrupts the ozone layer of the earth's atmosphere. Chemical companies are in the process of developing an acceptable substitute for the halon extinguisher.

A dry chemical fire extinguisher, on the other hand, is not appropriate when a laser is on fire because it emits a fine dust that could damage the optics or circuitry of a laser. A CO_2 fire extinguisher is usually not employed because its pressurized contents are extremely cold when discharged and can cause cryogenic tissue damage to the patient. The residue will also coat the inside parts of the laser and can cause tube fracture and other component damage. Pressurized water cannot be sprayed directly onto a laser system because of the high-voltage electrical current flowing through the unit. The water can provide a path for this electrical energy and thus lead to potential injury or death of anyone also in contact with the water.

If surgical drapes or other flammable items are burning, water or saline is usually available in the surgical or treatment room to douse a small fire. A halon fire extinguisher should not be used on flaming drapes. Water or saline can be used to keep sponges or towels wet during the procedure to prevent them from igniting.

Dry combustibles should never be placed in the immediate vicinity of the laser target area. Sponges or towels should be wet so that ignition cannot occur (Figure 3-13). The scrub nurse or assistant should constantly evaluate the moisture level of the sponges to prevent drying that could eventually support a fire.

Sample Safety Policy and Procedure:
Fire Safety During Laser Surgery

Purpose:

To provide guidelines that will reduce the hazard of a laser-induced fire.

General Statement:

By definition, a Class IV laser presents a fire hazard either from its direct beam or from its reflection.

Procedure:

1. Cloth and some paper drapes are flammable. To decrease the chance of fire, wet draping materials can be used around areas that are close to the laser interaction site that could possibly be ignited by a direct or indirect laser beam impact. Special laser-retardant drapes and fabrics have been developed to withstand limited laser beam impact. Careful attention must be paid to the drape fabric limitations.
2. Saline or water must be readily available in case of a fire.
3. During laser procedures on the lower bowel, the rectum may be packed with a wet counted sponge to reduce the chance of lower bowel methane gas explosion or fire.
4. During laser procedures on the trachea, special fire protection precautions must be followed to decrease the chance of an endotracheal tube fire.
   a. A special laser endotracheal tube or wrap may be used. Any limitations of this special tube or wrap must be communicated by the anesthesiologist or nurse anesthetist to the surgeon and laser team member (i.e., wattage per spot-size limitations).
   b. A red rubber endotracheal tube can be circumferentially wrapped with a special foil reflective tape in an overlapping fashion starting at the cuff. Each new roll of tape should be laser test-fired to note its resistance to laser impact.
   c. The endotracheal tube and cuff are protected with wet radiopaque sponges against laser impact.
   d. Nonexplosive anesthetic gases must be used during laser procedures.
5. The chance of accidental reflection of the laser beam can be decreased by using proper technique and nonreflective instrumentation in smaller areas where reflection is potentially high.
6. Flammable prep solutions must not be used during laser procedures (e.g., alcohol-based prep solutions).
7. A halon fire extinguisher should be available in the surgery suite or the laser center in case of fire. The laser team members must understand the operation of the fire extinguisher and know where it is stored.

Surgical Drapes

Surgical drapes can be ignited by laser impact. Cloth and some paper drapes are extremely flammable. Water-repellent paper drapes sometimes withstand more laser impact before they melt or react to laser energy. Studies have shown that polypropylene drapes are the least flammable compared with polyester drapes containing wood pulp (*Clinical Laser Monthly,* November 1993). Today there are many types of laser-retardant drapes on the market. The fire retardancy ratings of each drape should be noted.

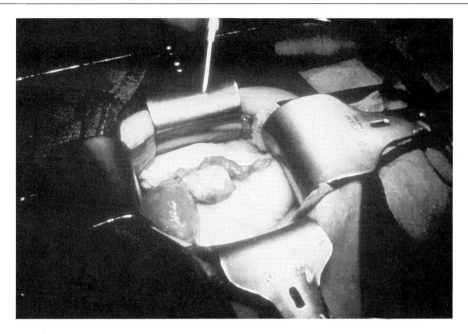

FIG. 3-13   Sponges near the laser-tissue impact site are kept wet throughout the procedure to minimize fire hazards.

Reflective drapes and coverings have been developed with a special surface that actually reflects the beam or causes the beam to scatter. These materials are used to cover anesthesia circuits and other highly flammable items near the laser impact site.

Laser surgery performed in the head and neck area can lead to surgical-drape fires if appropriate precautions are not taken. Around this area, the anesthesia nitrous oxide and oxygen concentrations can build up beneath the surgical drapes. This enriched environment can then help ignite materials that are usually not as flammable in normal room air concentrations. Nitrous oxide is a nonflammable anesthetic but can support combustion as readily as oxygen can. When laser energy is used through a bronchoscope or during a microlaryngoscopy, the oxygen concentration must be kept lower—between 21% and 30%—because it can become trapped beneath the drapes, creating a potential fire hazard (ANSI, 1988).

Flammable Materials

Flammable materials must not be used in the immediate vicinity of the laser-tissue impact site. Some skin preparation solutions are flammable, such as alcohol-based preps or acetone. During skin cleansing, an alcohol-based solution can pool under the patient, causing ethanol vapors to become trapped under the drapes. The volatility of these vapors increases the risk of surgical drape fires. Prep solutions should be pat-dried, because pooled fluids can retain the laser heat and subsequently burn the tissue. Dark-tinted prep solutions, such as iodine solution, should be rinsed off if the surgeon is incising the skin with a laser wavelength that is strongly absorbed by pigmentation.

Hair should be covered with wet sponges or towels to prevent ignition if close to the laser-tissue impact site. Facial hair is particularly vulnerable to bursting into flames because of its close proximity to anesthetic gases. Hair spray and styling gels or mousses also can increase the flammability of the hair and can easily ignite, causing an immediate flash fire. The patient should be instructed not to use hair spray or styling gels on the day of the procedure if the laser is to be used near the hairline.

During a microlaryngoscopy, a protector is placed over the teeth to guard against a stray laser beam pitting a tooth. The teeth protector should be able to withstand laser impact without causing a fire.

Other products that are flammable and can support combustion include oil-based lubricants, adhesive and plastic tapes, and plastic instruments. If flammability is in question, a product can be test-ignited in a controlled laboratory setting where an unexpected fire could easily be contained.

Methane Gas Explosion

A methane gas explosion potentially can occur from the presence of intestinal gas (flatus), which is composed mostly of methane and can be ignited when exposed to a laser beam. Laser surgery performed in the rectal area generally requires evacuation of the residual methane gas by gentle suctioning. Then the rectum may be packed with a counted saline-saturated radiopaque sponge. This will tamponade the area and decrease the chances of methane gas entering the surgical area. A cleansing bowel preparation (enema) is useful before rectal procedures to also minimize this hazard.

Airway Explosion

An airway explosion could occur during a microlaryngoscopy or an oral surgery involving an endotracheal (ET) tube. An unprotected polyvinyl chloride (PVC) ET tube must never be used during oral or laryngeal surgery because it can easily be ignited by a laser beam and will support combustion (Figure 3-14).

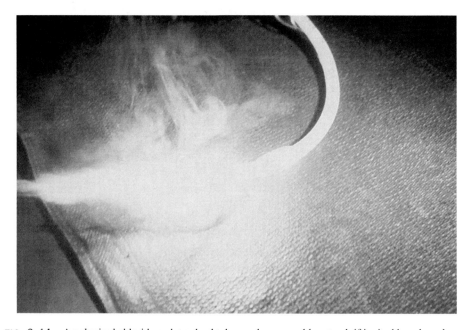

FIG. 3-14   A polyvinyl chloride endotracheal tube can become a blow torch if ignited by a laser beam.

Manufacturers have developed special ET tubes for laser use. These tubes are made out of materials that are not as flammable and will withstand limited laser impact. The manufacturer's instructions must be followed so that the amount of laser energy used does not exceed the recommendations. Special care must be taken to note these laser power limitations because the performance of the tube is not guaranteed for use with laser powers above the stated parameters.

A protective wrapping consisting of sponge-type material backed with corrugated silver foil is available to sheath a PVC or red rubber ET tube for protection (Figure 3-15). The tube wrap is then moistened and the hardened sponge material becomes soft, so trauma is not caused during intubation. This sponge material cannot be ignited by laser impact while it is wet, and the silver foil will not permit penetration of limited amounts of laser energy into the ET tube. Pledgets of the special sponge material are also moistened for placement around the ET tube to protect the tube's cuff from beam impact. Laboratory and clinical results have shown that this substance can withstand even very high laser powers at a variety of wavelengths.

If a special laser ET tube or wrap is not available, then a specially prepared red rubber ET tube may be used. This tube needs to be wrapped circumferentially with a foil or metal tape that will reflect a laser beam when inadvertently hit (Figure 3-16). Each new batch of tape should be test-fired at various settings to note the ability to withstand laser impact.

A flexible metal ET tube can be used to decrease airway combustion because the tube is not flammable. An external cuff can be attached manually to provide a sealed airway (Figure 3-17). Many physicians do not like to use these tubes because of the tracheal trauma that sometimes results during intubation.

When an ET tube is in place for a laser procedure, the cuff should be inflated with sterile saline. Often a drop of methylene blue is mixed with the saline to dye the solution

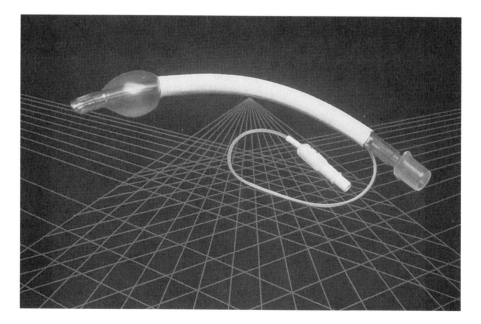

FIG. 3-15   A special wrap can be used to protect the endotracheal tube from laser beam penetration.

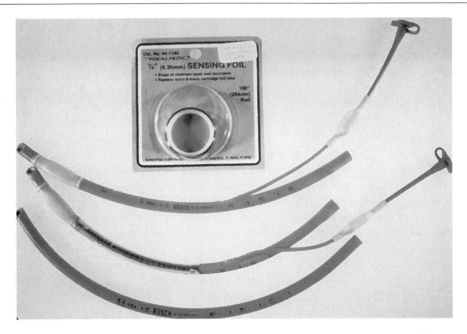

FIG. 3-16   Red rubber tubes can be wrapped with a foil tape to protect against laser beam impact.

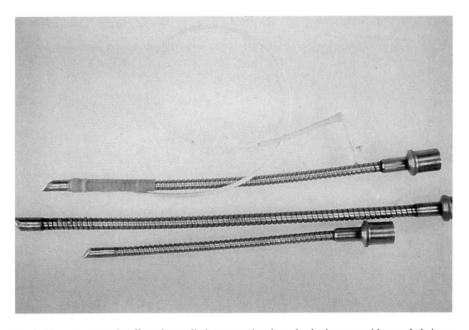

FIG. 3-17   An external cuff can be applied to a metal endotracheal tube to provide a sealed airway.

blue. Wet radiopaque cotton sponges are packed around the tube and cuff to provide a barrier against laser impact (Figure 3-18). If the cuff is inadvertently ruptured during the procedure, the presence of the blue solution on the sponges will alert the surgeon to the deflated cuff. The saline that escapes from the cuff absorbs the heat and decreases the chance of fire. A lengthy surgery may allow the sponges that are packed around the tube to become dry. The surgeon, assistant, or scrub nurse must make sure that the sponges are kept wet during the procedure to decrease the chance of ignition.

The laser team must constantly be prepared for an airway explosion or fire. If an ET-tube fire occurs, the following steps can be taken to minimize patient injury:

1. Remove the flaming ET tube and instruments. Stop the flow of oxygen by pinching the oxygen tube or shutting off the supply valve.
2. Reintubate immediately to prevent laryngospasm.
3. Inspect the mouth, oral cavity, and bronchial tree.

More detailed information is contained in the section on anesthesia precautions in Chapter 5.

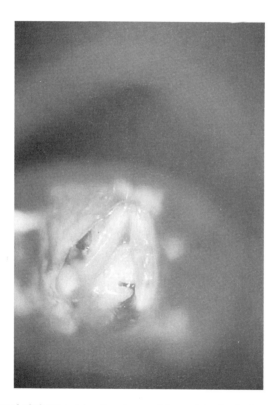

FIG. 3-18 Wet counted pledgets can be placed around the endotracheal tube to offer more protection against laser beam impact.

A study was conducted to determine which type of ET tube could be extubated the most quickly in an emergency. Results showed that red rubber tubes could be extubated faster than plastic tubes during model airway fires. If PVC tubes or other plastic tubes are used for laser surgery of the airway, then deflation of the saline-filled cuff is faster than cutting the pilot tube. However, unclamping the pilot tubes on red rubber ET tubes result in even quicker deflation because of their higher intercuff pressure (*Clinical Laser Monthly,* July 1993).

Jet ventilation may also be used during a laser microlaryngoscopy. A jet ventilator is a mechanical ventilation unit that delivers the anesthetic gases through a small metal needle used in conjunction with a rigid laryngoscope. Under pressurization, the jet ventilator is set to deliver a determined amount of anesthesia gas while the rate, pounds per square inch, and percent of inspiratory time are being set. The needle is positioned between the vocal cords on the side opposite the lesion. The needle extends into the trachea so that the proper amount of anesthesia gas can be delivered easily. After the surgery, the patient may be intubated to maintain an open airway if postoperative edema or tracheal spasm is anticipated (Meeker and Rothrock, 1995).

Nonreflective Instruments

Skin and eye injury can result from a reflected laser beam. Nonreflective instruments have been developed to decrease the chance of laser beam reflection when the instrument is used near the laser-tissue impact site. Also, instruments can be ebonized. Ebonization is the process of coating the instrument with a substance that decreases reflectivity, often producing a black surface. Many companies will ebonize existing instruments at a low cost. There is no need to ebonize an entire set of instruments; only those that will be used near the laser impact site need to be specially treated (Figure 3-19). These instruments should be inspected regularly to make sure that the integrity of the coating is not disrupted. Sometimes the instrument will need recoating after a period of time.

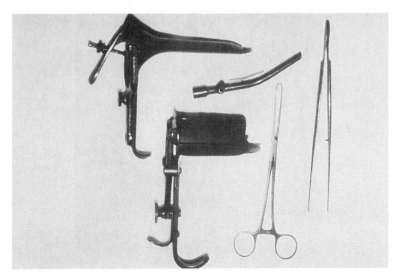

FIG. 3-19   Only the instruments that will be used near the laser-tissue impact site need to be ebonized to decrease reflection.

An instrument may also be anodized or have a matte finish to decrease the direct reflectivity of a laser beam. Often instruments used under the bright light of a microscope are anodized to decrease the direct reflection of the microscope light. Anodized instruments also scatter the light from a laser beam. Other coatings or surfaces have been introduced that cause a laser beam to scatter on impact thus not allowing the instrument to heat up from thermal absorption. A sample policy for proper use of instruments during laser surgery is provided below.

A study was conducted to determine which type of instrument coating or surface provided the best nonreflective surface. During the testing a series of 29 flat stainless-steel plates were treated with different surface finishes. The reflectance values were then mea-

---

Sample Safety Policy and Procedure: Proper Use of Instruments During Laser Procedures

Purpose:

To ensure proper use of instruments to decrease the chance of a laser-induced fire or inadvertent eye or tissue damage from direct or reflected laser-beam impact.

General Statement:

By definition, a Class IV laser presents a hazard either from its direct beam or from its reflection off a shiny surface.

Procedure:

1. Instruments can be ebonized or anodized (dulled) to decrease the risk of fire injury. Laser instruments should not be etched because the coating or surface will be disrupted, which may allow reflection.
2. Instruments (such as large retractors) may be covered with wet towels or sponges to decrease the chance of laser reflection.
3. Stainless steel mirrors used to purposely reflect the laser beam must be inspected regularly for cracks or damage that would decrease the reflective accuracy.
4. Glass rods should NOT be used during laser surgical intervention because of the shattering that can occur from the laser energy absorption and heat buildup. Metal rods should not be used because of the heat absorption and retention that could cause adjacent tissue damage. Teflon rods should not be used since they can melt and produce a toxic plume when struck by the laser beam.
5. Pyrex, quartz, or titanium rods can withstand laser impact and thus decrease the chance of laser reflection or damage to the rod material. Clear pyrex or quartz rods will allow transmission of the argon and Nd:YAG beams.
6. Proper endotracheal tube preparation should be performed to reduce the risk of endotracheal tube fires. A special laser endotracheal tube can be used that will withstand limited amounts of laser impact.
7. Plastic vaginal and rectal speculae should not be used as they usually burn or melt when struck by the laser beam. Test the laser impact on the material if there is any question as to the durability and flammability of the instrument when it is used near the laser-tissue impact site.

sured using CO_2, argon, and Nd:YAG laser beams. The results indicated that the best treatment to minimize reflection was a roughened, black surface finish with a fluoropolymer material (Wood, Sliney, and Basye, 1992).

OTHER SAFETY MEASURES

Backstops

Backstops have been developed that stop the laser beam from striking normal tissue. Titanium and quartz rods are effective backstops for the CO_2 laser and can be reprocessed easily. The argon and Nd:YAG wavelengths can be transmitted through clear rods, therefore titanium rods are preferred for use as backstops.

Mirrors

Mirrors may be used during laser surgery to actually reflect the beam to a hard-to-reach area, such as the undersurface of an ovary (Figure 3-20). Mirrors may be made of rhodium or stainless steel. Glass-surfaced mirrors are inappropriate because they will shatter as they absorb heat from the laser energy. The important point in using a mirror during laser surgery is to aim the beam at the image in the mirror and not at the mirror surface. This technique can be practiced in the laboratory setting.

Endoscope Precautions

Endoscope precautions are required when a fiber is used to deliver the laser energy through an endoscope. The end of the fiber must extend past the end of the endoscope at least 1 cm to decrease the chance of damage to the end of the scope (Figure 3-21). If the

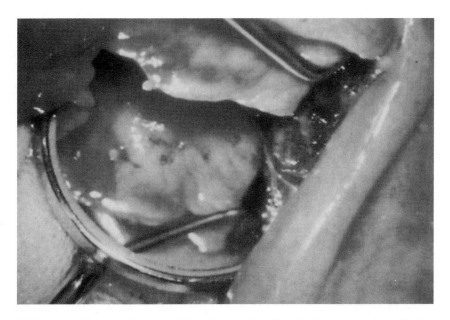

FIG. 3-20   A special laser mirror is positioned to directly reflect the laser beam onto a hard-to-reach area. (Courtesy of Grant Laser Center, Columbus, Ohio.)

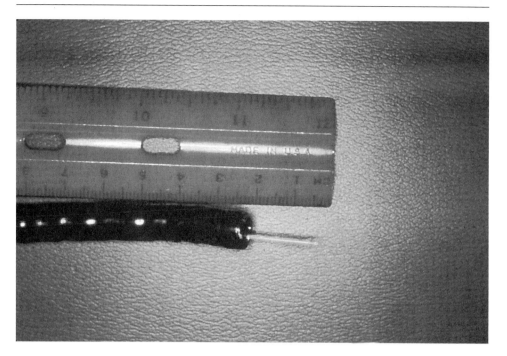

FIG. 3-21   The laser fiber should extend past the end of the endoscope before the laser is activated.

fiber is too close to the scope end, the backscatter from the laser beam can cause thermal damage, resulting in lens pitting, biopsy port trauma, and other related problems. Not only must the aiming beam be seen on the tissue, but the end of the fiber must be in view to ensure that the fiber is past the end of the endoscope. Often video cameras are used during laser endoscopy so that the laser team member can note that the fiber tip is in view before the laser is activated.

Also, the fiber can be marked before the procedure begins. The fiber is passed through the endoscope to position the tip past the end of the endoscope. A piece of tape is placed on the fiber at the biopsy port. The fiber is then withdrawn with the tape in place. During the procedure, when the fiber is passed through the endoscope, the location of the tape will alert the team that the fiber is extending past the end of the endoscope (Figure 3-22). This ensures that the fiber is fully extended before the laser is activated.

The end of a bare fiber is sharp and can damage the inside lumen of the biopsy port of a flexible endoscope. The end of the fiber can be protected by introducing the fiber into a length of medical-grade tubing with the sharp tip recessed inside the tubing. This unit is then passed into the biopsy port and through the channel. Once the fiber tip is past the end of the endoscope, the tubing is withdrawn to expose the fiber tip. This protects the inside lumen of the channel.

Foot Pedals

Foot pedals can present safety hazards if mistakenly activated during a procedure. Technology development is giving the physician more foot pedals to control the growing number of devices and other equipment used in today's complex surgical environment

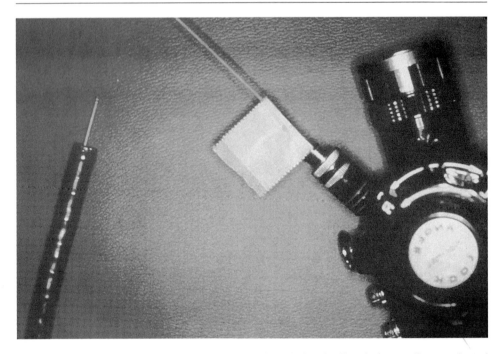

FIG. 3-22   By flagging the fiber, the team can determine whether the fiber tip is extending past the end of the endoscope.

(Figure 3-23). The laser foot pedal must be available to the physician who actually delivers the laser energy to the tissue. Laser surgery must not be performed with one physician activating the foot pedal while another physician guides the fiber or handpiece. Only one foot pedal should be available to the operating physician to decrease confusion during the procedure. Mistakes can easily be made when an electrocautery foot pedal and a laser foot pedal are next to each other under the surgical table. A sample policy for foot pedal placement is provided on page 92.

Electrical Hazards

Electrical hazards are constant during laser procedures. Solution bottles should never be placed on the laser unit because any spillage or splatter could cause internal short-circuiting within the laser. Connections to water-cooled lasers should be tight to decrease the chance of water overflow on the floor. This could present a problem if the laser or foot pedal is near the water overflow. The outside protective cover on the laser system should not be removed by unauthorized personnel because the potential for electric shock and electrocution is high.

Transportation Hazards

Transportation hazards are always a threat because lasers sometimes must be moved from one area to another. Lasers can be heavy and bulky, so manufacturers are making larger wheels for them to make transportation easier. Care must be taken not to jar the laser or hit it against a wall because laser components can easily be damaged. When mov-

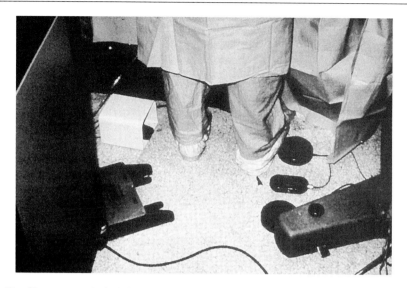

FIG. 3-23   Numerous technical devices operated by footpedals can be hazardous if mistakenly activated.

ing a laser system, proper body mechanics must be employed to decrease the chance of injury or damage (Figure 3-24).

LASER PLUME

When a laser beam strikes tissue, a plume of smoke is produced depending upon the laser wavelength, power, duration of exposure, tissue type, and amount of external fluid present on the tissue. Irritation by the laser plume (or plume produced by an electrosurgery unit) can cause burning, watery eyes for anyone near the impact site. Also, the odor from the plume can cause nausea. When surgical teams are subjected to this type of environment, they can become irritable and negative. Therefore, any smoke must be adequately removed to ensure clean, fresh air and a comfortable environment for the surgery team and the patient.

Laser Plume Research

Research studies have been conducted over the years that note the content of surgical smoke, particulate matter size, and potential viability.

During an investigation in Japan, Shigenobu Mihashi and his associates vaporized 1 g of excised canine tongue with a CO_2 laser and found that the amount of plume within the immediate surgical area was 52 times greater than that allowed by the government's environmental standards (Mihashi et al, 1975b). These results indicated that the air is definitely polluted by the smoke produced from laser irradiation.

Laser plume consists of particles, toxins, and steam. Particles include carbonized tissue, blood, and potential virus and bacteria. Toxins consist of polycyclic aromatic hydrocarbons, benzene, toluene, formaldehyde, and acrolein, which produce the offensive odor within the smoke. A highly important proven finding is that the contents of laser plume

**Sample Safety Policy and Procedure:
Foot Pedal Placement (Laser Surgery)**

Purpose:

To decrease the chance of accidental pedal activation during laser procedures.

Procedure:

1. Any foot pedal will be identified verbally by the laser team member as it is being placed on the floor for the operating physician to use.
2. The smoke evacuation foot pedal (if available) will be placed so that it can be activated by the scrub nurse.
3. All other foot pedals will be identified and placed in an appropriate area to decrease confusion during laser procedures.
4. No foot pedals will be placed on or near liquids so as to minimize electrical hazards.
5. All foot pedal electrical wiring must be inspected before each use for fraying or breaks that could lead to electrical shock or fire.

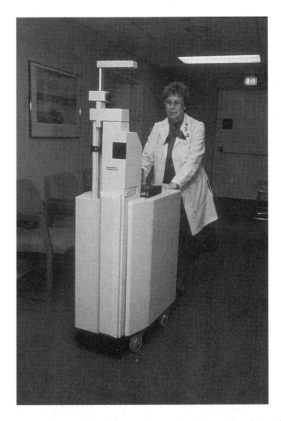

FIG. 3-24   Proper body mechanics must be used when moving heavy laser units.

and electrosurgery smoke are highly similar in particulate matter types and hazards (*Clinical Laser Monthly,* March 1993).

Two areas of concern must be highlighted regarding the content of any surgical smoke: the size of the particulate matter and the viability of the cells in the plume.

The size of the particulate matter found in surgical plume has been conclusively proven over the years. Studies have shown that 77% of the particulate matter in the laser plume is smaller than 1.1 μm (Mihashi et al, 1975b). This extremely small particulate matter can easily be deposited in the alveoli of the lungs if inhaled. This in turn causes chronic irritation that can lead to bronchitis or emphysema-like conditions. However, bacteria only colonizes on air particles that are 5 μm or larger. In contrast, viral organisms are smaller than 0.1 μm but are rarely found free-floating (Reeves, Forrest, and Nezhat, 1985). Viral organisms usually attach to larger cells, thus making their evacuation easier. Most smoke evacuation systems on the market will readily evacuate laser plume particulate matter down to 0.1 or 0.3 μm. Such systems must be employed to prevent bacterial or viral infection.

A study conducted by Baggish, Baltoyannis, and Sze (1988) compared the effects of laser smoke on rat lungs. Three groups of rats were forced to breathe in large amounts of laser plume from lased pigskin for different durations. All the rats developed hypoxia and pulmonary congestion with bronchial hyperplasia and hypertrophy. In further studies, the rats were subjected to plume that had been filtered. The researchers noted that the rats who breathed the air from the plume that filtered out particles down to 0.1 μm developed no lesions and remained identical to the control rats. Therefore, adequate plume filtering must be performed during a laser procedure. In 1988, Dr. Barry Wenig found that the conclusions from Baggish's study regarding the harmful effects of CO_2 laser smoke on lung tissue also applied to the use of the electrocautery and the Nd:YAG laser, (Stackhouse Inc., 1992a).

The controversial issue regarding laser plume is whether it contains viable cells that may be inhaled during a laser procedure and then transmit disease. Studies have been conducted over the years to address this dilemma. For example, the CO_2 laser wavelength is 10,600 nm in the invisible mid-infrared spectrum of the electromagnetic spectrum. The surface cells of the tissue absorb the beam readily depending upon the water content of the cells. In fact, 95% of the CO_2 beam is absorbed within the first 150 μm of tissue (Oosterhuis et al, 1982). The tissue absorbs the laser energy and causes a thermal buildup. Cells explode as the intracellular temperature increases to over 100° C. The viability of the cellular contents and the intact adjacent cells that are also spewn into the air needs to be determined.

Many studies were done to answer this question during the 1970s and 1980s. In 1975, Mihashi et al collected and cultured the laser plume. No cellular growth was found (Mihashi et al, 1975a). In a similar study in 1982, Oosterhuis et al were unsuccessful in obtaining any culture growth from plume produced by a CO_2 laser used on mice melanoma cells. In 1982, Bellina and his associates employed the CO_2 laser to excise condyloma, and the plume did not produce any viable virus cells or organisms (Bellina et al, 1982). In 1984, tumor cells in the brain were excised using a CO_2 laser, and no malignant cells were found in the laser plume or in the splatter (Voorhies et al, 1984).

In 1985, plume studies began to attract attention. Researchers discovered that when bacteria was placed on pigskin and was impacted by the CO_2 laser, viable bacteria could be found in the plume. Only 68 spores out of an original colony estimated at near

100,000,000 were noted, showing that this minuscule amount indicated no immediate danger (Mullarky, Norris, and Goldberg, 1985). In 1986, Walker and his associates noted cell clumps and erythrocytes in the laser plume. Their study also proved that viable cells could probably survive if the laser were operated at lower power settings (Walker et al, 1986).

In 1987, bacteria was successfully cultured from the plume, indicating that plume cell viability is determined by the power density of the laser beam on the tissue (Byrne et al, 1987). Later attempts to culture viral contaminants in the plume were unsuccessful in determining the plume viability. However, in 1988, Garden and his associates extracted viral material from cattle warts and exposed them to different laser power densities. Autoradiography was used to discover the presence of DNA. The research continued into the next phase, as the CO_2 laser with both high- and low-power densities was used to vaporize plantar warts on seven patients. Findings noted that the laser smoke contained intact strands of human papilloma virus (HPV) DNA. This study concluded that the target tissue can become aerosolized and could possibly be infectious. Research in 1991 (Baggish, Poiexz, 1991) detected human immunodeficiency virus DNA in laser smoke. There was no sustained viability, but there was positive tissue culture in the tubing of the evacuator. In 1989, Sawchuck, Weber, and colleagues found viral DNA in the vapor of warts when using the CO_2 laser and the electrocautery. This showed that the heat generated by the laser energy may not be enough to destroy all viable DNA from viruses.

Garden and Bakus continued this research by using pulsed and continuous laser energy at different wattages on excised bovine fibropapillomavirus. The plume contained intact DNA. This material was then reinoculated into the cows. The same viral lesions grew. This study concluded that the viral DNA can cause viral growth in the host (*Clinical Laser Monthly,* June 1993).

Further studies need to be performed to indicate whether these intact DNA strands can transmit disease or if the whole virus is needed. Therefore, more evidence through similar studies is needed to prove the viability of cells from the laser plume created by different laser wavelengths.

The type of laser plume depends on the type of laser used. The noncontact Nd:YAG lasers beam is absorbed by the tissue, causing a greater depth of penetration than that of most other lasers. The deeper cells can therefore be heated to the point of explosion. The surface cells may be thermally affected, but not to the point of destruction. The subsurface explosion of the deeper cells can cause the surface cells to be blown into the air also. This popcorn type of tissue effect can discharge potentially viable cells into the environment.

A study conducted in New Orleans found that this sequence can occur when tissue is impacted by a noncontact Nd:YAG laser beam; thus, viability may exist in the plume (Voorhies et al, 1984). Further research is needed to duplicate these findings.

HPV continues to be of great concern to laser team members and physicians because the laser (CO_2 and Nd:YAG) has become the preferred treatment for this virus in the excision and vaporization of condyloma. The prevalence of HPV in the general population continues to grow and now has attained epidemic proportions. A survey shows that between 1966 and 1983 the number of genital wart consultations grew 580% (169,000 in 1966 vs. 1.1 million in 1983) (Centers for Disease Control, 1983). Genital wart viral infection has been shown to be the most prevalent sexually transmitted disease in the United States (Becker, Stone, and Alexander, 1987). Noting these statistics, laser team members and physicians have considered the viability of the laser plume cells of crucial importance and have demanded that the laser plume be evacuated properly during these procedures.

The medical community's growing concern about the transmission of viral contaminants was illustrated in a retrospective survey conducted in 1988. This study was conducted to note the "incidence of acquired lesions among laser users and also the details predisposing them to the development of such lesions" (Lobraico, Shifano, and Brader, 1988). A questionnaire was sent to physicians and nurses. Results indicated that 26 possibly acquired verrucous lesions were reported, with four proven by biopsy. The highest incidence of acquired lesions existed among the dermatologists. An overwhelming number of lesions were reported to occur on the hands. Therefore, the question is whether the lesions resulted from direct contact with the verrucae or from the laser plume. The researchers stated that no lesions were reported in the buccal mucosa or larynx. Therefore, the risk of developing lesions by inhaling a possibly infective viral plume is insignificant according to this study. Conclusions from the survey indicate that strict adherence to wearing gloves and masks, plus controlling the plume through adequate smoke evacuation methods, is absolutely mandatory.

In 1991, a report was issued stating that a surgeon had performed a number of procedures with the Nd:YAG laser to vaporize anogenital condylomas. No smoke evacuator was used except for an in-line suction system. The physician developed a hoarseness that led him to seek medical attention. A biopsy of his laryngeal lesions showed the presence of the same viral types as those in his patients' warts. These findings suggested that the papilloma virus found in the physician's laryngeal lesions may have been caused by inhaled virus particles in the laser plume (Hallmo and Naess, 1991).

Smoke Evacuation

Smoke evacuators contain filters that remove the small particulate matter and the odor. Some smoke evacuation units have a three-phase system that works sequentially to remove the plume. Figure 3-25 describes how the prefilter, ultra-low particulate air (ULPA) filter, and charcoal filter work together to purify the plume. Sometimes the ULPA, high-efficiency particulate air (HEPA), and charcoal filters are combined within one unit to filter the plume.

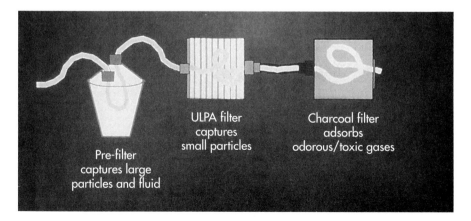

ULPA filter
captures
small particles

Charcoal filter
adsorbs
odorous/toxic gases

Pre-filter
captures large
particles and fluid

FIG. 3-25 Smoke evacuation may involve a three-step filtering process. (Courtesy Stackhouse, Inc., Riverside, CA.)

Smoke evacuation units currently on the market filter laser plume of 0.1 to 0.5 μm at 95% to almost 100% efficiency, depending on the system. Efficiency ratings are expressed in percentages, as follows (Stackhouse, Inc., 1992):

99.9%	1 in 1,000 particles gets through
99.99%	1 in 10,000 particles gets through
99.999%	1 in 100,000 particles gets through
99.9999%	1 in 1,000,000 particles gets through

A filter is rated by its ability to capture particles of a certain size at a specific efficiency using a certain flow rate. For example an ULPA filter has a filter rating of capturing particulate matter of 0.01 μm at 99.9999% efficiency at a flow rate of 30 cubic feet per minute (CFM). A HEPA filter has a filter rating of 0.3 μm at 99.97% efficiency.

ULPA and HEPA filters are made from depth media material usually consisting of a maze of glass or thermal plastic fibers. This substance forms a tortuous path that captures and entangles particulate matter within the mesh (Figure 3-26). Filtration occurs by three different methods as the particles come in contact with the fibers:

1. Direct interception: Particles of 1.0 μm and greater are too large to pass through the filter media (Figure 3-27).
2. Inertial impaction: Particles of 0.5 to 1.0 μm collide with the fibers and are held at the point of collision (Figure 3-28).
3. Diffusional interception: Particles of less than 0.5 μm are captured through the effects of Brownian motion (Figure 3-29). Brownian motion, or random thermal motion, is the indiscriminate movement of particles caused by collision with each other and with other molecules. Smaller molecules tend to have greater Brownian motion (Stackhouse, Inc., 1992a).

The mid-range particle is the most difficult to capture because it can pass through some of the 0.1- to 0.5-μm openings in the filter media. A particle this size is not small enough to have significant random thermal motion. A particle size of 0.12 μm is called

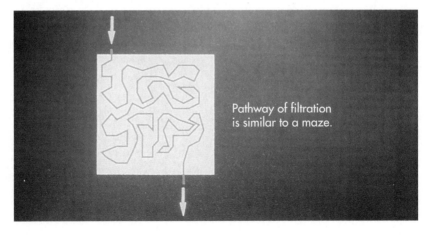

Pathway of filtration is similar to a maze.

FIG. 3-26   A depth filter is like a maze through which the plume is pulled. (Courtesy Stackhouse, Inc., Riverside, CA.)

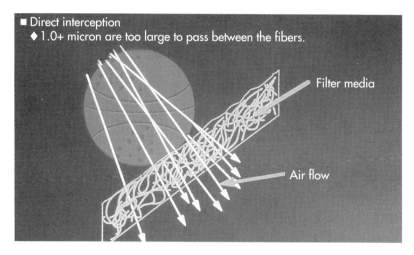

FIG. 3-27   Direct interception. (Courtesy Stackhouse, Inc., Riverside, CA.)

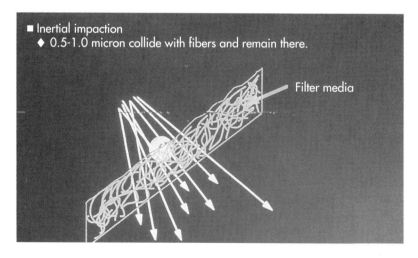

FIG. 3-28   Inertial impaction. (Courtesy Stackhouse, Inc., Riverside, CA.)

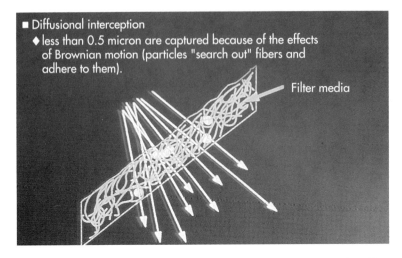

■ Diffusional interception
  ◆ less than 0.5 micron are captured because of the effects
    of Brownian motion (particles "search out" fibers and
    adhere to them).

Filter media

FIG. 3-29   Diffusional interception. (Courtesy Stackhouse, Inc., Riverside, CA.)

the most penetrating particle (MPP) and is the hardest size to capture (Stackhouse, Inc., 1992b). Particles of larger and smaller sizes are more easily captured through the methods described previously.

Another type of filtering absorbs the toxic gases, thus removing the odor. Charcoal from activated virgin coconut shell is effective in absorbing and deactivating the odor associated with the laser plume (Stackhouse, Inc., 1992b). "Activated" means that the charcoal was treated by a heating process to expose active absorption sites; "virgin" means that the charcoal has not been reprocessed. The coconut shell is more effective in absorbing particulate matter than wood charcoal because it has more internal pore area.

Some smoke evacuation companies also use special chemicals to treat the plume that circulates through the filters. These chemicals work by oxidizing and chemically interacting with the constituents of plume, thus significantly reducing the toxic carcinogenic and mutagenic elements of laser and electrosurgical plume. Neutralizing these harmful particles decreases the potential viability hazards associated with airborne contaminants.

There has been a movement to classify surgical smoke as able to harbor bloodborne pathogens. A bloodborne pathogen is a potentially infectious material that may be found in blood, body fluids, tissues, and organs (prior to fixation for pathological examination), or HIV and hepatitis B virus cultures (Johnson & Johnson Medical, Inc., 1992). Because research has proven the potential viability of the particulate matter in plume, logic could lead one to consider the possibility that plume contains bloodborne pathogens. Therefore, occupational exposure through skin, eye, and mucous membranes must be minimized. Universal precautions should be used when one is exposed to surgical smoke.

A concern during smoke evacuation is the noise of the smoke evacuation unit. Most units come with a foot pedal, so the scrub nurse or assistant can activate and deactivate the smoke evacuation system as needed. The condition of the foam padding inside some smoke evacuation systems also determines the amount of noise produced.

The proper timing of *changing filters* in the smoke evacuation unit is an important nursing consideration. The manufacturer's instructions regarding filter changing should be strictly followed. Usually, when a lingering odor is noticed in the air and the suction pressure has decreased, the filter needs to be changed. Some smoke evacuation units have an indicator light that notes when the filter needs to be changed. This signal is activated when the suction starts to decrease, signifying that the filter is becoming less effective. The laser team member can also note on the side of the filter the number of procedures or laser time during which the filter has been in use. This helps keep track of filter utilization for systems without an indicator light.

If the smoke evacuation filter needs changing, the contaminated filter should never be left in the unit for changing at a later time. The odor from the used filter can travel into the system and cause the foam padding, hoses, and other internal components of the unit to absorb this offensive smell. Therefore, constant surveillance of the filter protects the entire smoke evacuation unit and helps ensure proper plume elimination during the laser procedure. The laser team member should use gloves and clean technique in discarding the contaminated filter. The filter should be placed in a plastic bag and discarded in a general waste receptacle. A contaminated filter need not be treated as infectious or regulated medical waste.

Because many smoke evacuation systems are on the market today, they should be compared; the advantages and disadvantages of each system should be noted before purchase. Some of the considerations should include the following:

- Maintenance requirements
- Filtering capacity
- Noise level
- Size
- Portability
- Cost
- Reliability and ease of use
- Air movement or suction capability
- Cost of supplies

Special *in-line smoke filters* can be used if a small amount of plume is produced during a laser procedure (for example, during a microlaryngoscopy for vocal cord polyp removal). The in-line filter is connected to the existing ¼-inch wall suction line and is positioned between the wall connection and the suction canister (Figure 3-30). The suction canister is used to collect any fluids, and the air is purified by the filter. Care must be taken not to suction any fluids, through the in-line filter, because its effectiveness will be decreased if the filtering media gets wet. The suction canister must not have a filter in it, or the flow of air or the suction capability will decrease tremendously. If a laser procedure does not produce or require fluids that will be suctioned, the in-line filter can be used without the suction canister.

In-line devices usually filter out plume particulate matter of a size ranging down to 0.3 or 0.5 µm. Even if the plume seems to be invisible, an in-line filter should be used to prevent particulate matter from coating the inside of the wall suction line. Trace amounts of plume that are not filtered properly will continue to build up and lead to expensive repair bills for cleaning the inside of the clogged wall suction lines.

The flow rate of smoke evacuation is very important because it determines the amount of movement of the air or plume. A wall vacuum aspirates fluid through a ¼-inch tubing at approximately 2 CFM. Smoke evacuator units move plume through a ⅞-inch tubing up to about 50 CFM. This is another reason to use the wall suction only for small amounts of plume.

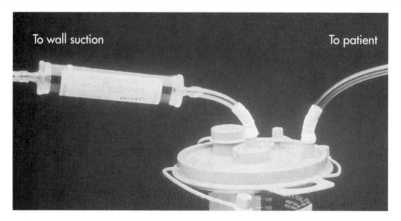

FIG. 3-30 An in-line filter is placed between the suction canister and the wall outlet and is used to evacuate small amounts of plume. (Courtesy Stackhouse, Inc., Riverside, CA.)

Smoke evacuation tubing is available in sterile or clean packaging. An astute nurse notes the cost differences in the packaging and opts to use clean tubing for procedures that do not require sterile technique (e.g., esophagoscopy for esophageal tumor vaporization). If reusable smoke evacuation tubing is used, careful cleaning is required to ensure proper removal of all accumulated debris that adheres to the inside lumen. High-pressure steam cleaners are often used to clean these tubes, but advances in technology have almost outdated this type of tubing.

Smoke evacuation tubing (usually ⅞ inch) has a smooth inner bore that allows suctioning to occur quietly even at the maximum speed setting (Figure 3-31). In an attempt to control costs, laser team members have tried to use anesthesia circuits as a substitute for smoke tubing. Since the inside lumen of anesthesia tubing is not smooth, a loud whistling noise is heard when anesthesia circuits are used. Therefore, this type of tubing is not practical for smoke evacuation purposes.

If a smoke evacuator is used with the ⅞-inch tubing, reducer fittings are available to connect the larger tubing to a ¼-inch suction line. The smaller suction tubing can then be attached to special laser instruments, such as the smoke tube on a vaginal speculum.

Positioning the smoke wand or tip is one of the most critical responsibilities for adequate smoke evacuation. Research has shown that as the smoke evacuation wand or tip is moved farther away from the laser-tissue impact site, a significantly greater amount of plume is allowed to escape into the air. When the plume wand is held within 1 cm of the laser impact site, approximately 98% of the smoke is eliminated. As the wand is held 2 cm away, the efficiency rate of plume evacuation is decreased to 51% (Mihashi et al, 1975b). Therefore, the scrub nurse or assistant must be constantly alert to ensure that the smoke hose or wand is held very close to the laser-tissue impact site. The wand or hose should be able to withstand an inadvertent impact by the laser beam. Some less expensive plastic suction tubes may burst into flames if impacted by laser energy.

If the CO_2 handpiece has purge gas flowing to keep the special focusing lens from becoming coated with debris and smoke, then smoke evacuation can become more difficult. The purge gas will also cause the plume to spread; therefore, the smoke evacuation wand must be held as close as possible to the target site.

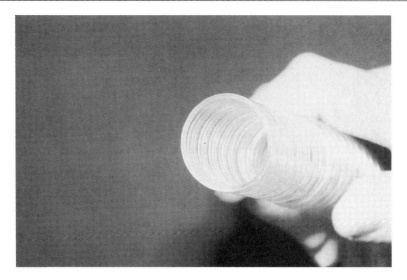

FIG. 3-31   The inside lumen of smoke evacuation tubes are smooth so as to decrease noise production.

A finger-controlled *low-pressure suction valve* can be used during laparoscopic and other endoscopic procedures if the presence of laser plume decreases visibility within the body cavity. This valve is attached to the suction line. When the valve is depressed manually, a gentle suction is provided to evacuate the unwanted laser plume (Figure 3-32). This low pressure suctioning is critical during laparoscopies so that the pneumoperi-

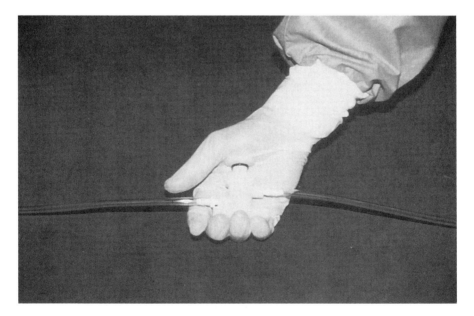

FIG. 3-32   A gentle suctioning of plume generated during laparoscopic procedures can be achieved by depressing a special suction valve.

toneum is not destroyed by allowing the insufflated gas to escape. Sometimes a high-flow gas insufflator is used during these procedures to help maintain the proper insufflation level when large amounts of smoke are anticipated.

Centralized smoke evacuation systems have been developed to accommodate the smoke evacuation needs simultaneously in a number of different surgery or treatment rooms. This type of system has advantages over portable systems, which are noisier, take up floor space, can only be used during one procedure at a time, and sometimes need a filter change with each procedure. One central smoke evacuation system pulls plume into disposable tubing through a permanent piping system and then into a centralized unit that spins the debris from the air through a centrifuge separator. The air is filtered and exhausted to the outside of the building while the debris is disinfected and disposed of with the medical waste. The system evacuates 98% of all airborne particles within surgical smoke (*Clinical Laser Monthly,* December 1993). A centralized system may cost more but its life expectancy is usually four to five times longer than that of portable units, and its filter does not have to be changed as often.

Smoke evacuation must be performed adequately during all laser procedures. Policies and procedures need to be written by each facility to provide guidelines for use during laser procedures. A sample smoke evacuation procedure is provided on page 103.

Masks

High-filtration masks should always be worn during surgical procedures that produce smoke to add further protection against unevacuated plume in the air. Most regular surgical masks filter particulate matter of 5 μm and larger. Double-masking leads to a false sense of security and does not provide adequate protection against microscopic plume particulate matter.

Some high-filtration masks filter particles down to 0.1 μm. The first high-filtration masks were extremely difficult to breathe through; today they are more comfortable and breathable. Since high-filtration masks are considerably more expensive than regular masks, they are usually identified by different colors or markings that readily distinguish them for use only during procedures that produce plume. This is an effective measure for minimizing the unnecessary use of more expensive masks. A sample policy for the use of high-filtration masks is provided on page 104.

Constant vigilance by everyone involved will ensure that the amount of laser plume escaping into the air will be minimized. Actions taken to protect the patient, physician, and surgical team from being exposed to the plume need to be refined. The quest for clean, safe air during laser intervention continues as researchers draw on available resources to solve this aggravating, annoying, and potentially hazardous problem. Maybe the solution is an individual breathing unit that must be worn by each member of the surgical team; maybe a device will be designed that will completely rid the plume of any viable or hazardous cells. More research is needed to prove the absolute viability of the plume cells so that uncertainty is diminished. But until then, the best way to control laser plume and decrease the hazard of inhaling the smoke is to follow these practices:

- Use an appropriate smoke evacuation system for the amount of plume produced.
- Change the filter(s) as often as required.
- Use filters that effectively evacuate plume particulate matter of at least 0.3 μm in size (ideally 0.1 μm).

Sample Safety Policy and Procedure:
Surgical Smoke Evacuation

Purpose:

To provide adequate smoke evacuation of surgical plume.

General Statement:

According to research studies, surgical smoke is potentially hazardous and must be evacuated effectively.

Procedure:

1. The smoke evacuation system must be adequate to handle the amount of plume produced during surgical procedures. For small amounts of plume, in-line suction filters may be used (e.g., for microlaryngoscopic vaporization of vocal cord polyps). For large amounts of plume, an individual smoke evacuator unit or a centralized system must be used.
2. An in-line suction smoke evacuation filter can become blocked by the particulate matter in large amounts of plume. This plume will then clog the wall suction lines.
3. An in-line filter is placed between the suction canister and the wall connection.
4. The smoke evacuation suction tube must be held close (less than 1 inch away) to the tissue interaction site to remove as much plume as possible. Surgical plume contains extremely small particulate matter and may contain viable cells.
5. When a purge gas flow is used with the CO_2 laser or a fiber delivery device, the smoke evacuation tube must constantly be held close to the laser-tissue interaction site because the gas flow will tend to spread the plume.
6. If a smoke evacuation foot pedal is available, the scrub nurse or first assistant can operate it.
7. Filters should be changed as recommended by the manufacturer. The contaminated filter should be bagged for disposal. Universal precautions, or at least gloves, should be used for filter changing.
8. Special efforts should be made to remove smoke during any endoscopic or laparoscopic procedure. Endoscopic smoke evacuation instruments, such as suction tubes, help decrease the presence and retention of plume inside a body cavity or organ. A low-pressure suction valve can be used to gently remove plume during a laparoscopic procedure without destroying the pneumoperitoneum.

- Ensure that the smoke evacuation wand or suction tubing is as close as possible to the site at which the plume is being generated.
- Ensure good room ventilation.
- Always wear high-filtration masks during smoke-producing laser surgery.
- Do not use the wall suction line for smoke evacuation without an in-line filter.
- Provide written smoke evacuation guidelines.

LASER SAFETY POLICIES

Complete and current laser safety policies are critical in providing guidance to ensure the safe and appropriate use of the laser. Safety policies and procedures must be reviewed annually to confirm relevance and practicality. Changes should be made as laser technology evolves.

Sample Safety Policy and Procedure:
High-Filtration Masks

Purpose:

To protect the surgical team members from inhaling possible viable and/or hazardous particulate matter during procedures that produce smoke.

Procedure:

1. High-filtration masks (with a filtering capacity of particulate matter at least 0.3 μm in size, ideally 0.1 μm) should be worn by the surgical team during any nonendoscopic procedure that generates plume.
2. The mask should be worn properly, covering the nose and mouth to decrease the chance of inhaling potentially viable hazardous matter. The sides of the mask should conform to the face adequately.
3. The laser should not be activated until all masks are on, the smoke evacuation tube is positioned near the laser-tissue interaction site, and the smoke evacuator is operating.

Laser team members and physicians are responsible for following and enforcing safety measures, such as wearing the appropriate eye protection for a particular wavelength being used. These practices should be documented in policy form so that everyone can easily reference them. Documentation of laser safety measures is valuable in providing a reference to guide practices if a question comes up or litigation occurs.

Laser service and preventive maintenance also must be documented routinely, as noted by the Joint Commission on Accreditation of Healthcare Organizations. This practice helps in recording measures taken to ensure the reliability and safe operation of a laser. Trends noting laser system problems can easily be detected and solved with appropriate follow-up.

Safety is the key ingredient in any laser program. Cooperative and continual efforts by the physician, laser team members, and other surgical personnel help ensure that safety measures are being followed. Laser accidents are caused by inattentiveness and a progressive relaxation in adhering to safety guidelines. As advances and changes in laser technology continue, the potential for hazards also may escalate. The surgery team is a vital element in monitoring and controlling these possible dangers.

REFERENCES

American National Standards Institute, Inc: American National Standard for the safe use of lasers in health care facilities, ANSI Z136.3, p 4, New York, 1988.

Association of Operating Room Nurses: 1989 AORN standards and recommended practices, Denver, 1989, The Association.

Baggish M: Laser plume danger? Questions remain, caution advised, *Clinical Laser Monthly,* pp 111-112, October 1988.

Baggish MS, Baltoyannis P, Sze E: Protection of the rat lung from the harmful effects of laser smoke, *Lasers Surg Med* 8:248-253,1988.

Baggish MS, et al: Presence of human immunodeficiency virus DNA in laser smoke, *Lasers Surg Med* 11:197-203,1991.

Becker TM, Stone KM, and Alexander ER: Genital human papillomavirus infection: A growing concern, *Obstet Gynecol Clin North Am* 14:389-394, 1987.

Bellina JH, Stjernholm RL, Kurpel JE: Analysis of plume emissions after papovavirus irradiation with the carbon dioxide laser, *J Reprod Med* 27:268-270, 1982.

Byrne PR et al: Carbon dioxide laser irradiation of bacterial targets in vitro, *J Hosp Infect* 9: 296-273, 1987.

Centers for Disease Control: Condylomata acuminata-United States, MMWR 32:306-308, 1983.

Central laser smoke evacuator is up and running in one hospital, *Clinical Laser Monthly,* pp 185-186, December 1993.

Eyewear optical density accurate, but the direct beam exposure risky, *Clinical Laser Monthly,* pp 114-115, July 1992.

False alarm in concern over halon fire extinguishers, *Clinical Laser Monthly,* pp 28-29, February 1993.

Garden JM, O'Banion K, Shelnitz L et al: Papillomavirus in the vapor of carbon dioxide laser-treated verrucae, JAMA 8:1199-1202, 1988.

Hallmo P and Naess O: Laryngeal papillomatosis with human papillomavirus DNA contracted by a laser surgeon, *Eur Arch Otorhinolarygol,* pp 425-427, March 1991.

Johnson & Johnson Medical, Inc.: Bloodborne infections: A practical guide to OSHA compliance, p 4, Arlington, TX, 1992, Johnson & Johnson Medical, Inc.

Lobraico RV, Schifano MJ, and Brader KR: A retrospective study on the hazards of the carbon dioxide laser plume, *Journal of Laser Applications,* pp 6-8, Fall 1988.

Meeker MH and Rothrock JC: *Alexander's care of the patient in surgery,* ed 10, St. Louis, 1995, Mosby.

Mihashi S et al: Laser surgery in otolaryngology: Interaction of CO_2 laser and soft tissue, *Ann NY Acad Sci* 267:263-294,1975a.

Mihashi S et al: Some problems about condensates induced by CO_2 laser irradiation, Karume, Japan, Department of Otolaryngology and Public Health, 1975b, Karume University.

Mullarky MB, Norris CW, and Goldberg ID: The efficacy of the CO_2 laser in the sterilization of skin seeded with bacteria: Survival at the skin surface and in the plume emission, *Laryngoscope,* 95:186-187, 1985.

New research confirms laser plume can transmit disease, *Clinical Laser Monthly,* pp 81-84, June 1993.

Non-compliant docs confound eyewear safety policies, *Clinical Laser Monthly,* pp17-21, February 1993,

Oosterhuis JW et al: The viability of cells in the waste products of CO_2 laser evaporation of cloudman mouse melanomas, *Cancer* 49:61-67, 1982.

Reeves WG, Forrest D, and Nezhat C: Smoke from laser surgery—Is there a health hazard? 1985.

Rubber tubes allow quicker removal during airway fires, *Clinical Laser Monthly,* pp 110-111, July 1993.

Sawchuck WS, Weber PJ et al: Infectious papillomavirus in the vapor of warts treated with carbon dioxide laser or electrocoagulation: Detection and protection *J Am Acad Dermatol* 21(1):44-49, 1989.

Stackhouse, Inc.: The hazards of surgical smoke, video study guide, pp 4-6, Riverside, CA, 1992a, Stackhouse.

Stackhouse, Inc.: The hazards of surgical smoke, video, Riverside, CA, 1992b, Stackhouse.

Study rates polypropylene drapes least likely to go up in flames, *Clinical Laser Monthly,* pp 168-169, November 1993.

Two years after passage, device act leaves confusion in its wake, *Clinical Laser Monthly,* pp 27-28, February 1993.

U.S. Department of Health and Human Services: Regulations for the administration and enforcement of the Radiation Control for Health and Safety Act of 1968, HHS Publication FDA 88-8035, April 1988, Part 1040, sections 1040.10 and 1040.11.

U.S. Department of Health and Human Services: Highlights of the Safe Medical Device Act of 1990, p 3, 1991.

U.S. Department of Health and Human Services: Medical Device Reporting for User Facilities: Questions and Answers Based on the Tentative Final Rule, December, p 5, 1991.

U.S. Department of Health and Human Services: Suggested state regulations for the control of radiation, Vol. II, Nonionizing radiation, *Lasers,* 1983.

Use smoke evacuators during electrosurgery, laser procedures, *Clinical Laser Monthly,* pp 36-37, March 1993.

Walker NPJ, Mathews J, and Newsom SWB: Possible hazards from irradiation with the carbon dioxide laser, *Lasers Surg Med* 6:84-86, 1986.

Wood RL, Sliney DH, Basye RA: Laser reflections from surgical instruments, *Lasers Surg Med* 12:675-678, 1992.

Voorhies RM et al: Does the CO_2 laser spread viable brain-tumor cells outside the surgical field? *J Neurosurg* 60:819-820,1984.

CLINICAL LASER APPLICATIONS

In today's health care environment, many surgical procedures and medical treatments are being enhanced by laser technology. This amazing tool has simplified many surgeries, allowing them to be performed on an outpatient basis under local anesthesia or no anesthesia at all. The advantages of hemostasis, precision, and quicker recovery are being realized with the introduction of new laser techniques. The nurse is constantly challenged to understand new laser wavelengths and delivery systems, innovative laser applications, safety practices, instrumentation, and perioperative patient care. This part describes the impact of laser technology on different specialties and focuses on the perioperative course and nursing intervention for each area.

4

OPHTHALMOLOGY LASER APPLICATIONS

L aser use in ophthalmology has expanded tremendously since it was first introduced in the early 1960s. The laser has become such a useful and standardized tool for the ophthalmologist that laser technology is now being taught as part of the medical school curriculum. Applications are continually being refined, and new wavelengths are being introduced that provide precision and predictability.

Advances in ophthalmology laser systems continually enhance surgical procedures. Lasers that produce more than one wavelength offer precision because specific wavelengths are selectively absorbed differently by the various types of tissue in the eye.

One laser combines video capabilities with illumination and laser technology. Through a single 20-gauge probe, surgeons can illuminate and view every aspect of the inner eye while simultaneously delivering diode laser energy to any intraocular structure (Figure 4-1). This system is extremely useful during eye procedures that require a clear view of the internal structures. Sometimes the retina may be difficult to see because of miosis, loss of corneal clarity, opacification of the posterior capsule after a cataract extraction, or other clinical conditions. This laser system provides direct visualization by inserting the probe into the interior of the eye. Video recording is also possible during diagnosis and the actual surgical treatment (Uram, 1992).

Other laser systems combine diagnostics with the therapeutic laser unit. For example, computerized fluorescein angiography is now possible through the diagnostic part of the system. The adjacent laser is then used to perform the needed retinal treatment.

Another laser system combines a sophisticated imaging system, an automated tracking and positioning system, a topography corneal mapping system, a pachymeter (for true three-dimensional corneal modeling), and a laser unit. This technology provides a tracking system to lock on to the target site while maintaining precise focusing even with the constant, rapid natural eye movements and involuntary motions such as breathing. The accuracy of the laser is much greater if the target site is controlled; therefore, delicate eye surgery can be performed with optimal results.

New laser wavelengths are being used to treat a variety of ophthalmic conditions. For example, a small, compact ophthalmic erbium:YAG laser at 2940 nm can be conducted through a metal halide fiber to perform a number of various ophthalmological surgeries.

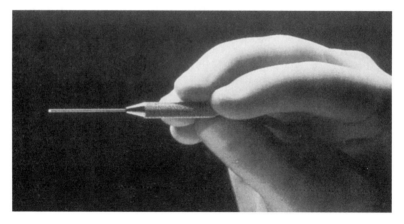

FIG. 4-1   A 20-gauge probe inserted into the eye provides video imagery, illumination, and laser energy. (Courtesy Endo Optiks, Inc., NJ.)

This type of wavelength has been approved or is being investigated for anterior capsulotomy, cyclophotocoagulation, excision of pupillary membranes, oculoplastic applications, sclerostomy, cataract emulsification, and refractive surgeries. The ophthalmological applications of laser technology are under constant evaluation as new equipment is developed, new approaches are discovered, and older techniques are refined.

Before discussing detailed ophthalmological laser applications, one must understand the anatomy of the eye.

ANATOMY

The three major layers of the eye are the retina, uvea, and sclera (Figure 4-2). The central cavity of the eye is filled with a gelatinous substance called vitreous humor. The anterior chamber (in front of the iris) and the posterior chamber (behind the iris) are filled with a watery aqueous humor.

Retina

The retina is composed of 10 layers containing rods and cones, which sense light, and nerve fibers, which conduct the impulse to the optic nerve. The color of the retina is usually a uniform reddish orange, caused by the deeper vascular supply and pigmented layers. The optic disc can be observed on the retina with four sets of retinal vessels that emerge and travel medially and laterally. Near the optic disc is a small depression known as the fovea centralis. The cones are the most concentrated at this point of central vision and intense color detection. The macula is the yellowish area surrounding the fovea centralis.

Uvea

The uvea consists of the choroid, ciliary body, and iris. The choroid is the vascular layer of the eye and is situated between the retina and sclera. The ciliary body is located in the anterior chamber and produces aqueous humor that is constantly circulated in this area. The aqueous humor flows from the ciliary body through the pupil before reaching the trabecular meshwork at the intersection of the iris and cornea. Schlemm's canal, situ-

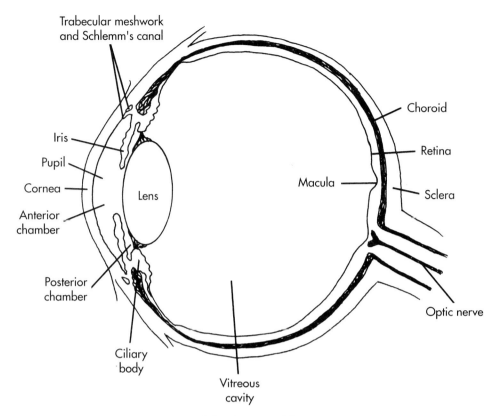

FIG. 4-2 Anatomy of the eye.

ated in the trabecular meshwork, then conducts the aqueous humor to the systemic circulation. The balance of aqueous production and elimination maintains the intraocular pressure of the eye. The iris is a circular pigmented structure that acts as a diaphragm to vary the size of the pupil as light is sensed by the retina. The lens is encapsulated within an elastic capsule and is located behind the iris. The thickness of the lens is controlled by the muscles of the ciliary body as the lens focuses light on the retina.

Sclera

The sclera is the tough white outer layer that serves as structural support, maintains ocular integrity, and forms the transparent cornea at the front of the eye.

RETINAL PHOTOCOAGULATION FOR RETINOPATHIES
Types of Retinopathies

Diabetic retinopathy is classified into two categories: background diabetic retinopathy or proliferative diabetic retinopathy.

Background diabetic retinopathy is thought to be caused by chronic damage to small retinal blood vessels produced by the diabetic condition. Retinal microaneurysms, intraretinal edema, small retinal hemorrhages, exudates, and vascular occlusive disease characterize this process. Loss of vision is usually caused by macular edema, blood or exudates in the fovea, or occluded vessels. Localized laser photocoagulation is performed to decrease leakage from the vessels. Macular edema is treated by placing laser spots in a grid pattern to stabilize the acuity.

Proliferative diabetic retinopathy involves the development of new blood vessels on the retina because of the metabolic changes produced by diabetes. This proliferation of blood vessels is thought to be caused by the hypoxic retinal pigment cells that produce a neovascular growth factor that stimulates vessel growth. These vessels eventually lead to retinal and vitreal hemorrhage, retinal traction, and detachment. The patient's visual acuity is severely compromised at this point.

To stop the stimulation of the hypoxic retinal pigment cells from forming fragile blood vessels, laser photocoagulation is performed. The laser energy impacts these ischemic areas by debriding the retinal layer and destroying the ischemic retina that produces the factor responsible for the growth of new, fragile blood vessels. This in turn allows for increased oxygenation from the choroid layer to enhance retinal perfusion.

Other ischemia-producing retinal conditions can also be treated with laser photocoagulation. These include retinal vein occlusion, sickle-cell disease, leukemia, and radiation retinopathy. All of these conditions are associated with a decreased perfusion of the retina, leading to ischemia. Thus, new blood vessels are formed to accommodate the decreased retinal tissue oxygenation. Hemorrhage can occur from the neovascularization of these fragile blood vessels. Ischemic retinal disease can lead to rubeosis iridis, in which new vessels form on the iris that can eventually cause glaucoma as the flow of the aqueous humor is obstructed.

Choroidal neovascularization may occur because of age-related (senile) macular degeneration, ocular histoplasmosis, and other related conditions. An overgrowth of new blood vessels spread from the choroid into the retinal layers. Neovascularization expands rapidly towards the fovea. Serous fluid or blood may accumulate between the retinal layers, which may lead to fibrotic changes and disastrous retinal detachment. If the abnormal vessel formation has progressed to under the fovea, localized foveal photocoagulation must be performed to arrest this condition. This specific treatment is still being investigated for its effectiveness as complications may lead to loss of sight.

Treatment

Before using the laser for retinal conditions, a detailed assessment of the pathology must be made. A fluorescein angiogram can be performed by injecting a special dye intravenously. This dye quickly circulates through the ophthalmic vessels, and a series of images is recorded on 35-mm film or by computerization (Figure 4-3). The results of the fluorescein angiogram will show any vessel abnormalities, leakage, edema, or circulation problems. An ophthalmological ultrasound can be done to test for retinal detachment.

Historically, the argon laser has been the most popular laser used for retinal photocoagulation. In the past several years, the diode laser has become a popular choice for this procedure. The laser energy can be applied in one spot (focal) or all around the retina (panretinal) to seal new blood vessels or debride the retina to improve or stabilize vision (Figure 4-4).

The argon wavelength is transmitted through the clear structures of the eye, such as the cornea, lens, and vitreous humor. This beam is composed of blue-green light and is highly absorbed by the retinal pigmentation's hemoglobin and melanin. The blue compo-

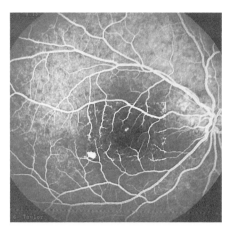

FIG. 4-3   Fluorescein angiography.

nent of the argon beam is highly absorbed by the yellow xanthophyll pigment of the macula. This action may cause retinal damage because of the high degree of absorption and may decrease the effectiveness of laser beam penetration. Therefore, a filter may be used to deliver green-only light to the macular area to provide more selective laser beam absorption. Most clinicians prefer the green-only to the combined blue-green laser energy because of this precision. Argon laser energy is also absorbed by cataracts and vitreal or retinal blood, sometimes decreasing the effectiveness of the procedure.

The diode laser produces wavelengths such as 810 nm. Solid-state laser systems, such as the diode laser, are much more compact and easier to move. These systems are very reliable and do not require a lot of maintenance. Diode lasers are challenging the larger lasers that require tubes of gas.

The krypton red laser is sometimes used for localized retinal photocoagulation in conjunction with argon application. This wavelength is absorbed less by the macular yellow

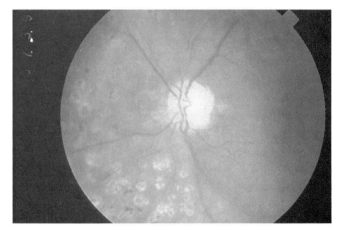

FIG. 4-4   Panretinal photocoagulation for retinopathy.

xanthophyll pigment, allowing for high penetration. Therefore, the krypton laser beam more effectively photocoagulates the macular area of the retina without damaging delicate structures. The krypton laser also is less absorbed by a cataract lens or vitreal blood. The disadvantage associated with the krypton laser is that because of the deeper penetration into the choroidal layer, an increase in pain and possibly choroidal bleeding can result. The pain can be controlled by administering a retrobulbar anesthetic injection to help the patient tolerate the procedure. The hemorrhaging can be controlled by increasing the duration of the beam exposure to the tissue. Currently, the tunable dye yellow laser and the frequency doubled Nd:YAG laser are also being used for photocoagulation treatments.

Panretinal photocoagulation is usually performed with the patient under local anesthesia. Dilating drops are usually instilled before the procedure to widen the pupil so a larger surgical field is provided and the retinal pathology and vasculature can be visualized. The laser energy can be delivered to the retina via a slit lamp. The patient's head is stabilized by straps connected to the slit lamp or by the nurse assisting with the procedure (Figure 4-5). Thorough preoperative education is critical for the local-anesthesia patient, who needs to understand the importance of immobility during the procedure.

Retinal procedures may also be performed using an indirect ophthalmoscope, which is attached to a headband worn by the physician. The laser energy is delivered from the ophthalmoscope (Figure 4-6). A lens is positioned near the patient's eye to focus the beam on the appropriate target. This type of delivery requires acute eye, hand, and head coordination.

When laser energy is directed through a microscope slit lamp, a special focusing lens may be placed directly on the anesthetized surface of the eye. This lens is cushioned with a drop of methylcellulose before it is placed on the eye. The lens is rotated to focus the laser energy on the retinal area to be treated (Figures 4-7 and 4-8). Recently there has

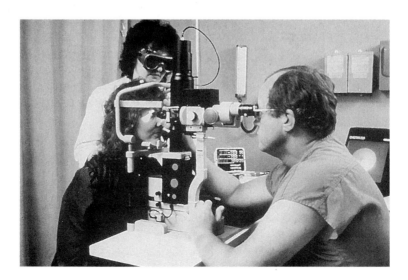

FIG. 4-5   The nurse helps stabilize the patient's head during a retinal laser procedure.

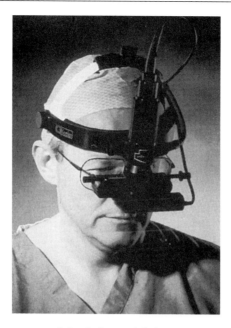

FIG. 4-6   Indirect ophthalmoscope.

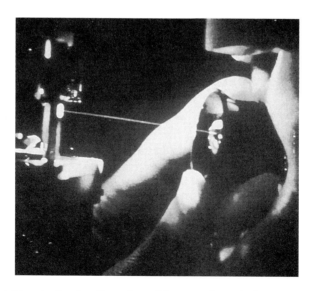

FIG. 4-7   A special lens is placed on the surface of the eye to focus the laser energy on the retinal area to be treated.

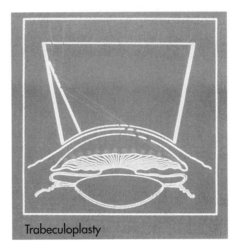

Trabeculoplasty

FIG. 4-8   The lens directs the laser energy to the target tissue. (Courtesy Coherent, Inc., Palo Alto, CA.)

been much discussion on the appropriate care of these lenses between their use on different patients. A sample policy is provided on page 117.

Many times panretinal photocoagulation is performed in a series of treatments to accommodate the patient's tolerance level. Sometimes the patient may complain of more discomfort during subsequent treatments because the retina may become more sensitive to the laser energy.

Laser spots are placed in specific areas using a larger spot (approximately 250 μm), less than 1-second pulses, and 200 to 500 mW of energy. These laser parameters and the number of spots should be recorded on the patient's record. Evaluation of the retinal response to the laser energy should be monitored in the physician's office during regular postoperative visits.

Immediately after surgery the patient may suffer from macular edema, which could cause a decrease in vision. This macular edema may continue to persist postoperatively. Vision change is usually temporary, but the patient may also experience a more permanent alteration in peripheral or night vision. Sometimes an ice bag is applied to the eye immediately after surgery to decrease edema. A small bag of frozen peas wrapped in a thin cloth or tissue may be substituted for ice because it weighs less, conforms to the eye socket, and can be refrozen (Figure 4-9). Retinal traction may become evident if fibrotic changes occur in the macular area. This could eventually lead to retinal detachment.

A new procedure known as dye-enhanced laser photocoagulation is being investigated to treat choroidal neovascularization. This procedure involves intravenous administration of indocyanine green dye followed by diode laser therapy. The dye circulates through the body and is absorbed into the optic neovascular supply. The laser light at an infrared wavelength is readily absorbed by the dye but not by the retinal pigment epithelium. Therefore, when the diode laser energy impacts the vessels that have retained the light-sensitive dye, specific vascular injury occurs using less laser energy than is required with other photocoagulation techniques. The goal of this therapy is to minimize the amount of energy required to produce closure of neovascular membranes, preserve visual acuity, and reduce recurrences (Puliafito, 1991).

Sample Policy and Procedure for Care of Ophthalmic Focusing Lens

Purpose:

To decrease the risk of nosocomial infection among patients by providing a patient-safe prepared lens.

Policy:

1. All ophthalmic focusing lenses will be prepared in the same manner for patient use.
2. The cleaning process for the focusing lenses must result in a patient-safe lens.

General statements:

1. Patient-safe preparation involves a high-level disinfectant.
2. High-level disinfecting is recommended for medical devices that come in contact with mucous membranes, such as ophthalmic focusing lenses.

Procedure:

1. As soon as the lens is removed from the patient's eye, rinse it in cold or tepid water.
2. Clean the lens with a few drops of mild soap on a moistened cotton ball. Gently clean with a circular motion to remove mucus, sebaceous deposits, or other debris.
3. Rinse the lens carefully with cool water and blot dry with a non-lint-forming tissue.
4. Soak the lens in a 2% aqueous glutaraldehyde solution according to the manufacturer's instructions.
5. Rinse the lens thoroughly in cool water several times to remove all of the disinfectant solution.
6. Dry the lens carefully with a non-lint-forming tissue.
7. Store the lens in a dry storage case.

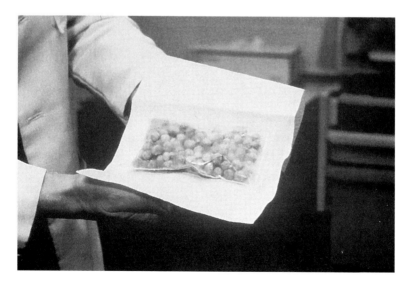

FIG. 4-9   A small bag of frozen peas can provide a cold compress for the eye after laser surgery.

LASER REPAIR OF RETINAL TEARS AND DETACHMENTS

Retinal detachment can result from an injury, intraocular neoplasm, or degeneration. The vitreal body can separate from the retina, causing a tear. Vitreous fluid may seep through this tear, causing it to enlarge and possibly detach the retina. The patient may complain of seeing floating spots, which are caused by pigmentation or blood cells in the vitreous humor. The patient may also complain of a distinct shadow, which is caused by a loss of function in the portion of detached retina. The detachment may progress as more and more fluid leaks into the retinal layers. Visual loss also continues as the detachment becomes more severe.

Argon or diode laser energy is delivered to the area around the retinal tear through a slit lamp or with an intraocular probe introduced directly into the eye. Laser photocoagulation is performed to prevent permanent loss of central vision by controlling the extent of a tear. Photocoagulation sealing spots placed strategically around the tear cause an adhesive scar to form. This adhesive action stops the tear from progressing into a detachment (Figure 4-10). Therefore, the laser is used to prevent rather than treat a retinal detachment. If more than one area of the retina has become detached, a conventional nonlaser retinal detachment procedure should probably be performed.

Postoperatively, the patient's activities are limited while the retinal tear heals. The eye may be covered with a patch to encourage complete rest for a period of time.

LASER PROCEDURES FOR GLAUCOMA

Glaucoma is a disease characterized by an increase in intraocular pressure, which can lead to optic nerve atrophy and blindness. After the aqueous humor is produced by the ciliary body, it travels through the pupil to Schlemm's canal, deep in the trabecular meshwork. It then returns to the systemic circulation (Figure 4-11). When the aqueous humor

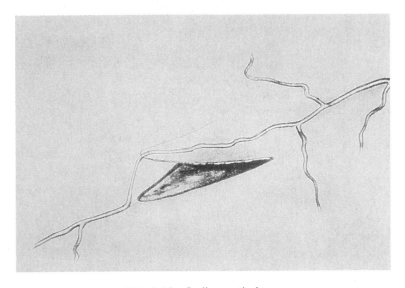

FIG. 4-10   Sealing a retinal tear.

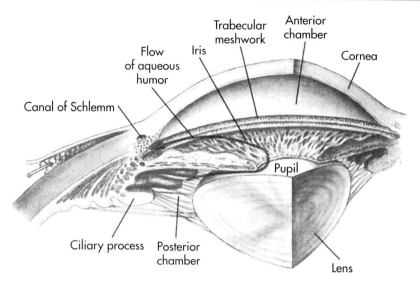

FIG. 4-11   Flow of aqueous humor. (From Thompson JM et al: *Mosby's clinical nursing,* ed 3, St. Louis, 1993, Mosby.)

is prevented from flowing into the systemic circulation, fluid builds up, leading to a rise in the intraocular pressure. A tonometry reading of over 24 mm Hg suggests glaucoma.

Open-Angle Glaucoma

Open-angle glaucoma occurs when the angle between the iris and the cornea is open, but an obstruction in the trabecular meshwork or in the Schlemm's canal area prevents the aqueous humor from returning to the systemic circulation. This condition develops slowly and is characterized by impaired peripheral vision. The patient may complain of headaches and seeing halos around lights.

Topical and systemic medications usually help control open-angle glaucoma. Argon laser trabeculoplasty has proven to be highly beneficial when used in conjunction with these medications; sometimes the medications may even be eliminated. This procedure decreases the intraocular pressure by accommodating the fluid flow.

For the argon laser trabeculoplasty, a three-mirrored contact lens is placed on the anesthetized eye to provide visualization of the chamber angle and retraction of the eye lid. The physician determines a landmark as a starting point for the laser spots. Using a small spot size of 50 µm and approximately 850 mW of energy in 0.1-second pulses, carefully spaced argon photocoagulation spots are placed along the pigmented zone of the midtrabecular meshwork (Figure 4-12). Sometimes a patient cannot tolerate the entire procedure, so two or more treatments may have to be scheduled. The ophthalmic Nd:YAG laser has also been used to produce holes along the trabecular meshwork.

The mechanism of action of this procedure has not been specifically determined. It has been theorized that the laser energy causes a shrinkage in the meshwork that accommodates the flow of the aqueous humor to Schlemm's canal. Postoperatively, an ice bag may

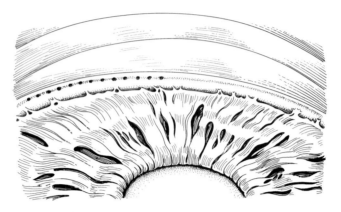

FIG. 4-12   Laser trabeculoplasty.

be applied to the closed eye to minimize swelling. Previous glaucoma-controlling medications are continued to ensure a decrease in intraocular pressure. Repeat laser therapy may be needed at a later date if the pressure increases again.

Closed-Angle Glaucoma

Closed-angle glaucoma is less common than open-angle glaucoma. This condition involves the closure of the angle between the iris and the cornea, which blocks the flow of the aqueous humor to the trabecular meshwork. Closed-angle glaucoma may be caused by a pupillary block that results in aqueous accumulation behind the iris. The iris then is pushed forward and the angle is closed, stopping the flow of the fluid. This condition is associated with age-related lens thickening, medications used to dilate the pupil, side effects of antihistamines, or trauma.

This type of glaucoma usually has a sudden onset and is associated with severe pain in and around the eye. Artificial lights may appear to have a rainbow of colors around them, and vision may become blurred. The pupil mid-dilates, and the patient may experience nausea and vomiting. This condition must be treated immediately to avoid irreversible damage and blindness.

To control this condition, an iridectomy is usually performed to facilitate the fluid flow in the anterior chamber. The patient is positioned at the slit lamp after a topical anesthetic agent is administered to the eye via drops. An ophthalmic lens is placed on the eye to focus the laser energy on the target. A thin area of the iris is selected for the laser interaction. Either the argon or the Nd:YAG laser beam can be used to perform the iridectomy. Short-duration pulses are used with either laser to make a small hole in the iris to allow the aqueous humor to flow from the posterior chamber (Figure 4-13).

Sometimes the argon laser uses a larger spot size (200 µm) with low power (200 to 300 mW) to place a coagulative spot on the iris. The spot size is then decreased to 50 µm, and the laser power is increased to 600 to 1000 mW to make an adequate opening in the center of the initial argon spot. The Nd:YAG laser can be used instead of the argon laser to pop the hole in the center of the coagulated area. This technique decreases the chance of bleeding from the iris and helps ensure that the iridotomy will stay open. An Nd:YAG laser may also be used alone to perform this procedure.

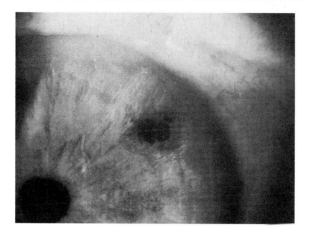

FIG. 4-13 Laser iridectomy.

After any laser glaucoma procedure, a tonometry reading will be performed to note the intraocular pressure. In addition to the procedure, topical prednisolone or dexamethasone drops should be instilled to help control the glaucoma.

Other Laser Treatment Techniques for Glaucoma

Contact Nd:YAG laser technology has been used to effectively decrease intraocular pressure using synthetic sapphire delivery tips during transscleral cyclophotocoagulation and internal sclerostomy. These procedures have been successful with patients who have not responded well to other treatments or who have a poor prognosis.

Transscleral cyclophotocoagulation involves the application of a special convex probe to the external surface of the eye above the ciliary body (Figure 4-14). The laser energy is transmitted through the cornea and sclera and is absorbed by the melanin pigmentation of the ciliary body, where the aqueous humor is produced. Through controlled coagulation, the ciliary body begins to atrophy and produce less aqueous humor. There are virtually no thermal effects to the sclera or conjunctiva.

This procedure can be performed in the physician's office or in the operating room. The patient is placed in a supine position. A retrobulbar or peribulbar injection is administered to decrease discomfort during the procedure. A lid speculum is placed in the eye to be treated; the other eye is usually patched. During the procedure the cornea is kept moist with drops of balanced saline solution.

The probe is positioned over the ciliary body perpendicular to the surface of the eye. Approximately 7 W of Nd:YAG laser energy is delivered through the convex probe at 0.7 seconds per pulse. Usually 28 to 32 spots are applied circumferentially about 0.5 to 1.0 mm from the limbus (the site at which the cornea and sclera meet.) The 3- and 9-o'clock positions are avoided to protect the long ciliary arteries from thermal damage.

Immediately after the procedure, the eye is patched for 4 to 6 hours, and anti-inflammatory medications are administered topically. Intraocular pressure may rise immediately after the procedure, but a decrease in pressure is noticed soon after that. The physician sees the patient in follow-up visits to regulate any miotic medication used to enhance the

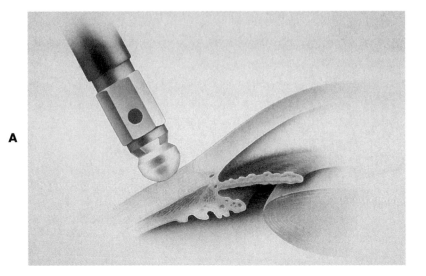

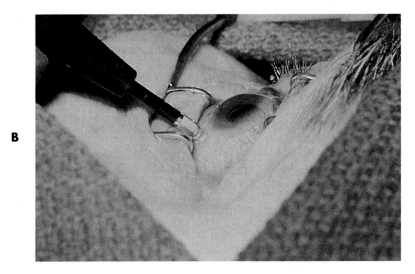

FIG. 4-14   **A** and **B** Transscleral cyclophotocoagulation. (Courtesy Surgical Laser Technologies, Inc., Oaks, PA.)

surgical effects. The procedure may be performed again after 2 weeks if pressure reduction is not adequate.

Patients with darker pigmented eyes may require less laser energy to achieve acceptable results. Darker pigmentation actually may absorb and distribute the laser energy, thus increasing the process of cyclodestruction. Therefore, less wattage is needed for these patients (Schuman, et al 1990).

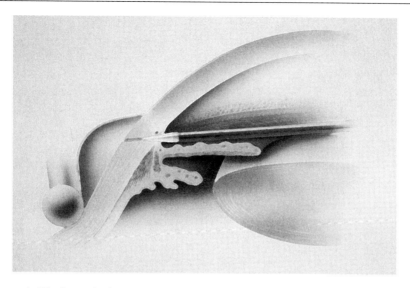

FIG. 4-15   Internal sclerostomy. (Courtesy Surgical Laser Technologies, Inc., Oaks, PA.)

Internal sclerostomy, a full-thickness filtering procedure performed under local or general anesthesia, can also control glaucoma. During this procedure, a very slender contact Nd:YAG scalpel is introduced through the cornea (Figure 4-15). The scalpel traverses the anterior chamber to an angle of 180 degrees from the opening to be made in the trabecular meshwork. A conjunctival bleb is made using balanced salt solution to protect the conjunctiva by pulling it away from the impact area. A muscle hook is used to raise the bleb to change the angle of the trabecular meshwork. The laser is activated at 10 W for 0.1 to 0.2 seconds for one or two firings. An opening is then made through the trabecular meshwork, thus providing full-thickness filtration. A simultaneous peripheral iridectomy can be performed during this procedure.

Internal sclerostomy can also be performed using the holmium laser in an office type of surgical environment. Since adjacent tissue damage is limited to 300 µm and less, great precision is afforded. Thermal holmium laser sclerostomy is performed by first making a 1-mm conjunctival stab about 12 to 15 mm from the intended sclerostomy site. A narrow probe is inserted and advanced to the limbus. Laser energy is delivered at an approximate 90-degree angle, enabling the sclerostomy to be created without an incision in the overlying conjunctiva. The creation of the sclerostomy is confirmed with visualization of small bubbles in the anterior chamber and movement of the iris. This treatment facilitates the flow of aqueous humor, and the intraocular pressure decreases.

In another procedure, which is used to treat glaucoma conditions that are more difficult to control, diode laser energy is directed through a microendoscope. Approximately 200 to 300 mW of diode laser energy is delivered directly to each visualized ciliary body for about 1 to 2 seconds until shrinkage and whitening is visualized. The sclerostomy site and conjunctiva are closed, and antiinflammatory drops are instilled. Intraocular pressure drops 2 to 4 weeks after treatment (Uram, 1992).

POSTERIOR CAPSULOTOMY

The crystalline lens is located directly behind the iris and is surrounded by a cellophane-like membrane called a capsule. A cataract or cloudy lens can be caused by a number of conditions, including trauma, age, certain diseases such as diabetes, and genetic or hereditary conditions. Usually the lens becomes cloudy from a natural change in the lens chemical composition.

The most popular approach for cataract extraction today is the extracapsular technique. This procedure removes the lens but leaves the posterior capsule (secondary membrane) shell in place. An artificial intraocular lens is then placed in the eye and is supported and stabilized by the posterior capsule. This secondary membrane also provides a barrier, keeping the vitreous humor from escaping into the front portion of the eye during the healing process.

After 1 to 3 years, many patients who have had cataract surgery may again experience cloudy vision. This cloudiness does not involve the artificial lens, though most patients believe that the cataract has formed again since vision is decreased. Instead, the posterior capsule has become clouded from a migration of cells that cause opacification.

The conventional method of treatment before the advent of the laser was to perform a capsular discission. This technique involves introducing a needle-tipped knife into the eye to cut a small opening in the clouded membrane. Hospitalization was necessary because this procedure required surgical entry into the eye.

Today the Nd:YAG pulsed laser is used to destroy the clouded posterior capsule. Preoperatively, a pupillary dilating drop may be administered to widen the field of vision. This medication is contraindicated for patients who have glaucoma because dilating the pupil may further increase intraocular pressure. The patient is positioned at the slit lamp with the chin supported on the frame. The nurse may help stabilize the patient's head during the procedure, especially if small tremors cause the patient to move inadvertently.

Posterior capsulotomy can be performed using the Q-switched or mode-locked Nd:YAG laser. These lasers produce a powerful thermal-acoustical effect within a very small spot using a minimal amount of energy and a short-pulse duration. The Nd:YAG beam is focused on the clouded secondary membrane. Photodisruption occurs as the laser energy causes electrons to be stripped from the atoms, creating a plasma shield of electrons and ions. This energy reaction produces a shock wave, or acoustical effect, that rips apart the clouded membrane (Figure 4-16). The impact of the laser is confined to the focal area of the beam. A series of holes is placed in the membrane as it begins to fold back to be reabsorbed into the body. When the physician has determined that the opening in the capsule is adequate for vision, the procedure is complete. The patient has no pain but sees a bright light and hears the clicking noise of the laser. The total laser time may vary between 1 and 5 minutes depending upon the thickness of the capsule and the skill of the physician (Figure 4-17).

There are a few complications associated with the posterior capsulotomy. The surface of the implanted lens may be pitted from unfocused laser energy because the lens is very close to the laser-tissue interaction area. A slight increase in intraocular pressure may occur postoperatively but is usually temporary. Other complications, including bleeding, iritis, and retinal problems are very rare but can occur.

Postoperatively, a topical steroid may be prescribed to reduce inflammation. As soon as the effects of the dilating medication subsides, an examination is performed to note the

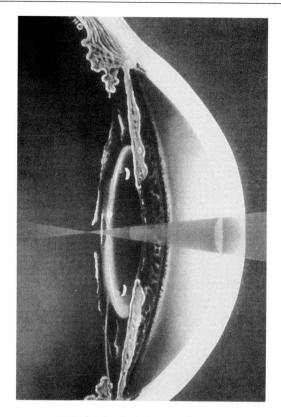

FIG. 4-16   Posterior capsulotomy.

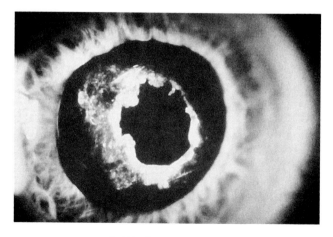

FIG. 4-17   Posterior capsulotomy.

patient's visual acuity. Usually a postoperative tonometry reading is taken to ensure that the procedure has not caused an increase in intraocular pressure. A follow-up examination is scheduled to evaluate the true results of the procedure.

RECENT OPHTHALMOLOGICAL LASER APPLICATIONS

Laser Photocoagulation for Trichiasis

Occasionally an aberrant eyelash growing on the undersurface of the eyelid will cause great discomfort as it irritates the surface of the eye. The cause of this condition may be idiopathic, congenital, posttraumatic, or inflammatory. Chronic conjunctival and corneal irritation can lead to more severe consequences that may affect vision.

Conventional surgery for trichiasis involves a full-thickness wedge resection of the abnormal area of the eyelid where the misdirected eyelash is growing. This surgery may be followed by associated scar formation and continued irritation.

With topical anesthesia, the argon laser has been proven effective in destroying the trichiatic cilia. With minimum adjacent tissue damage, the argon laser energy is directed through the slit lamp to the abnormal follicle using a 50- to 200-μm spot, 0.1- to 0.2-second duration, and 1000 to 1200 mW of power. A crater of at least 2 mm is created along the intradermal shaft of the eyelash to adequately destroy the hair follicles (Awan, 1988).

Capsule Contraction Syndrome

After a cataract extraction, the implanted lens may become displaced even if it has been correctly positioned in the capsular bag. The lens may move out of alignment with the central zone when the lens capsule shrinks asymmetrically . The ophthalmic Nd:YAG laser has been used successfully to perform a relaxing anterior capsulotomy at 2 to 3 weeks after cataract surgery. Active capsular fibrosis and contracture of the anterior capsule can be influenced with early treatment (Davison, 1993). This procedure is still being refined to provide even better results.

Photorefractive Surgical Procedures

The excimer laser is currently being investigated for correcting refractive eye disorders such as myopia, hyperopia, and astigmatism. The precision of this wavelength is valuable because one cell at a time can be affected with no significant thermal buildup.

The conventional radial keratotomy procedure is performed using a diamond-tipped knife to make a series of cuts in the periphery of the cornea. These cuts must penetrate 90% of the cornea to correct the refractive disorder. Weakening the cornea in this manner makes further complications possible. The incisions may heal too vigorously, causing some regression of corneal flattening and therefore some loss of corrective effect.

The argon fluoride (ArF) excimer laser, at 193 nm, is being used for photorefractive keratectomy (PRK) (Figure 4-18). PRK is performed to ablate the central portion of the cornea, thus sculpting the cornea to the desired thickness. The accuracy of this laser allows excision or incision of the cornea precisely at predetermined depths. The excimer laser, using short pulsations, does not significantly impair the corneal transparency or cause optical degradation. A computer-controlled scanning system has been combined with the laser to provide ultimate precision. A corneal topography unit has been added to many of the excimer lasers to provide immediate corneal measurements, which are vital to the success of this procedure. Since the ablation of corneal tissue is directly over the pupil, a postoperative complication of corneal hazing may result from this removal of tissue on the optical zone. A sample of postoperative discharge instructions is provided on pp. 128-129.

A technique called corneal reprofiling seems to be an effective alternative to this procedure. Reprofiling the cornea involves shaving through only 10% of the corneal thickness with the excimer laser to shape a corneal contact-lenslike correction on the surface of the eye. Since the cornea is primarily responsible for 60% to 70% of focusing, changing the shape of the cornea curvature allows a change in the focusing of the light on the retina. Therefore, poor eyesight caused by refractive disorders can be corrected.

Excimer systems are being refined and coupled with scanning units to enhance PRK. Other lasers wavelengths are being investigated for performing refractive surgery. Most of these lasers are solid-state systems that do not require the toxic gases that excimer lasers use. Some lasers are equipped with a tracking system to reduce decentration and make complex ablation patterns.

A solid-state Nd:YLF laser that generates picosecond pulses is being investigated for intrastromal procedures to refractive surgery. The cornea consists of five layers: the epithelium, Bowman's membrane, the stromal layer, Descemet's membrane, and the endothelial layer. An applanation system is used to flatten the cornea to permit correction of refractive disorders by removing intrastromal corneal tissue without cutting the surface of the cornea or disrupting the epithelium or Bowman's membrane. This technique is expected to eliminate corneal scarring, hazing, and fluctuations in visual acuity.

The holmium:YAG laser is also being used to perform intrastromal refractive procedures. With a wavelength of 2100 nm, approximately 20 to 30 short laser pulses of about 10 ms each gently heats the stromal layer of the cornea. This causes localized shortening of the stromal collagen fibers, resulting in the shortening of the simultaneous flattening of the cornea. The optical center of the cornea is left untouched. The postoperative goal is to ensure that the cornea remains stable from 3 to 6 months after the postoperative healing process is complete.

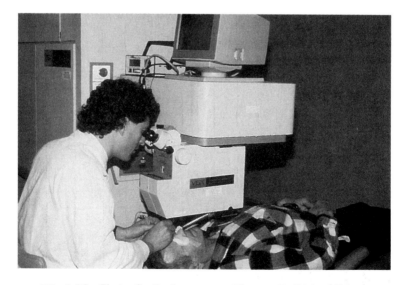

FIG. 4-18   Photorefractive keratectomy. (Courtesy Dr. Richard Erdey.)

Sample Postoperative Discharge Instructions:
Photorefractive Keratectomy

IMMEDIATELY AFTER SURGERY:

Go home and place 1 drop of antibiotic solution and 1 drop of antiinflammatory solution in the operated eye. Take a sleeping pill, if needed, to help you relax so you will go to sleep. If you cannot sleep, try to rest and keep your operated eye closed.

General cleanliness:

Do not get anything in your eye during the first 2 weeks, especially particulate matter such as mascara. If you do, your eye will hurt, and you will greatly increase the risk of infection. Keep all foreign matter out of your eye, including soap and water. Avoid swimming for 2 weeks. Wear protective eyewear for racket sports at all times.

The first day after surgery:

The morning after surgery, your eye may still be somewhat sore and sensitive to touch. Do not touch or rub your eye. Your vision will probably be somewhat blurry, especially if you are over age 40. You can expect your vision to clear by mid-afternoon. The redness and irritation will subside after you begin using the drops.

Drops:

You will be using an antibiotic drop in the operated eye. Put 1 drop in your eye four times a day for 2 weeks or as otherwise directed. Expect the drops to sting when you put them in. Lubricating drops can be used to relieve the dry, irritated feeling in your eye. Use the antiinflammatory drops as directed.

THE SECOND DAY AFTER SURGERY:

By the second day, you should be feeling quite well except for a sense of scratching of your cornea that will be somewhat relieved by the drops. You will again have morning blurriness, which will clear by afternoon. You can also expect some dimming of your vision in the evening. You may use artificial tears for the scratchiness. These may be repeated as often as necessary.

THE FOLLOWING DAYS:

Expect your vision to fluctuate during the first few weeks. It will probably be blurry in the mornings but clear in the afternoons. However, the reverse pattern might also occur. You can expect dimming of vision in the evening for awhile. You may also notice some sensitivity to light. These symptoms and any pain you might have will decrease each day. Get plenty of rest.

FOLLOW-UP VISITS:

You will need to come in for a checkup periodically. If you have any questions or unusual problems after the surgery, please call the office during office hours. After office hours, the answering service will contact the physician for you.

Sample Postoperative Discharge Instructions:
Photorefractive Keratectomy—cont'd

SURGERY OF THE SECOND EYE:

If the initial surgery is not performed on both eyes, then surgery for the second eye can be scheduled. If you are wearing a soft contact lens, remove the lens 3 days before surgery. If you are wearing a hard contact lens, remove the lens 3 weeks before surgery.

Discharge instructions courtesy of Dr.Richard Erdey.

Cataract Extraction

The excimer laser is also being investigated for use in cataract extraction. The excimer wavelength is delivered directly to the lens through a very small puncture site to decompose and fragment the nucleus of the cataract. This procedure has been computerized for accuracy and complete fragmentation of the lens. A tiny corneal-scleral incision is made in the eye to extract the cataract debris through an aspiration tube. Intracapsular hydrogels or a foldable silicone intraocular lens is then inserted through the small incision.

The erbium(ER):YAG laser, at 2940 nm, has also been introduced to perform an anterior capsulotomy during the cataract extraction. A circle is inscribed on the surface of the anterior capsule using the Er:YAG laser. The tactile sensation offered by the special handpiece enhances maneuverability and accuracy. The lens is then removed through the capsulotomy, decreasing the risk of radial tears. The capsulotomy then allows for smooth insertion of a posterior chamber intraocular lens (IOL). Postoperatively, there is less chance of displacement of the IOL since there has been minimal trauma to the capsule. Investigations have also used the Er:YAG laser to facilitate nucleus extraction (laser emulsion) of the cataract lens and lysis of vitreous bands.

Oculoplastics and Other Ophthalmological Procedures

The CO_2, contact Nd:YAG, holmium:YAG, and other lasers are used during oculoplastic surgeries because of the needed precision and hemostasis. Tissue can be cut, coagulated, and vaporized with minimum damage to the surrounding healthy tissue. For example, the laser can be used to remove an eyelid tumor. Ocular tumors, such as retinoblastoma, malignant melanoma of the choroid, and retinal angioma, have been treated with laser photocoagulation.

Treating retinoblastoma usually requires a combination of laser therapy and chemotherapy or radiation therapy. Sometimes laser therapy is used as the sole treatment for smaller tumors. The focus of the laser procedure is aimed at the tumor's blood supply and not at the tumor itself.

Malignant melanoma of the choroid has been effectively treated with argon laser photocoagulation. The tumor is treated directly to coagulate and destroy it. The thickness of the tumor determines the effectiveness of the argon beam's penetration. Laser photodynamic therapy has also been employed investigationally to selectively destroy the tumor. A light-sensitive dye is injected systemically into the patient. The tumor retains the dye; the other body cells eliminate the dye. When a laser light of a specific wavelength is exposed to the tumor, the dye is activated, and a reaction occurs that destroys the tumor cells very selectively. There is little damage to the adjacent normal cells.

The laser can also be used to treat an abnormal formation of new blood vessels on the cornea. Sometimes this condition is promoted by the use of contact lenses or is associated with a corneal growth known as a pterygium. The laser is used to seal off the progression of these new blood vessels before vision is obscured.

Other uses of laser technology in ophthalmology include using laser energy to cut stitches in the cornea or other areas of the eye after surgery. The laser has also been employed to treat dry eyes. The beam of light narrows or closes tear duct drains in the eyelids to help retain moisture on the surface of the eye.

REFERENCES

Awan KJ: Laser photocoagulation-vaporization therapy of trichiasis, *Ophthalmic Laser Therapy* 3(1):3, 1988.

Davison JA: Capsule contraction syndrome, *Journal of Cataract Refract Surg,* 19:582-589, Sept 1993.

Puliafito, CA: Choroidal neovascularization: Dye-enhanced diagnosis and treatment, Wayland, MA, 1991, Candela Laser Corp.

Schuman JS, et al: Contact transscleral continuous wave Neodymium:YAG laser cyclophotocoagulation. *Ophthalmology* 97:571-580, 1990.

Uram, M: Ophthalmic laser microendoscope ciliary process ablation in the management of neovascular glaucoma, *Ophthalmology* 99(12):1829-1832, 1992.

SUGGESTED READINGS

Apfelberg DB, editor: *Evaluation and installation of surgical laser systems,* New York, 1987, Springer-Verlag.

Geyer O and Lazar M: Laser therapy of eye diseases, *Lasers Surg Med* 6:423, 1986.

Iscoff R, editor: Excimer lasers in ophthalmology, *Lasers and Optics* 65, Nov 1987.

Langseth FG: Transscleral cyclophotocoagulation, a laser treatment for glaucoma, *AORN* 48(6):1122, 1988.

Meeker MH and Rothrock JC: *Alexander's care of the patient in surgery,* St. Louis, 1995, Mosby.

5

EAR, NOSE, AND THROAT AND RELATED LASER APPLICATIONS

L aser application in the field of otorhinolaryngology began in 1967 when Dr. Geza Jako coupled the use of the laser with the use of the microscope (Jako, 1986). The laser has become the instrument of choice for many benign lesions of the upper aerodigestive tract, including polyps, papillomas, and other benign conditions. The laser has also significantly proved its worth in cancer treatment. Advances continue as the laser's precision and convenience is realized by ear, nose, and throat (ENT) and head and neck specialists.

LASER PROCEDURES FOR THE EAR

Laser Stapedectomy

The middle ear contains three small bones or ossicles called the malleus, incus, and stapes (Figure 5-1). The footplate of the stapes fits into the oval window, which leads into the inner ear. The ossicles of the middle ear conduct sound vibrations from the eardrum to the oval window. The sound waves are then conducted to the round window to be changed into electrochemical impulses within the cochlea.

Otosclerosis causes immobility of the stapes footplate as an overgrowth of spongy bone forms around the stapes. The sound vibrations cannot be transmitted from the stapes into the oval window, and a decrease in auditory sensation results. The cause of this condition is not known, but hereditary trends have been indicated. Slow progressive hearing loss characterizes this condition, and the patient may complain of buzzing or ringing, usually in both ears.

The treatment of choice is to remove the stapes and insert a prosthesis that will conduct the sound waves into the oval window. Many times the footplate is left in place, and a hole is drilled in it to position a stapes prosthesis. A mechanical drill can cause vibrations that may disrupt the footplate during the procedure. The laser has been introduced to refine this procedure because it can be used to delicately drill a hole in the stapes footplate or loosen the stapes for removal. Since the laser energy does not actually cause vibratory movements, the procedure can be performed much more precisely, thus leading to better results.

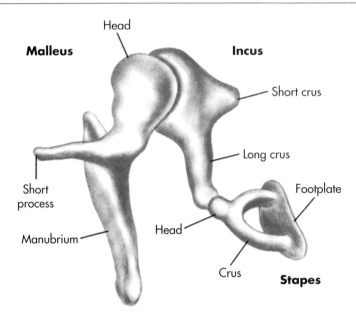

Malleus

Head

Incus

Short crus

Long crus

Short
process

Footplate

Manubrium

Head

Crus

Stapes

FIG. 5-1   Anatomy of the ear. (From Thompson JM et al: *Mosby's clinical nursing,* ed 3, St. Louis, 1993, Mosby.)

Laser stapedectomy is usually performed under local anesthesia supplemented with intravenous sedation if needed. The tympanomeatal flap is turned, using the conventional methods, to expose the middle ear bones.

Argon, frequency doubled YAG, or CO_2 laser energy is delivered to the tissue during this procedure in two different ways. The laser can be connected to the microscope and delivered to the tissue via a micromanipulator. The disadvantage of this method is that the laser beam must be in the same visual axis as that of the microscope, therefore positioning is sometimes a problem. The laser energy can also be delivered to the tissue using a handpiece chosen from a selection of handpieces of various sizes and angle shapes. With an angled handpiece, the laser energy can be delivered from different positions.

The stapedial tendon is sometimes vaporized using laser energy (Figure 5-2). After exposing the bones of the middle ear, the stapes is disarticulated using low settings of laser energy, and the superstructure of the stapes is removed (Figure 5-3). A fenestration is made in the footplate with the laser light approximately 0.4 to 0.8 mm in diameter (Figure 5-4). Since the laser does not produce vibratory movements, a hole in a loose or floating footplate can be precisely made. This cannot be accomplished as easily using any other tool. The fine bone char is removed by gentle suctioning through a microsuction instrument.

A stapes prosthesis is secured to communicate between the incus and the oval window (Figure 5-5). The patient's hearing may be evaluated at this time (if local anesthesia is used) by whispering to the patient, by gently touching the malleus to produce a vibratory sensation, or through intraoperative audiometry. Finally, tiny squares of moistened absorbable gelatin sponges are placed around the prosthesis to stabilize it. A tissue seal of fascia or perichondrium may also be used for stabilization. The tympanic flap is returned

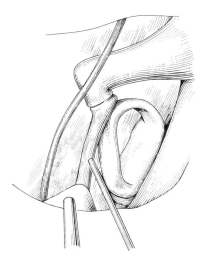

FIG. 5-2   Laser vaporization of the stapedial tendon.

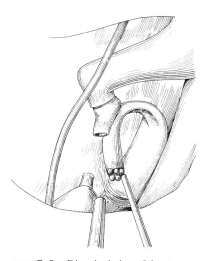

FIG. 5-3   Disarticulation of the stapes.

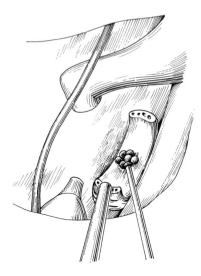

FIG. 5-4   Using laser energy to drill a hole in the footplate.

to its normal position, and the external ear canal is packed with a cotton ball or more gelatin sponge material.

Patient education involves instructing the patient not to lie on the operative ear for the first 24 hours after the surgery. Vertigo should be expected because the inner ear, where balance is controlled, has been invaded. The patient should be instructed to move slowly to alleviate these unpleasant symptoms. Coughing, sneezing, and nose-blowing should be avoided because the pressure buildup from these actions could dislodge the prosthesis. Hearing will probably decrease temporarily as healing occurs but should improve gradu-

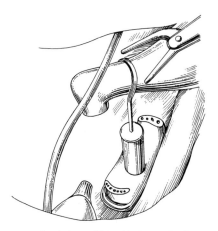

FIG. 5-5   A stapes prosthesis is positioned between the incus and oval window.

ally, usually over a 6-week period. The patient should not swim for several months after the procedure so that contaminants are not introduced into the ear. Flying is not recommended because the pressure changes may alter the results of the surgery.

Other Otological Laser Applications

Argon, frequency doubled YAG, contact Nd:YAG, and CO_2 lasers have been used to vaporize, cut, and coagulate during different ear procedures. The technological advances achieved with each of these lasers have offered delivery systems that provide extremely small spot sizes and high accessibility for application.

Vaporization of scar tissue, granulomas, cholesteatoma, and mucosal bands has been performed precisely without causing damage to surrounding healthy tissues.

Cutting has been achieved by increasing the power and decreasing the spot size of the beam. The laser has been used to divide the vestibular nerve for patients who have severe vertigo with nausea and vomiting. The argon and frequency doubled YAG lasers have been used to divide the vestibular portion of the eighth nerve with great precision without damaging adjacent auditory fibers.

Coagulation with the laser during otological applications controls bleeding during a procedure. The power of the beam is decreased and the spot size is increased to provide hemostasis. Hemostasis has been achieved during a variety of procedures, such as stopping microbleeding on the facial nerve sheath with argon laser energy during facial nerve decompression.

New laser applications continue to be explored for use in more common procedures. Studies are being conducted to compare the success of laser myringotomy with that of the cost-effective conventional method. Researchers are attempting to determine how long the hole will stay patent so as to eliminate the need to insert myringotomy tubes.

LASER PROCEDURES FOR THE NOSE AND SINUS

Different laser wavelengths, delivery systems, and techniques have expanded the use of laser technology for nasal and sinus procedures. The anatomy of the nose and sinuses is illustrated in Figure 5-6.

Laser Surgery for Sinus Conditions

The laser has been combined with the sinuscope to provide access into sinus cavities and treat a variety of conditions. The CO_2, holmium, argon, frequency doubled YAG, and the contact Nd:YAG lasers are being used to precisely vaporize and excise sinus tissue and lesions.

Sinus conditions are identified by symptoms such as headaches, congestion, facial pain, chronic infections, and difficult breathing. Initially, sinus conditions are usually treated with medications, such as antibiotics and decongestants. Other treatment alternatives need to be considered when medications become ineffective and the symptoms become chronic.

Endoscopic sinus surgery can be performed using the conventional dry environment or by using a fluid medium. When the contact Nd:YAG laser is used in a fluid environment, the depth of tissue penetration is precisely controlled. Warm saline can be used to continually lavage the sinus cavity. Hemostasis is achieved because the warm fluid causes vasoconstriction of the mucosa. Also, the continuous irrigation removes debris, thus providing

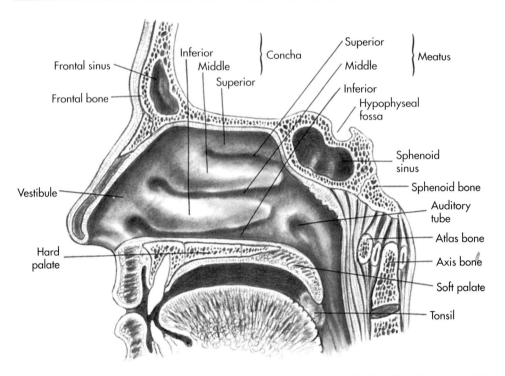

FIG. 5-6   Anatomy of the nose and sinuses. (From Thompson JM et al: *Mosby's clinical nursing,* ed 3, St. Louis, 1993, Mosby.)

clear vision of the anatomical structures and pathology. The irrigant flow helps keep the lens of the endoscope clean and free of tissue buildup. A special lens cleaner pad may be used before the scope is inserted, to keep the lens clean and defogged during the procedure. This eliminates the need to constantly withdraw the scope to wipe the end and enables the surgeon to maintain constant visual contact with landmarks within the sinus cavity. The laser energy causes hemostasis; therefore, postoperative packing is not needed.

The laser has been used to perform sinus polypectomy, to treat deformities to improve sinus drainage, and for revision sinus surgery. Many other techniques are being developed that use the combined technologies of laser energy and endoscopy.

Laser Surgery for Allergic Rhinitis

Allergic rhinitis is a common otolaryngological condition that is usually treated with antiallergenic drugs or desensitizing injections. Argon, CO_2, Nd:YAG, and frequency doubled YAG lasers have been used to treat this disease, with significant results.

The patient with allergic rhinitis complains of sneezing, watery eyes, continual nasal discharge, and nasal stuffiness. The patient qualifies for laser treatment if other conventional methods have failed and the patient has a positive allergic response to certain environmental contaminants, such as house dust. Sometimes the laser procedure is performed in a series of treatments or in one surgical treatment. Postoperative complications such as bleeding and swelling are sometimes reduced when the laser applications are performed in a series of multiple superficial treatments.

Laser surgery for allergic rhinitis is performed on an outpatient basis. A local anesthetic is administered to the nasal mucosa. Pieces of gauze soaked with epinephrine are applied to the mucosa to shrink the turbinates.

A CO_2 laser can be used to vaporize the entire surface of the inferior turbinate through special hand-piece tubes designed specifically for this procedure. The tube delivers the CO_2 laser energy to the inferior turbinate area, which is thought to be the area of sensitivity to irritants. The CO_2 laser causes superficial coagulation that prevents bleeding; therefore, postoperative packing is not necessary. Scar tissue forms in the superficial submucosal area of the inferior turbinate and thus eliminates or decreases the allergic reaction. A subsequent alteration has also been thought to occur in the autonomic nervous system, which controls the vasoactive response and prevents changes in turbinate size and secretions.

The frequency doubled YAG or argon laser is also being used to treat allergic rhinitis. A flexible endoscope is positioned to visualize the inferior turbinate. The mucosa is photocoagulated with traversing sweeps across the areas from anterior to posterior and then from superior to inferior. If the middle turbinate appears to be involved, then this area is also treated. Complications that could occur include hemorrhage, atrophy, and synechia. Edema may occur immediately after surgery but usually subsides within 3 to 5 days. Complete reepithelialization of the turbinate occurs within 2 to 4 weeks.

Laser Turbinectomy

A turbinectomy is performed to provide adequate ventilation. Polyps may also be removed to enhance airway passages. By removing a section of the turbinate or polyps, drainage is promoted and pressure against the floor of the nose is relieved.

The CO_2 laser was initially used to reduce the size of turbinate bodies. This tool allows for ablation and vaporization of the turbinates with significantly less blood loss. Postoperatively, the patient has less pain during the healing process. The drawbacks of using the CO_2 laser for this application are the awkward delivery systems needed to access the turbinate area, interference from the reflected helium-neon aiming beam on the mucosal lining, sometimes questionable hemostasis, and the tremendous skill required to control the CO_2 beam in this restricted area. With the development of CO_2 waveguides and smaller handpieces, easier access is now possible.

The synthetic sapphire contact probe used to deliver Nd:YAG laser energy is also being used for laser turbinectomy. This technology allows actual tissue contact with the delivery device and decreased adjacent tissue damage as a result of the localization of the laser energy. The Nd:YAG laser energy is directed to the turbinate through a cone-shaped laser probe. The back part of the turbinate is vaporized, and the laser moves towards the front until most or all of the turbinate has been treated.

Postoperative instructions for laser turbinectomy include reminding the patient to avoid coughing, sneezing, nose-blowing, and even bending over. Any of these activities can increase the intranasal pressure and can cause coagulated vessels to be disrupted. Intraoperative bleeding and postoperative complications have sometimes decreased with the use of contact Nd:YAG technology.

Laser Treatment of Nasolacrimal Duct Surgery

The frequency doubled YAG, contact Nd:YAG, and holmium:YAG laser have been used to treat nasolacrimal duct obstructions. These obstructions inhibit the flow of tears from the eyes, resulting in recurrent infections and chronic tearing. The traditional treatment has been to perform a dacryocystorhinostomy (DCR) by first making an external incision near the medial canthus. Dissection to the lacrimal bone and nasal mucosa produces a rhinostomy and a passage for tear drainage. The disadvantage of this procedure is that an external incision has to be made, and there is a potential risk of damaging the external lacrimal system.

With the use of a small nasal endoscope (30 degrees) to view the superior nasal cavity, the intranasal approach to DCR can be visualized. Usually the combined skills of an ophthalmologist and an ENT specialist are needed. The procedure is performed under general anesthesia, topical anesthesia, and topical vasoconstriction (4% cocaine nasal pledgets). The eye is protected with a special scleral protector. Low-wattage settings at interrupted pulses are used to ablate nasal mucosa and the underlying bone to form a rhinostomy. A stent is inserted into the rhinostomy and sometimes is left in place for 6 months. The stent can be removed in the physician's office (Peterson and Finch, 1992).

Laser Treatment for Other Nasal Conditions

Epistaxis (nosebleed) is being treated with the argon and the frequency doubled YAG (KTP) laser. The selectivity of these beams to vascular tissue causes the laser energy to be selectively absorbed into the tissue, but not into the underlying cartilage or bone. Scar tissue then helps decrease the incidence of epistaxis.

Hereditary hemorrhagic telangiectasia is being successfully treated by spraying the laser energy onto the involved areas of the septum, turbinates, and nasal walls. Because the depth penetration of these wavelengths is controlled, the septum is preserved.

The laser is being used to debulk intranasal polyps so that a dry field is maintained throughout the surgery. The procedure can be performed under local anesthesia with minimal blood loss.

Laser intervention can be used to treat patients who have granuloma formations in the nose from chronic infection resulting from cocaine abuse. The laser coagulates and vaporizes the abnormal nasal mucosa, leading to a return of normal nasal mucosa and function within 6 to 8 weeks.

Symptoms of chronic sinusitis, tearing, and nasal obstruction can be associated with scarring from previous nasal surgeries. The scars can be vaporized with laser energy without much incidence of rescarring.

LASER MICROLARYNGOSCOPY

Laser application during a microlaryngoscopy has become the standard of care for endoscopic treatment of many benign and malignant lesions in the larynx. Advances in this area have refined the delivery systems and enhanced exposure for better visualization.

Indications for Laser Microlaryngoscopy

Laser microlaryngoscopy is performed for a variety of disorders, including papillomatosis, laryngeal and subglottic stenosis, granulomas, nodules, paralysis of the vocal cords, and carcinomas.

Papillomatosis is a condition involving widespread formation of papillomas, which are benign epithelial tumors. The laser is used to precisely shave the papilloma from the vocal cord while preserving the normal laryngeal structures. Since laser intervention cannot cure this recurrent disease, the goal of laser therapy is to maintain the airway and voice. Many times the rate of regrowth is tremendously decreased when the laser is used. The frequency of laser treatments depends on the rate of regrowth of the papillomas.

Laryngeal and subglottic stenosis is also treated with laser microlaryngoscopy. Scar tissue can be effectively removed with laser energy, but the recurrence of this scarring remains a problem. The timing of supplemental therapy involving laser vaporization, lesion steroid injections, periodic dilatations, stents, and microtrapdoor flaps seems to be the key to successfully treating this condition. Anterior lesions sometimes respond better to laser therapy than do posterior lesions. If the severity of the condition does not subside within two or three laser applications, then future laser treatment will probably fail also.

Granulomas are vaporized when the source of irritation cannot be removed and continues to intensify the condition. The granuloma is grasped and then excised from the vocal cord using the lowest possible power density. Any charred material must be removed so that irritation does not foster regrowth of the granuloma.

Nodules are excised with the laser using the lowest power settings and the shortest exposure time to decrease adjacent tissue damage. A backstop is held behind the nodule so that the beam will not strike other areas accidentally. Voice rest is important to decrease the chance of nodule recurrence.

Paralysis of the vocal cords is successfully treated with endoscopic laser arytenoidectomy. The arytenoid cartilage supports the posterior portion of the true vocal cords. Surgery to excise and vaporize this area has helped improve the airway by moving the vocal cords. Postoperatively, the formation of webs or fibrosis that could compromise the airway is a complication that must be recognized.

Excision of carcinomas with the laser is performed in selected cases with success and precision. More research is required to validate the advantages of using the laser in this application.

Before anesthesia induction, steroids are administered intravenously to decrease the chances of postoperative edema secondary to excisional biopsy or laryngoscopy. The biopsy specimen to be excised is outlined and removed with laser energy. Depending on its pathology, the specimen is evaluated immediately to determine the status of the margins. If the margins are positive for malignancy, then another biopsy specimen is excised and sent to the pathology department for evaluation. The procedure is continued until the margins are free from tumor, or the inner perichondrium of the thyroid or arytenoid cartilage is encountered. If the procedure is stopped for the latter reason, then adjunctive radiation treatment therapy or an external surgical approach may be recommended. Patients are followed closely after surgery for early detection of any recurrence.

When the laser is used for malignant tumor removal during microlaryngoscopy, many advantages can be noted. The hemostatic effects of the laser result in less bleeding both during and after surgery. The precision of the laser preserves the integrity of the normal healthy tissue. There is less spread of malignant cells to other areas of the body because of the sealing effect of the laser energy on the lymphatic system. The laser procedure is repeatable in the future, in contrast to radiation therapy. The surgical field is sterilized from the thermal effect of the laser energy. There is minimal tissue trauma, leading to a decrease in postoperative edema and other complications. The laser also helps to debaulk neoplasms that can cause swallowing disorders and airway obstruction, and may eliminate the need to perform a tracheostomy.

Anesthesia Concerns and Safety Precautions

When the laser is being used in the patient's airway, extreme caution must be taken to avoid airway fires. A sample policy addressing airway safety is provided on page 141.

Since the laser produces concentrated power, an unprotected polyvinylchloride (PVC) endotracheal tube can easily be ignited (Figure 5-7). The gases flowing through the tube can easily support combustion during administration of the anesthetic. An unprotected PVC endotracheal tube must never be used because it can immediately be converted into a "blow torch" if ignited by a laser beam and will then emit offensive hydrogen chloride fumes. The patient could sustain extensive burns, suffer from airway obstruction, and even die. Teamwork among the nurse, surgeon, anesthesiologist, and nurse anesthetist is critical to ensure safe and appropriate use of the laser during microlaryngoscopy.

The *type of endotracheal (ET) tube* selected for the laser microlaryngoscopy should be documented. There are special ET tubes currently on the market that will withstand specific amounts of laser impact. These tubes either have been coated with a laser-resistant material or are made of a substance that does not readily ignite. There are also flexible metal ET tubes that will withstand limited laser impact. Special attention must be paid to how much laser energy each tube can withstand. These limitations must be strictly followed.

A special fire-retardant wrap has been introduced to promote laser safety. The wrap is applied to the surface of a red rubber PVC ET tube. The wrap has a foil layer that withstands certain amounts of laser energy. The rough external surface of the wrap is moistened before intubation for softening to decrease potential tracheal trauma on intubation. Manufacturer's recommendations on laser power limitations must be followed.

A red rubber ET tube wrapped with 0.25-inch, self-adhesive foil or metallic tape protects the ET tube from higher laser powers. Reports have noted that up to 70 W of CO_2 laser energy or up to 50 W of Nd:YAG energy have struck the foil-wrapped tubes without penetrating the tape. Exposure to the beam of continuous energy occurred for 1 minute with 100% oxygen flowing through the tube (Sosis, 1989). Most manufacturers of this type of metal or foil tape do not guarantee the performance their products.

Each new batch of metallic or foil tape must be test-fired to note its reaction to the laser energy. Limitations must be communicated to the surgery team to prevent fire hazards. Lead tape should never be used because it is easily broken or melted, and the vapors are toxic.

Special metal or foil tape is wrapped circumferentially from the cuff up the shaft of the tube. At least 6 to 10 cm of the most distal portion of the tube should be covered. The edges of the tape should smoothly overlap at least one third to one half of the tape width with each consecutive turn. Ragged tape edges can cause tracheal trauma during intubation. The tube can be sterilized with ethylene oxide and stored for later use.

The Norton metal ET tube with a supplemental cuff can be used because it readily withstands laser impact. The trachea can easily be traumatized when this tube is inserted; therefore, metal ET tubes are not very popular.

Laser Safety in the Airway

Purpose:

To provide methods to protect the airway during laser surgery.

Procedure:

Action	Rationale
1. A special laser endotracheal (ET) tube or wrap can be used during laser procedures of the airway.	To decrease the chance of laser beam penetration of the ET tube.
• Special commercial laser ET tube	
• Special laser resistant ET tube wrap placed on red rubber or polyvinyl-chloride (PVC) tube	
• Red rubber tube wrapped with metal foil tape that has been test-fired to note laser beam resistance	
Manufacturer's instructions must be carefully followed regarding laser energy limitations.	
The ET tube is never taped in place.	To allow for rapid extubation if needed.
2. The ET tube cuff must be inflated with the appropriate amount of sterile saline or water.	The inflated cuff provides a sealed airway. The sterile saline or water provides a heat sink barrier that will decrease the chance of fire if the cuff is accidentally ruptured by the laser beam.
3. After ET tube placement, small counted sponges soaked in sterile saline or water are placed around the ET tube by the anesthesiologist or nurse anesthetist.	The wet sponges provide a barrier to decrease the chance of laser beam penetration. Counted sponges decrease the chance that the surgeon will lose a sponge in the airway.
The sponge strings are positioned away from the laser impact path.	To decrease the chance of the laser beam igniting the strings.
4. The sponges are kept wet throughout the procedure.	Wet sponges decrease the chance of ignition.
5. If airway combustion occurs, the anesthetic gases are stopped, and the flaming ET tube is immediately withdrawn. Oxygen is administered, and the patient may be reintubated with a smaller PVC ET tube. The extent of damage is assessed (possibly by bronchoscopy). Further treatment depends upon the extent of the injuries.	To respond quickly to prevent further patient injury and to maintain the airway.
6. Bronchoscopy equipment must be immediately available.	The airway may be compromised by ET tube particles or eschar.

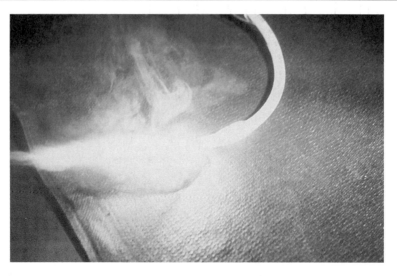

FIG. 5-7   An unprotected polyvinylchloride tube can be easily ignited with a laser beam.

The ET tube cuff should be inflated with sterile saline or water to provide a heat sink barrier if the cuff is inadvertently ruptured. If the cuff were punctured, the fluid would be released to squelch the fire. Adding a drop of methylene blue dye to the insufflation solution has also been advocated. Then, if the cuff were ruptured, the dye solution would immediately indicate that the cuff was no longer inflated and that the airway was not sealed.

After intubation, the ET tube should be protected by placing wet counted small sponges or pledgets around the area. This packing will stop the laser energy if an inadvertent beam hits the wrong area. The strings that are connected to the pledgets must be moved to one side so that the laser beam will not ignite them or cut through them. During the procedure, the pledgets must remain wet so that they will not dry out and support combustion. This can be achieved by keeping a syringe of sterile saline or water in the surgical field for use when needed.

Several *ventilation methods* can be used to administer the anesthetic gases during laser microlaryngoscopy.

First, the anesthetic gases can be delivered through a special laser-retardant ET tube.

Second, spontaneous ventilation can be used while the anesthetic gases are administered through a nasal catheter. This allows for a complete view of the surgical area without obstruction by an ET tube. This is usually the preferred method for pediatric patients. The disadvantage is that there is no control of the airway, so apnea, laryngospasm, and hypoventilation can occur. Scavenging the anesthetic gases through exhalation via the mouth can be hazardous to the laser team.

The third method is jet ventilation. The anesthetic gases are administered with intravenous sedation, muscle paralysis, and nitrous oxide. The oxygen and nitrous oxide gases are administered under high pressure through a metal jet ventilation needle that can be passed through a channel of the laryngoscope (Figure 5-8). These parts are ebonized or treated with a nonreflective surface to decrease laser beam reflection. Correct placement of the needle is critical, as it usually is placed between the vocal cords on the side oppo-

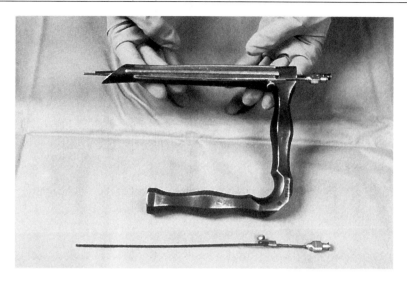

FIG. 5-8   Jet ventilation is passed through a metal tube attached to a metal laryngoscope.

site the lesion and into the upper part of the trachea. The needle should be in the trachea lumen and parallel to the trachea.

When the laser procedure is completed, an ET tube may be inserted through the laryngoscope. The jet ventilation needle is removed and the patient is awakened with the ET tube in place. The tube is left in place until spontaneous breathing begins (Mechenbier, 1992).

The advantage of this method is that the view of the surgical area is unobstructed. Disadvantages include the difficulty in positioning the jet ventilation needle adequately to direct the pressurized gas into the trachea, stomach distention, the possibility of causing such complications as pneumothorax or pneumomediastinum, and the difficulty in achieving adequate perfusion in obese patients or those with chronic obstructive pulmonary disease. Complications decrease with the increased skill level of the physicians. Accumulations of high concentrations of oxygen produced by the system can be hazardous, therefore combinations of gases are recommended.

The anesthetic gases must not support combustion. Nitrous oxide is contraindicated because it will support combustion as readily as oxygen will. Helium or nitrogen can be used with the lowest possible level of oxygen concentration. When the patient's oxygen saturation is maintained at 93%, adequate perfusion is maintained. Volatile anesthesia agents such as halothane, enflurane, and isoflurane can be used during laser microlaryngoscopy because they will not burn at clinical concentration levels. Intravenous anesthetics can be used for laser surgery, and muscle relaxants are important for patient immobility.

Other protective measures should be employed during laser microlaryngoscopy. The patient's eyes are protected by taping them shut (during general anesthesia procedures) and then covering them with moistened gauze sponges (Figure 5-9). Wet towels are then placed over the patient's face so that only the oral cavity is exposed (Figure 5-10). This protects the face from the inadvertent impact of a stray laser beam.

The patient's teeth must be protected from inadvertent beam impact during CO_2 laser procedures. The teeth can easily be in the line of fire when the laser is activated. The teeth

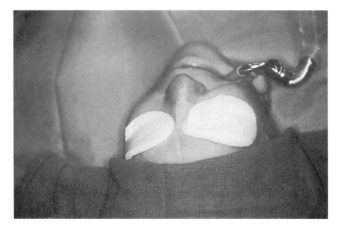

FIG. 5-9   The patient's eyes are protected with moistened gauze sponges.

protector must be made of material that can withstand laser impact without bursting into flames (Figure 5-11). If there is a question of flammability, the teeth protector could be lased in the laboratory environment to note its reaction at different power settings. Sometimes physicians have a teeth protector customized to provide maximum protection against the pressure of the laryngoscope. The mechanism of this device is based on the equal distribution of the pressure to all the maxillary teeth and hard palate.

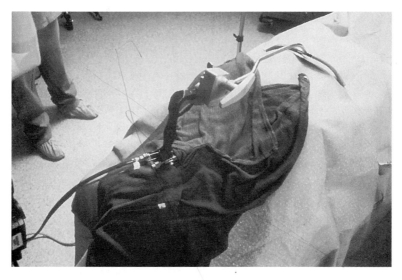

FIG. 5-10   Wet towels placed on the patient's face provide protection from an accidental laser impact. (Courtesy Dr. James Mechenbier.)

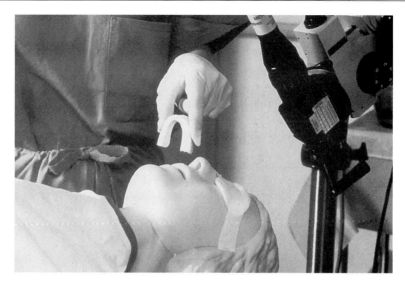

FIG. 5-11   A teeth protector must be made of material that can withstand laser beam impact. (Courtesy Dr. James Mechenbier.)

Emergency measures for airway fire must be understood thoroughly by everyone involved in the procedure. If an airway fire occurs, all anesthetic gases must be stopped. The flames must be immediately doused with saline while the ET tube is removed. The patient is ventilated by mask with pure oxygen. Anesthesia is continued with the narcotic muscle relaxant technique to facilitate evaluation of patient injury and responses. Reintubation is performed using a small ET tube, if needed. An unprotected PVC tube can be used at this point since the laser will not be used again.

Bronchoscopic equipment should always be immediately available since the patient's airway may be compromised by ET tube particles or charred tissue. Bronchoscopy can be performed to determine the effects of the airway fire; any charred tissue or remnants of the ET tube are removed. Flexible bronchoscopy is performed to evaluate distal airway status. The mouth, face, and other involved areas are examined for injury. A chest x-ray should be obtained as soon as possible.

In some cases, a tracheotomy is necessary to ventilate the patient. High-humidity ventilation is needed to maintain secretions that can be aspirated easily. A pulmonologist is usually notified for consultation. Each patient's treatment is individualized according to the extent of the injury.

Laser Microlaryngoscopy Procedure

The patient is positioned on the operating room table with support to maintain the head in full neck extension. The operating room table is aligned with the microscope for adequate visualization. The laser is then connected to the microscope. The CO_2 laser has been the most popular laser for microlaryngoscopy, but other wavelengths have been employed, including the Nd:YAG laser using the contact technique, frequency doubled YAG laser, and the argon laser.

The rigid laryngoscope is positioned using the Mayo stand or padding on the patient's chest to support the suspension arm. A Ziv laryngeal depressor can be connected to the suspension arm if desired. This instrument was designed to provide gentle external pressure on the larynx for better exposure of the anterior half of the larynx and anterior commissure. Using this device decreases the chances of overextending the patient's neck in an attempt to gain better visualization (Figure 5-12).

The lesions to be removed or treated are visualized, and the laser is activated using the lowest possible power density and the shortest exposure time. The tissue removed should always be sent to the pathology department for evaluation.

The laser allows precise tissue removal without significant damage to adjacent healthy tissue. Small blood vessels are sealed and the surgical area remains hemostatic. Lymphatic tissue is also sealed, decreasing the chances that malignant cells will spread to other areas of the body.

Any lased tissue is removed immediately to prevent aspiration or occlusion in the distal airway. Smoke is evacuated as it is generated to decrease the chance of smoke inhala-

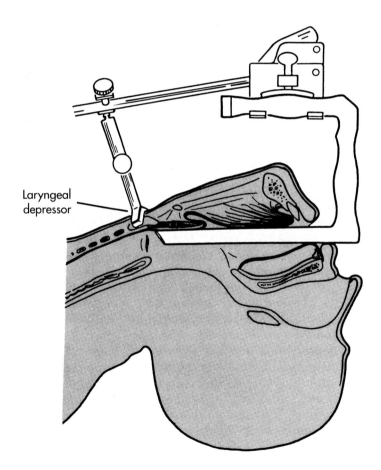

Laryngeal
depressor

FIG. 5-12   The laryngeal depressor enhances visualization during laser microlaryngoscopy.

tion by the patient and to increase the visibility of the surgical site. The total time required to perform laser microlaryngoscopy can be much shorter than that required for conventional methods.

During the procedure the patient may experience tachycardia and hypertensive periods from the placement of the laryngoscope in the airway. Patients with heart problems should be monitored closely for signs of myocardial ischemia.

After laser microlaryngoscopy, the anesthesiologist should be prepared for possible laryngeal spasm and edema. Steroids can be administered to decrease the chance of laryngeal edema. The chance of postoperative edema is much less when the laser is used during a microlaryngoscopy than when the electrocautery is used. The patient should still be closely evaluated for hypoxia during the postoperative phase.

Most patients are comfortable after laser microlaryngoscopy for procedures such as vocal cord polyp removal and do not require analgesics. Healing is complete within 2 to 3 weeks. The patient will probably be somewhat hoarse until the vocal cords have had time to heal. Voice rest fosters quicker healing. Steam or mist inhalation may also be helpful during the first week after surgery.

LASER BRONCHOSCOPY

Laser use during bronchoscopy was first described in 1974. Since then, the technology has advanced to the point of reducing the need to perform major surgical procedures and providing palliation for patients who would not otherwise experience a satisfactory quality of life.

Laser Systems

Laser technology has opened up new avenues for the treatment of certain diseases in the tracheobronchial tree that are accessible through the endoscope. The most popular lasers used for bronchoscopy are the CO_2 and the Nd:YAG lasers. Because of reports of tissue necrosis, unpredictability, substantial postoperative edema, and low-grade inflammation, the argon laser is still being challenged as an instrumental tool in this application. Photodynamic therapy is currently being used with laser bronchoscopy to selectively destroy or shrink bronchial tumors. The different delivery systems and the tissue response must be considered when the appropriate laser for laser bronchoscopy is being determined.

The *CO_2 laser*, with its extremely long wavelength, must be conducted to the tissue by bouncing the beam off a series of mirrors in the joints of the articulated arm. Therefore, the CO_2 laser must be used through a rigid bronchoscope. Proper alignment is mandatory because the laser must be coupled to the rigid endoscope.

CO_2 laser energy is readily absorbed by soft tissue because the beam has a very high water-absorption coefficient. Absorption does not depend on color, so a uniform impact can be expected on tissues of all colors. The tissue effect is precise because the lateral zone of damage is less than 0.5 mm from the impact point. The CO_2 beam also seals blood vessels, so the operative site remains hemostatic, and minimal edema and scarring occur.

The CO_2 laser beam is the wavelength of choice for treating diseases that are not highly vascular. Some of these conditions are recurrent respiratory papillomatosis, stenosis, granulomas, and web formations. A disadvantage of using the CO_2 laser is that only vessels of less than 0.5 mm in diameter are sealed. Many of the tracheobronchial neo-plasms are highly vascular; therefore, bleeding can become a problem.

The *Nd:YAG laser* beam is characterized by a high degree of scattering. The uniform zone of thermal coagulation may extend from 2 to 6 mm from the point of impact. This allows the laser to bring about hemostasis during the procedure. The Nd:YAG laser func-tions best when used for diseases requiring high penetration of laser energy. Examples of these conditions are tracheobronchial adenomas and obstructing carcinomas. Because of its short wavelength, the Nd:YAG laser energy is usually conducted through a flexible quartz fiber, so either a rigid or a flexible endoscope can be used.

One disadvantage of the noncontact Nd:YAG laser is lack of precise cutting. Because of its scattering effects, the beam cannot focus on one area for cutting. The introduction of contact Nd:YAG technology is currently addressing this dilemma. Another disadvan-tage of the noncontact Nd:YAG laser is the deep absorption of the beam. There is always a chance that the beam could perforate the tracheal or bronchial wall or a major artery during the laser intervention.

Bronchoscope Systems

The *rigid bronchoscope* was the original type of bronchoscope used for visualization of the tracheobronchial tree. Since hypoxemia and hemorrhage are of major concern dur-ing this procedure, the rigid bronchoscope is often the instrument of choice. Larger tissue specimens can be removed through the rigid endoscope during direct visualization. Be-cause tissue that has been excised is rapidly removed, the airway is not compromised and the chance of hypoxemia is minimized. Suctioning can occur during laser intervention through multiple ports to help evacuate smoke, secretions, or irrigants. ET tubes are usu-ally not used today during laser bronchoscopy because of the introduction of the ventilat-ing bronchoscope. A special port for anesthesia gases provides an unobstructed flow (Fig-ure 5-13). The tip of the rigid bronchoscope is often used to help bluntly dissect bulky tumors; it is also used to mechanically compress a bleeding tumor bed for hemostasis.

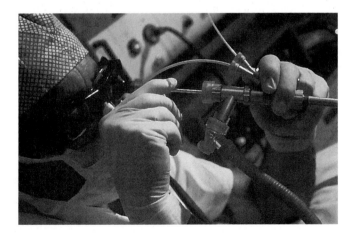

FIG. 5-13   A ventilating bronchoscope that delivers anesthetic gases can be used with the laser with no need for an endotracheal tube.

A disadvantage of the rigid endoscope is that the patient must be anesthetized for comfort and airway control during the procedure. The rigid endoscope can be used only in the tracheal and proximal endobronchial areas. Also, the physician must become adept at gently manipulating the rigid endoscope to access the areas to be lased.

The *flexible bronchoscope* allows sufficient flexibility to reach areas in the distal endobronchial tree and upper lobe. Local anesthesia can be used because the flexible endoscope has a smaller diameter than that of the rigid endoscope and can be tolerated more easily. The flexible endoscope can be introduced through the rigid scope to reach those areas not accessible through the rigid system.

One of the disadvantages associated with the flexible endoscope is that large tissue removal is not possible, and quick removal of debris is a challenge because the airway can easily become obstructed. Since the number of ports is limited on the flexible bronchoscope, suctioning while using the laser is difficult. Special bronchoscope adapters that allow suctioning, laser fiber introduction, and oxygen administration have been developed by some endoscope manufacturers. The flexible endoscope cannot be used for blunt dissection of tumor masses and cannot provide direct compression against bleeding vessels. There is always the risk of fire because the endoscope is made of flammable materials.

Safety during Laser Bronchoscopy

One of the most critical safety measures that must be employed during laser bronchoscopy is eye protection for the patient and the physician. A wet towel can be placed over the patient's eyes to protect against accidental laser impact. When using the Nd:YAG laser, the physician should wear appropriate eyewear or use a special lens cover to protect against backscatter. The Nd:YAG beam is transmitted through the clear structures of the unprotected eye and is refocused by the lens onto the retina. The power density of the beam is then changed significantly, and injury to the physician's retina can occur.

Flammable materials used during laser bronchoscopy must be recognized. The surface of the flexible bronchoscope can catch fire, especially if used in an oxygen-rich environment (concentrations greater than 50%). By increasing the power of the laser beam, the possibility of ignition is increased. Other potentially combustible materials are the laser fiber sheath and the plastic suction catheter. The laser settings should be kept low, with intermittent exposure times to further prevent fires. This also allows the tissue time to cool so that unanticipated perforation is not usually a problem.

Everyone involved in the laser bronchoscopy procedure must react quickly if a fire occurs. Policies must be written with input from the physician, anesthesiologist, nurse anesthetist, and nursing staff and reviewed annually for appropriateness.

Laser Bronchoscopy Protocol

Before the procedure, the patient's respiratory system is thoroughly evaluated, including blood work and x-rays. General anesthesia or local anesthesia with intravenous sedation is administered depending on the type and location of the pathology, the patient's general condition, and the patient's tolerance to the procedure. The bronchoscope (flexible or rigid) is inserted over the tongue and through the vocal cords into the trachea. When a rigid bronchoscope is used, the patient's head is turned to the right to visualize the left bronchi and to the left to visualize the right bronchi.

Secretions are suctioned as needed during the diagnostic phase of the procedure. After the pathology has been visualized, laser energy is delivered to the tissue. The oxygen concentration should be kept lower than 30% to prevent development of an oxygen-rich environment that would support combustion.

During a local anesthesia procedure, the laser therapy is usually done in a series of sequential steps. The oxygen is turned off, the laser energy is emitted, the smoke is evacuated, and the oxygen is turned back on. The procedure progresses using this format until the treatment of the pathology has been completed. The patient must be monitored closely throughout the procedure, including monitoring of blood gases, oxygen saturation, and cardiac function.

Complications Associated with Laser Bronchoscopy

Since laser bronchoscopy is often performed on patients with severely compromised respiratory functions, complications can occur quickly and easily. Hypoxemia is the most common problem associated with laser bronchoscopy. This condition is caused by respiratory depression from accumulated secretions or charred tissue, anesthetic agents, persistent oozing of blood, or an obstructive tumor. Therefore, the laser procedure must be stopped at intervals to ensure that the patient is getting enough oxygen.

Hemorrhage is a concern, especially for patients with a massive incurable cancer. If hemorrhage does occur, the rigid bronchoscope can be used to tamponade the area. The laser energy can be used to help coagulate the active bleeding vessel after the bleeding is under control. If the hemorrhaging cannot be stopped, the patient is placed with the uninvolved lung up, so that aeration can be maintained. The bleeding side is placed in the dependent position. Usually the bleeding will subside. Occasionally, the bleeding area will be packed with gauze soaked in topical thrombin. If the bleeding persists, an open emergency thoracotomy may be indicated. If the patient has incurable cancer, this type of heroism is not appropriate. Careful preoperative discussions about complications is very important because if hemorrhaging occurs, the patient may die.

Perforation with laser energy may occur, especially if the tumor is very friable. Excessive laser energy applied to the bronchial wall will eventually cause a perforation. This condition must be treated immediately.

LASER TONSILLECTOMY

Using the laser to perform a tonsillectomy continues to be controversial. The CO_2, argon, frequency doubled YAG, and contact Nd:YAG lasers have been used for tonsillectomies. Three major complications are associated with conventional tonsillectomy: intraoperative bleeding, postoperative pain, and postoperative bleeding; thus, comparative studies must address these issues. Some reports have noted that the laser seals the smaller blood vessels and significantly decreases the intraoperative bleeding. Decreased postoperative pain has been attributed to the possible sealing of the nerve endings by the laser energy. The postoperative bleeding complication, caused by tissue sloughing, has also been reported to be reduced because of the laser's sealing effect. These reports have not been conclusively supported with scientific research.

The patient is positioned supine, with the surgeon at the patient's head. A headlight worn by the surgeon helps illuminate the tonsillar area. A special laser retardant ET tube may be used; it is inserted and packed with moistened gauze sponges. The specially prepared or laser-retardant ET tube is inserted to minimize the chance of airway fire from an inadvertent impact of the laser beam. If contact Nd:YAG laser technology is used, the anesthesiologist and surgeon may opt not to use a special ET tube since this laser energy is confined and easily controlled. The patient's face and eyes are protected with wet sponges and towels.

The tonsil is grasped with a forceps or a tonsil schnidt and traction is maintained while the laser beam cuts the tonsil from the tonsillar bed. A wet sponge acts as a backstop to prevent the beam from impacting other tissue. Sometimes it is difficult to create a plane of dissection between the tonsil and the superior constrictor muscle of the pharynx underneath because of scar tissue around the tonsil. The procedure is usually completed within 20 to 30 minutes depending upon the surgeon's expertise. Since there is no current accepted method of removing the adenoids, the adenoidectomy (if needed) is performed using the conventional protocols. Some physicians are exploring the technique of removing the adenoids transnasally with a contact Nd:YAG rounded tip with mirror control or using the CO_2 laser beam bounced off a mirror. These investigational techniques could be extremely important for patients with coagulopathies.

The laser tonsillectomy technique has been refined to the extent that the procedure can be performed on an outpatient basis. The patient can eat solid foods on the same night of the surgery instead of the traditional clear liquid diet or soft foods because postoperative pain is minimized and intraoperative bleeding was controlled. The patient experiences less postoperative complications and returns to work quickly.

LASER PROCEDURE OF THE TEMPOROMANDIBULAR JOINT

The temporomandibular joint (TMJ) connects the mandible with the skull and through its rotational movement allows such activities as eating, speaking, and yawning. The TMJ motion can become limited with arthritis, malocclusions, or trauma. If an open treatment procedure is recommended, the traditional electrosurgery pencil can be replaced with the contact Nd:YAG scalpel.

After the initial small incision is made in the preauricular area, the contact Nd:YAG laser is used to dissect down to the temporalis fascia and on to the joint capsule. Adhesions are then ablated, or diseased tissue can be excised. There is significantly less bleeding during this procedure than during the traditional procedure. A drier operating field enhances visibility within this small surgical area; therefore, the anatomy can be easily recognized. Delicate structures, such as the temporal branch of the facial nerve, can be preserved. Ultimately, the surgery time is less than with the traditional procedure because of the increased hemostasis. Postoperatively, the patient has less pain and edema because of the minimal damage to adjacent tissue (Pasqual, 1992).

The contact Nd:YAG laser combined with endoscopic technology results in an extremely small initial incision. And using smaller instruments results in a shorter postoperative recovery period.

LASER TREATMENT FOR SNORING

Because approximately 40% of adults snore, the development of a procedure to address this problem has been greatly appreciated by many people (*Clinical Laser Monthly*, May 1993). The snoring sound comes from the vibration of soft-palate tissue. When at rest, the muscles that elevate the soft palate relax, causing this tissue to fall into the major airway of the throat. When the mouth is open, the sound of the snoring is even louder.

A treatment for snoring is a laser-assisted uvula palatoplasty (LAUP). The goal of this procedure is to stiffen and recontour the soft palate, using the laser (CO_2, contact Nd:YAG, or frequency doubled YAG) to cut away tissue that surrounds the uvula. This in turn alters the soft palate and reduces its vibration.

The procedure is performed on an outpatient basis with the patient under local anesthesia. This is very important for patients who are obese and have a snoring problem since they are poor anesthesia risks.

The surgery is usually performed with the patient sitting. The laser is used to trim and reshape the soft-palate tissue. The CO_2 laser is used at approximately 20 W of superpulse power; the contact Nd:YAG laser is used with a scalpel tip at about 15 to 20 W.

The procedure lasts about 10 minutes. Because the goal is to remove no more tissue than necessary, a more conservative approach is taken. Repeated treatments are usually needed until the amount of tissue removed is adequate to stop or decrease the snoring. Usually two to seven sessions are required. Postoperative pain is relieved by oral analgesics and antiinflammatory medications. A sample of postoperative discharge instructions is provided below. Most insurance companies or reimbursers do not pay for this procedure unless it is related to sleep apnea.

Obstructive sleep apnea occurs when loud episodes of snoring are interrupted by periods of completely obstructed breathing. If sleep apnea progresses, the condition can be fatal. As the cumulative effect of the sleep apnea progresses, reduced oxygenation to the brain causes the snorer to tighten the muscles of the breathing passage. Thus the patient is robbed of a good night's sleep and may fall asleep during the day. This could be disastrous if the person were operating hazardous machinery or an automobile.

Sample Discharge Instructions:
Laser Treatment for Snoring

Resume regular activities after surgery.

Maintain a soft diet for the first 2 to 3 days (avoid citrus fruits and spicy foods).

Drink plenty of liquids, but do not drink any alcohol for 2 to 3 days.

Gargle gently with diluted salt water every 6 hours for 1 week (2 tablespoons of salt in 1 cup of water).

Brush your teeth and use diluted mouth wash as necessary.

You may experience a sore throat for 5 to 10 days and possibly an earache from day 2 to day 4.

Take all medications as directed:

    Antibiotic

    Steroid or antiinflammatory medication

    Analgesics (pain relievers)

Use analgesic lozenges as needed to relieve sore throat.

Call the office if you have excessive pain or fever.

Please keep follow-up appointments.

From instructions given by J. Bert Davis, MD, FACS, Fort Myers, FL.

LASER PROCEDURES IN THE ORAL CAVITY

The laser has been used effectively in the oral cavity for conditions such as benign tumors, scar release, tongue release, leukoplakia, superficial carcinoma, and palliation for recurrent carcinoma.

Tongue surgery performed with the laser has many advantages. Since the tongue is so highly vascular, any incision into the tongue produces a lot of bleeding. The laser helps to seal the smaller blood vessels of the tongue, thus decreasing blood loss during surgery and fostering a dry surgical field.

Wedge resection of the tongue can be performed under local anesthesia and/or intravenous sedation on an outpatient basis. Xylocaine with epinephrine is injected into the tongue to provide local anesthesia and vasoconstriction. The patient's face and eyes are covered with moistened sponges or towels.

The laser may be used to superficially mark or blanch the tongue mucosa to outline the intended excisional area. The excision then is performed while the laser cuts and coagulates the tissue. The specimen is evaluated by a pathologist for the presence of abnormal tissue on the margins. The wound is usually left open because the laser seals off blood vessels, and sometimes an avascular surface will not heal as readily if sutured. The surgical area will heal by granulation within 2 to 3 weeks.

Postoperative pain is reportedly decreased and other complications are minimized in contrast to conventional surgery. The amount of lingual swelling is also minimized.

Benign lesions of the oral cavity are easily excised using laser energy. The CO_2 laser is particularly useful for treating denture-induced hyperplasia of the gums. Minimal discomfort is experienced postoperatively, frequently allowing the dentures to be worn comfortably. There usually is little scarring or distortion of the soft tissues that may cause future problems.

Mucoceles or ranulas can be eliminated with the CO_2 laser. The cyst sac is vaporized or excised with a minimal amount of bleeding, allowing the surgeon visualization during the procedure. Pyogenic granulomas are very vascular and respond well to CO_2 laser vaporization. Adenomas of the soft palate are also easily removed with laser energy with no limitation of palate mobility.

Leukoplakia can be treated with the laser in the defocused mode to vaporize the affected epithelial layer and some of the underlying connective tissue. It is theorized that vaporizing the deeper layer minimizes the recurrence rate because the subepithelial layers may be responsible for the formation of leukoplakia.

Healing is enhanced when the laser vaporizes the leukoplakia. Newly regenerated epithelium appears to be healthy. This procedure helps minimize the chance of benign leukoplakia progressing into a malignant lesion; therefore, a biopsy is important to diagnose the pathology before vaporization is performed.

Malignant lesions have also been successfully treated with laser energy. Larger lesions found in the posterior region of the oral cavity and those that have spread to the lymph nodes should probably be excised using the conventional methods. When a malignant lesion is excised with pulsed laser energy, the pathologist usually can identify the margins to verify the absence or presence of malignant cells. Swelling, inflammation, contraction, and scarring is often minimized when the laser is used.

After removal of an oral lesion of less than 3 cm, the wound is usually not sutured. Healing is accomplished by secondary epithelialization, and this process is usually complete from 3 to 6 weeks after the laser procedure. During the discharge instruction teaching, the patient is advised to use a hydrogen peroxide mouthwash four times during the day and again at bedtime. Mild analgesics are prescribed for postoperative pain if needed.

SOFT-TISSUE LASER PROCEDURES

The laser's hemostatic value is greatly appreciated during procedures involving soft tissue. The CO_2 and the contact Nd:YAG are the most popular lasers for these procedures. Radical neck dissection and thyroidectomy/parathyroidectomy are procedures that require a lot of attention to hemostasis since the neck area is so vascular.

The contact Nd:YAG laser can provide precise dissection of a lesion since the depth of penetration of the laser energy is very shallow. There is controlled lateral damage to adjacent tissue. The tip size concentrates the laser energy and provides an excellent cutting tool. Decreased bleeding allows for better visualization of vital structures, such as nerves, glands, or vessels. Since laser energy does not involve an electrical current, the muscles and nerves are not innervated, and the tissue does not move unexpectedly during the procedure. This benefit is extremely important when skin flaps are being made.

As the many benefits of laser technology become proven and identified, the laser will become a standard tool with which to cut, coagulate, and vaporize soft tissue. The main stumbling block appears to be the cost of lasers compared with other tools. Even this disadvantage can be challenged as the many patient benefits are validated and the procedures can be moved to less costly environments, such as laser centers, clinics, or physicians' offices.

LASER APPLICATIONS IN DENTISTRY

Dentistry is one of the youngest disciplines to explore the use of laser technology. New applications are being discovered because the laser affects all aspects of the dentist's modalities of care. Controversy exists within the dental community as to the actual merits of laser technology. More scientific research needs to be conducted with reproducible results to justify laser technology in dentistry.

Education is paramount in ensuring the success of a dental laser application. In some areas, dentists without appropriate education are using lasers on their patients (see chapter on laser education). Patient injuries can easily slow the progression of any new technology, no matter how beneficial the application may seem.

The CO_2, Nd:YAG, argon, holmium, and erbium lasers are the most used lasers today in dentistry. These wavelengths are being used on soft tissue to excise tumors and lesions, vaporize excess tissues, control bleeding of vascular lesions, and remove or reduce hyperplastic tissue. Hard-tissue applications include vaporizing dental cavities, desensitizing exposed root surfaces, glazing teeth, smoothing rough surfaces in preparation for bonding procedures, stopping demineralization of enamel surfaces, promoting remineralization, and debonding ceramic orthodontic brackets (Miller and Truhe, 1993). Many other procedures are being investigated.

Aphthous ulcers are being treated with laser energy. The CO_2 laser beam is defocused and debrides the necrotic tissue. The procedure can be performed without an anesthetic. The results are remarkable as painful symptoms are minimized; almost immediately after the procedure, the pain is relieved.

Herpetic lesions are also being treated with laser applications. The pain relief is just as significant as with aphthous ulcers, and these lesions tend to heal more quickly than when conventional methods are used. The smoke must be adequately evacuated during herpetic lesion vaporization because the plume has the potential to contain viable particulate matter.

Gingival overgrowth is being treated with the CO_2 laser by precisely shaving away the excess tissue. Some patients may experience an overgrowth of gum tissue when certain drugs, such as Dilantin (phenytoin sodium), are taken over extended periods. Conventional treatment requires the excision of this tissue with a knife. Postoperative pain can be intense; therefore, patients are reluctant to have the procedure performed again if the tissue regrows.

The CO_2 laser can be used in the focused mode at approximately 10 W of power to excise the bulk of the excess gum tissue. The defocused beam is then used to remove the remaining residual tissue. Bleeding is easily controlled because the laser energy seals the smaller blood vessels. Postoperative pain may be significantly less with the laser procedure. Tooth protection can be achieved by using a periosteal elevator or a wax spatula to provide a backstop to prevent etching of the tooth.

One of the newest applications is *gingival toughening*. A laser can be used to make a trough around a tooth before an impression is taken to replace the need for a retraction cord, electrosurgery, or the use of a hemostatic agent. Bleeding and postoperative problems are minimized. The results have been highly significant in that they are predictable, and less time is needed for the procedure.

The laser is also being used in *exposing implants*. The noncontact Nd:YAG laser should not be used because it could damage titanium implants. The CO_2 laser is the most popular for this application. The laser energy is used to vaporize the overlying tissue until the implant is visualized.

Diagnosing dental caries is usually performed using a tool called the explorer that catches as it moves across a tooth with a cavity. This method of detection has many limitations, including the instrumentation, the preciseness required in performing the technique, and the tactile and subjective judgment required by the dentist.

The laser is currently being investigated for dental caries detection. When a tooth is subjected to low powers of CO_2 laser energy, normal dental surfaces retain their natural color. Any demineralized areas caused by dental caries produce carbonized residue when exposed to laser photovaporization. These blackened areas indicate potential dental caries.

One disadvantage of this diagnostic system is that the dentist cannot rely on familiar tactile sensation to diagnose caries. Another disadvantage is that higher laser powers or extended exposure to laser energy could damage a healthy tooth or surrounding tissue.

One advantage of this laser diagnostic method is that the determination of dental caries is objective and verifiable. Also, this system can reduce the amount of time needed to diagnose dental caries. False-positives are minimized because the laser correctly detects cavities in normal grooves or indentations, in contrast to the explorer method.

Dental cavities are being treated with the CO_2 laser. The laser, at low power settings, is used to drill out the decayed area. The top layer of the decay is vaporized and then removed with a mechanical instrument. The next layer is then vaporized and also removed mechanically. This sequence is repeated until all of the decayed area is removed. The tooth is then filled using conventional methods. Further research is investigating this application. Patients appear to appreciate not having to listen to the sound of the conventional drill as dental decay is removed. The laser is also being investigated for use in desensitization of root surfaces.

Enamel replacement has always been a problem because enamel wears off the surface of the tooth with age. The next layer down is the dentin, but this layer is much softer and is subject to much quicker infection with dental caries. Research is investigating the use of low-power CO_2 laser and other wavelengths to provide a glazing over the dentin layer wherever the enamel has worn off. The glazing tends to form a very hard surface, and this new surface responds to dental caries much as an enamel surface does. The laser's ability to glaze enamel and thus seal occlusal grooves to prevent dental caries is also being investigated.

Curing composite is being done with the argon laser. When the laser is used, the process is shortened, and the physical properties of the resin restorative materials are enhanced (Pick, 1993).

Recent research has shown the value of the erbium:YAG laser in treating hard tissue. It has shown great promise as a cutting tool for the dentist because it is the most effective wavelength for removing dentin and enamel. When the erbium laser is used on pulpal tissue, the dentin layer adjacent to the laser interaction site thickens. There has been some thought that this wavelength stimulates reparative dentin formation, but further research is needed. When the CO_2 or Nd:YAG lasers are used on hard tissue, there is a greater chance that they will harm the pulp or surrounding tissue (Wigdor et al, 1993).

Finally, the use of *dental spectroscopy* to diagnose dental problems is being explored. The laser is being used to spectroscopically determine normal vs. diseased dental tissue. This area of diagnosis is quickly expanding as laser spectroscopy rapidly evolves.

REFERENCES

Jako GJ: State of the art otolaryngology, *Lasers Surg* 6:389, 1986.

Lasers make treatment for snoring more accessible, *Clinical Laser Monthly,* p 78-79, May 1993.

Mechenbier JA: Jet ventilator in microlaryngoscopy reduces anesthesia risks, *Clinical Laser Monthly,* p 23-26, Feb 1992.

Miller M and Truhe T: Lasers in dentistry: An overview, *JADA* 124:33, Feb 1993.

Pasqual HP: Contact Nd:YAG laser surgery of the temporomandibular joint, *Clinical Laser Monthly,* p 175-177, Nov 1992.

Peterson RJ and Finch R: KTP successful with nasolacrimal duct surgery, *Clinical Laser Monthly,* p 109-110, July 1992.

Pick RM: Using lasers in clinical dental practice, *JADA* 124:45-46, Feb 1993.

Sosis MB: Minimize risk of catastrophic airway fires during laser surgery, Laser practice report, *Clinical Laser Monthly,* p 1S, March 1989.

Wigdor H et al: The effect of lasers on dental hard tissues, *JADA* 124:69-70, Feb 1993.

SUGGESTED READINGS

Benedetto MD: Detect caries quickly, objectively by using a pulsed CO_2 laser, *Clinical Laser Monthly,* p 3S, July 1988.

Dumon JF et al: Principles for safety in application of Nd:YAG laser in bronchology, *Chest* 86:163, 1984.

Fukutake T, Kumazawa T, and Nakamura A: Laser surgery for allergic rhinitis, *AORN J* 46(4):756, Oct 1987.

Kirschner RA: Laser turbinectomy quicker, less painful using Nd:YAG, *Clinical Laser Monthly,* p 1S, Nov 1988.

Levine HL: Endoscope and the KTP/532 laser for nasal sinus disease, *Ann Otol Rhinol Laryngol* 98:46, 1989.

Lim RY: CO_2 laser used for management of airway and swallowing disorders, *Clinical Laser Monthly,* p 2S, July 1988.McCaughan JS, Hawley PC, and Walker J: Management of endobronchial tumors—A comparative study, *Semin Surg Oncol* 5:38, 1989.

Meeker MH and Rothrock JC: *Alexander's care of the patient in surgery,* ed 10, St. Louis, 1995, Mosby.

Shapshay SM and Beamis JF: Safety precautions for bronchoscopic Nd:YAG laser surgery, *Otolaryngol Head Neck Surg* 94(2):175, Feb 1986.

Wigdor HA: CO_2 and Nd:YAG lasers may provide potent new modality for dentists, *Clinical Laser Monthly,* p 3S, Sept 1987.

Ziv M: Laryngeal depressor for laser surgery, *Otolaryngol Head Neck Surg* 94(3)411, 1986.

Ziv M: Saving teeth from the tube, *Wellcome Trends,* p 6, Nov 1981.

6

DERMATOLOGY AND PLASTIC SURGERY LASER APPLICATIONS

Dermatologists have found the laser to be an integral part of the surgical instrument armamentarium. Dermatological conditions respond favorably to laser energy, and many times the laser is the only instrument needed for a procedure.

Most dermatological procedures can be performed on an outpatient basis, usually with local anesthesia. As contrasted with conventional dermatology techniques, laser applications are uncomplicated and almost bloodless. These procedures are very easily tolerated, and patients complain less of postoperative discomfort and edema. The laser is also used to debride ulcerations or necrotic tissue with a thermal effect that has been described as similar to sterilizing infected tissue. The laser's intense heat almost eliminates the spread of infection. When laser energy is used to excise malignant disease, small blood vessels and the lymphatics are sealed, thus leading to a decreased chance of malignant cells spreading to other areas of the body.

The first dermatological procedures were performed by Dr. Leon Goldman using the ruby laser in the 1960s. This wavelength was soon replaced by CO_2 and argon laser wavelengths. Today these two lasers are being challenged by new wavelengths that precisely treat cutaneous lesions. Lasers used for dermatological conditions are briefly reviewed below, starting with the longest wavelengths. A comparison of the depth of penetration of different lasers is illustrated in Figure 6-1.

CO_2 (10,600 nm) laser energy is absorbed readily by water. Since the body contains 75% to 90% water, the CO_2 beam penetrates very superficially to approximately 0.1 to 0.2 mm in depth. The laser can cut, vaporize, and coagulate at the point of the focused or defocused beam, leaving adjacent tissue practically unaffected. The CO_2 laser seals smaller blood vessels as it cuts through tissue. This laser energy also can be used for surface vaporization to ablate superficial lesions with great precision. Laser dermabrasion can successfully remove the superficial skin layers to the depth desired with excellent healing results. Postoperative scarring parallels that of conventional procedures, but with the laser, postoperative pain and edema are significantly reduced.

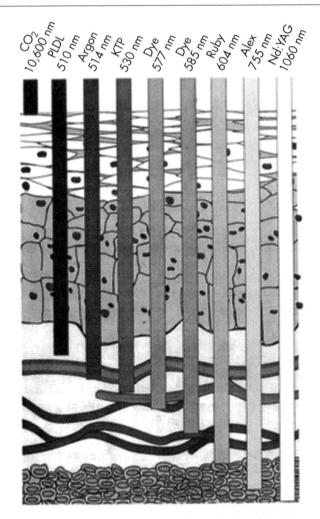

FIG. 6-1   Approximate levels of penetration for various lasers: candela pigment lesion dye laser (PLDL), neodymium-yttrium-aluminum-garnet (Nd:YAG), carbon dioxide (CO_2). (From Goldman MP and Fitzpatrick RE: *Cutaneous laser surgery,* St. Louis, 1994, Mosby.)

Use of contact Nd:YAG (1064 nm) technology has gained acceptance in the areas of dermatology and plastic surgery. Various configurations of the synthetic sapphire probes and scalpels enable the Nd:YAG beam to be tremendously localized. The smaller diameter of the tip on the scalpel concentrates the Nd:YAG laser energy into a tiny spot for cutting and vaporization. Rounded or flat-surfaced probes distribute Nd:YAG energy over a larger area to provide greater hemostatic effects. When a special frosted contact scalpel is used, the laser beam is still focused at the tip, but small amounts of laser energy also escape along the frosted areas. This design allows the Nd:YAG energy to precisely cut at the tip while vaporization and coagulation is provided along the frosted areas. Less plume is produced with contact technology, making it sometimes the preferred tool for cutting and coagulating soft tissue.

Noncontact Nd:YAG (1064 nm) laser energy has been used to effectively treat capillary hemangiomas. This laser energy penetrates deep into the lesion to arrest the abnormal growth. A noncontact Nd:YAG laser has also been designed that produces an extremely short pulse duration through Q-switching. This short pulsation provides less thermal spread, thus preserving surrounding tissue.

A Q-switched Alexandrite laser (760 nm) has been developed to treat tattoos without breaking the dermal layer. This laser energy may be delivered to the tissue via a liquid-filled light guide connected to a lens-coupled hand piece. This special fluid-filled delivery device is used to achieve a uniform dispersion of the light, thus decreasing the chance of creating an intense hot spot. The laser light is delivered in short pulsations with a larger spot size (3 mm). A red helium neon laser beam is coupled with the therapeutic beam to provide an aiming light.

The Q-switched ruby laser produces a very short pulse duration with a wavelength of about 694 nm. This beam is highly absorbed by black, blue, and green pigmentation; therefore, this laser is highly appropriate for treating vascular lesions and tattoos.

Lasers that produce yellow light in the range of 577 to 585 nm have been rapidly accepted for many dermatology applications. A variety of lasers—including copper vapor, tunable dye, and pulsed dye lasers—can produce a yellow wavelength. This laser energy is remarkably well absorbed by vascular structures. Yellow laser energy is being used for very selective destruction of the vasculature beneath the skin with no significant effect or damage to the overlying or adjacent dermal tissue. Yellow light, especially at 585 nm, is better absorbed by oxyhemoglobin and exhibits much less absorption by melanin. This allows the beam to penetrate deeper, causing less damage to adjacent tissue than occurs with argon energy. Therefore, yellow wavelengths are preferred today because of the superior results obtained compared with those of argon laser technology for vascular lesions.

The frequency doubled YAG laser, also known as the KTP laser, produces a wavelength of 532 nm that has gained more popularity in recent years for a variety of facial plastic surgeries, including face and neck lifting, blepharoplasty, and excising small lesions. This laser energy is delivered to the tissue via a quartz contact probe that allows for increased control of the amount of thermal energy emitted. KTP laser energy is extremely effective for excising tissue and elevating skin flaps. Because the face is extremely vascular, the laser's coagulative properties are useful in increasing visibility through a drier field, thus decreasing the surgery time.

A krypton laser has been developed that produces two wavelengths: green (520 nm) and yellow (568 nm). With the combination of these two wavelengths, vascular and epidermal-pigmented lesions can be effectively treated. The energy is delivered to the tissue via a fiber that is connected to a hand piece or an automatic scanning device.

A laser that generates a wavelength of 510 nm with a pulsed mode (about 300 ms) has also been developed for dermatology treatments. This wavelength is selectively absorbed by melanin. Since the pulsed mode produces a very short pulse that impacts the tissue, thermal damage is confined to the target. Penetration into the dermis is limited to less than 1 mm unless high energies are used.

The argon laser's intense blue-green beam, at 488 and 514.5 nm, is strongly absorbed by hemoglobin and melanin. Argon light can penetrate intact overlying skin from 0.5 to 2 mm to be absorbed by deeper pigmented areas or vascular structures. The laser energy absorbed is then converted to heat to coagulate the abnormal vessels or vaporize pigmented tissue. Normal adjacent tissue is left relatively unaffected, thus allowing healing to occur rapidly.

New laser systems are being developed that combine two or more laser wavelengths, thus giving the operator the option of using more than one wavelength during a procedure. This promotes greater efficiency and precision and more significant results.

Many of the laser systems that have been introduced to the dermatology and plastic surgery arena can be connected to an automatic scanning device that precisely delivers a preset amount of laser energy to the tissue. The duration of exposure can be extremely short, thus decreasing the thermal spread and damage to surrounding tissues. The pattern or area of laser impact can also be designated to provide consistency to foster optimal results. For example, the Hexascanner delivers laser energy spots within octagon-shaped areas of various sizes. Each pulsation delivers the same amount of energy at the same depth of penetration (Figures 6-2 and 6-3).

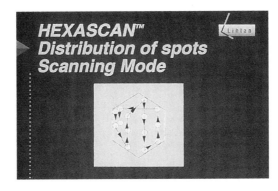

FIG. 6-2   The automatic scanner delivers the laser energy in a specific preset pattern. (Courtesy Lihtan Technologies, Inc., San Anselmo, CA.)

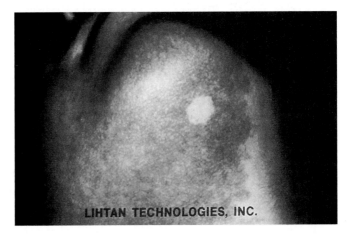

FIG. 6-3   Immediate lightening of a port-wine stain with the laser energy delivered by the Hexascan device. (Courtesy Lihtan Technologies, Inc., San Anselmo, CA.)

LASER SURGERY FOR VASCULAR LESIONS

Because yellow light and argon laser energy are highly absorbed by pigmentation and melanin, these wavelengths are popular for use in treating vascular lesions. Because the depth of penetration is approximately 0.5 to 2 mm, vascular lesions located deeper in the dermis do not respond well to this laser energy. However, vascular lesions in the upper dermal layer respond readily to yellow light or argon laser treatment. Other laser systems continue to be researched for use in various vascular applications.

Port-Wine Stain

Port-wine stains occur in 0.3% to 0.5% of newborns and represent a superficial dermal capillary malformation. Most port-wine stains are superficial, with an average vessel depth of 0.46 mm (Goldman and Fitzpatrick, 1994, pp. 32-33). Port-wine stains not only cause cosmetic concerns but are sometimes related to other medical conditions, such as glaucoma. Usually the extent of the stain does not correlate directly with neurological disease; however, patients with bilateral port-wine stains often display neurological problems, such as seizures. In the natural evolvement of a port-wine stain, the vessels become progressively ectatic over time, which leads to gradual thickening and darkening. Tissue hypertrophy may occur, and nodules usually develop; physical deformity results, and bleeding often occurs. In addition to the physical problems, the patient can have lasting psychological, social, and interpersonal detrimental effects (Figure 6-4).

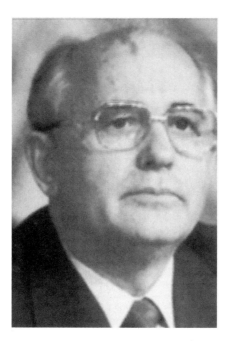

FIG. 6-4   Mikhail Gorbachev's port-wine stain was airbrushed off for many published photographs by the Soviet news agency until perestroika.

Before the development of the argon laser, there was no treatment that produced a significant outcome. Today the argon wavelength and yellow light laser energy can be used successfully to lighten the color of port-wine stains approximately 50% to almost 100%. Absorption of this laser energy by the pigmented areas causes a blanching effect that selectively lightens the area. Hypertrophic growth and thickening of a lesion can be decreased if the lesion is smoothed to the level of the normal surrounding skin.

Preoperatively, the patient must be advised that the color of the stain may not be removed completely. Several sessions may be required to obtain acceptable results. Normal expectations of the surgery are a reduction in the color intensity of the lesion, decreased friability and number of surface blebs, and improved skin texture. The patient must thoroughly understand the anticipated results before the procedure is performed.

Controversy exists as to when laser treatment should be performed. Researchers have tried to prove that lightening port-wine stains is more successful when the procedure is performed before vs. after puberty. Many physicians believe that treating lesions earlier will decrease the progression of the condition. Also, treating the patient at a younger age will minimize any negative psychological effect. Advantages of early treatment include quicker resolution with fewer treatments, less need for anesthesia, and fewer laser pulses because the area is smaller. Sometimes pediatricians and family practitioners are reluctant to refer their patients for treatment because they are not aware of the most recent literature that describes the success of laser therapy. Also, the failures of earlier laser treatments still may be embedded in the minds of these physicians.

Preoperatively, an anesthetic cream may be applied to the lesion to decrease pain. A dressing usually is placed over the cream to enhance the action of the medication (Figure 6-5). Sensation of the skin surface is decreased by using this cream, so that increased power settings can be employed. An injection of a local anesthetic is not always used since it increases the distance the laser beam must travel to impact the vessels. Epinephrine is not recommended because it constricts the target vessels. If the patient is too young to tolerate the procedure, then a light anesthetic may be administered.

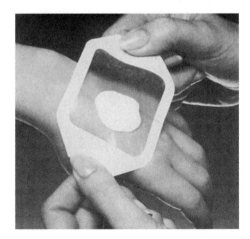

FIG. 6-5   A dressing is placed over the anesthetic cream to enhance the action of the medication. (Courtesy Astra USA, Westborough, MA.)

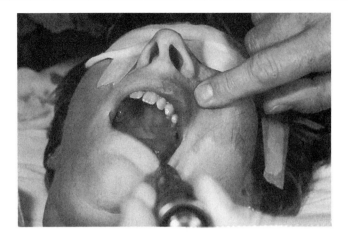

FIG. 6-6   The patient's eyes are covered with gauze pads while the laser is used to treat the port-wine stain, which has extended into the mouth. (Courtesy Dr. James Mechenbier.)

The patient's eyes are protected with the appropriate goggles or glasses, or they may be covered before the treatment to protect against retinal damage from laser energy (Figure 6-6). If periorbital tissue or the eyelid is being treated, a protective eye shield is used to protect the eye. Eye shields made of lead can be autoclaved to provide sterility. They must be thoroughly cooled before being placed on the eye. Topical ophthalmic anesthetic is instilled to numb the surface of the eye. The eye shield is then placed under the upper and lower lids in a way that ensures patient comfort.

Sometimes a pretreatment test (test spots) is performed on part of the most involved area of the stain. This is done to determine the most appropriate laser settings for the severity of the stain. Any immediate blanching merely represents a coagulum of the surface epithelium and not the true desired vascular thrombosis. Permanent lightening occurs after 3 to 4 months. Then the lesion test area is evaluated to determine the most appropriate settings for treating the rest of the lesion. Today many physicians opt to perform the procedure without testing the area first because of the tremendous experience they have gained over the years in treating these lesions.

Different techniques are used to treat the port-wine stains. Vessels may be traced using magnification and a 100-μm spot size while the laser is activated in a continuous wave mode. This method is time-consuming and tedious. Recent studies have shown that increasing the spot size to 1 mm or greater causes the vessel to absorb 2.5 times more energy to achieve photocoagulation, thus decreasing the surgery time (Goldman and Fitzpatrick, 1994, p. 35). Also, automatic scanning devices are being used to deliver a preset amount of energy in a designated pattern using a larger spot size to treat the stain.

During the lightening procedure, the lowest possible power density that will produce acceptable blanching is used. Thus pain is decreased because the thermal buildup within the tissue is not felt. When higher settings are used for longer exposure times, the patient experiences a burning sensation from the thermal impact of the beam. If the patient can tolerate the lower settings, no local anesthetic is needed for the procedure. The automatic scanning devices help decrease intraoperative discomfort because the laser energy is delivered in very short pulsations. Patients have described the laser impact sensation as feeling like a stretched rubber band snapping the skin.

Lightening a port-wine stain may be done in a series of treatments if the lesion is large. Smaller areas may only require one session. The patient must understand that true lightening does not occur for several months after the surgical procedure. The lesion usually does not continue to blanch after 12 to 18 months. Spot retreatment may be performed 1 year after the initial treatment for areas that appear darker than most of the lesion.

Different types of laser systems produce different immediate results. For example, the flashlamp pulsed dye laser explodes the smaller blood vessels, leading to postoperative bruising that subsides after a short time. The tunable dye laser, with longer pulse durations, coagulates the superficial vessels with less postoperative bruising. Each type of laser technique produces the same end result, that is, lightening the unwanted pigmentation.

Overlapping the impact areas 10% to 15% helps avoid the mottled egg-crate effect and ensures that the entire lesion is treated (Figure 6-7). The darker, purple lesions may be less responsive to laser energy since they are usually located deeper in the dermis. Patients with darker skin pigmentation may require more laser sessions because the increased melanin alters the absorption of some of the laser energies, such as argon.

The degree of response to the laser energy is dependent upon the anatomical location of the stain. Lesions in the midfacial area involving the medial cheek, upper lip, and nose respond more slowly with lightening than do other facial areas (Goldman and Fitzpatrick, 1994, p. 36). A stain on the extremities also responds slowly. It has been theorized that this may be related to gravitational or deoxygenation effects on circulation. Distal vessels also have a thicker wall than those of the face, thus making them more difficult to treat with laser energy.

After the laser intervention, ice may be applied to the surgical area to decrease swelling and thus minimize pain. Superficial erosion of the skin usually resolves within 7 to 10 days. During this time the wound may be cleansed with 3% hydrogen peroxide and

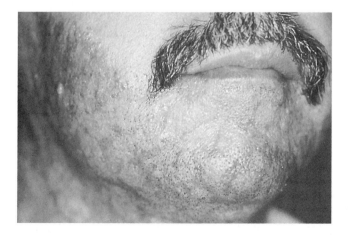

FIG. 6-7   The laser impact sites must overlap, or a mottled egg-crate appearance will result.

followed with an application of an antibiotic ointment. This postoperative care continues until the wound has completely reepithelialized. The patient must understand the home care that is needed to ensure proper healing. A sample of home care instructions is provided below.

Complications that may result from lightening port-wine stains with laser energy are scarring, hypopigmentation, and changes in skin texture. Hypertrophic scarring is the most significant complication. It is theorized to be caused by the laser's thermal spread and zone of destruction. Although this complication is not common, the areas most affected are the thin tissue of the lateral and anterior neck, the mustache portion of the upper lip, and the eye lid margins.

Sample Discharge Instructions:
Laser Port-wine Stain Lightening

You have just had laser surgery. The treatment area may appear to have no changes, but tiny blisters or bruising may normally develop within 24 hours. The blisters will break down and form a crust on the surgical area. Eventually, this scab will fall off as the skin heals. The skin underneath may appear pink, but the color will begin to fade within 3 months. Usually complete lightening may not be apparent for up to 1 year after the treatment. Retreatment may be necessary to help lighten specific areas.

The care you give to your surgical area is important to ensure proper healing. The following measures should be observed after your surgery.

1. Keep the surgical site clean and dry for 24 hours.
2. Ice compresses may be applied during the first 24 hours to decrease the swelling. Frozen peas may be placed in a small plastic bag for use as a cold pack. If the treatment has been on the facial area, then swelling can be minimized if you sleep with your head elevated on a few pillows.
3. Clean the area daily with hydrogen peroxide. Then apply a thin layer of antibiotic ointment one to two times per day for 5 days or until the surface is totally healed. Cover the area with a clean dressing.
4. If bleeding occurs, cover the area with a clean gauze pad and apply pressure for 3 to 10 minutes.
5. Do not break any blisters or remove scabs. The scabs will fall off as the healing process continues. A protective dressing should be applied if the area is irritated by jewelry or clothing.
6. When the scabs have fallen off and new skin has formed, cosmetics and creams can be used.
7. You may take acetaminophen (Tylenol) to control pain or discomfort.
8. If you have excessive bleeding, pain, or infection (tenderness, redness, swelling, or pus) of the surgical area, contact the physician's office.
9. You must avoid direct sunlight for 2 to 6 months because the sunlight will cause discoloration of the surgical site. Apply a sunblock of at least 15 SPF (sun protection factor) if you cannot avoid direct sunlight.

With successful lightening of a port-wine stain, some patients notice a decrease in the fullness of the facial features or improvement in the symmetry of the face. This is due to the resolution of the underlying blood-vessel distention.

The CO_2 laser has also been used to treat port-wine stains. For very superficial lesions, CO_2 laser energy can provide significant lightening by vaporizing the surface epithelium and sealing the superficial dermal plexus of the distended small blood vessels. The surgical area is anesthetized with an injectable local anesthetic. A defocused beam is passed over the area; then the char is removed using a sponge soaked in 3% hydrogen peroxide. A second pass is made to vaporize the superficial blood vessels. Again, the area is cleansed with hydrogen peroxide. At the completion of the procedure, an antibiotic ointment is applied. The wound heals by secondary intention within 2 to 4 weeks.

The CO_2 laser is also used to treat nodular lesions of the port-wine stain by sculpting the tissue to reestablish a normal facial contour (Figures 6-8 and 6-9). An injection of a local anesthetic decreases the pain of the laser pulses. An ultrapulse or very quick pulse duration is needed to prevent char buildup. After the nodules are leveled, the argon, yellow light, or other color selective wavelength can be used to lighten the stain.

Research is being conducted to treat extensive port-wine stains with photodynamic therapy. An injection of a light-sensitive drug is absorbed by the dysfunctional vasculature of the stain. When these vessels are exposed to special laser energy, coagulation occurs; the blood flow therefore is altered and the stain lightens. This research is being con-

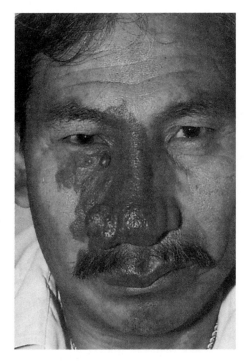

FIG. 6-8   This patient has a congenital port-wine stain with hypertrophied tissue and nodules. (From Goldman MP and Fitzpatrick RE: *Cutaneous laser surgery,* St. Louis, 1994, Mosby.)

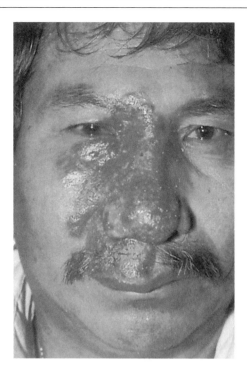

FIG. 6-9 The ultrapulse CO_2 laser is used to smooth the surface of the port-wine stain hypertrophied tissue and nodules on the right inner canthus and the right lateral distal nose. (From Goldman MP and Fitzpatrick RE: *Cutaneous laser surgery,* St. Louis, 1994, Mosby.)

ducted on more extensive stains that sometimes do not respond well to the conventional laser therapy.

Pigmented Lesions

A *hemangioma* is a benign vascular tumor of dilated blood vessels with proliferative plump endothelial cells. It can occur in the skin, mucous membranes, and other soft tissues. A hemangioma may infiltrate the skin without elevating it, thus giving it an appearance similar to a port-wine stain. Hemangiomas are the most common tumor in infants; 60% occur on the head and neck, 25% on the trunk, and 15% on the extremities. Females are three times more likely than males to have a hemangioma (Goldman and Fitzpatrick, 1994, p. 52).

Hemangiomas located closer to the surface appear raised and bright red, while more deeply embedded lesions may have a smooth skin surface with overlying telangiectasia. (Telangiectasia is discussed later in the chapter.) A characteristic of an infant hemangioma is the rapid proliferation that occurs during the first 6 to 12 months of life. Complications during this phase are ulceration, bleeding, and infection. Gradual spontaneous involution then occurs at 6 to 10 months of age. The first sign of involution is the color change from crimson to dull purple. Lesions on the lips and nose usually involute more slowly. Studies have shown that complete involution occurs in 50% of children by age 5 and 70% by age 7, with continued improvement until the age of 10 to 12 years. Lesions that do not begin to involute by age 6 are not likely to completely regress. The rate of involution and extent of resolution are not related to the size of the lesion (Goldman and Fitzpatrick, 1994, p. 55).

Laser treatment usually involves waiting until natural regression is complete, but current research notes that effective treatment has been accomplished during the proliferative phase (Goldman and Fitzpatrick, 1994, p. 57). Since yellow laser light and argon laser are selectively absorbed by hemoglobin from the blood in the vessels, these wavelengths can very effectively lighten these lesions.

Strawberry (capillary) hemangiomas on infants have been treated with a variety of laser energies, including the copper vapor laser, the flashlamp pulsed dye laser, and the noncontact Nd:YAG laser. Yellow laser light usually penetrates the upper 1 mm of dermis, causing a superficial thrombogenesis. This action stimulates spontaneous involution and shrinkage of the lesion. The lesion fades significantly over 3 to 4 months because of the blanching effect and shrinkage. However, some physicians advise parents against laser treatment to allow the lesion to resolve itself.

Early aggressive treatment of superficial vascular lesions has been found to improve the eventual cosmetic results as well as prevent complications that can occur because of the expansion of the lesions impinging on other structures. Early involution is promoted, irregular skin surfaces are smoothened, enlargement is arrested, and scarring is minimized (Taylor, 1993).

Cavernous hemangiomas that appear on infants cause the family a great deal of emotional trauma. The old wisdom of leaving it alone until it naturally disappears in 6 to 8 years is often not acceptable when an obvious facial deformity is involved. Cavernous hemangiomas do not involute at this age as the strawberry hemangiomas do.

Deep cavernous hemangiomas can be resected with the CO_2 laser because the argon or yellow light laser energy cannot penetrate the lesion to the fullest extent. The procedure is relatively bloodless unless large vessels are encountered; these require either cautery or ligation. When a superpulse or ultrapulse mode is used, the incidence of scarring is decreased.

The flashlamp pulsed dye laser that emits a yellow wavelength can be used on hemangioma vasculature that is 1.5 mm from the surface. Many times the involution phase will be enhanced when this treatment is used. Other color-selective wavelengths can also be used to provide coagulation with a limited depth of penetration.

When treating a capillary hemangioma in an infant, general anesthesia is used because infants cannot tolerate the procedure unanesthetized. The noncontact Nd:YAG laser has been used successfully to treat this condition. A cold or iced slide may be used to compress the lesion to reduce its height. The cold temperature of the slide helps to minimize a greater surface thermal response to the laser energy. The Nd:YAG laser beam is delivered perpendicular to the tissue, and the depth of penetration extends from 5 to 7 mm. The scattering effect of the laser energy causes a thermal response of coagulation, necrosis, and hemostasis through a large volume of tissue. Using a polka-dot method, the mass of the hemangioma is treated. Obvious blanching and shrinking of the lesion can usually be observed during the procedure.

Immediately after laser intervention, a steroid is sometimes injected into the lesion at multiple sites to decrease the incidence of scarring. The amount of steroid injected depends on the size of the lesion. An antibiotic ointment is applied, and an ice compress is used to decrease postoperative swelling. The patient (or parents of an infant patient) should be instructed that some swelling will be experienced in the first 5 days.

Healing occurs first with the formation of a superficial crust. Later healing involves blanching of the color and shrinkage of the lesion. Complete healing is noticed from 2 to 5 months later (Apfelberg, 1989).

A *nevus* is a congenital discoloration of the skin caused by pigmentation. This lesion may be excised with the CO_2 laser or treated with argon lasers. The argon laser wavelength is readily absorbed by the pigment or melanin in the dermis of the skin. When the laser energy is selectively absorbed by the melanin, destruction of the melanocytes occurs followed by a lightening of the area. Currently this method of treatment has been limited to benign pigmented lesions. More research is being conducted on photoradiating primary and metastatic melanomas.

Café-au-lait (coffee with milk) macules are light tan to brown hypermelanotic flat lesions that range from 2 to 20 cm in diameter. It has been estimated that 13.8% of the population has one or more of these lesions (Goldman and Fitzpatrick, 1994, p. 115). The 510-nm pulsed laser has been found to be very successful in treating these benign epidermal pigmented lesions. After the first treatment, the lesion responds with approximately 50% lightening; subsequent treatments, usually two to three, lighten the spot completely. Because of the short pulse duration, about 300 ms, a local anesthetic is not needed because there is no significant thermal buildup. The pulses feel like the snap of a rubber band on the skin, resulting in a burning sensation similar to that of a sunburn. An ashwhite discoloration of the epidermis occurs immediately. Because the wavelength interacts with hemoglobin, superficial capillaries coagulate and purpura occurs.

After the surgery, mild edema and reactive erythema may occur. An ice pack helps prevent swelling and soothes the burning sensation. Patients are instructed not to use cosmetics for 2 to 3 days but to apply an antibiotic ointment to the area. Usually crusts last from 2 to 10 days depending upon the treatment site. (Facial lesions require about 10 days for the crusts to peel off.) Retreatments can be done at intervals of 4 to 6 weeks. Temporary hypopigmentation may occur during the first 2 to 3 weeks. Hyperpigmentation may also occur and usually resolves after 2 to 4 months. The 510-nm pulsed laser minimizes scarring by preventing thermal damage beyond the intended epidermal target (Fitzpatrick, 1992). The krypton laser has also produced similar results.

Telangiectasia

Telangiectasia is caused by the dilatation of capillaries and sometimes terminal arteries. This lesion is visible on the surface of the skin as the vessels can measure between 0.1 to 1.0 mm in size. Telangiectasia involving arteries at the origin is small, bright red, and does not protrude above the skin surface. Telangiectasia involving veins at the origin is wider, blue, and often protrudes above the skin surface. Telangiectasia originating from capillaries is initially fine and red but becomes larger and turns purple or blue after a time because of the venous backflow. All telangiectasias are thought to be caused by the release or activation of vasoactive substances that are precipitated by anoxia, hormones, infection, chemicals, and physical factors. Telangiectasia may appear as a birthmark and is most frequently found on the face and thighs.

Different laser wavelengths can be used to treat this condition, including CO_2, argon, and yellow or green light. Because of the CO_2 laser's nonselective absorption, this technology is no different from electrosurgery. Argon laser energy has been used with settings of 0.8 to 2.9 W, at exposure times of 50 ms to continuous, and spot sizes of 0.1 to 1 mm. Success rates of 65% to 99% have been reported, but scarring, hypopigmentation, hyperpigmentation, and recurrence have also been noted (Goldman and Fitzpatrick, 1994, p. 71). These adverse consequences are caused by the high absorption by the epidermal melanin and the radiation and dissipation of the thermal energy. An automatic scanning device can be used to limit this heat diffusion.

The tunable dye laser or flashlamp pulsed dye laser that produces a yellow light, from 577 to 595 nm, is being used successfully to treat telangiectasia. The beam size can be varied from 50 μm to 6 mm. A tracing technique to coagulate the small vessels directly has been advocated by many physicians. The endpoint of this technique is when the vessel disappears because of a disrupted blood flow but before blanching, blistering, or charring occurs. This laser may also be attached to an automatic scanning device to deliver the laser energy (Figure 6-10).

A local anesthetic is usually not injected because it will increase the volume of the tissue and temporarily obliterate the vasculature, thus decreasing the laser beam absorption. The patient can easily tolerate the procedure without the local anesthetic if the tissue is allowed to cool between the pulses. The patient will feel a mild, warm sensation with this technique. By decreasing the time that the beam is in contact with the tissue, thermal spread is controlled, thus decreasing the pain response. Also, a preoperative anesthetic cream may be applied to help control pain during the procedure.

Healing is significant after 6 to 8 weeks. Facial telangiectasia responds more favorably to this therapy than lesions on the extremities or trunk do.

Spider angiomas or superficial varicosities are caused by dilated, branched capillaries on the skin that resemble a spider. Lesions of this type have been successfully treated on the face and neck, but superficial varicosities on the leg have not responded well to treatment. When located on the lower extremities, these lesions are difficult to control because of the increased hydrostatic pressure that recanalizes the vessels that supply blood from a number of other vessels. Approximately 29% to 41% of women and 6% to 15% of men in the United States have this condition. Even though 53% of these patients also have asso-

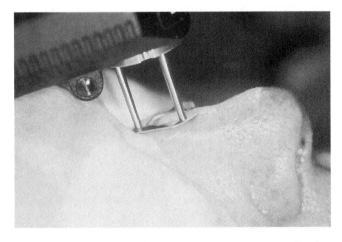

FIG. 6-10 Hexascan device delivers the yellow light laser energy to treat telangiectasia on the nose. (Courtesy Dr. James Mechenbier.)

ciated conditions, the reason they seek treatment is usually cosmetic (Goldman and Fitz-patrick, 1994, p. 82).

Many techniques have been investigated over the years to treat spider veins of the legs. The argon, CO_2, contact YAG, green-only argon, and frequency doubled YAG laser systems have been used with moderate success.

Yellow light laser energy has shown the most promise in the treatment of spider veins on the legs. The beam is delivered to the tissue using high-power magnification with spot sizes ranging from 100 μm to 5 mm in diameter (Figure 6-11). The first pulse may be de-livered to the central vessel, which usually results in partial or complete blanching of the peripheral part of the lesion. The yellow light is absorbed selectively by the hemoglobin of the vessel, causing coagulation and lightening. The overlying tissue of the skin remains unaffected. An ice pack is applied to the treatment area until the laser heat has resolved (5 to 15 minutes). A compression bandage is often used to enhance coagulation of the smaller vessels so that blood will not flow into these vessels (the legs are usually in the dependent position after surgery).

Studies are noting better results using this technique with patients over age 30 and with vessel sizes under 1 mm in diameter (Apfelberg, 1987). Larger vessels are treated with a combination of a sclerosing agent injection using a 33-gauge needle and laser en-ergy. Other studies are exploring delivering the laser energy directly to the vessel via a

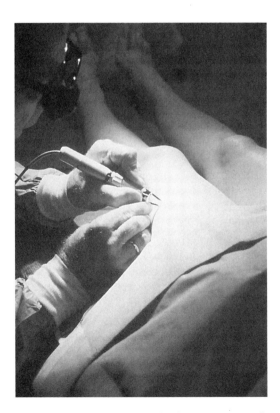

FIG. 6-11   Spider veins on the legs do not respond to laser energy as well as facial lesions do.

hypodermic needle. The skin surface is cooled with ethyl chloride spray. Scarring is minimized and the vessel is coagulated. Continuing studies are being conducted to refine these techniques, but preliminary results are proving the value of the yellow light laser in the treatment of spider veins of the legs.

LASER SURGERY FOR CUTANEOUS LESIONS
Skin Incisions

Different laser wavelengths have been used for skin incisions. Today the laser is not usually used for the sole purpose of making the skin incision. However, if a laser procedure is to be performed during surgery, then the laser may also be used to make the skin incision.

The healing of a laser wound is similar to that of a wound caused by a conventional scalpel incision. Three anatomical layers are involved in the normal healing process. At the epithelial level the cells grow rapidly, with new epithelial cells migrating along the edge of the dermis layer. In the subcutaneous layer, fibroblasts and capillaries repair the connective tissue of the skin. The deeper fibroblasts then progress toward the dermis and epidermis and form a bulge. Collagen fibers then bridge the incised dermis to fill the area.

When the laser is used to make the incision, there is an earlier migration of the new epithelial cells toward the dermis. Also, slower collagen formation occurs, making the tensile strength of the healed area less strong than that of a conventionally healed wound until the healing is complete, in approximately 3 weeks. These findings are insignificant histologically when comparing the two incisions. Therefore, the laser can be used effectively to make skin incisions.

When the CO_2 laser is used to make the skin incision, any skin prep solution must not be allowed to pool or accumulate in areas where the incision will be made because the thermal energy of the laser will heat the solution and possibly cause a skin burn.

When making an incision with the CO_2 laser, the hand piece is held at a specific distance from the skin so that the beam is in focus on the tissue. At this point all of the laser energy is concentrated within a small spot, thus increasing the power density. The surgeon can control the depth of penetration of the beam by varying the wattage, exposure time, and spot size. To take advantage of the hemostatic properties of the CO_2 laser, the hand piece is defocused on the tissue (by moving the hand piece away from the target) and the laser energy coagulates blood vessels up to 0.5 mm in diameter. Larger blood vessels may be ligated.

The CO_2 laser beam does not allow for tactile sensation, which surgeons have depended upon for years. This may be a disadvantage for physicians until they attain a high level of skill and comfort with this nontouch technique.

When used for cutting, the CO_2 laser energy also provides a certain sterilizing effect to the tissue from the thermal energy that is generated. Therefore, the chance of producing an infected wound is minimized when the laser is used. The CO_2 laser also has been theorized to seal the cutaneous sensory nerve endings of the skin, as contrasted with the frayed ends resulting from a scalpel incision. This usually minimizes postoperative pain. The CO_2 beam can also seal the lymphatic channels, leading to a reduction in postoperative swelling and decreasing the spread of malignant cells to other areas of the body.

Currently, contact Nd:YAG scalpels are also being used to cut skin. Their advantages and healing effects are similar to those of the CO_2 laser, but tactile sensation is returned to the physician because the contact tip must touch the tissue.

The tunable dye laser producing a yellow light wavelength is being investigated for use to excise small skin tags. Anesthesia is not necessary since the patient does not appear to experience any major discomfort as with the CO_2 laser.

Tissue welding is currently being investigated for producing sutureless tissue fusion. Skin incisions are being welded back together with the use of laser energy. These studies are being refined so that someday the laser may be used not only to open the skin, but also to close it.

Keloids and Scars

A keloid tends to recur when excised by conventional methods using a scalpel. Scars and keloids are being successfully removed with the CO_2, Nd:YAG, argon, and yellow light lasers. Laser energy is delivered to remove the areas containing the hypertrophied tissue. If the keloid is near the hairline, the patient must be instructed to not use hair spray or styling gels because any highly flammable material will easily ignite from the laser interaction (Figure 6-12).

When the laser is used, wet towels are placed around the lesion. A local anesthetic is administered, and the laser energy excises the keloid down to the level of the normal skin. Additional, deeper layers are ablated if fibrotic tissue is palpated at the base. Sutures are not recommended because tension across the wound could lead to reformation of the keloid. The wound heals within 3 to 6 weeks, depending on the size of the area involved. Some theories state that the laser energy suppresses the collagen reformation that is associated with the regeneration of the keloid.

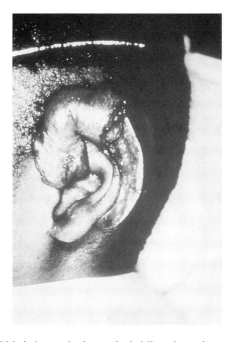

FIG. 6-12   When a keloid is being excised near the hairline, the patient must be reminded not to use hair spray, styling gels, or other products that could increase the risk of fire.

The flashlamp pulsed dye laser of 585 nm has been used to treat scars, but the exact mechanisms of tissue reaction is not completely understood yet. Research has shown that there is an apparent improvement of the clinical appearance of erythematous and hypertrophic scars when this type of laser is used (Alster, 1993).

When the Nd:YAG laser is used to treat keloids, significant results have been noted in the effect on collagen metabolism. Studies have shown that the collagen production is selectively inhibited, while normal fibroblast DNA replication and cell viability are spared. Therefore, the Nd:YAG laser wavelength appears to be the laser of choice today in treating keloids (Goldman and Fitzpatrick, 1994, p. 82).

Research using the argon laser to treat keloids notes that because this laser light is highly absorbed by the oxyhemoglobin of blood, coagulation occurs in the capillary plexus. Localized anoxia then leads to lymphatic plugging and vasculature disruption at the laser site. Glycolysis produces excessive amounts of lactic acid. The granulocytes are lysed from this low pH environment and release their enzymes, including collagenase. With increased levels of collagenase, lysis of collagen increases, thus altering the recurrence of collagen and keloid formation (Goldman and Fitzpatrick, 1994, p. 82).

Dermabrasion with the Laser

Dermabrasion can be performed using the CO_2 laser for conditions such as psoriasis. The laser energy in a defocused mode is delivered to the tissue. Superficial effects are observed as the heat from the laser absorption causes the surface tissue to be supraheated leading to a sterilization effect. A thin layer of antibiotic ointment is applied to enhance the healing process. Reepithelialization takes place within 2 weeks as the inflammation subsides.

Dermabrasion has been used for other skin conditions, such as acne problems and even wrinkles. Laserbrasion, as it is termed, precisely removes superficial skin layers to the desired depth in the dermis. Postoperative pain and swelling are reduced, and healing usually occurs without complications. The CO_2 laser, in the superpulse or ultrapulse mode, may be used alone or in combination with trichloroacetic acid as a chemical peeling agent to precisely resurface the skin.

The use of the automatic scanning device coupled with the CO_2 laser allows the laser energy depth to be controlled so that a uniform and smooth depth of penetration can be obtained. The area to be treated is outlined by the scanner, and this information is stored in the computer. The physician selects the laser spot size, power, and speed of the movement of the laser scanner that will deliver the energy to the tissue. The laser is then activated, and the scanner delivers a predetermined amount of laser energy over the lesion. The physician evaluates the depth and extent of the tissue reaction at the end of each pass to decide whether another pass is needed. The computerized scanner allows the laserbrasion to be accomplished very precisely with a uniform depth of penetration. This technique results in decreased intraoperative bleeding and postoperative pain.

When the CO_2 laser is used to smooth wrinkles, great experience and expertise is needed because the depth of destruction is difficult to judge. The laser is activated over the wrinkle until the tissue color turns to a light gray tone. Usually hydrogen peroxide is not used as it causes a distinctive whitening of the surgical site that obscures tissue detail. Normal saline leaves the tissue detail intact so that the level of destruction can be evaluated adequately. Thus, normal saline is the irrigant of choice for this delicate procedure (Goldman and Fitzpatrick, 1994, p. 227).

The laser is also being used for burn therapy. Charred skin can be precisely and accurately ablated down to the normal tissue level. With a special high-power, very-short-pulse (100 ns) CO_2 laser, burn debridement can be performed without interfering with graft survival. This type of laser can be used to remove the necrotic tissue rapidly with less than 100 μm of thermal damage. Research is coupling spectroscopic analysis with burn treatment to provide computerized imaging to help determine the depth of tissue damage. The laser can then be used to debride the charred tissue to this level. Continued research is needed to refine the technique so as to achieve optimal results.

Treatment of rhinophyma can be accomplished through laser dermabrasion. The procedure is easy to perform with the use of a local anesthetic and provides precise tissue removal and nasal sculpting. Rhinophyma is caused by hypertrophied nasal tissue resulting from clogged sebaceous glands (Figure 6-13). Patient preparation must be thorough because the patient is awake during the procedure. The eyes are covered with a wet towel, and the smoke evacuation wand is held close to the laser-tissue impact site to prevent inhalation of the plume by the patient. The patient is reminded about the importance of not moving during the procedure as the nose must be sculpted precisely.

The excess nasal tissue is vaporized layer by layer until the desired level of contouring is achieved (Figure 6-14). As the CO_2 laser impacts the tissue, the dermis contracts and causes sebum from the sebaceous glands to be expressed. As this is observed, and if the nose is squeezed and sebum is extruded, then the sebaceous glands are intact and postoperative scarring is minimized. If the laser excision is below the level of the glands, scarring will occur.

The patient is allowed to see the surgical site before the dressing is applied to promote compliance with the postoperative instructions (Figure 6-15). The patient is instructed how to provide proper home care to the surgical site. Changing the dressing, cleaning the surgical site properly, and reapplying the antibiotic ointment are critically important to prevent postoperative infection. Reepithelialization occurs within 2 to 4 weeks as the skin cells from the nasal pores assist with the healing process (Figure 6-16). A skin graft is not needed.

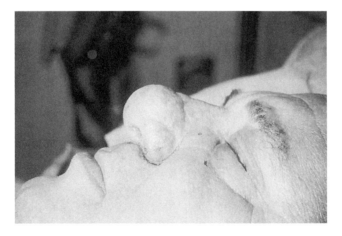

FIG. 6-13   Rhinophyma causes an overgrowth of nasal tissue.

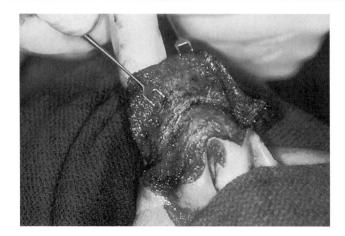

FIG. 6-14   The CO_2 laser is used to excise excess nasal tissue.

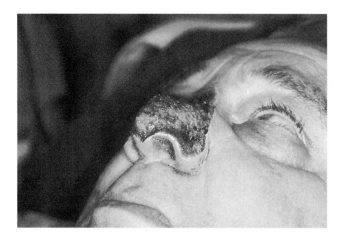

FIG. 6-15   The patient is allowed to see the surgical site before the dressing is applied.

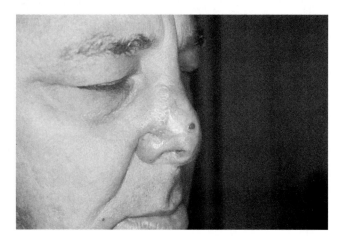

FIG. 6-16   The nose is reformed after the CO_2 laser procedure.

Verruca

The CO_2 and contact Nd:YAG lasers are being used to treat verruca lesions. Since these warts are caused by a virus, the high temperatures that the laser energy generates aids in the elimination of the wart virus.

A local anesthetic is administered around the verruca, which is vaporized using a defocused CO_2 beam. The surface char produced is removed with 3% hydrogen peroxide, and the depth of the laser penetration is evaluated. The laser is used again to remove a deeper layer of the verruca, and again the charred material is removed. This sequence continues until all of the wart tissue is gone. The use of a microscope is valuable in assessing the texture and appearance of the underlying normal dermal layer as the wart is being removed. Any viral tissue that is left will cause recurrence of the verruca.

Healing occurs within 10 to 14 days. Usually there is minimal postoperative pain and a reduced rate of recurrence, compared with conventional surgical wart removal procedures using the scalpel or cautery. Scarring is usually not a problem, except when the verruca is on the back of the hand (Figure 6-17). This is a common area for scarring, and care must be taken not to vaporize this area too extensively. Hypertrophic scars tend to resolve with time.

Contact Nd:YAG laser energy is also being used to remove verruca lesions. The physician appreciates the tactile sensation as a probe or scalpel is held in contact with the wart. The depth of penetration is easily assessed to ensure that all of the viral tissue has been destroyed so the verruca will not reform.

Actinic Cheilitis

Actinic cheilitis is a premalignant condition of the lower lip that resembles chapping. It is caused by chronic sun exposure and is associated with squamous cell cancer. It can appear in variegated red, brown, and white blotchy colors, with blurring of the vermilion border; focal thickenings are present; and it can flake or crust. Many physicians advocate removal of the entire surface of the vermilion of the lower lip to prevent the development

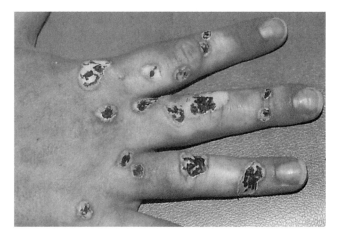

FIG. 6-17   Multiple warts of the dorsum of the hand are treated with a continuous CO_2 laser at 10 W. Obvious scarring of the tissue is visible immediately after the treatment. (From Goldman MP and Fitzpatrick RE: *Cutaneous laser surgery,* St. Louis, 1994, Mosby.)

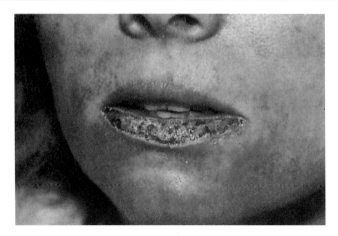

FIG. 6-18   Actinic cheilitis is treated with CO_2 laser energy. (From Goldman MP and Fitzpatrick RE: *Cutaneous laser surgery,* St. Louis, 1994, Mosby.)

of squamous cell cancer. Approximately 11% of squamous cell carcinoma of the lip metastasizes (Goldman and Fitzpatrick, 1994, pp. 240-241).

The CO_2 laser is used at 4 to 5 W to vaporize the epidermis with a spot size of about 2 to 3 mm in diameter. The surgical site will whiten and bubble as the laser energy debrides this area (Figure 6-18). A saline-soaked gauze is used to wipe away any charred tissue. The depth of penetration is controlled to surface ablation to avoid scarring and allow for faster healing. The usual healing period can extend to 5 weeks when continuous CO_2 laser energy is used. The quicker the pulsation of the laser beam, the faster the healing takes place. For example, the ultrapulse CO_2 laser ablation will heal within 13 days (Goldman and Fitzpatrick, 1994, p. 242).

Other Laser Applications

The CO_2 laser has been used successfully to treat seborrheic keratoses of the face, scalp, and torso. Using the CO_2 in combination with a facial chemical peel usually allows the procedure to be completed in one session. The ultrapulse or superpulse CO_2 laser allows the lesion to be treated and decreases the thermal damage below the lesion. When the seborrheic keratoses are on the scalp, hair even tends to regrow in the treated area.

The ultrapulse CO_2 laser is also being used to facilitate hair transplants. The hair follicle plugs are excised with a special delivery device specifically made for this purpose. The margins of the plug are preserved since significantly less thermal energy is spread through the tissue. The implanted plug tends to heal very quickly, sustaining the hair in the transplanted area. Refinements of this technique are helping to make this application very popular today.

LASER SURGERY FOR TATTOO REMOVAL

There are two types of tattoos: decorative and accidental.

Decorative tattoos can be applied by an amateur or a professional. A tattoo is made by injecting pigmentation into the skin. Professionally made tattoos are more uniform in depth of penetration than amateur tattoos, which are irregular in depth of penetration.

Sometimes tattoos are made by radiation oncologists to mark treatment sites of cancer patients to make localization of radiation ports more accessible. Many patients want to remove this reminder of their unpleasant experience in cancer treatment.

Accidental tattoos are caused by the mechanical penetration of the skin with a particle of foreign matter. An explosive tattoo involves gunpowder or other volatile substances, such as fine particles that can be embedded deep within the skin. An abrasive tattoo is a result of friction, such as dragging along a road surface during an automobile or motorcycle accident. A traumatic tattoo occurs when foreign substances such as dust, sand, dirt, glass, wood, or metal are forced into the skin.

The CO_2, argon, pulsed ruby, Alexandrite, Nd:YAG, and 510-nm lasers have been effective in removing decorative tattoo pigmentation from the skin layers. The patient must understand that with some of the tattoo treatment techniques, the texture of the skin after the procedure may change and that ghost scarring may result. Many patients are pleased with the results if they understand this information preoperatively so that realistic postoperative expectations can be anticipated.

Cosmetic tattoos are also being removed with laser energy. For example, an unwanted eyeliner tattoo can be removed. This procedure can become complex because of the need to avoid damage to the eyelash follicles and scarring of the lid margin. The CO_2 laser can provide the precision needed to perform this procedure. Healing is by secondary intention, and results note a scar line that is not noticeable. Other facial cosmetic tattoos, such as red lip liner, simulated rouge on cheeks, and eyebrows can be treated with other wavelengths that provide color-selective absorption.

The CO_2 laser is used to abrade the layers of skin that contain the pigmentation (Figure 6-19). After injections of a local anesthetic, the CO_2 laser energy is directed at the tattoo using a large spot size (defocused beam) at power settings from 4 to 25 W. Less hypertrophic scarring is noted if the laser is used in the pulsed mode. One layer of tissue is vaporized using overlapping sweeps in a circular or linear manner. The tattoo must be vaporized not only where the pigmentation exists because ghost scarring will form the exact shape of the tattoo. Rather, the pigmentation and some of the normal skin must also be treated so as not to duplicate the original tattoo's shape. The surface char and debris is aggressively scrubbed from the area with 3% hydrogen peroxide on a sponge or soft brush. Any residual pigmentation is retreated for removal. Careful examination of retained pigmentation is complemented with the use of magnification loupes or a microscope.

A combination of superficial CO_2 laser vaporization and 50% urea paste has shown significant results. The tattoo is vaporized at pulsed or continuous modes with 10 to 15 W of energy. The goal is to remove only 30% to 40% of the tattoo pigment. The urea paste is applied liberally over the wound and is covered with a Telfa dressing. The urea paste is reapplied and the dressing replaced daily. The action of the urea paste is to assist with the leaching of the tattoo dye. Tattoo pigment will be present in the wound exudate on the dressing. When the tattoo pigmentation is no longer present (usually after 1 to 2 weeks), treatment is discontinued. Usually 95% of the pigment can be removed using this method (Goldman and Fitzpatrick, 1994, p. 157-158).

Hypertrophic scarring often occurs when the CO_2 laser is used to remove tattoo pigmentation. The degree of scarring depends on the anatomical location of the tattoo. One study showed that 25% of patients who had tattoos removed from the deltoid and chest area had hypertrophic scarring, while only 10% of those with tattoos in other areas healed with this complication (Goldman and Fitzpatrick, 1994, p. 158). Cosmetic results are

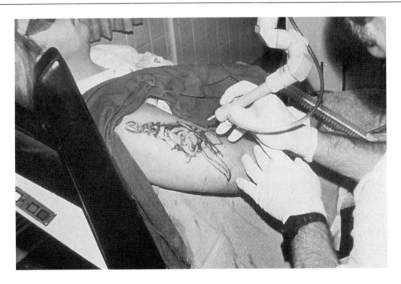

FIG. 6-19   The CO$_2$ laser is used to remove a decorative tattoo. (Courtesy Dr. James Mechenbier.)

somewhat unpredictable when the CO$_2$ laser is used. The more superficial the tattoo, the more promising the results. Newer tattoos tend to respond better than the older ones do.

Retin A (tretinoin) is being researched for minimizing postoperative scarring after CO$_2$ laser treatment. This substance has been used to treat acne patients and to reduce wrinkles. It works by irritating the skin, thus causing the top layers to peel off. It also increases circulation to the skin and enhances collagen formation to fill skin indentations, thus smoother skin results. Before treating a tattoo with the laser, pretreatment with Retin A one to three times per day causes new vessels to be formed to enhance circulation, helps bring the pigmentation closer to the skin surface, and thickens the epidermis. Then the CO$_2$ laser is used to ablate the tattoo. Retin A is also being researched for postoperative use. This research has not been conclusive but shows promising results (*Clinical Laser Monthly,* May 1992).

Traumatic tattoos can be treated using laser energy, such as the CO$_2$ laser, to ablate the surface of the skin to allow the foreign matter to escape from the skin surface. After ablating the area, aggressive scrubbing of the wound with a peroxide solution helps to debride the pigmentation. A steroid may be injected around the operative site to decrease the chance of hypertrophic scarring, an antibiotic ointment is administered to the wound, and a pressure dressing is applied. Patients are given instructions for changing dressings and caring for the wound.

Because some of the laser treatments, such as the CO$_2$ laser, require that the surface of the skin be broken, the chance of contracting hepatitis B virus, HIV, or other viral conditions is increased. Therefore, new procedures that do not break the epidermal barrier are becoming more popular.

The argon laser is also used to remove decorative tattoos. The pigmentation readily absorbs the argon wavelength, causing an inflammatory reaction (by the body's phagocytes). This in turn leads to the residual pigmentation leaching from the skin. The melanin of the skin also absorbs this argon wavelength, thus leading to unacceptable postoperative scarring.

The pulsed (microseconds) or Q-switched (nanoseconds) ruby laser produces a wavelength that is highly absorbed by blue, black, and sometimes green pigmentation in a tattoo. The pigmentation breaks into pieces that are absorbed by the body. This laser wavelength is not effective with other pigmentation colors, such as red and yellow. Sometimes this laser induces punctate bleeding and tissue-splattering at the laser-irradiated site. This side effect can be minimized by covering the surgical site with a plastic wrap or transparent film to protect the operator from tissue and blood contact. But usually the overlying skin is left intact. Delayed pulse delivery (one pulse every 2 seconds) can make this laser procedure very tedious. Postoperative complications include hypertrophic scarring and hypopigmentation. The laser must be used in a series of treatments to achieve the desired effects of tattoo removal.

The Q-switched (10 nanoseconds) Nd:YAG laser is being investigated for use in tattoo removal. Professionally made tattoos appear to respond better to the Nd:YAG energy because they uniformly absorb the beam. Healthier, lighter skin with less melanin seems to heal better after tattoo removal with the Nd:YAG laser than with other lasers. This wavelength is highly absorbed by black and blue pigmentation. The Q-switched Nd:YAG laser energy causes the skin to billow up to expose the pigment instead of actually vaporizing it. Tissue-splattering and bleeding may occur. When the tattoo appears most intense in color, the procedure is complete. The pigmentation is then allowed to leach from the skin cells. After 3 months the pigmentation is gone, and the skin texture remains much like normal skin. Hypopigmentation is minimized after the procedure. A series of treatments is needed to treat the tattoo.

Since the Q-switched Nd:YAG laser is limited to the treatment of black and dark blue pigments, another laser wavelength can be produced by this laser system. A frequency doubling crystal can cause the incident 1064-nm Nd:YAG beam to become a 532-nm wavelength. This beam is highly absorbed by red pigmentation and thus allows more colors in the tattoo to be treated.

The Q-switched Alexandrite laser at 755 or 760 nm at 100-ns pulsations has been introduced to treat tattoos by allowing the epidermal layer to remain intact. No anesthesia is required as laser energy at a pulsed 50- to 100-ns duration is delivered through a larger spot, 3 mm in diameter. The tattoo dye (black, blue, and green) is fragmented and reabsorbed, and the epidermis remains intact. Purpura or bleeding may occur from the rapid thermal expansion and shock waves that also fracture capillaries. The treated skin remains normal in color, texture, and elasticity. Sequential treatments are needed to resolve the tattoo to an acceptable appearance. Hypopigmentation is a common side effect that occurs in approximately 50% of patients but may not be apparent until after the fifth treatment. This side effect usually resolves within a year (Goldman and Fitzpatrick, 1994, p. 177). Usually resolution of the tattoo pigmentation occurs after four to ten treatment sessions performed at 1- to 2-month intervals.

The flashlamp pulsed dye laser that produces a wavelength of 510 nm at 300-ns pulses can be used to treat red, purple, orange, and yellow pigmentations. When the beam is absorbed by these colors in the epidermal layer, the pigmentation fragments. Macrophage engulfment of the pigmentation follows, with resolution of these colors. Postoperative hypopigmentation, textural change, and scarring has not been a reported problem.

Whichever laser wavelength is used, the patient should see the results of the surgery before an antibiotic ointment is applied and the wound is patched. This helps the patient understand the extent of the lased area and encourages compliance with postoperative instructions. Sometimes a steroid is injected to decrease the chance of scarring.

After the tattoo is removed, strict adherence to the postoperative care regimen is required to decrease the chances of infection. The patient should be instructed to clean the surgical area daily with 3% hydrogen peroxide and then apply a thin layer of antibiotic ointment. A sterile dressing (and usually an elastic wrap) is applied to provide a barrier against infection. The pressure of the elastic wrap helps decrease the formation of a hypertrophic scar, especially in the upper extremities, and also helps decrease postoperative pain. A sample patient-information sheet is provided on page 183.

The patient should *not* expose the surgical area to direct sunlight because ultraviolet rays may cause hyperpigmentation of the area. Light-skinned patients seem to have better healing results than do olive- or dark-skinned patients. Tattoos on the upper arm and shoulder do not respond as well to tattoo removal because these areas have a poor prognosis for healing. The success of the healing depends upon the patient's compliance with instructions involving daily wound care, massaging the area gently to promote circulation, external compression to decrease scarring, and sunlight restriction to reduce hypopigmentation.

The patient usually feels less pain after the laser procedure because the laser energy, it has been thought, seals the nerve endings in the skin. The wound heals in approximately 2 to 4 weeks, depending upon the area that was treated, the depth of the pigmentation, and the laser wavelength used. Healing is complete within 12 to 18 months.

The complications associated with laser tattoo removal are skin-texture changes, hypertrophic scarring, and residual pigmentation. The patient must understand these complications so that expectations will be realistic.

LASER BLEPHAROPLASTY AND OTHER PLASTIC REPAIR PROCEDURES

Creative procedures are being performed with the laser. The dermatologist and the plastic surgeon are discovering new applications to benefit the patient that result in less time spent in the hospital, less blood loss during surgery, less pain after the procedure, and better cosmetic results.

Laser Blepharoplasty

Laser blepharoplasty is a new technique used to eliminate bulges under the eyes to promote a more youthful appearance. The conventional method of blepharoplasty is performed with a scalpel. This technique results in increased bleeding, surgical time, bruising, swelling, and pain. Patients appreciate laser blepharoplasty because it can be performed quickly and easily, with the patient under local anesthesia, in an outpatient clinic or the physician's office, with minimal complications or side effects.

Preoperative patient education is paramount to ensure that the patient fully understands the procedure, the anticipated results, and what is expected for home care after the procedure. Preoperative photographs are usually taken so comparisons can be made postoperatively. A simple eye examination is performed to provide baseline information in case complications occur.

Sample Patient Instructions:
Laser Tattoo Removal

Dear patient,

The following information is to help you understand the laser tattoo treatment and the after-surgery care for the area where your tattoo has been removed. Complying with these simple instructions will ensure the best cosmetic results and success of the treatment.

1. No guarantee can be given for complete removal of the tattoo because of the variability of the depth of the tattoo pigmentation and the different chemical compositions of the tattoo dyes.
2. Photos will be taken before and after surgery to help document the results of your treatment.
3. You may need more than one treatment to eliminate your tattoo.
4. If you experience discomfort during the procedure, a topical or local anesthetic may be used.
5. After the treatment, you must not expose the treated area to direct sun exposure for at least 6 months. Daily use of a sunscreen of at least 15 SPF (sun protection factor) will help protect the area if exposure cannot be avoided.
6. You will be instructed on how to apply the antibiotic ointment to the treated area and how to change the dressing on the wound. A compression bandage may help decrease swelling and discomfort after the surgery.
7. Do not rub, scratch, or pick at the treated area.
8. Avoid contact sports while the surgical area is healing.
9. If you experience discomfort after the procedure, you can take an oral analgesic (such as Tylenol) and use an ice compress. Apply the ice compress for 20 minutes and remove it for 20 minutes in sequence for the first 24 hours after surgery to reduce swelling.
10. If the treatment area shows signs of infection (tenderness, redness, swelling, or pus), contact the physician.
11. Subsequent treatments and evaluations will be scheduled with you. Follow-up can be very critical.
12. Your insurance will probably not pay for this treatment because it is not medically necessary. Therefore, you will be expected to pay for each treatment at the time of the service. Terms of payment can be discussed at your request.

Light sedation can be administered to anesthetize the patient. A marking pen is used to outline the lower eyelid where the bulges are located. A local ophthalmological anesthetic is instilled in each eye, and wet sterile towels are placed around the operative site. The conjunctiva is infiltrated with local anesthetic solution.

A special plastic instrument called a Jaegar plate is used to protect the eye and provide access to the conjunctival area. CO_2 laser energy at 5 to 8 W of power is used to incise the conjunctival area of the lower lid. An incision of 1.0 to 1.5 cm is made, and the muscle is manipulated to raise the fat through the incision. The fat is removed using gentle traction and the laser beam to free it. Care must be taken not to provide too much traction because bleeding can occur. When the bulk of fat has been pulled through the incision, the fat is then excised using laser energy.

No sutures are necessary because the laser incision in the conjunctiva will heal by primary intention. Ophthalmic antibiotic ointment is applied to the conjunctival area. A sterile gauze sponge soaked in saline is placed over each eye, followed by ice compresses. Frozen peas placed in a small plastic bag can be used as an ice compress. This pack tends to follow the contour of the surgical area better, it weighs less, and the peas can be refrozen.

The patient recovers for approximately 1 hour with the head elevated at a 45-degree angle. Home discharge instructions include maintaining ice packs as much as possible over the first 24 hours and elevating the head when lying down. This helps decrease the amount of swelling after the procedure. Acctaminophen can be taken for any discomfort. Antibiotic ointment is applied to the conjunctiva for approximately 5 days. An oral antibiotic may also be prescribed. Vigorous exercise should be avoided during the first week after the procedure to decrease any chance of injury, infection, or undue pressure.

At the first follow-up visit, 3 days after the surgery, a comparative eye examination is performed. Photographs are usually taken during subsequent postoperative visits at 2 weeks, 30 days, 3 months, and 6 months.

Complications are rare if the procedure is performed properly and if the patient adheres to the postoperative instructions. The most devastating complication is blindness attributed to hemorrhage during or after the surgery. Ecchymosis and hematoma formation can be avoided by ensuring intraoperative hemostasis.

Repair of Pierced Ear

A pierced ear from trauma can be repaired using the CO_2 laser. Patients have complained that the pierced hole in the earlobe has become enlarged or is a slit instead of a hole (Figure 6-20). Repair is needed to provide an attractive appearance. The earlobe is injected with an anesthetic. The CO_2 laser is used to deepithelialize the slit (Figure 6-21).

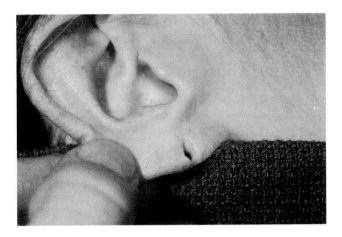

FIG. 6-20   An enlarged hole caused by trauma to the pierced ear.

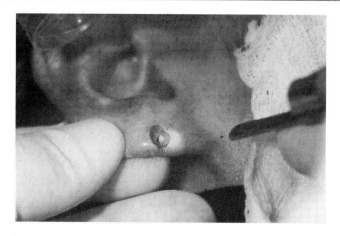

FIG. 6-21   The CO_2 laser deepithelializes the tissue so that healing can occur to repair the hole.

The wound is then closed with absorbable sutures. Either a large-bore suture or an earring is placed in the area where the hole is desired. An antibiotic ointment is applied postoperatively, and healing occurs within 2 to 3 weeks, and the suture or earring is removed. The patient should be reminded to not wear heavy earrings because the weight could destroy the surgical results.

REFERENCES

Alster R: Pulsed dye laser gives hope to scar patients, *Clinical Laser Monthly,* pp 155-156, Oct 1993.

Apfelberg DB: Newer lasers can treat varicosities in legs with few adverse reactions, *Clinical Laser Monthly,* p 1S, June 1987.

Apfelberg DB: Nd:YAG laser, direct steroid instillation used to treat hemangiomas, *Clinical Laser Monthly,* p 3S, Jan 1989.

Fitzpatrick RE: Candela laser eliminates scarring after treatment of benign pigmented lesions, *Clinical Laser Monthly,* pp 75-76, May, 1992.

Goldman MP and Fitzpatrick RE: *Cutaneous laser surgery,* St. Louis, 1994, Mosby.

Retin A pretreatment may reduce scarring after tattoo vaporization, *Clinical Laser Monthly,* pp 73-74, May 1992.

Taylor MB: Can early therapy make a difference in treatment of strawberry hemangiomas? *Clinical Laser Monthly,* pp 87-90, June, 1993.

SUGGESTED READINGS

Achauer BM, Vander Kam VM, and Burns MW: *Lasers in plastic surgery and dermatology,* New York, 1992, Thieme.

Milstein HG: CO_2 laser is practical, economical tool for dermatology office, *Clinical Laser Monthly,* p 3S, Dec 1988.

Pfister JI, Kneedler JA, and Purcell SK: *The nursing spectrum of lasers,* Denver, 1988, Education Design.

Ratz JL: *Laser in cutaneous medicine and surgery,* Chicago, 1986, Year Book.

Schliftman AB: Argon, copper-vapor lasers used to treat port wine stains, *Clinical Laser Monthly,* p 1S, July 1988.

Spadoni D and Cain CL: Laser blepharoplasty, *AORN J,* 47(5):1184, May 1988.

7

GASTROENTEROLOGY AND COLORECTAL LASER APPLICATIONS

LASER ENDOSCOPY

In the mid 1970s, the marriage between the endoscope and the laser finally became a reality with the development of the quartz fiberoptic delivery system. The inside of the gastrointestinal (GI) tract could be visualized while active bleeding was stopped. The first type of laser to be used was the argon system to photocoagulate bleeding gastritis. This was a major breakthrough in gastroenterology because various disorders of the digestive tract could be managed without an invasive surgical procedure.

Today, the Nd:YAG system is the most popular laser used in the GI tract through an endoscope. The noncontact Nd:YAG beam scatters on impact and is not as readily absorbed by the red pigmented areas as is the argon beam. Instead, the Nd:YAG wavelength penetrates deeper and can provide coagulation and greater destruction of large tumor masses. The contact Nd:YAG laser is used to precisely excise lesions or ablate other GI conditions. The argon laser is used when shallower penetration is desired or when color selectivity is critical. Since this blue-green wavelength is highly absorbed by red pigmentation, treating angiodysplasias in the thin wall of the intestine with argon energy is highly effective and safe. The final results obtained with either of these lasers are not immediately observable at the time of the lasing, even though initial changes are seen. This disadvantage of not being able to witness the true tissue responses at deeper levels could cause delayed postoperative bleeding or fistula formation. The CO_2 laser cannot be used through the flexible endoscope because this wavelength cannot be conducted through quartz fibers.

Endoscopy Protocol

Upper or lower endoscopic procedures are safely and effectively performed today for diagnostic and therapeutic procedures. No matter which part of the GI tract is viewed, these endoscopic procedures have common elements. Basic GI endoscopic protocols need to be reviewed.

Many times the patient is awake or lightly sedated during an endoscopic procedure, so thorough preparation of the patient helps relieve anxiety. Preoperative patient education includes a discussion of endoscopy and laser technology and what the patient can expect before, during, and after the surgery. The rationale for wearing protective eyewear is simply explained so that the patient will not feel uncomfortable when the special glasses are applied.

The patient may be positioned on the left side so that aspiration is minimized if the patient vomits. The procedure is usually performed with the patient under intravenous sedation. Vital signs are monitored closely throughout the procedure. Protective eyewear is placed on the patient. The endoscope is introduced into the orifice and manipulated through to the diseased area. Landmarks are identified and a diagnostic assessment is made of the severity of the disease process. Often a video system is used to record the procedure and provide visualization for the rest of the surgical team.

When the laser fiber is inserted into the endoscope, great care must be taken not to puncture the inside lumen of the biopsy port with the sharp tip of the fiber (Figure 7-1). The endoscope should be as straight as possible during this insertion. If a bare fiber is used without a catheter sheath, a length of medical-grade tubing can be used to avoid contact with the sharp tip. The fiber is placed inside the tubing with the tip recessed. The entire unit of the fiber and tubing is inserted into the biopsy port until it extends past the end of the endoscope. The tubing is then pulled back far enough to expose the end of the fiber before the laser is activated. Care must be taken to position the tubing far enough from the end of the fiber because it can burn if it gets too close.

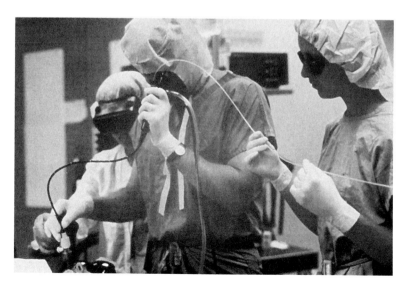

FIG. 7-1   The laser fiber is passed through the biopsy port of the endoscope.

The physician will see the aiming beam on the tissue but must also observe the end of the fiber before activating the laser. If the laser is activated while the fiber is inside the endoscope, the lens and end of the scope will be easily damaged by the laser's thermal energy. The end of the laser fiber should extend past the end of the endoscope at least 1 to 2 cm (Figure 7-2). The laser team member can help the physician monitor the position of the end of the fiber if a video system is used. The laser should only be taken off standby when the fiber tip is seen by the physician and the laser team member.

Irrigation can be performed during the endoscopy procedure to clear the laser target area. Any fluids can be eliminated through wall suction or a suction device connected to the smoke evacuation unit.

The smoke must be evacuated during the laser procedure to allow for optimal visibility. Care must be taken not to suction the smoke directly into the wall suction system because the particulate matter will coat the inside of the suction lines. An in-line filter or individual smoke evacuation system is needed.

Postoperatively, after the patient is able to resume a regular diet, high-roughage foods are avoided to allow the GI tract to heal. The patient is reevaluated periodically to assess the results of the procedure and note any recurrence of the original problem.

During *upper endoscopy,* an anesthetic spray is used to suppress the gag reflex. Therefore, the patient should take nothing by mouth for at least an hour after the procedure to reduce the chance of aspiration.

During the endoscopy procedure, gastric distention may occur due to gas insufflation. Allowing the patient to move to a more comfortable position will help expel these gases and relieve the pressure on the respiratory system. The patient may even belch smoke after the procedure. This is a normal but unpleasant side effect of laser therapy.

Perforation is a major complication that can occur during upper endoscopic laser procedures. If perforation occurs at the cervical level of the esophagus, the patient will have

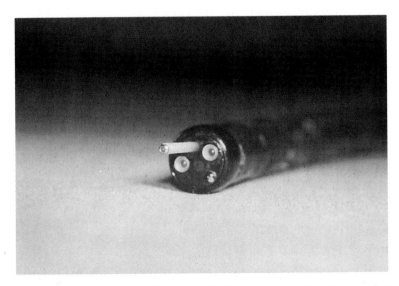

FIG. 7-2   The laser fiber must extend past the end of the endoscope before the laser is activated.

pain while swallowing and moving the neck. Pain in the substernal or epigastric area may indicate perforation of the thoracic area. Perforation of the thoracic level results in dyspnea and shoulder pain. Back pain, abdominal pain, cyanosis, pleural effusion, or fever can indicate gastric perforation. These symptoms can appear immediately when the perforation occurs, or over a 4-day period as the extent of the tissue necrosis expands.

Postoperatively, complications such as hemorrhage, hematemesis, or hypovolemic shock may occur. A slow-bleeding vessel in the GI tract may be indicated by a drop in hemoglobin or hematocrit levels or by blood in the stool. Sepsis may be a complication of laser endoscopy, so a temperature over 100° F for more than 24 hours should be reported.

During *lower endoscopy,* the patient may feel a burning sensation and some discomfort because the rectal area is more sensitive to thermal laser energy than the rest of the GI tract. The colon is also thinner than the rest of the GI tract, so the laser power should be turned to a low setting when treating this area to avoid perforation.

When a CO_2 gas is used to inflate the bowel for better visualization, the gas is easily absorbed by the colon. Excess blood levels of CO_2 should be monitored, especially in patients with chronic heart conditions. This insufflation gas may also cause distention of the bowel and cramping. The patient can be moved to a more comfortable position to accommodate the expelling of this gas. A rectal tube may be inserted if necessary. Postoperative pain usually results from overdistention of the bowel and not from the laser surgery.

One of the major complications of laser lower endoscopy is perforation. The first signs of perforation are usually overdistention, pain, and rectal bleeding; later signs are mucopurulent discharge and fever. Therefore, initial complaints after the laser procedure should be evaluated closely.

Laser Treatment for Esophageal Obstruction

One of the primary uses for lasers in gastroenterology is for palliation of malignant tumor obstruction of the esophagus. Many times patients cannot even swallow their own saliva. Patients with a neoplasm of the esophagus usually have a poor prognosis; many are incurable at the time of diagnosis. The alternative treatments for this disease are major surgery for esophageal resection or the placement of a gastric feeding tube to detour the passage of food from the mouth into the stomach. Most patients with this condition are geriatric and cannot withstand an extensive surgical procedure. Therefore, more conservative approaches must be taken.

Advances have refined the technique for relieving the esophageal obstruction by using laser energy through an endoscope to vaporize, excise, or debaulk the tumor. Squamous cell and adenocarcinoma, melanoma, and lymphoma of the esophagus can be treated using Nd:YAG laser energy with or without chemotherapy or radiotherapy. When laser intervention is used, the quality and length of life improve. Nd:YAG contact tip technology is also being implemented because it offers the precision needed to shave a tumor away from the esophagus without perforating the wall.

There are many advantages to using the laser to vaporize a tumor obstructing the esophagus. The procedure does not require an operating-room environment because it can be performed in a laser center or clinic with the patient under local anesthesia or intravenous sedation. Laser esophageal tumor ablation can be used repeatedly when surgical excision, radiotherapy, or chemotherapy have failed.

There are no major systemic effects of laser endoscopy as there are with chemotherapy or radiotherapy. Palliation can be expected within days rather than weeks as a patent lumen is restored. Tumors at all levels of the esophagus can be treated, but the most technically difficult area to lase continues to be just below the cricopharyngeal sphincter. Therefore, increased risk of perforation in this area can be a problem.

The *prograde technique* of esophageal tumor vaporization is the initial method that was used to relieve esophageal obstruction with the laser. With this technique the endoscope is introduced to the proximal margin of the tumor, and laser photocoagulation is performed to a depth of 1 to 2 cm. From 1 to 2 days pass before the necrotic tumor area can be mechanically removed. Another 1 to 2 cm of tumor is again photocoagulated. After another 1 or 2 days the procedure is repeated. This sequential method involves laser intervention over several treatments until the obstruction is relieved.

The *retrograde method* is the more accepted technique for treating esophageal obstruction and requires only one treatment. If the esophageal lumen is small, a guidewire may be passed through the tumor. Fluoroscopy should be used to note the placement of the guidewire to avoid perforation of the esophageal wall. Dilators are then passed over the guidewire to sequentially dilate the area to allow the endoscope to be passed into the stomach. Dilators may also be used without a guidewire. Diagnostic evaluation of the stomach is performed, and then the endoscope is withdrawn to the distal end of the tumor. With the laser fiber tip in full view, the lesion at the end of the scope is vaporized from the distal end to the proximal area (Figure 7-3). Usually higher power settings of Nd:YAG laser energy are used (80 to 100 W) since the fiber is not being fired at right angles to the target tissue. If a right-angle noncontact fiber is used, then the laser energy should be lowered to control the depth of penetration. A contact Nd:YAG chisel probe or other type of tip at lower power settings may be used to directly vaporize or excise tumor in the esophagus.

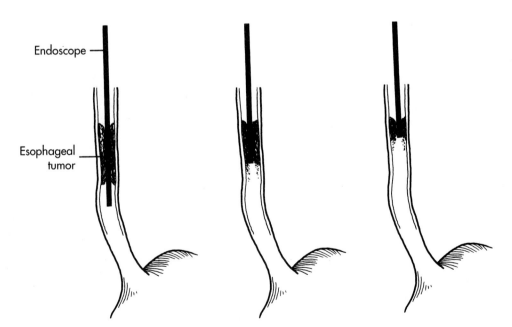

FIG. 7-3   The retrograde method of esophageal tumor vaporization requires that the endoscope be passed through the tumor. The tumor is vaporized from the distal end to the proximal area.

The surgical site is irrigated to remove charred tissue during this tumor vaporization. The smoke should be evacuated along with any excess gas used for insufflation to prevent gastric distention. The goal of this method is to produce a lumen large enough to easily accommodate the endoscope and possibly to allow the passage of solid foods.

The thermal energy produced during this procedure can cause postoperative edema. Therefore, the patient may be able to swallow immediately after the surgery, but 12 hours later swallowing may be prevented by the edema. Usually the swelling will resolve itself within 3 days. The patient can graduate from liquids to soft foods and then to a regular diet as tolerated. The patient must understand thoroughly that this treatment is for palliation and that the tumor will probably regrow and may have to be treated again at a later date. Many patients are extremely grateful to be able to eat and drink again even though the metastatic disease is still present.

Photocoagulation of GI Bleeding Lesions

The initial use of the argon and Nd:YAG laser in the GI tract was to control bleeding lesions in the gastric area. Ulcerations from erosion of the mucosal lining can cause the exposure of an underlying vessel branch that can begin to actively bleed (Figure 7-4). An endoscope is used to evaluate the active bleeding site. Copious amounts of lavage may be used to irrigate the area. Adequate suction is necessary. Protecting the airway against aspiration is of paramount importance during this assessment phase. Repositioning the patient may be helpful in shifting the blood or clots away from the bleeding site.

The actual bleeding site is never attacked directly. Rather, a coaptation technique is used to control this condition. This method involves placing laser spots circumferentially around the bleeding site to cause subsurface edema that will compress the underlying vessel thus indirectly stopping or slowing the bleeding (Figure 7-5). The Nd:YAG laser is usually the laser of choice because of the greater depth of tissue penetration, ranging from 2 to 6 mm. Approximately 60 to 90 W of noncontact power is delivered to the tissue in exposure times of 0.5 to 1.0 seconds.

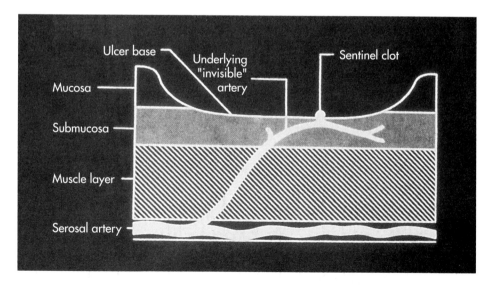

FIG. 7-4   Anatomy of a bleeding ulcer in the stomach.

When the pattern of laser spots is made around the bleeding site, the laser energy heats the tissue from 45° to 60° C, causing protein coagulation and denaturation to occur. As the duration of exposure to the laser beam continues, the temperature of the tissue continues to rise to 90° to 100° C. Tissue desiccation then occurs with an increased rise in the intravascular temperature, and procoagulation factors are released from the damaged endothelial vessel lining. As the surrounding tissue is heated to over 100° C. The blood inside the underlying vessel is coagulated, and further shrinkage of the vessel occurs. A thrombus forms and the bleeding stops. The actual bleeding site is not directly treated with laser energy because this stimulation could lead to further bleeding. The site can be lavaged with cold irrigant to help control the bleeding. If oozing or rebleeding occurs, retreatment may be performed in the same manner.

Areas that are extremely difficult to treat because of their location are those in the gastric cardia, the posterior wall of the upper gastric body, and the superior flexure of the duodenum. A flexible right-angle fiber may be used to treat these areas. Bleeding sites in the duodenal area are hard to treat because of decreased visibility and maneuverability as the endoscope enters this tubular structure.

The patient is observed postoperatively for bleeding symptoms. The hemoglobin level is monitored regularly to note any further loss of blood. Usually a nasogastric tube is not inserted after treating a gastric ulceration because of the mechanical trauma that this device could cause to the area. A nasogastric tube can be inserted if the ulceration is in the duodenal area.

The patient is not allowed to eat or drink for the first 24 hours until healing begins to occur. If there is no evidence of bleeding, a bland liquid diet is then prescribed. As the patient's condition is evaluated for stability, the diet will be gradually changed until a more general diet is allowed. The patient's recovery course is determined by the severity of the condition and compliance with postoperative instructions.

The main complication associated with laser treatment for GI bleeding is perforation. The patient may develop symptoms immediately or shortly after the laser procedure. The risk of perforation becomes higher as the severity of the disease increases. Another complication is hemorrhage. If this occurs, a surgical laparotomy may have to be performed immediately to directly control the bleeding before too much blood is lost.

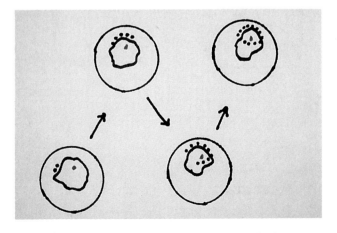

FIG. 7-5   Laser coaptation of a bleeding gastric ulcer.

Linear tears in the mucosa of the gastroesophageal juncture, called Mallory-Weiss syndrome, are usually characterized by bleeding. The argon and Nd:YAG lasers are being used successfully to treat this condition. Since this juncture site is rather thin, the laser energy is lowered to decrease the chance of perforation. The tear is not treated directly but circumferentially around the lesion to cause swelling to decrease the bleeding. One area should be treated, with a pause after the laser activation. This pause allows for accurate evaluation because there may not be an instantaneous cessation of the bleeding from the laser interaction.

Massive esophageal bleeding has a high mortality and morbidity rate. There are several alternative treatments for stopping or slowing esophageal bleeding. The laser has been used to control this bleeding, but injection sclerotherapy has been proven to be a very popular procedure for this condition during the acute phase. The advantage of this procedure over laser use is the immediate hemostasis that it achieves.

Laser Treatment for Malformations in the GI Tract

Hereditary hemorrhagic telangiectasia is characterized by chronic slow bleeding from mucocutaneous lesions in the GI tract. Patients with this disorder are usually on a long-term regimen of iron preparations and occasional hospitalization to treat the symptoms.

The argon laser has been effectively used to treat this condition because the beam is strongly absorbed by hemoglobin-pigmented areas (such as the telangiectasia areas). Since the lesions are located in the submucosal layer, only shallow penetration of the beam is required. Approximately 5 W of argon energy or 50 W of noncontact Nd:YAG energy is delivered to the tissue in pulse durations of 0.5 to 1.0 seconds. The area is photocoagulated until blanching is achieved. If larger blood vessels of over 2 to 3 mm in diameter are encountered, then the lesion is coapted indirectly, with pulsed laser spots placed circumferentially around the lesion, causing edema to decrease bleeding.

The patient takes nothing by mouth postoperatively for at least 6 hours and then has liquids for the next 24 hours. A standard diet can be resumed after the next day. Hospitalization is usually required for only 1 day unless the treatment is performed on an outpatient basis.

Arteriovenous malformations are most common in the cecum and ascending colon and can result in recurrent blood loss. These malformations usually occur in older persons because of the aging process and are often related to aortic valve disease, postural hypertension, or renal disease. The lesions may be solitary or multiple and range in size from microscopic to 2 cm in diameter.

The laser treatment procedure is performed on an outpatient basis with the patient under intravenous sedation. Close monitoring of the patient's condition is necessary because many of the patients also have other medical problems. The bowel is prepared with enemas given at home before the procedure. A clean bowel ensures that the physician will be able to adequately evaluate the lower GI tract to avoid missing any lesions. The laser surgery is usually performed when there is no or little active bleeding from the arteriovenous malformation. There is always a chance that the laser intervention could suddenly precipitate active bleeding during the procedure.

Approximately 60 to 80 W of Nd:YAG laser energy in pulses of 0.5 to 1.0 seconds are placed around the lesions. The argon or KTP laser is used at lower power settings of approximately 4 to 10 W to treat areas in the cecum because the cecum is thin, and these wavelengths do not produce as great a depth of penetration. The treatment is performed circumferentially first to decrease the inflow of blood by producing an edema cuff. Then the lesion area is treated directly with laser energy for complete coagulation. The Nd:YAG laser tends to create a larger edema cuff because of its greater depth of penetration compared with that of the argon or KTP lasers.

The purge gas is kept at a low flow level to decrease the chance of overdistending the bowel. When the bowel becomes overinflated, the colon walls become thin, and the incidence of perforation is greater.

Laser Colonoscopy

Argon and Nd:YAG lasers have been successfully used to treat *colon or rectal polyps* in patients with polyposis. In patients who are poor surgical risks, the physician can insert the laser fiber through the colonoscope without having to perform major surgery. Bleeding is stopped and obstructions are relieved in colon tumors treated with the laser, to avoid surgery in these unstable patients. The argon or KTP laser energy is adequate for tumors or polyps smaller than 1 cm in diameter, whereas the Nd:YAG laser is more effective for the larger lesions (Figures 7-6 and 7-7).

Fistulas are being treated with argon, KTP, or Nd:YAG laser energy. The contact Nd:YAG laser can also be used for a fistula repair. A small-tissue curette is used to clean out the material in the fistula tract. Then the area is ablated with the laser energy. Usually no bleeding, infection, or perforation occurs postoperatively. Healing occurs within 6 weeks.

Colorectal tumors are treated with laser energy as a palliation to relieve obstruction and control bleeding. Nonsurgical candidates, such as elderly patients or those with multiple system disorders, benefit from laser therapy when major surgery is not recommended.

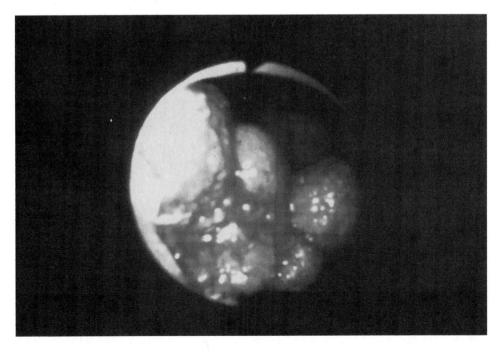

FIG. 7-6   Polyps in the colon obstruct the lumen. (Courtesy Surgical Laser Technologies, Inc., Oaks, PA.)

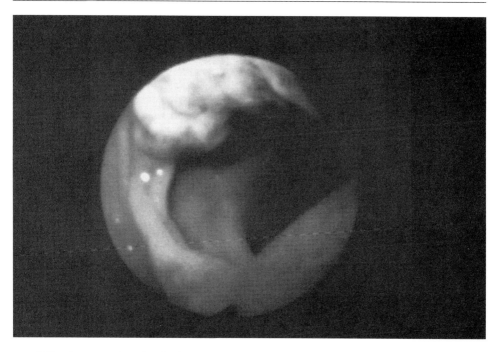

FIG. 7-7   A patent colon after the laser was used to remove the polyps. (Courtesy Surgical Laser Technologies, Inc., Oaks, PA.)

Colorectal tumors are treated in a manner similar to that for esophageal tumors. The procedure is usually performed on an outpatient basis with the patient under intravenous sedation. A bowel prep is performed before the procedure. The tumor is vaporized with the Nd:YAG laser set at 30 to 70 W beginning at the lumen and moving toward the bowel wall. An adequate margin of tumor should be left adjacent to the bowel wall to prevent perforation. The coagulated tumor tissue will slough off and be passed out through the GI tract. Treatments are repeated as necessary.

Contact Nd:YAG technology is being used to precisely shave tumor away from vessels or the bowel wall. Because less Nd:YAG laser light is required, there is less thermal penetration by the energy and less damage to adjacent normal structures.

Lower bowel stenosis is also being treated with laser energy. After a major surgical resection of the sigmoid or rectosigmoid areas, stenosis may occur. The laser can be used to open a patent lumen in these stenotic areas.

LASER SURGERY FOR RECTAL AND PERIANAL CONDITIONS
Laser Hemorrhoidectomy

A hemorrhoid is a collection of dilated and tortuous vessels and capillaries that are located in the anorectal area. External hemorrhoids involve vessels that are distal to the anorectal demarcation, whereas internal hemorrhoids involve vessels that are proximal to the anorectal line.

Internal hemorrhoids occur in four different degrees. A first-degree hemorrhoid may extrude slightly into the anal canal and may also bleed. A second-degree hemorrhoid will protrude from the anus on straining but will spontaneously reduce. A third-degree hemorrhoid will prolapse out during straining but can be manually pushed back into the anal canal. A fourth-degree hemorrhoid cannot be pushed back and will remain prolapsed. When internal and external hemorrhoids are present together, they are called mixed hemorrhoids.

When symptomatic, first- and second-degree hemorrhoids are usually treated conservatively with warm soaks and compresses, antiinflammatory medications, analgesics, and rubber-band ligation. Third- and fourth-degree hemorrhoids are treated by rubber-band ligation, cryosurgery, or operative hemorrhoidectomy using scalpel or laser surgery. A variety of laser wavelengths have been used successfully to treat hemorrhoidal disease.

Laser hemorrhoidectomy is an outpatient procedure that may be performed using intravenous sedation and a long-lasting local anesthetic. The patient should be instructed to self-administer a preoperative enema to clean the lower bowel. Before activating the laser, the physician can use suction to evacuate any methane gas, which could cause a lower bowel explosion or fire. The physician may also pack a wet counted sponge into the lower rectal area to decrease the chance of methane gas from escaping into the surgical area and creating a fire hazard.

The anticipated results of the surgery are communicated realistically to the patient before the procedure. When the laser is used, there usually is less intraoperative bleeding. The laser procedure sometimes allows the patient to return to work earlier than the nonlaser treatment because healing appears to be faster. Postoperative pain is sometimes less than with conventional methods. The laser also has been known to require less surgical time than is needed for the traditional hemorrhoidectomy procedures. These benefits still need to be supported by further research.

When the CO_2, argon, and KTP lasers are used, third- or fourth-degree hemorrhoids are treated by excision with laser energy used as a cutting tool. Conventional suturing methods are used to close the incision area.

Third- and fourth-degree mixed hemorrhoids can be treated by using a contact Nd:YAG scalpel to excise the hemorrhoidal tissue (Figure 7-8). After the physician exposes the hemorrhoid by maintaining gentle traction, an incision is made through the mucosal and submucosal layers. The hemorrhoid is dissected from the underlying internal sphincter muscle. Any bleeding is treated by contact with the laser probe or scalpel. The vascular pedicle is sutured close to the base, and laser energy is applied distal to the ligature for final sealing effects. The mucosa may be closed with absorbable suture or left open (Figure 7-9).

Second- and third-degree internal hemorrhoids are sometimes treated by using the noncontact Nd:YAG laser beam or the contact probe to coapt the hemorrhoidal tissue. The power of the Nd:YAG beam is kept at lower settings to ensure that the zone of damage is not overly extensive, which could lead to necrotic debris that could later cause rectal discharge. Laser spots are placed in a rosette fashion around the hemorrhoid, causing deeper tissue coagulation and shrinkage of the hemorrhoidal plexus. The hemorrhoid itself is then treated directly to ensure coagulation and shrinkage of the tissue. Coaptation is complete when the hemorrhoidal tissue blanches and a white membrane develops.

After the hemorrhoidal tissue is treated by either excision or coaptation, the anorectal area may be packed with a large moistened gauze pad for compression hemostasis. The

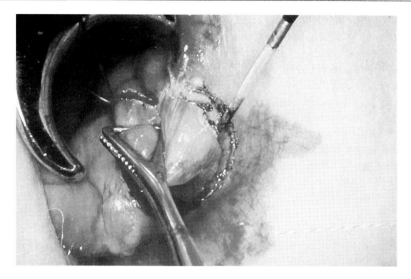

FIG. 7-8   Hemorrhoidal tissue is excised using a contact Nd:YAG scalpel. (Courtesy Surgical Laser Technologies, Inc., Oaks, PA.)

packing is removed 1 hour after the procedure. The patient is discharged when the vital signs are stable and there is no sign of bleeding.

Postoperative home care after a laser procedure is similar to the care needed after a conventional hemorrhoidectomy. The surgical site is gently cleansed with warm saline or water. Soap is not recommended to cleanse the rectal area because it will cause irritation. Warm (not hot) 10-minute sitz baths are recommended every 2 hours to decrease discom-

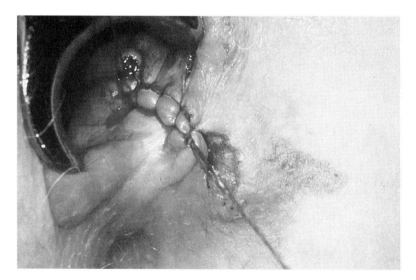

FIG. 7-9   The mucosa is closed with suture after the hemorrhoid is excised. (Courtesy Surgical Laser Technologies, Inc., Oaks, PA.)

fort. A steroid ointment may be prescribed for insertion into the immediate internal os and the external area. Dry cotton balls are placed over the surgical site. The patient is instructed to take acetaminophen for pain and to adjust the diet to include high-fiber foods. Regular well-balanced diets with adequate bulk and fluids are needed to promote the passage of normal-sized, well-formed stools. Alcohol, spices, fried or fatty foods, coffee, and citrus juices should be avoided during the healing process. Stool softeners can be prescribed to decrease trauma to the healing site caused by hardened fecal material. The patient may experience some burning and a slightly bloody or mucoid discharge. The patient is usually seen at the physician's office after 1 to 2 days for evaluation of the surgical site. Repeated visits may be scheduled at weekly intervals until healing is complete within 3 to 4 weeks. Heavy labor and lifting should be avoided for 1 month after the procedure.

Complications that can occur from this procedure include bleeding, sphincter spasm, urinary retention, perianal tags, impaction of fecal material, or recurrence of the hemorrhoid. More comparative research is needed to justify actual results and incidence of complications connected to laser hemorrhoidectomy before many physicians praise its merits. With more emphasis on cost today, physicians sometimes challenge using the laser for soft-tissue procedures such as hemorrhoidectomies. Cost should not be the only deciding factor because patient issues such as postoperative pain and missed workdays must also be addressed. This controversy will continue until significant research is published.

Fissures

Fissures are usually associated with the presence of hemorrhoids. If asymptomatic hemorrhoids are left untreated at the time of a fissurectomy procedure, they often become painful after surgery. Therefore, a fissurectomy often is performed with a hemorrhoidectomy.

A CO_2 laser can be used to vaporize the fissure and its adjacent drainage area rather than actually excising them. As a result, postoperative pain is minimized and healing is quicker. Postoperative care is similar to that for hemorrhoidectomy.

Fistulas and Abscesses

To treat the traditional fistula, a probe is passed from the external to the internal opening along the fistula. This tract is then incised with the CO_2 laser with approximately 15 W of superpulse energy with a spot size of 2 to 3 mm (Joffe, 1989, pp. 155-6). A V-shaped area is excised with the fistula tract as the base to provide adequate drainage and healing from the inside to the outside areas. With a high anal fistula, the sphincter must be preserved so that fecal incontinence does not result. The contact Nd:YAG laser can also be used.

Abscesses can be opened using the CO_2 laser at about 15 W in the superpulse mode. A wide opening is recommended to promote continuous draining, which decreases the chance of infection. Postoperatively, a steroid ointment is applied, and cotton balls are placed over the area without pressure or packing. Postoperative care is similar to that for a hemorrhoidectomy.

Pilonidal Cysts and Sinuses

The pilonidal cyst and sinus tracts are excised and laid open with CO_2 or contact Nd:YAG laser energy. The goal is to remove all of the affected sinus tracts to avoid recurrence after the surgery (Joffe, 1989, p. 156). The laser seals the smaller blood vessels, but larger ones must be ligated.

When comparing laser energy with electrocautery, the laser becomes the preferred tool. Electrosurgery involves the use of electrical current; thus local muscle contractions are observed at the surgical site. Since laser energy does not cause this condition, there is less chance of inadvertent injury to the rectal sphincter. The patient has less pain when the laser is used, therefore the procedure can be performed using a local anesthetic. The laser's hemostatic value is appreciated because anatomical structures can be easily identified in this bloodless field. The patient can usually be discharged on the day of surgery or the next day.

REFERENCES

Joffe SN, editor: *Lasers in general surgery,* Baltimore, 1989, Williams & Wilkins.

SUGGESTED READINGS

Aguilar PS: Lasers in colorectal diseases (from the laser conference manual of the Seventh Annual Laser Medicine and Surgery Symposium), Columbus, OH, March, 1988, Grant Laser Center.

Pietrafitta JJ and Dwyer RM: Endoscopic laser therapy for malignant esophageal obstruction, *Arch Surg* 121:395, 1986.

Zadch AT and Kirchner B: Outpatient hemorrhoidectomy—Laser treatment and case results, *AORN J* 44(6):966, Dec 1986.

8

GYNECOLOGY LASER APPLICATIONS

Gynecologists were among the specialists who first truly appreciated the potential of the laser. One of the first lasers they used was the CO_2 laser, which they found tremendously effective in treating patients with erosion of the cervix. New gynecological applications were introduced, and with instrumentation refinements, the laser advanced laparoscopic surgery to a fine art. The laser was then found useful for cutting, coagulating, and vaporizing during intraabdominal procedures. Also, the laser was coupled with the hysteroscope to perform surgery within the uterus. Other clinical applications continue to be developed by innovative gynecologists who strive to provide less invasive, less complicated procedures to benefit their patients.

During the past few years, laser technology has been challenged by electrosurgery. Several reasons explain this trend: greater accessibility to an electrosurgery unit, (sometimes) less cost to the patient, successful patient outcomes, and no need for specialized training. Laser technology has declined in popularity as gynecologists increasingly favor the electrosurgery unit. However, comparative research is beginning to convince many gynecologists that the laser is preferable for many procedures. Additional research is being conducted to note the extent of adjacent tissue damage, incidence of recurring lesions, time required to return to normal activities, intraoperative and postoperative discomfort, and patient charges. Thus laser technology is not dead for the gynecologist but merely in transition. Already more physicians are reconsidering the need to use laser energy for a number of gynecological conditions.

Many different wavelengths are being used effectively for a variety of gynecological applications, including lower tract, laparoscopic, hysteroscopic, and intraabdominal procedures. A review of gynecological anatomy, shown in Figure 8-1, will enhance understanding of the various laser applications.

LOWER TRACT LASER APPLICATIONS
Cervical Conditions

Cervical intraepithelial neoplasia (CIN) is an abnormal growth of cells in the squamous epithelium of the cervix. It occurs secondarily to the human papilloma virus (HPV). CIN is limited to the surface epithelium but also can involve the endocervical crypts.

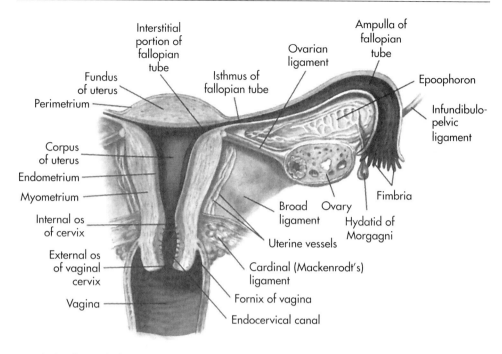

FIG. 8-1   Gynecological anatomy. (From Bobak IM, Lowdermilk DL, Jensen MD: *Maternity nursing,* ed 4, St. Louis, 1995, Mosby.)

Most CIN conditions extend to a depth of less than 4 mm from the surface into the cervical crypt. CIN involves a spectrum of cellular abnormalities from CIN I (mild cervical dysplasia) to CIN III (severe dysplasia and carcinoma in situ). A severe form of CIN is known as carcinoma in situ, which may require treatment by hysterectomy. When a more radical approach is necessary, however, conization of the cervix often is adequate, particularly for women who wish to maintain childbearing potential.

The laser has introduced an alternative treatment for CIN that involves eradicating the entire lesion while preserving the patient's sexual, anatomical, and reproductive integrity. The key to this procedure is to locally remove all of the abnormal tissue so that the dysplasia will not progress to carcinoma in situ and eventually invasive cancer.

The abnormal squamous cells form in the transformation zone of the cervix. When the transformation zone can be defined colposcopically, cervical ablation or vaporization is sufficient. When the transformation zone is poorly delineated, excisional conization is appropriate. When the abnormal cervical tissue is removed, the transformation zone and the cervical dysplasia must be destroyed adequately to decrease recurrence. But overly aggressive destruction will cause injury to healthy tissue and lead to poor results and possible future reproductive problems. Successful CIN treatment requires controlling the amount of tissue ablated and preserving the normal anatomy. Laser intervention seems to adequately address these concerns.

Traditionally, knife, cryosurgery, or electrosurgery conization techniques have been used to excise the abnormal tissue of the cervix. The conization knife procedure is performed on an outpatient basis and requires general anesthesia. Its complications include hemorrhage, infection, subsequent infertility, and cervical stenosis. Also, the physician may have difficulty identifying the squamocolumnar junction after healing is complete. The success of cryosurgery depends on complete destruction of the entire transformation zone. The depth of damage is hard to control during this procedure and is usually followed by profuse postoperative vaginal discharge. Postoperative scarring is also a frequent complication of cryosurgery and knife conization.

Electrosurgery LLETZ (large loop excision of the transformation zone) conization has gained in popularity over the past few years. This procedure is accomplished by using high-frequency alternating current flowing through wire loop electrodes. An insulated speculum must be used so that the speculum will not conduct the electrical energy. The loop is pushed into the cervix and a rounded specimen is obtained. Larger lesions require more than one pass. Healthy tissue may be removed along with the diseased tissue. A specimen is always obtained, even if this seems unnecessary. (When the laser is used, a specimen may or may not be obtained.) The procedure is cost-effective and can be performed quickly, but the rate of cervical stenosis is higher (Dibler, 1994).

The CO_2 laser can be coupled with the operating microscope or colposcope to treat cervical disease. The superficial mucosal cells are heated to the point of boiling and then explode and evaporate, producing vaporization. The thermal energy produced in the superficial layer is then conducted to the deeper layers until there is complete vaporization of a cervical cylinder of tissue. Cervical conization and ablation are two of the most commonly performed laser procedures in gynecology today.

Laser cervical conization can be performed on an outpatient basis, with the patient receiving a light general anesthetic or a paracervical block. During conization the laser excises the tissue to the depth adequate to remove the specimen, which can be submitted to the pathologist for diagnosis. Only very minimal thermal damage will occur at the cone margin.

Laser vaporization of the cervix usually can be performed without the administration of any anesthetic. Because the number of pain receptors on the cervix is somewhat limited, this procedure usually produces only mild to moderate discomfort. The patient may complain of a burning sensation but can tolerate the procedure without anesthesia. The physician can minimize the patient's discomfort by controlling the amount of heat buildup in one area of the cervix. With the laser applied in interrupted pulses, the tissue is allowed to cool, and the pain is reduced. Tactics are often used to help divert the patient's attention away from the surgery and thus decrease discomfort, such as hanging a picture of a mountain scene over the operating table.

Laser cervical vaporization can also be performed with the patient under local anesthesia, using a paracervical block. Injections of the anesthetic agent are made at the 3- and 9-o'clock positions.

Before the cervical conization or ablation procedure begins, the cervix is dabbed with a swab to remove any mucous film. Sometimes an injection of vasopressin is administered to the cervix to cause the small blood vessels to constrict and therefore reduce the amount of bleeding during the procedure. A solution of 4% acetic acid (vinegar) is applied to the cervix so that the borders of the lesion will be delineated as abnormal cells turn white. An outline of the dysplastic area is made using the CO_2 laser in a pulsed mode at 10 to 30 W of power.

During laser cervical ablation, the outlined area is divided into quadrants, the beam is defocused, and the vaporization continues within the lower quadrants first (Figure 8-2). The depth and width of the laser-vaporized area is measured with lateral and vertical mi-

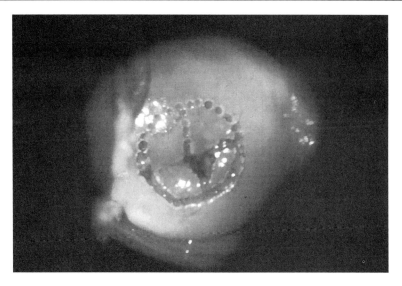

FIG. 8-2 CO_2 laser pulses outline the area on the cervix to be ablated.

crocalipers and documented on the operating-room record. Bleeding and oozing are controlled with the CO_2 beam in the defocused mode or by painting the cervical area with ferric subsulfate solution. Any charred tissue from the ablation or conization is removed by gently rubbing the surgical site with a wet sponge. Lasing may then continue on the newly exposed tissue.

After the procedure, the patient may have uterine cramping due to a prostaglandin release that occurs in response to the laser energy. Sometimes premedication with prostaglandin inhibitors helps minimize this discomfort.

Postoperatively, the patient is instructed not to douche, use tampons, or have sexual intercourse for 4 weeks to allow the cervical area to heal. The patient should wear an external pad to absorb any discharge during the healing process. Daily application of an antibiotic cream or acidifying gel is usually recommended to decrease the chances of infection. The patient should be told to notify the physician if she experiences heavy bleeding, fever, or pain. Vaginal discharge may occur and is usually a sign that healing is taking place. A Pap smear should be performed annually to note any recurrence of disease, and colposcopy should be performed every 6 months to note any observable tissue changes.

Contact Nd:YAG technology also is used for cervical procedures. The contact Nd:YAG scalpel makes a clean incision while providing coagulation to control bleeding during the conization (Figure 8-3). Traction is achieved with a small hooked instrument to provide tension on the cervix. The base of the specimen can be excised with a steel scalpel or curved scissors so that the margins are not destroyed if disease is present in the endocervical canal. The contact Nd:YAG probe also can be used to lightly rub over the cervical area to ablate the tissue.

Argon and frequency doubled YAG lasers also are used for cervical vaporization and excisions. The tip of the fiber is held just off the surface of the cervix and is moved in rapid circular motions. The cervix is vaporized while bleeding is controlled. The ablation crater should be 7 mm deep. Another 1.5 to 2.0 mm of tissue is necrosed under the surface of the crater. The cervix heals quickly, within 2 weeks, with reepithelialization.

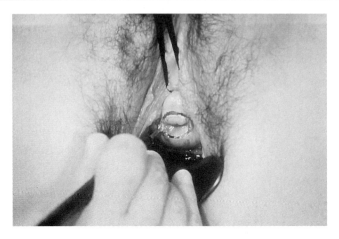

FIG. 8-3   The contact Nd:YAG scalpel is used to perform a cervical conization. (Courtesy Surgical Laser Technologies, Inc., Oaks, PA.)

The advantages of using the laser over conventional methods for cervical procedures continue to be debated. Supporters of laser technology state that laser energy seals blood vessels to reduce the amount of bleeding during surgery. The laser's precision is valuable because it allows for excision of the dysplastic tissue only. This reduces the amount of adjacent tissue damage to the cervix, thus decreasing the chance of cervical stenosis. This in turn reduces the risk of infertility and complications of pregnancy. A lower tract laser procedure can be performed quickly and easily on an outpatient basis. The patient requires minimal anesthesia, has little postoperative discomfort, and can return to normal activities quickly.

Vaginal Conditions

Carcinoma of the vagina is rare, but there has been an increase in the incidence of vaginal intraepithelial neoplasia (VAIN) that is thought to be secondary to HPV infection. Treatment of VAIN is difficult because of the large surface area of the vagina, the irregular rugae on the surface of the vagina, and the inaccessibility of some of the vaginal areas.

The CO_2 laser is being used to ablate the vaginal tissue. General anesthesia is necessary because of the sensitivity of the vaginal mucosa, especially in the deeper areas of the vagina. Because rather large areas are usually affected, local anesthesia is not appropriate. The procedure is usually performed on an outpatient status.

The vaginal area is painted with 4% acetic acid to delineate the involved areas. The depth of penetration by the laser energy must be visualized to ensure complete vaporization of the diseased tissue, thus the laser is coupled with an operating microscope or colposcope. Approximately 15 to 30 W of continuous or superpulse CO_2 laser power is used in a defocused mode sweeping over the involved vaginal area. Great care must be taken not to perforate the vaginal wall and affect other structures, such as the colon or the bladder. The epidermis is vaporized off the underlying dermis. The surgical plane of dissection must be identified so that the depth can be monitored. The top layer of the dermis is then vaporized. Throughout the vaporization, charred tissue is wiped away with a wet sponge to determine the adequacy of the penetration depth.

Because treatment of VAIN often includes multiple areas in the vagina, vulva, and cervix, postoperative pain stems from the various surgical sites. A regimen of oral analgesics and sitz baths in a mild salt solution helps decrease discomfort. Applications of estrogen, sulfa, or antibiotic cream are usually prescribed. The patient is normally evaluated weekly for a time to avoid vaginal coaptation and to gently clean away secretions and medications to permit proper assessment of the surgical areas. The vagina heals quickly and usually without scarring. Retreatments are sometimes needed to completely control the disease.

Vulvar Conditions

Vulvar intraepithelial neoplasia (VIN) is an unpredictable disease that sometimes spontaneously regresses. Simple vulvectomy was the conventional therapeutic procedure but is no longer acceptable. Today, laser skinning is performed, on an outpatient basis, to superficially remove the diseased tissue without the need for a skin graft.

A biopsy is performed to confirm that the disease is not invasive. Anesthesia is necessary for the biopsy and surgery because the vulvar area is very sensitive. This procedure can be performed with the patient under local anesthesia if only a few lesions are present. General anesthesia is always necessary for patients with more extensive disease.

The laser is coupled with the operative microscope or the colposcope. A 4% acetic acid solution is applied to the vulva to delineate the areas with VIN. The depth of VIN involvement is usually not uniform because VIN can produce raised areas on the surface. Once the margins have been established, the plan is to vaporize 0.5 mm more from the edge of the margins. Approximately 15 to 20 W of defocused CO_2 laser energy is used in the continuous or superpulse mode to rapidly brush over the vulvar area to remove the epidermis while identifying the dermis. Charred tissue is mechanically removed with a wet sponge and the top layer of the dermis (the papillary dermis) is superficially vaporized to the level of the reticular dermis. Preserving the reticular dermis precludes the need for skin grafting.

Postoperative healing occurs within 10 to 14 days if the reticular dermis is preserved. Sometimes the patient does not have immediate postoperative pain because the laser seals the nerve endings. However, pain frequently occurs on the third or fourth postoperative day because of urine contamination of the area. Vulvitis is common because of urinary salts. Often a catheter is placed postoperatively for 1 to 2 weeks to decrease the chance of urine contamination.

The patient is instructed to take regular sitz baths, blow-dry the surgical area with a hair dryer, and apply a thin layer of sulfa or antibiotic cream to the wound. Frequent evaluation of the results will enable the physician to detect a recurrence that can be treated if necessary.

Chronic vulvovaginal pain has been treated successfully with a flashlamp-excited dye laser; recovery time is shorter and recurrence rates are lower compared with conventional treatment methods. The 585-nm wavelength is selectively absorbed by the blood vessels in the irritated vulvar tissue, and smaller vessels in the superficial dermis are destroyed. The pain fibers begin to degenerate, and the patient's symptoms resolve. This treatment has also been successful in the treatment of idiopathic or unexplained vulvar pain that can lead to painful intercourse.

The procedure is usually performed in the operating room with the patient under general or regional anesthesia. This type of anesthesia is necessary because adequate visualization is required to effectively treat all areas. Therefore, the vestibular epithelium is usually everted using traction sutures. The laser energy is delivered to the erythematous tissue until visible changes are noted.

After the surgery a topical antibiotic is applied to the vulva and intravaginally, and an occlusive dressing is placed. Zinc oxide paste is sometimes used three times per day to decrease the chance of postoperative bacterial cellulitis (*Clinical Laser Monthly,* Nov 1993).

Condyloma Acuminata Vaporization

Condyloma acuminata (genital or venereal warts) is an infection of the human papilloma virus (HPV) that is sexually transmitted. The lesions can range from flat pigmented lesions to polypoid clusters. Condyloma may be localized to one area or extend from the vulva into the vagina or rectum. Conventional treatment methods include application of podophyllin to the solitary lesions and fulguration for multiple lesions. Postoperative pain and local recurrence are often associated with the electrocautery treatment. The laser has been effectively used to vaporize these warts with minimal postoperative pain and recurrence.

The laser procedure is usually performed on an outpatient basis. If few lesions are noted, injections of a local anesthetic will suffice, but extensive condyloma usually requires general anesthesia. The area is painted with 4% acetic acid to delineate the margins of the lesions. A colposcope, operating microscope, or loupes are used to enhance visualization and identification of the lesions.

The CO_2, frequency doubled YAG, argon, and Nd:YAG lasers have all been used successfully to treat condyloma acuminata. The disease process is limited to the epidermal layer, so vaporization of the deeper layers of the dermis is unnecessary. Laser energy is used to vaporize the superficial tissue, and the charred surface is removed with a wet sponge. The vaporization is continued until the dermal layer of the skin is identified. Deeper vaporization is recommended if intraepithelial neoplasia is suspected.

After the surgery, the physician often prescribes sitz baths in a mild salt solution to reduce discomfort. A salt-solution mix such as Instant Ocean can be obtained at a pet store where synthetic salt-water aquarium supplies are sold. Postoperative instructions for the patient include oral analgesics for discomfort; keeping the area clean and dry when not taking a sitz bath (a hair dryer can be used to blow-dry the area); using an antibiotic ointment if prescribed; and contacting the physician if severe pain, elevated temperature, or bleeding occurs. The patient must be instructed to advise her sexual partner to be evaluated for condyloma acuminata. Even though the woman has been treated, the HPV can remain, thus she can still spread the virus.

Laser vaporization of condyloma acuminata offers many advantages over conventional methods, including precise tissue removal, preservation of normal adjacent structures, minimal scarring and blood loss, less postoperative pain, rapid healing, and reduced recurrence.

LAPAROSCOPIC LASER APPLICATIONS

The CO_2 laser was first coupled with the laparoscope in the late 1970s, many problems were encountered with the delivery system and instruments. The aiming beam was difficult to align adequately, and the intensity of its light reflected off the inside of the endoscope lumen, making visibility a problem. Evacuating the plume produced during the laser interaction resulted in loss of the pneumoperitoneum and necessitated a pause in the procedure for reinsufflation. Instrumentation was cumbersome because of the size of the

CO_2 laser and the awkward articulating arm. Procedures took longer because the physician was usually inexperienced.

Refinements have advanced laser laparoscopy to a superior and preferred method of treatment. The laparoscope has been modified to accommodate different wavelengths and delivery systems. Smoke evacuation methods have allowed plume to be eliminated without destroying the pneumoperitoneum. Physician expertise has progressed, and the procedure can be performed in a short time.

The laser has converted many inpatient open abdominal procedures to outpatient laparoscopic procedures with more successful results and fewer complications. The advantages of laser laparoscopy include precision, minimal adjacent tissue damage, hemostasis, and less postoperative adhesion formation. Moreover, the physician can cut, coagulate, and vaporize within the abdominal cavity without making a large incision.

The procedure is usually performed on an outpatient basis with the patient under general anesthesia. A straight catheter is inserted to deflate the bladder so as to minimize the chance of bladder perforation or injury. The patient is placed in the Trendelenburg position to allow the abdominal organs to gravitate toward the chest. A probe is placed inside the uterus to allow uterine manipulation during the procedure. A special large-bore needle is introduced immediately below the umbilical area, and the pelvic cavity is insufflated with a gas (usually medical-grade CO_2). After adequate pneumoperitoneum is established, the sheath and trocar are inserted. The trocar is then withdrawn and the laparoscope is introduced. Other puncture sites may be used to permit passage of ancillary instruments, such as suction devices or probes, to assist with the procedure.

The CO_2 laser is attached to a special laser sidearm laparoscope with a coupling device (Figure 8-4). The manufacturer's instructions must be followed for the care, cleaning, and maintenance of the coupler to ensure its proper functioning. The laser's articulated arm may also be coupled with a trocar sheath that is introduced through another puncture site. This setup eliminates the need to purchase a special CO_2 sidearm laparoscope since the beam is being introduced through another puncture site.

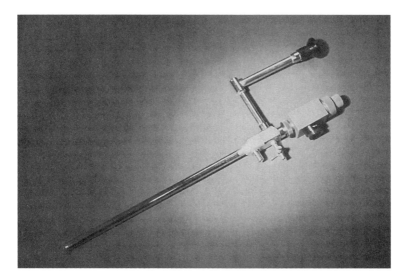

FIG. 8-4   A special coupler connects the laparoscope to the CO_2 laser's articulated arm.

A CO_2 waveguide may be used through an operating port of a regular sidearm laparoscope or a second puncture site. This narrow tube conducts the laser energy directly to the tissue, thus the beam is not reflected off the inside lumen of the laparoscope (Figure 8-5). The spot size can be made smaller for more precision and accuracy. The various delivery tubes have different ends that provide suctioning, beam backstop, or beam deflection.

A study was conducted to determine why the CO_2 beam could not be focused into a small spot during laparoscopy. The results showed that the CO_2 insufflation gas within the laparoscope acted as a negative focusing lens, causing a "blooming effect" in the beam. Therefore, optimal cutting cannot be achieved because an intense, high-power-density, pinpoint beam of coherent CO_2 laser radiation cannot be maintained. As the laser power is increased, the beam gradually becomes enlarged. This observable phenomenon is directly related to the laparoscope channel size and the gas used (Reich, MacGregor, and Vancaillie, 1991). Further studies note that this blooming effect can be minimized when the CO_2 insufflation gas is forced through the laparoscope at a rate of at least 8 L/min, which is possible with modern insufflators.

Argon, frequency doubled YAG, Nd:YAG, and holmium wavelengths can be conducted through fibers, thus special laparoscopes are not needed during laser laparoscopy. The fiber is introduced into the biopsy port of the standard laparoscope and is directed toward the diseased area.

To eliminate surgical smoke that obscures the physician's vision, a special low-pressure suction valve can be attached to the suction tubing connected to the laparoscope. By depressing the valve when plume is produced, the physician can initiate gentle suction to remove the smoke without evacuating the insufflated gas. A high-flow insufflator is needed to maintain the level of insufflation required for optimal visualization.

After the laparoscope is inserted, landmarks are identified and the disease is assessed. The laser energy is delivered to the surgical sites, while the normal tissue is preserved. Any charred tissue is removed with irrigation or lavage. A video system is often used so that the nurse or assistant can view the procedure and anticipate any needs.

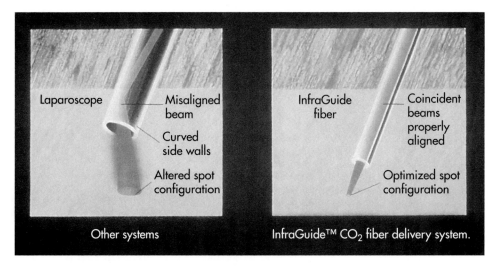

FIG. 8-5   The CO_2 laser can be directed through a waveguide during laparoscopy thus avoiding reflection of the beam off the inside lumen of the laparoscope. (Courtesy Lasersonics, Milpitas, CA.)

After the laser intervention but before the removal of the trocar sheath, the insufflation gas is removed to reduce postoperative pain caused by the pressure of the gas on the internal organs. To decrease the chance of possible contamination from the insufflation gas, suction is used to minimize airborne particulates that could contain HIV matter. The puncture sites are closed using traditional subcuticular methods.

Postoperatively, the patient is instructed to take mild oral analgesics for discomfort, keep the skin incisions clean and dry, and apply a thin layer of an antibiotic ointment daily. The patient may return to normal activities within 2 to 3 days. The prognosis for laser laparoscopy depends upon the location and extent of the diseased area. The physician and nurse must give the patient realistic expectations of the procedure.

New instruments and endoscopes are being introduced that will affect the traditional laparoscopic procedure. Microendoscopes from 0.5 to 1.6 mm have been developed that contain 10,000 to 15,000 tiny microfibers. These fibers not only provide illumination but also transmit a video image. The gynecologist does not have a panoramic view of the abdominal organs but must view each organ individually. Laser energy can then be delivered to the target site. The many advantages of this microsystem include shorter surgery time, quicker recovery, and significantly less postoperative pain (Lomano and Grochmal, 1992).

New techniques are challenging the need for insufflation during laparoscopy. One laparoscopic system that has received much attention uses a special instrument that is inserted into a small puncture site and positioned beneath the peritoneum. The instrument then lifts the abdominal cavity so that the physician can view the organs (Figure 8-6). The physician can pass instruments through other small incisions to perform surgery from within the abdomen without having to make a larger incision. There is no need for gaskets or other attachments to decrease the chance of insufflation gas escaping. Advances continue as the advantages and potential for this gasless laparoscopy method are realized.

Endometriosis Vaporization

Endometriosis is rapidly becoming a common condition in young women today. The disease is caused by ectopic endometrial cells migrating out of the uterus to various sites throughout the pelvic and abdominal areas. The main symptom is pain, especially during

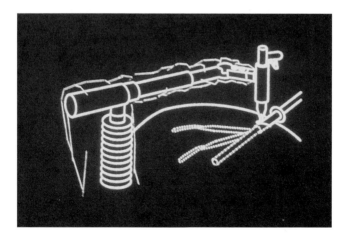

FIG. 8-6   This laparoscopic instrument lifts the abdominal cavity to allow visualization, thus eliminating the need for insufflation. (Courtesy Origin, Inc., Menlo Park, CA.)

the premenstrual phase and during menstruation, when the ectopic endometrial cells also bleed. As the condition progresses, the endometrial cells form implants that can advance into bands that may constrict or impair organs and structures. This condition can easily lead to reproductive problems if left untreated.

Because the initial diagnosis of endometriosis is often made on young women, hysterectomy and bilateral salpingo-oophorectomy are not acceptable treatments in all cases. Conservative measures such as oral contraceptives and danazol (Danocrine) hormone therapy may help relieve the symptoms by causing a temporary resorption of smaller endometrial implants. This therapy is being questioned today, and it is not effective for extensive endometriosis. Most patients cannot easily tolerate long-term hormone therapy.

Traditional surgical treatment for endometriosis is laparotomy to directly excise the endometrial implants. The procedure involves hospitalization and a relatively lengthy recovery period. Most patients prefer to avoid this more invasive treatment, which can usually be performed with the laparoscope.

Physicians as well as patients appreciate a less invasive method, and they can easily use the laser through a laparoscope to precisely vaporize and excise endometrial implants from the normal tissue. Bleeding is minimal during the procedure because the laser energy seals smaller blood vessels. Hard-to-reach areas inside the pelvic region are accessed with the endoscope for potential vaporization. There is less recurrence of endometriosis with this method because the laser energy accurately destroys most of the implants.

Argon, frequency doubled YAG, and Nd:YAG lasers are also being used effectively to treat endometrial implants because of the color selectivity of the beams. The fiber is held about 0.5 to 1.0 cm from the lesion. The implant is coagulated until the area is blanched to approximately 1 mm beyond the margins of the lesion. The darkened implant more readily absorbs the laser energy, whereas the lighter, underlying tissue is relatively unaffected. This provides great precision during the removal of the implants. The contact Nd:YAG tips are also being used for precise treatment of endometrial implants (Figure 8-7).

Postoperatively, the patient may be maintained on a regimen of danazol or other hormone for a time to ensure that the symptoms subside. Hormone therapy to control en-

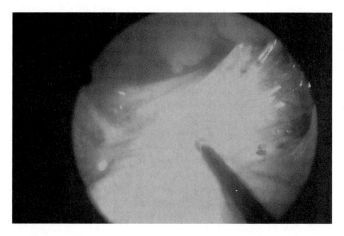

FIG. 8-7   Endometriosis is treated with contact Nd:YAG laser energy. (Courtesy Surgical Laser Technologies, Inc., Oaks, PA.)

dometriosis is being challenged today. Pregnancy incidence after the laser vaporization of endometrial implants has been favorable. The hormones produced during pregnancy may help decrease the progression of the disease.

Neosalpingostomy

Chronic hydrosalpinx is conventionally treated with open abdominal surgery. The results have not been favorable. Laser laparoscopy has been introduced to treat this condition, and the results are promising. The ability to diagnose and treat the condition during the same surgical procedure is attractive to the gynecologist.

In neosalpingostomy, the laparoscope is passed through the primary puncture site, and accessory instruments are passed through secondary puncture sites. A grasping instrument is used to stabilize the distal tube; another instrument is used to retract the end of the tube. A probe may be used to assist with tissue manipulation and exposure.

The laser energy is directed to the tissue at lower power settings in a defocused beam to reduce the possibility of injury to adjacent thermal tissue. The laser beam coagulates the serosal layer of the end of the tube, which results in shrinkage and causes eversion of the fimbria. Radial incisions are made in the avascular areas of the ampulla to create the fimbria-like structures. This flowering technique does not require the use of sutures to evert the distal cuff of the tube.

The advantages of neosalpingostomy are that the patient can return to normal activities quickly because the procedure is performed through the laparoscope, and less time usually is required to achieve conception if the surgical intervention is successful. The disadvantage is that the procedure is tedious and difficult to perform and requires tremendous skill. Pregnancy rates are related to the extent of the tubal disease.

Uterosacral and Presacral Transection

Primary dysmenorrhea and central dysmenorrhea associated with endometriosis can be controlled with transection of the afferent limb of the pain fibers of the uterosacral ligament or more completely at the superior hypogastric plexus. The goal of this surgery is to decrease the pain usually associated with the menstrual cycle.

Transection of the hypogastric plexus, or presacral neurectomy, was introduced in 1899. The procedure was performed through a laparotomy incision to control pelvic pain and dysmenorrhea. During the 1960s this treatment was replaced by nonsteroidal antiinflammatory drugs, oral contraceptives, and other hormonal medications. But this therapy had a 20% to 25% failure rate (Perez, 1990).

Laparoscopic uterine nerve ablation (LUNA) was introduced in the 1980s. With this procedure the laser energy transects the neurons so that conduction of pain stimulation is not permitted. The laparoscope is introduced and the uterosacral ligaments behind the cervix are identified. The laser energy is used to vaporize and incise the ligaments close to the posterior cervix. Bleeding is easily controlled, and adjacent tissue damage is minimized. The success of the procedure depends on complete transection of the nerves. The immediate results with this technique are significant. However, pain may recur in up to 75% of these patients, so long-term results still could be improved.

In 1987 Dr. Jim Perez, in Columbus, Ohio, performed the first successful presacral neurectomy through the laparoscope, hoping to improve long-term pain relief compared with that of the LUNA procedure. During laparoscopic presacral neurectomy, all suspected lesions are excised with laser energy. After adjacent structures are identified, the superior hypogastric plexus is bluntly dissected from the sacral promontory. A 3-cm segment of the nerve is resected with the contact Nd:YAG laser. This technique has promising results because it is minimally invasive, and 70% to 80% of patients experience long-term pain relief.

Ovarian Procedures

The laser is being used to treat a variety of ovarian conditions through the laparoscope. Benign cysts can be drained by placing a laser hole through the thin wall of the cyst. Polycystic ovaries are treated by drilling holes into the ovary to reduce its size to relieve the excess androstenedione and destroy a portion of the stroma. After 30 to 40 small indentation holes are symmetrically drilled, the ovary looks like a golf ball. Ovulation usually occurs spontaneously, and conception can follow. The results of this technique are usually temporary because the patient frequently reverts to the anovulatory phase after 9 months to 1 year if conception has not occurred. Also, a portion of the ovary can be precisely excised with the laser through the laparoscope (Figure 8-8).

Laparoscopic oophorectomy can also be performed. If the patient complains of persistent unilateral pain and has no other medical problems, oophorectomy may be attempted through the laparoscope after the diagnosis has been confirmed. This technique requires 2 to 3 puncture sites to introduce the instruments needed for the procedure. Suture ligatures or staples are placed around the ovary and laser excision is performed, leaving a generous pedicle. The physician then vaporizes the pedicle base to reduce its size, making sure to leave just enough to ensure ligature safety. The ovary is then removed in pieces through the 10-mm laparoscopic trocar. The patient must be instructed that a laparotomy may be performed if the laser laparoscopic oophorectomy cannot be accomplished. Another technique involves using the bipolar cautery to desiccate the infundibulopelvic ligament; the ovary is then resected with the laser.

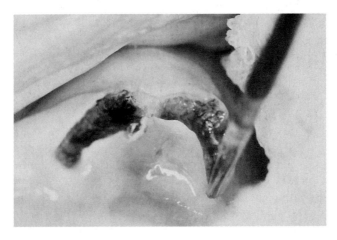

FIG. 8-8 A portion of the ovary is excised using a contact Nd:YAG scalpel. (Courtesy Surgical Laser Technologies, Inc., Oaks, PA.)

Laser Treatment of Ectopic Pregnancy, Fibroids, and Adhesions

The laser can be used through the laparoscope to remove ectopic pregnancies in the tube. If tubal pregnancy is suspected from clinical observation and the results of beta-hCG (human chorionic gonadotropin) testing and ultrasound, the uterus may be examined with a safe and simple hysteroscopy. The persistence of a positive beta-hCG and an empty intrauterine cavity suggest an extrauterine pregnancy.

Laparoscopy is performed to note the location of the ectopic pregnancy. Argon, holmium, CO_2, frequency doubled YAG, or contact Nd:YAG laser wavelengths can be used for this procedure. If the pregnancy is in the ampullar portion of the tube, a linear salpingotomy is made with the laser energy. Dilute vasopressin may be administered trans-abdominally with a spinal needle into the fallopian tube to reduce blood loss. The products of gestation are removed and the tube is irrigated. Any bleeding vessels are coagulated with laser energy as the tube is inspected for integrity. The linear incision is not sutured but left open to heal by secondary intention. A follow-up beta-hCG test is performed a week later to determine whether any products of conception are still within the tube.

Fibroids can be excised using a variety of wavelengths. The contact Nd:YAG laser can excise a fibroid from the uterus while controlling the bleeding (Figure 8-9). To treat larger fibroids, a zone of coagulation, ligatures, or staples are placed around the base of the fibroid; the mass is then cut into pieces for easy removal through the trocar sheath. The base of the fibroid is coagulated to ensure hemostasis. Vasopressin may be injected trans-abdominally with a spinal needle to help control any significant bleeding. Smaller fibroids can be directly vaporized with laser energy.

Adhesions can also be cut with laser energy delivered through the laparoscope. Care must be taken to protect the normal tissue behind the adhesion. Backstops can be used to prevent laser impact on normal tissue. Some waveguides for CO_2 lasers are designed with backstops (Figure 8-10).

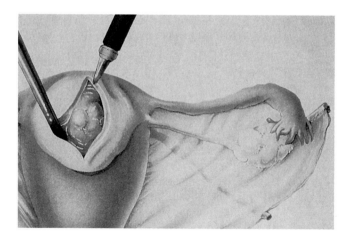

FIG. 8-9   A fibroid is excised laparoscopically using the contact Nd:YAG laser. (Courtesy Surgical Laser Technologies, Inc., Oaks, PA.)

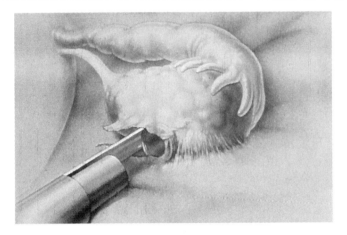

FIG. 8-10   Adhesions around an ovary are cut with a CO_2 laser waveguide backstop. (Courtesy Laser-sonics, Milpitas, CA.)

HYSTEROSCOPIC LASER APPLICATIONS

The hysteroscope has recently been coupled with the laser to treat conditions inside the uterus. Excision and vaporization of uterine septa, sessile polyps, and smaller fibroids can be performed through the hysteroscope. Refined instruments are now available to help direct the laser fiber to the disease site. This surgical procedure is less invasive and more cost-effective, fewer complications occur, and the patient can return to normal activities sooner than with an open procedure.

Endometrial Ablation for Menorrhagia

Chronic menorrhagia (excessive bleeding) or metrorrhagia (irregular bleeding) can be caused by a number of factors, including infection, tumors, polyps, and hormonal imbalances. If the bleeding is not treated, further complications, such as anemia, may occur. These conditions usually cause a severe disruption in the woman's normal lifestyle. Conservative treatments with hormone therapy or dilation and curettage may be effective, but sometimes hysterectomy is warranted.

Between 570,000 and 735,000 hysterectomies are performed in the United States each year (Wingo et al, 1985). The risk of morbidity and mortality affects a significant number of patients who undergo these procedures. Approximately 600 women die each year from complications from hysterectomies (*Clinical Laser Monthly,* July 1992). Approximately 30% to 40% of hysterectomies are performed to treat dysfunctional uterine bleeding (Lomano, 1986).

At the end of the nineteenth century, Asherman's syndrome was first described as the presence of posttraumatic intrauterine adhesions that result in amenorrhea (absent menses) or hypomenorrhea (light menses). This concept was the foundation of a procedure called endometrial ablation because a pseudo-Asherman's syndrome could be safely produced inside the uterus of the female patient who had menorrhagia.

The development of the hysteroscope allowed the physician to access the inside of the uterus for diagnosis and surgical treatment. Laser or electrosurgical energy can be used to cut, coagulate, and vaporize within the uterine structure, and therefore allows endometrial ablation to be performed easily and quickly. Menorrhagia is the usual symptom warranting endometrial ablation. Menorrhagia can be defined as heavy menstrual periods requiring more than 20 pads or tampons per month, clotting or gushing that keeps the woman home from work, or a menstrual flow that soils the underwear despite the use of pads or tampons and cannot be controlled with hormone therapy (*Clinical Laser Monthly,* July 1992).

The patient first visits the physician's office for evaluation of her menstrual bleeding problems. A Pap smear, hysteroscopy, and endometrial biopsy (if indicated) are performed to rule out any other problems that might be causing the symptoms. The treatment alternatives are discussed, and the benefits and risks of endometrial ablation are described.

The endometrial lining must be suppressed before the surgery to increase the effectiveness of the procedure. An atrophic endometrium decreases bleeding during the procedure. Three types of drugs have been used for endometrial suppression, including progestins, danazol, or depot leuprolide acetate. Leuprolide acetate requires only one injection; by comparison, oral therapy lasts 4 to 6 weeks. This drug appears to be the most effective in suppressing the endometrium (Saver, 1992). Side effects are usually minimal with this hormone therapy, but the patient may complain of facial blemishes or weight gain.

Sometimes a laminaria stent is inserted into the uterine cervix in the physician's office the day before the surgery. The purpose of this stent is to facilitate cervical dilation, thus decreasing the risk of cervical laceration during the procedure. The laminaria may cause cramping, so oral analgesic can be prescribed.

General, epidural, or intravenous sedation with paracervical block may be used for this outpatient procedure. Glycopyrrolate (Robinul) may be administered to decrease the potential for bradycardia, which may be caused by the uterine manipulation and vagal nerve stimulation. The patient is placed in the lithotomy position using knee crutch stirrups. A straight catheter is inserted to drain the bladder.

After the skin and vaginal prep, the draping is completed. A special drape with a collection bag located under the vaginal orifice is applied. The suction line is connected to the spout at the end of the collection bag so that the overflow of the hysteroscopy fluid can be measured. Accurate calculations of the fluid instilled compared with the fluid collected will determine the amount of fluid absorbed during the procedure. This number is critical because fluid absorption is enhanced as the ablation may open capillaries that will absorb the fluid. Usually the fluid absorption is less than 1 L. Any greater absorption may require the administration of a diuretic postoperatively to prevent fluid overload. Because fluid is absorbed, the patient's temperature must be monitored; external warming will probably be needed. A warming blanket placed on the surgery table will help control the patient's body temperature. During and after the procedure, nursing care should include maintaining the patient's thermal comfort.

Two 3000-ml bags of 0.9% sodium chloride solution are hung on a broad-based irrigation fluid stand. Glycine, sorbitol, or Ringer's solution have also been used. The gravitational pull is usually strong enough to promote the flow of the solution because of the increased height of the stand. Large-bore tubing is also used to provide adequate flow of the solution to the hysteroscope (Figure 8-11).

The normal irrigation chosen for use during a routine hysteroscopy is 32% dextran 70 in dextrose (Hyskon) because it allows for clear examination of the intrauterine cavity even if bleeding occurs. This solution should not be used during a hysteroscopy because

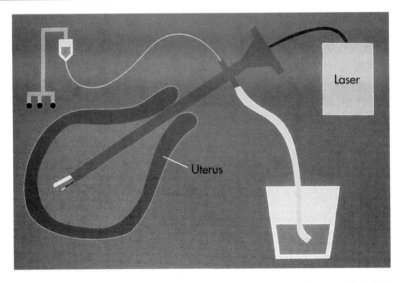

FIG. 8-11   Setup for a laser endometrial ablation. (Courtesy Dr. Leonard Schultz.)

the systemic effects of this solution, should significant absorption occur, have not been determined. Also, the heat generated by the laser energy tends to cause the dextrose to caramelize. Recently, surgeons have been using 10% dextrose in water because this solution flows like water and provides a clear surgical view.

The patient is placed in the Trendelenburg position, and a weighted speculum is inserted into the vaginal vault to dilate the opening. The cervix is grasped with a single-toothed tenaculum, and the uterine sound is inserted to determine the size of the uterus. The cervical canal is dilated to accommodate the passage of the hysteroscope. A hysteroscope with a 30-degree angle is introduced into the uterus as the solution irrigation flows. A 70- or 90-degree hysteroscope is used later to completely inspect the inside of the uterus. Landmarks are identified throughout the procedure for orientation.

Endometrial ablation can be performed using an electrosurgical roller-ball or a laser fiber to deliver the energy that will cause coagulation and ablation of the endometrial lining. The choice of tool depends upon the physician's skill level and preference as well as on cost. Endometrial ablation was first introduced using the laser, but today many physicians prefer to use the electrosurgery device. Reports have documented patient injury with the electrosurgery device. The electric current can traverse the uterine wall and impact adjacent bowel, causing a serosal burn and perforatio (Kivnick and Kanter, 1992). Research continues to compare the results of these techniques.

When laser technology is chosen, usually the noncontact Nd:YAG laser is used. The laser fiber is introduced through a stopper to prevent the escape of fluid from the biopsy port (Figure 8-12). The fiber is then directed to the guiding bridge at the distal end of the hysteroscope. Usually the Nd:YAG noncontact method is preferred because the depth of penetration of this beam allows successful coagulation of the endometrium. The contact method with the Nd:YAG laser has been used but tends to be slower. The argon and the frequency doubled YAG lasers are also being used, but their depth of penetration is not as great as that of the noncontact Nd:YAG laser.

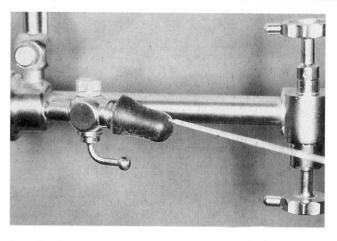

FIG. 8-12   The laser fiber is passed through a stopper to prevent fluid escape during a laser endometrial ablation.

The fiber used with the noncontact Nd:YAG laser is a bare quartz fiber coated with a Teflon and silicon material. If a fiber with a sheath is used to conduct a coaxial fluid or gas, one special reminder is extremely important: The fiber is *never* to be purged with a gas because an air embolism could easily be introduced through the vasculature. The catheter fiber must always be purged with solution when in a fluid environment.

Laser energy should not be delivered to the internal cervical os because of the large vessels in this area; thus, a marking tape may be placed on the hysteroscope 4 cm from the distal end to indicate the scope position inside the uterus. When the scrub nurse sees the tape, he or she informs the physician so that the laser will not be activated in this area.

A special lens cover to protect the physician's eye against laser backscatter can be placed over the lens of the endoscope. Ideally, protective glasses or goggles should be worn to provide the best protection. Even though the fiber is activated within the uterus, appropriate eye protection is still recommended for everyone in the room.

The Nd:YAG laser energy is delivered to the endometrial lining at 60 W in a continuous mode. In a sequential manner, the endometrial lining is totally ablated. The physician must be especially careful near the tubal ostia because this area is the thinnest portion of the myometria.

The blanching technique is used throughout most of the procedure with the fiber tip perpendicular and approximately 3 to 5 mm from the lining (Figure 8-13). The tissue is ablated until a blanching reaction is observed. This technique does not directly open the small vessels, therefore fluid absorption is minimized.

The laser is activated while the fiber is moved from side to side or from back to front. If bleeding occurs, the laser is used to coapt or directly coagulate the blood. The high pressure of the irrigant also helps compress the bleeding vessel.

The dragging technique is used for the hard-to-reach areas located immediately inside the uterine cavity. The laser is activated while the fiber is dragged through the endometrial tissue (Figure 8-14). The chance of perforation is greater with this technique because the fiber, with its small diameter, can easily be pushed through the uterine wall. The laser

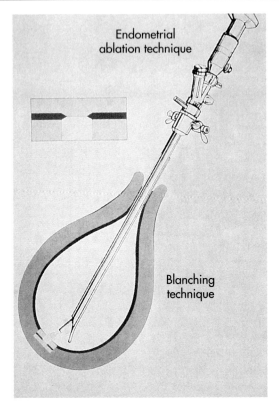

FIG. 8-13   Blanching technique used during laser endometrial ablation. (Courtesy Dr. Jack Lomano.)

energy should never be delivered while the fiber is being advanced to minimize the hazard of perforation.

After the endometrial lining has been treated, the physician reinspects the cavity for any missed areas or areas that may need to be retreated. The excess solution is drained from the uterus, and the procedure is completed.

For the first 12 hours after the procedure, the patient may experience some abdominal discomfort due to the prostaglandin release resulting from trauma to the uterine lining. This release of hormones causes the uterus to cramp. Oral analgesics can be taken to control this pain. The patient is discharged as soon as she is alert.

The patient is instructed to notify the physician if she has severe pain, excessive bleeding, or a temperature over 100° F. She is told not to douche, have sexual intercourse, or engage in strenuous exercise for 2 weeks. She should not use tampons for at least 2 weeks to decrease the chance of infection. A small amount of watery, bloody discharge is normal for the first 6 weeks after the procedure. The patient may return to work within 1 to 2 days. Reevaluation in the physician's office is scheduled for 6 weeks after the procedure.

Endometrial ablation does not prevent pregnancy, even though the endometrial lining has been destroyed and a fertilized egg cannot easily implant itself in this tissue. The

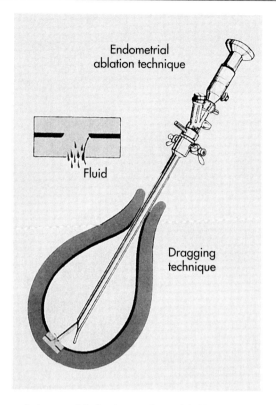

Endometrial
ablation technique

Fluid

Dragging
technique

FIG. 8-14   Dragging technique used during laser endometrial ablation. (Courtesy Dr. Jack Lomano.)

chance of pregnancy after an endometrial ablation is similar to that after a tubal ligation (*Clinical Laser Monthly,* July 1992).

Possible complications from laser endometrial ablation include fluid overload, uterine perforation, and gas embolism. At least two deaths due to laser endometrial ablation have been reported (*Clinical Laser Monthly,* July 1992). One patient had fluid overload that led to pulmonary edema and death; the other died of a gas embolism from a catheter fiber that was being purged with CO_2 gas. The laser energy opened a vessel, and the purge gas flowed into the vessel, causing a fatal embolism. Both of these deaths could have been avoided if the surgical team had been properly educated about safety measures needed during the procedure. Fluid absorption must be monitored, and a nonpurge or bare fiber must be used to prevent complications such as these.

There has been concern that endometrial cancer would be difficult to diagnose after an endometrial ablation. After the procedure the endometrial lining becomes scarred. According to popular opinion, endometrial cancer would cause increased bleeding, which would alert the woman to be evaluated. A hysteroscopy and pelvic ultrasonography can be performed to assess this type of abnormal bleeding. To date, there have been no reports of endometrial cancer in patients who underwent endometrial ablation (Saver, 1992).

A hysterectomy requires a 3- to 5-day hospital stay for abdominal or vaginal procedures. The patient usually cannot return to work for 4 to 6 weeks. Endometrial ablation has proven to be a successful alternative to hysterectomy for chronic menorrhagia. Ideally, the menstrual period is completely stopped, but a greatly decreased menstrual flow is also very acceptable. The patient appreciates the less invasive procedure, the ability to return to normal activities quickly, the decreased chance of complications, and the cost savings with laser endometrial ablation.

INTRAABDOMINAL LASER APPLICATIONS FOR INFERTILITY

Gynecologists have expanded the use of the laser to open intraabdominal procedures. Whether handheld or coupled with the operating microscope, the laser is an accurate tool for cutting, coagulating, and vaporizing tissue with a minimal amount of bleeding and adjacent tissue damage. Because of this precision, the laser is being used for complex and delicate surgeries to correct infertility. A variety of methods are being used, depending upon the location and cause of the disease.

Adhesiolysis

Adhesion formation is the most identifiable condition that produces infertility. Causes of adhesion formation include pelvic infections (especially from chlamydia), endometriosis, and previous surgery.

Adhesions affect fertility when they form bands that constrict the tubes, or when they restrict the mobility or motility of the reproductive organs. An adhesion can obstruct a tube by not allowing passage of a fertilized ovum, thus causing an ectopic pregnancy.

Laser lysis of adhesions (adhesiolysis) is usually performed when the patient is in the early proliferative phase of the menstrual cycle. Adjunctive medication therapy should be initiated if pelvic infection is present so that the medicinal substance will be at high levels in the tissue when the surgery is performed. Other surgical considerations include washing off the surgical glove powder before handling the organs so that the residual powder will not initiate adhesion formation.

Adhesions are treated with CO_2, argon, frequency doubled YAG, holmium, or contact Nd:YAG energies. These laser beams can precisely cut through adhesions while the integrity of the normal adjacent structures is maintained. A quartz rod, titanium rod, or similar backstop can be used when the laser beam cuts through the tissue (Figure 8-15). Otherwise, the beam will continue forward until it strikes and injures the normal underlying tissue.

Mirrors are often used to identify and access adhesions in hard-to-reach areas. The mirror should be warmed to body temperature before it touches the tissue. A mirror that is cooler than the body tissue will fog easily. The mirror must be held away from the impact site because the vaporization will also fog the lens. The laser beam should be focused on the tissue and not the mirror to prolong the integrity of the mirror. The physician must become adept at using the mirror during laser surgery because the images are reversed.

Salpingoplasty, Reanastomosis, and Tubal Reimplantation

The integrity of the fallopian tube may be the cause of infertility. A salpingostomy may be performed by first distending the distal tube to protect the endosalpinx from laser radiation. Laser energy is then used to incise the ampulla and make radial incisions to

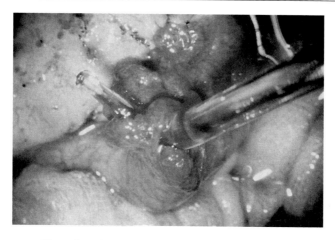

FIG. 8-15 A quartz rod is used as a backstop for CO_2 laser energy during an open abdominal procedure.

flower or evert the ends. This is easiest to perform on a thin-walled tube. A titanium or quartz rod backstop is used to protect the underlying tissue when the radial incisions are made. The surgeon can then evaluate the tubal patency by performing tubal insufflation to note any obstructions in the flow of the solution.

Because tissue trauma is a major cause of adhesion formation, the surgeon should manipulate the tissue as little as possible to decrease the chance of adhesion and scar formation caused by the operation itself. Studies have shown that laser-induced tissue necrosis does not promote secondary adhesion formation (Klink et al, 1978). Since the operative field remains relatively hemostatic when the laser is used, adhesions are less likely to reform.

The CO_2 laser is commonly used for tubal reanastomosis. The success of the procedure depends upon the site of the reanastomosis and the length of the tube. Anastomoses at the isthmic area near the uterus with at least 5 cm of tube have the best results. The tube is transected with the focused laser energy, and moist packing serves as a backstop behind the surgical area. The surgeon evaluates the patencies of the distal and proximal tubes to make sure all of the obstructed tube is removed. The diameters of the two tube ends are made to correspond with each other, and the ends are approximated (Figure 8-16). The different layers of the tubes are closed with fine suture, and the procedure is completed according to traditional protocols.

Tubal reimplantation is performed when the tube needs to be repositioned to communicate with the uterus. The laser serves as a drilling device, boring a hole in the uterus to reimplant the tube. The size of the hole is determined by the diameter of the proximal tube. The tube is sutured in place and the patency is evaluated.

Myomectomy and Endometriosis Vaporization

The most common pelvic tumor is a uterine leiomyoma or uterine fibroid. The conventional treatment for this condition is hysterectomy. For women who may want to preserve their reproductive capabilities, palliative surgery or laser myomectomy can be performed.

The fibroid is visualized in an open abdominal procedure. The CO_2 laser is commonly used for this surgery, but the argon, frequency doubled YAG, holmium, and con-

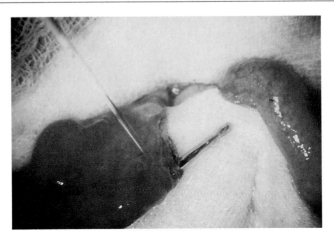

FIG. 8-16   The CO_2 laser is used to prepare the ends of the fallopian tubes for reanastomosis.

tact Nd:YAG are also used. If CO_2 laser energy is employed, approximately 50 W of continuous power is used to make the incision over the fibroid. The serosa and myometrium usually retract after the incision is made, exposing the capsule of fibroids. Traction is applied as the CO_2 laser energy circumferentially resects the tumor. Small tumor seedlings are vaporized with a defocused CO_2 beam. Bleeding is controlled with the laser in a defocused mode, coagulating the vessels. The uterine repair proceeds with the placement of absorbable sutures, and the area is irrigated completely before the abdominal cavity is closed.

Postoperative pain after the first 24 hours is easily controlled with oral analgesics. The patient is usually discharged on the third day after the surgery and resumes unrestricted activity after 3 or 4 weeks. Most patients experience abatement of preoperative symptoms of dyspareunia and pelvic pressure. The initial goal of maintaining reproductive status is usually very successful. Reports have noted that recurrence of uterine fibroids is minimal when laser surgery is used (Reyniak, 1988). Because of refinements in technique and instrumentation, this procedure is performed through the laparoscope today.

Extensive endometrial implants are treated during an open abdominal procedure in the same manner as during laser laparoscopy. The patient may be given hormone suppression therapy preoperatively to facilitate the procedure. The surgeon treats smaller implanted areas with laser vaporization while trying to preserve the normal healthy adjacent tissue. Larger implants may require resection with the laser energy and suturing of the underlying structure. The laser is advantageous because the deeper penetration of its beam allows it to vaporize all of the endometriosis and because the sealing effect provides hemostasis.

REFERENCES

Dibler J: Study compares laser vs. cautery for the treatment of CIN, *Clinical Laser Monthly*, p 8-10, Jan 1994.

Endometrial ablation: Should it ever be elective? *Clinical Laser Monthly*, pp 101-105, July 1992.

Flashlamp-excited dye laser relieves chronic vulvar pain, *Clinical Laser Monthly*, p 175-7, Nov 1993.

Kivnick S and Kanter MH: Bowel injury from roller-ball ablation of the endometrium, *Obstet Gynecol*, 79(5):833-835, Part 2, May 1992.

Klink F, Grosspietzsch R, Klitzing LV et al.: Animal in-vivo studies and in-vitro experiments with human tubes for end-to-end anastomotic operation by a CO_2 laser technique, *Fertil Steril* 30:100, 1978.

Lomano JM: Ablation of the endometrium with the Neodymium:YAG laser: A multicenter study, *Colposc Gynecol Laser Surg* 2(4):203, 1986.

Lomano JM and Grochmal SA: New micro-endo-scopic techniques reduce scars, recuperation time, *Clinical Laser Monthly*, p 125-7, Aug 1992.

Perez JJ: Laparoscopic presacral neurectomy, *J Reprod Med* 35(6):625, June 1990.

Reich H, MacGregor TS, and Vancaillie TG: CO_2 laser used through the operating channel of laser laparoscopes: In vitro study of power and power density losses, *Obstet Gynecol* 77(1):40-47, Jan 1991.

Reyniak JV: Abdominal myomectomy with CO_2 laser, *Laser Med Surg News Adv* 6(6):26, Dec 1988.

Saver CL: Rollerball endometrial ablation: New treatment options for women, *Today's OR Nurse*, pp 11-14, June 1992.

Wingo P et al: The mortality risk associated with hysterectomy, *Am J Obstet Gynecol* 152:803, Aug 1, 1985.

SUGGESTED READINGS

Ball KA: Laser endometrial ablation, treatment for dysfunctional uterine bleeding, *AORN J* 48(6):1153, Dec 1988.

Daniell JF: Advanced operative laparoscopic laser techniques, *Laser Med Surg News* 5(3):15, June 1987.

Lomano JM: Laser hysteroscopy: New benefits, new risks, *Contemporary OB/GYN*, p 71, Aug 1988.

Lomano JM: Photocoagulation of early pelvic endometriosis with the Nd:YAG laser through the laparoscope, *J Reprod Med* 30(2):77, Feb 1985.

Nezhat C, Winer WK, and Nezhat F: A comparison of the CO_2, argon, and KTP/532 lasers in the videolaseroscopic treatment of endometriosis, *Colposc Gynecol Laser Surg* 4(1):41, 1988.

9

UROLOGY LASER
APPLICATIONS

L asers were first experimentally used in urology within gas-filled bladders. The laser was inserted through conventional rigid cystoscopes with special deflecting prisms or shutoff windows to conduct the laser energy. Advances have led to the development of cystoscope accessories and quartz fibers to conduct the beam through a fluid-filled bladder. In the 1970s, Dr. A. Hofstetter successfully performed Nd:YAG laser cystoscopy to irradiate bladder tumors. This accomplishment led to tremendous advances in treating recurrent bladder tumors and initiated the development of other urological laser applications.

A variety of laser wavelengths are used today to successfully treat many urological conditions. The CO_2, Nd:YAG, frequency doubled YAG, argon, and holmium lasers are commonly used for different procedures. Reviewing the anatomy of the urinary system shown in Figure 9-1 will enhance understanding of the clinical applications described in this chapter.

ENDOSCOPIC LASER APPLICATIONS
Bladder Tumors

Conventional surgery to remove bladder tumors involves admitting the patient to the hospital for 3 to 5 days. A general or spinal anesthetic is administered while the bladder tumor is removed through an external incision or through transurethral resection using an electrocautery device. Muscle relaxation is imperative because the electrical current from the electrocautery unit will stimulate the obturator nerve. Complications associated with the conventional procedures include perforation, bleeding, and probable scar formation that will reduce the bladder capacity. If a significant amount of blood is lost during the procedure, the patient will need a blood transfusion. A postoperative catheter with a large balloon is placed to help compress the blood vessels and thus decrease bleeding. The presence of the catheter increases the chance of urinary tract infection.

When conventional methods are used to resect bladder tumors, the recurrence rate is estimated at 50% to 70%. This high incidence is attributed to the failure of the physician to vaporize all of the underlying tumor cells and the possible implantation of tumor cells to other areas after these cells are dislodged during the procedure. The lower recurrence

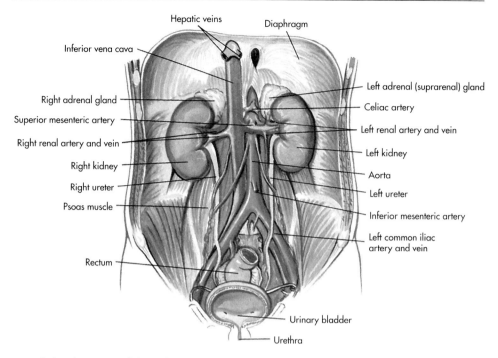

FIG. 9-1   Anatomy of the urinary system. (From Thibodeau GA and Patton KT: *Anatomy & Physiology*, ed 2, St. Louis, 1993, Mosby.)

rates reported with laser surgery explicitly demonstrate the laser's ability to provide deeper and more thorough tissue destruction, with a possible decrease in tumor seeding.

The laser procedure to treat bladder tumors can be performed on an outpatient basis. A topical anesthetic is administered to the urethra. An anxious patient may also require intravenous sedation. Usually a 21 French panendoscope is introduced into the bladder; the condition of the urethra is evaluated during insertion. The small size of the endoscope minimizes urethral trauma and reduces the rate of urethral stricture.

Physiological saline or a comparable fluid is used as the irrigating solution to distend the bladder for visualization. An electrolyte-free flushing solution is not needed because the laser does not create an electrical current that would conduct this energy. Care must be taken to avoid overdistending the bladder because the bladder wall will become thin, and the chance of perforation by laser energy will increase. The physician identifies landmarks during the cystoscopy and notes the overall condition of the bladder.

A biopsy is usually taken to diagnose the disease. A pathologist must examine the tumor base to determine the stage or involvement of the lesion. Patients with recurrent superficial bladder tumors are excellent candidates for laser tumor vaporization. Research is being conducted to determine the role of the laser in removing invasive bladder tumors.

Usually the Nd:YAG laser is used to treat bladder tumors because of its greater depth of penetration. The argon or frequency doubled YAG lasers are chosen to treat more superficial lesions. The contact Nd:YAG at approximately 15 W of power is often used because its controlled depth of penetration affords more precision.

A laser guiding bridge placed over the endoscope can direct the end of the flexible laser fiber to deliver the laser energy to a specified area (Figure 9-2). The laser fiber tip should be positioned perpendicular to the tissue to achieve ideal impact. Sometimes a bridge is not used and the scope is merely turned to reposition the fiber; however, this technique increases the chance of trauma to the urethra.

Superficial bladder tumors can be vaporized with noncontact Nd:YAG energy using approximately 35 to 45 W of continuous energy. The argon settings are lower, at 4 to 10 W. The peripheral area of larger tumors are attacked first, followed by the central portions. Smaller tumors are impacted directly.

Necrosis of the bladder tumor is achieved by blanching the abnormal areas. The depth of penetration is determined by the duration of exposure of the laser energy to the lesion. A 0.5-cm margin around the bladder tumor is also coagulated to ensure penetration into all of the involved areas.

During laser vaporization of bladder tumors, the light energy seals the blood vessels, thus impressively reducing the amount of blood loss and eliminating the need for a postoperative catheter. The laser energy also seals the lymphatics, decreasing the chance of tumor spread. The obturator nerve is not stimulated when laser energy is delivered because an electrical current is not present. Patients usually have less pain after the laser procedure than after conventional procedures, and they recover very quickly. The procedure is easily and rapidly performed and thus costs significantly less than conventional procedures.

The hardest areas to reach are immediately inside the bladder neck, where the appropriate angle of fiber positioning cannot be achieved. The contact Nd:YAG laser, the right-angled noncontact fiber, or direct contact with the argon or frequency doubled YAG laser fiber can be used to effectively treat these areas. The contact Nd:YAG laser probes are also being used to excise and coagulate pedunculated and sessile tumors. Figures 9-3 to 9-6 illustrate the sequence in laser ablation of bladder tumors.

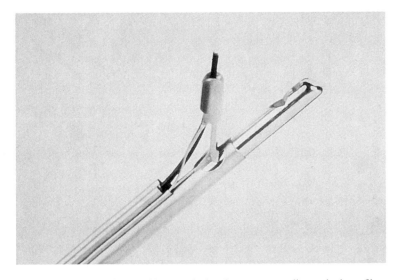

FIG. 9-2　A laser guiding bridge attached to the cystoscope directs the laser fiber.

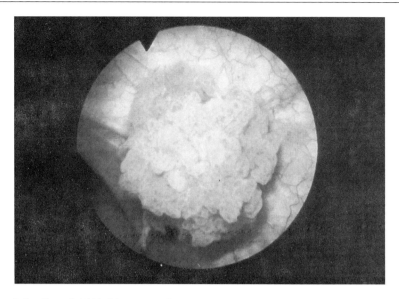

FIG. 9-3   Superficial bladder tumor. (Courtesy Surgical Laser Technologies, Inc., Oaks, PA.)

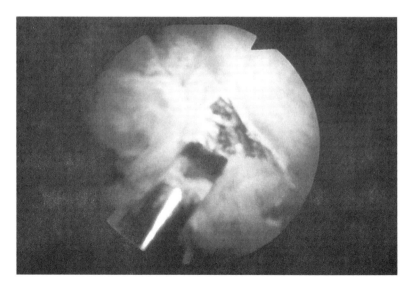

FIG. 9-4   Ablation of the bladder tumor with a contact Nd:YAG laser probe. (Courtesy Surgical Laser Technologies, Inc., Oaks, PA.)

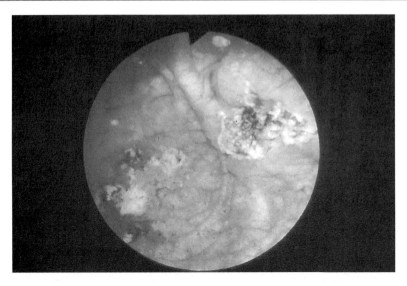

FIG. 9-5   Immediate postoperative results show a small charred area where the bladder tumor was removed. (Courtesy Surgical Laser Technologies, Inc., Oaks, PA.)

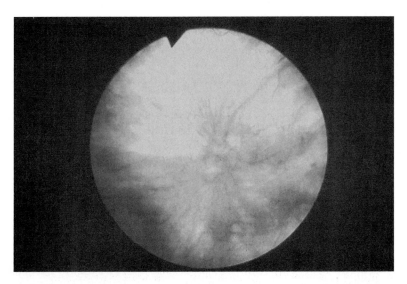

FIG. 9-6   Evaluation 3 months after the laser procedure indicates no tumor regrowth. (Courtesy Surgical Laser Technologies, Inc., Oaks, PA.)

After the laser surgery, the patient is instructed to drink a lot of fluids but avoid alcoholic beverages. Rest and relaxation are recommended for 24 hours after the procedure. The patient may experience hematuria for 48 hours; gross bleeding or severe abdominal pain should be reported to the physician immediately.

The complications associated with laser vaporization of bladder tumors are bleeding, pain, perforation, and bladder-wall instability. The incidence of complications is directly proportional to the experience and skill of the physician performing the procedure.

Laser treatment of malignant bladder tumors is also being performed as an adjunctive therapy to chemotherapy or radiation therapy. Responses indicate that these combined attempts significantly decrease the chance of recurrence. Further research is being conducted to determine the effectiveness of laser methods to treat malignant bladder tumors.

Urethral Strictures

A urethral stricture is a contraction of fibrous tissue that decreases the lumen of the urethra. Most urethral strictures are benign and occur secondarily to inflammation, scarring, or trauma.

Conventional methods of treating urethral strictures involve a steel scalpel or an electrosurgery device. These procedures are associated with postoperative scarring, the need for postoperative catheterization, and high rates of stricture recurrence.

The CO_2 laser can be used to precisely remove scarred or fibrotic tissue. However, because the CO_2 beam cannot easily be delivered through a cystoscope and is highly absorbed by the cystoscopy irrigating solution, this wavelength is not practical for treating urethral strictures.

The Nd:YAG laser can be used successfully to excise urethral strictures through the endoscope because the beam can be delivered through solutions via a quartz fiber. The Nd:YAG wavelength fosters healing by decreasing collagen formation and increasing the preservation of internal elastic fibers. Therefore stricture recurrence is minimized.

A topical urethral anesthetic is administered for patient comfort, and the stricture is viewed through a standard cystoscope. A stainless steel guidewire may be passed through the stricture into the bladder to allow for proper orientation throughout the procedure. Plastic or teflon guidewires should not be used as they could melt or burn if impacted by the laser beam.

The Nd:YAG fiber is positioned approximately 0.5 cm from the fibrous stricture. From 40 to 50 W of energy are delivered on a continuous-pulse duration. When thermal changes are noted or blanching of the strictured tissue is visible, the treatment is complete.

Some disadvantages have been associated with the use of the noncontact Nd:YAG laser beam to treat urethral strictures. Because of the greater depth of penetration of the Nd:YAG beam, deeper tissues are affected, possibly leading to scarring and stricture recurrence. Sloughing of the necrotic tissue continues for almost 6 weeks after the procedure, so the patency of the urethra must be monitored and maintained. Postoperative dilation of the urethra may be needed to provide short-term relief of urinary retention.

Contact Nd:YAG laser technology has gained popularity because it offers the physician tactile feedback similar to that provided by the conventional methods. Scattering of the Nd:YAG energy is decreased when it is delivered through a contact tip. This in turn leads to less adjacent tissue damage and stricture recurrence.

Different geometrical configurations of the contact probes can be used to incise the strictured areas strategically to provide patency. Various techniques involve making an incision at the 12 o'clock position only; making incisions at the 3, 6, 9, and 12 o'clock positions; or circumferential vaporization of the stricture.

Postoperatively, the need for a catheter to help maintain the patency of the urethra can be avoided if the patient is instructed to perform hydrodilation. When the patient feels the need to void, he holds the head of the penis while the pressure of the urine dilates the urethra. The expansion allows the urethra to dilate before the orifice is released. Catheterization should be avoided if at all possible because a catheter is a source of irritation that can lead to stricture recurrence. The catheter also provides a route for bacterial invasion that can lead to postoperative edema and stenosis from stricture formation.

Other wavelengths, such as the argon, frequency doubled YAG, and holmium, are being used to treat stenosis and strictures. Significant outcomes show promising results with these laser systems.

Ureteral Calculi

Various methods have been used to fragment urinary calculi depending upon the location of the stones. Stones embedded in the kidney are being successfully fragmented using extracorporeal shock-wave lithotripsy. This procedure cannot be performed as effectively when the stone begins to travel from the kidney into the ureter because the sound waves can easily damage ureteral walls. Therefore, laser energy delivered through a ureteroscope to vaporize stones inside the ureteral area is the procedure of choice.

A flashlamp pulsed dye laser of 504 nm in duration pulses of approximately 1 ms is delivered through a small fiber introduced through the biopsy port of the ureteroscope. Constant irrigation is used to flush the area during the procedure. The fiber is held in contact with the calculi. This specific wavelength is absorbed by the yellow or black stone, and the temperature of the calculi is elevated only 10° C. The hemoglobin of the surrounding tissue absorbs little of this laser energy, thus decreasing any temperature changes and damage to the ureteral walls. The ultrashort bursts of laser energy also decrease the chance of trauma to normal tissue.

The photoacoustic effect causes a mechanical shock wave to occur at the end of the fiber; the shock wave fragments the stone without damaging the ureter. The precision of this laser can be demonstrated in the laboratory by holding the fiber almost in contact with an egg. The pulsed laser energy will fragment the outer shell of the egg, leaving the peripheral membrane intact (Figure 9-7).

A special laser stone basket has been developed that will hold the stone within the basket. The laser fiber is introduced through the shaft of the stone basket to communicate with the stone. The laser energy is directed to the stone to reduce its size for easier extraction or for spontaneous passage of the fragmented pieces. The smaller stone fragments are flushed out with the irrigation solution, whereas the larger pieces must be mechanically removed using the conventional stone basket technique.

A wide variety of stones can be treated with this laser energy. Yellow stones consisting of calcium oxalate dihydrate easily break into small fragments with laser irradiation. Sometimes these stones have a central portion of black calcium oxalate monohydrate that is more resistant to laser fragmentation. These cores may have to be removed using the stone basket after being reduced in size by laser energy.

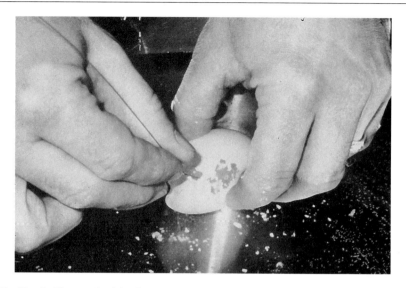

FIG. 9-7   The flashlamp pulsed dye laser energy precisely fragments the shell from an egg while the inner membrane remains intact.

At the conclusion of the procedure, the physician inspects the ureteral walls for mucosal trauma from the sharp fiber tip or from the introduction of the ureteroscope. If ureteral injury is suspected, or if edema at the stone impact site is probable, a ureteral stent is inserted for 24 to 48 hours depending upon the extent of injury.

Postoperatively, the patient is instructed to drink a lot of fluids and carefully observe complications such as bleeding or pain. The physician reevaluates the patient in 6 weeks to note the status of the lumen of the ureter and to check for the recurrence of any urinary calculi.

One of the advantages associated with laser stone fragmentation is that a stone that is completely obstructing the ureter can be chipped away effectively using laser energy, while trauma to the ureter is minimized. The extremely small fiber can easily be passed through a ureteroscope, compared with the larger ureteroscope needed for ultrasonic lithotripsy. Flexible endoscopes and instruments are available to enhance and facilitate this procedure.

Prostatectomy

The Nd:YAG, KTP, and other laser wavelengths are now commonly used during procedures to treat bilateral prostatic hypertrophy (BPH). The prostate gland encircles the bladder neck and proximal urethral outflow tract (Figure 9-8). Benign glandular and stomal hyperplasia may cause this gland to enlarge, causing voiding dysfunction in 50% of men by the sixth decade of life (Tuttle, 1993).

Surgery to relieve this obstruction is the second most common procedure in the older male population (second to cataract surgery). This traditional procedure is performed through an endoscope using electrosurgery to resect the hypertrophied prostate. Approximately $4.8 billion is spent to perform the estimated 400,000 transurethral resection of the prostate (TURP) procedures (Tuttle, 1993). The conventional TURP surgery usually

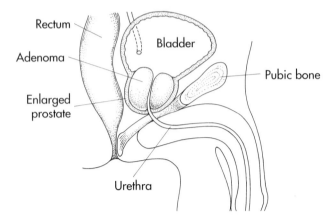

FIG. 9-8   Hyperplasia of the prostate gland.

requires a 3- to 5-day hospital stay. Complications associated with the procedure include hematuria, urinary tract infection, retrograde ejaculation, recurrence of prostate enlargement, and impotency. Other methods to treat BPH include medication, hyperthermia, balloon dilation, and stent placement; however, the success of these treatments has been questioned.

The concept of visual laser ablation of the prostate (VLAP) was introduced in the late 1980s using the Nd:YAG laser. Today two Nd:YAG laser methods are used to treat BPH that decrease intraoperative bleeding and postoperative complications. Laser treatment of malignant prostate problems has not been successful; research continues in this area.

One of the Nd:YAG laser procedures used to treat BPH involves a noncontact flexible fiber or a noncontact side-firing fiber that delivers the laser beam to the tissue at almost a 90-degree angle. The other involves sophisticated Nd:YAG contact laser probes that ablate the gland. Both delivery devices are introduced through the operative cystoscope, which permits visualization of the hypertrophied gland.

Before a laser procedure can be performed, the patient must have a complete evaluation to determine the extent of the condition. Preoperative assessment includes obtaining the patient's medical history, a physical examination, blood tests, urodynamics, and cystoscopy. If the patient has no significant symptoms, such as voiding problems and retained urine, then surgery is delayed until symptoms become notable. The size of the prostate does not always correlate with the severity of symptoms. The American Urologic Association Treatment Guidelines for BPH are usually followed, meaning that the patient should score more than seven points on the American Urologic Association Symptom Index before surgery is suggested. A prostatic ultrasound is usually performed to rule out cancer and to note the size of the gland. Laser prostatectomy has the best results on glands of 30 to 50 g, but advances in technique and delivery devices have made it possible to successfully treat glands larger than 75 g.

In preparation for the procedure, the patient receives a light general anesthetic or is sedated. During the noncontact Nd:YAG laser procedure, the light energy is delivered to the prostatic tissue via a right-angled fiber (Figure 9-9). Different types of fibers have been developed with a deflecting device to allow the beam to exit the fiber and impact tissue at

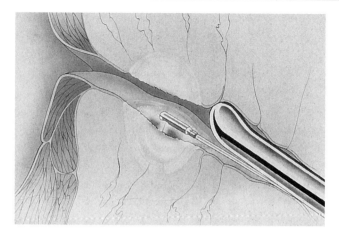

FIG. 9-9　The laser energy is delivered to the tissue via a right-angled fiber. (Courtesy Myriadlase, Inc., TX.)

an angle. As the beam exits the fiber, it also diverges, increasing the spot size and thus allowing the beam to impact a larger area.

The standard 30-degree cystoscope (17-23F) or a panendoscope is inserted through the urethra into the bladder. Normal saline or other solutions can be used to irrigate the area to permit optimal visualization. Because a lot of irrigation solution may be used, the laser foot pedal is covered with a plastic bag to protect it from spillage.

Urinary landmarks are identified through the cystoscope. Some urologists begin the laser procedure by delivering 40 to 60 W of Nd:YAG laser energy at the bladder neck level at the 5 and 7 o'clock positions for 60 seconds. The purpose is to relieve any bladder neck obstruction while preserving antegrade ejaculation.

The laser energy is then delivered to the hypertrophied tissue in pulses of 40 to 60 W for 30 to 90 seconds each. Usually the prostatic gland is visually divided into a number of sections, and the laser energy is delivered equally to each section. For example, the gland may be visually divided into quadrants. The noncontact Nd:YAG laser energy at 60 W for 60 seconds is delivered to each quadrant at the 2, 4, 8, and 10 o'clock positions. Depending upon the size of the gland, another around-the-clock treatment sequence may be needed. The fiber is aimed at one area and is not moved around in a painting manner. The painting method is used only for coagulation, such as to coagulate a small vessel that is bleeding. The fiber must not touch the tissue during this procedure, and charring should be avoided.

If the median lobe of the prostate is significantly enlarged, lower wattage (less than 40 W) is carefully delivered to the tissue at the 5, 6, and 7 o'clock positions. Additional sequences may be needed depending upon the size of the lobe.

Sometimes a transurethral incision of the prostate (TUIP) with the KTP or contact Nd:YAG laser is made at the 5 and 7 o'clock positions to open the bladder neck, thus allowing quicker removal of the urinary catheter during the recovery period. If the lateral lobes are so enlarged that they touch in the midline, a TUIP may be performed at the beginning of the procedure to permit relaxation of the lobes, making the procedure easier to complete.

A postoperative catheter is positioned to maintain patency of the urethra as edema may occur at the surgical site. The catheter is left in place depending upon the amount of laser energy used. As a guideline, for every 10,000 J of laser energy used, the catheter is left in place for 1 day. The patient may be taught how to safely remove the catheter at home.

The gland will reepithelialize and slough the necrotic tissue for about 6 weeks. At the end of this period, the patency of the urethral lumen is restored, and symptoms subside.

The advantages of VLAP over the traditional TURP are significant. VLAP is performed on an outpatient basis in less than 30 minutes. The procedure is bloodless since vessels are not impacted, thus fluid absorption and electrolyte shifts are not problems. VLAP also preserves antegrade ejaculation and sexual function in most patients. Bladder-neck contracture is minimized. Because the procedure is relatively noninvasive, it is less expensive. The patient can usually return to work or other normal activities the next day.

VLAP has a few disadvantages. Because tissue is not actually removed, a pathological evaluation is not possible unless a biopsy is performed. An indwelling postoperative catheter is placed because urethral swelling occurs from the heat transmission of the laser energy.

A transurethral ultrasound-guided laser-induced prostatectomy (TULIP) procedure has also been introduced using noncontact Nd:YAG laser energy. This system consists of an ultrasound imager and a transurethral probe that are used in conjunction with the laser. The ultrasound provides guidance for the laser delivery. A control handle moves the ultrasound probe and laser delivery window longitudinally along the length of the urethra where the prostate gland is located. The entire prostate can be imaged and treated.

To begin the procedure, the physician performs a cystoscopy to examine the bladder and urethra. The bladder remains full when the cystoscope is removed. The physician then introduces the transurethral probe into the prostate area, using a fluid-filled balloon to correctly position the probe. An ultrasound image allows the physician to examine the prostate anatomy and note the depth of the tissue. Under constant ultrasound guidance, the laser energy is delivered precisely to the tissue. The treatment begins at the bladder neck and safely stops before reaching the thinner tissue at the apex of the prostate. The number of laser passes is determined by the size of the prostate. Usually 30 to 35 W of laser energy is delivered at a penetration rate of 1 mm per second. The tissue is allowed to cool between passes (Gordon, 1993).

Postoperatively, a cystoscopy is performed to evaluate the results. A small suprapubic catheter may be inserted along with a Foley catheter. The patient is discharged the next day after the Foley catheter is removed. Usually the suprapubic catheter is left in place for approximately 7 days for precautionary measures if obstruction occurs. The patient can resume full activities after discharge.

Research continues on the techniques associated with the VLAP and TULIP procedures. Amount of laser energy, target sites, delivery methods, use of postoperative catheters, and other factors are being explored and refined to provide optimal methods for treating BPH.

The contact Nd:YAG method is also being used to treat BPH. The procedure is similar to the noncontact method in patient preparation, intraoperative considerations, and postoperative course. The main difference is that with the contact method, immediate results are visible as the hypertrophied prostatic tissue is actually vaporized. Tactile sensation is restored for the physician as the contact probe delivers the laser light directly to the prostate. The laser energy provides shallow penetration, so ultrasonography is not needed to determine how deep the energy extends.

The irrigant helps cool the laser probe. Different sizes and configurations are available to vaporize the prostatic tissue. A catheter may not be needed as postoperative edema of the urethra may not occlude the lumen. The patient can usually be discharged on the day of surgery or on the next postoperative day.

One method with promising results involves a combination of the conventional transurethral resection with adjunctive laser intervention. The electrosurgery method of debulking the prostate is performed with a resectoscope. The contact or noncontact Nd:YAG laser energy is then delivered to the base of the prostate to vaporize and coagulate the remaining tissue.

The advantage noted with this combination procedure is less intraoperative and postoperative bleeding. Also, there is less edema, which can lead to postoperative urinary retention. Refinements and advances continue to be introduced that will enhance or even replace traditional prostatectomy.

Another combination method used to ablate the prostate involves first performing a VLAP with the noncontact Nd:YAG laser and then using the contact Nd:YAG method to actually remove some of the tissue. The prostate will slough for 6 weeks. This combination method decreases the problem of postoperative edema because tissue is removed, and thus a postoperative catheter may not be needed. Technology is striving to make this combination method cost-effective since it requires two laser delivery devices.

Chronic Cystitis

Many patients suffer from chronic cystitis that is difficult to control or treat. The most notable symptoms include bladder pain, urgency, and frequency. Contact Nd:YAG laser techniques have been introduced to control this condition. A flat probe is used to provide superficial blanching of the involved parts of the bladder lining. This technique arrests inflammation and decreases the severity of the symptoms.

EXTERNAL AND OPEN LASER PROCEDURES
Condylomata Acuminata

Condylomata acuminata of the genitalia are viral-induced lesions that are transmitted through sexual contact. Smaller lesions usually are treated with the chemical podophyllin to arrest the viral spread. Electrosurgical fulguration may also be used to control the disease process, but there usually is an associated increase in postoperative pain and scarring. Condylomata, especially larger or recurrent conditions, are being successfully treated with laser energy, including CO_2, Nd:YAG, frequency doubled YAG, argon, and holmium. Even the more difficult lesions of the meatal or periurethral areas respond very well to laser intervention.

When a male has had sexual contact with someone who may have exposed him to condylomata, early assessment can determine whether the virus has been transmitted before obvious growths are noted. This assessment is performed by wrapping the penis in a sponge moistened with 4% acetic acid (vinegar). The sponge remains around the penis for at least 2 to 3 minutes. When the sponge is removed, any condyloma lesions will appear white from interaction with the solution. Sometimes a microscope or optical loupes are used to help the physician detect any evidence of the disease. The lesions are then identified and are treated with laser energy.

If the viral implants are tiny, the laser may be used in short pulsed durations; anesthesia is not necessary because an injection may cause the patient more discomfort than the laser impact. For significant lesions, a local injection of an anesthetic agent is administered subcutaneously around the condylomata. A smaller, 30-gauge needle is used for the injection because this area is so sensitive. For multiple lesions, a penile block may be used. For larger patches of condylomata in the perianal area, a regional anesthetic may be needed. Intraurethral condylomata or extensive condylomata may require general anesthesia.

CO_2 laser energy has often been the wavelength of choice to vaporize smaller condylomata using 5 W of power for continuous impact. Adjacent tissue is protected with wet sponges. The CO_2 beam is initially delivered in the focused mode to remove the major bulk of the lesion. The beam is then defocused to vaporize and coagulate the base. Three-dimensional passes—vertical, horizontal, and oblique—are made over the dysplasic tissue to ensure uniform depth of penetration.

Larger lesions are treated with 10 to 20 W of CO_2 energy to remove the major mass of the condylomata. The wattage is then decreased and the beam defocused to vaporize the base.

As CO_2 laser energy interacts with the condylomata, the superficial tissue undergoes carbonization and volume loss. The laser plume produced must be evacuated adequately because the potential for transmission of viable particulate matter is great. The laser smoke wand must be held close to the laser-tissue impact site to decrease the chance of particulate matter floating into the air. A smoke evacuation wand cover should be used so that tissue is not suctioned into the device.

The carbonized tissue is gently removed with a moist sponge to expose the deeper tissue layers. If more condylomatous layers are present in the deeper tissues, repeat three-dimensional passes are made. Again, the charred tissue is removed. As normal tissue is exposed at the base, care must be taken not to destroy any of the healthy areas with laser energy.

Bleeding is minimized during the laser intervention because the laser energy coagulates the smaller blood vessels. Gentle direct pressure also helps control any localized bleeding.

The noncontact Nd:YAG laser also is used to treat condylomata. Low powers of approximately 40 W are used to sweep over the lesions. The lesions will turn white when adequate thermal coagulation has occurred. Because of the deeper penetration of the Nd:YAG wavelength, care must be taken to prevent deeper injury to the dermis. The lesions then are mechanically removed or allowed to undergo secondary sloughing.

Urethral condylomata are being successfully treated using the Nd:YAG laser through the cystoscope. The disadvantage of using noncontact Nd:YAG laser energy is that its greater scattering and penetration can lead to postoperative scarring.

Contact Nd:YAG laser energy is also being used to treat condylomata. With this technology physicians can use contact probes and scalpels to accurately cut and vaporize the lesions while producing a minimal amount of smoke. Since contact Nd:YAG laser energy produces limited forward and lateral scattering, there is minimal adjacent tissue damage and less postoperative scarring.

After the procedure, the patient is instructed to keep the surgical area dry, which can be achieved by using a hair dryer after showering or bathing. A thin layer of an antibiotic ointment is applied daily. Complaints of postoperative pain are minimal after laser treatment compared with traditional methods because of the theorized sealing of nerve endings in the surgical site by the laser. Discomfort can be controlled with acetaminophen if needed. Healing occurs within 2 to 3 weeks with good cosmetic results.

The recurrence rate of condylomata is tremendously reduced when the laser is used because the thermal energy helps to destroy the surrounding viral contaminants. The patient is instructed to use a condom during sexual relations to decrease the chance of becoming reinfected if there is any question as to the partner's infective status. The patient should be instructed to advise his sex partner to be checked for condylomata and treated if needed.

Penile Carcinoma

Penile carcinoma, a rather uncommon disease, usually requires partial or complete penile amputation. Because most lesions occur around the glans penis, local surgical excision of the tumor is difficult. Laser intervention is used successfully to locally control penile carcinoma with good cosmetic results.

Histological diagnosis requires a biopsy of the penile lesion before laser intervention. The Nd:YAG laser is often used because of the increased depth of penetration and tissue destruction achieved with this wavelength. From 20 to 40 W of noncontact Nd:YAG laser energy is directed at the tumor until its base discolors and becomes white due to thermal coagulation of the tissue. The contact Nd:YAG laser can also be used to precisely excise the tumor. Bleeding is minimized and easily controlled.

Postoperative pain is less than with traditional techniques because of the laser's theorized sealing effect on the nerve endings. The necrotic tissue sloughs for up to 6 weeks. Reepithelialization occurs after the sloughing is complete. Periodic follow-up evaluations are vital for early detection of any recurrence.

Circumcision

Contact Nd:YAG technology is being used during adult circumcisions. From 12 to 15 W of laser energy is directed from the small-diameter tip of a nonfrosted laser scalpel to excise the foreskin while coagulating the superficial blood vessels (Figure 9-10). Large major vessels are easily identified, clamped, and ligated because of the dry hemostatic surgical field. After the foreskin is excised, the edges of the wound are approximated and sutured in the traditional manner.

Postoperative pain and bleeding are less with this procedure than with conventional procedures. The patient is instructed to keep the area clean and dry and apply a thin layer of antibiotic ointment daily to decrease the chance of infection. Healing occurs with good cosmetic results within 1 month.

Vasectomy Reversal

Vasectomy reversal has been attempted using a variety of techniques. Different lasers are being researched for use with a laser welding technique. One approach involves using a modified Nd:YAG laser coupled with a personal computer to provide precise fusion of the vas deferens. When the laser energy heats the tissue, the cellular contents coagulate and bond. Therefore, a strong anastomotic site is produced, and the vas deferens is resealed. Other methods involve the use of different glues or bonding materials that provide an anastomotic bond when impacted with the laser energy. Research continues to develop delivery devices and laser wavelengths, refine techniques in vas deferens welding, and introduce new bonding materials to advance this procedure. The success rate continues to increase as advances are made.

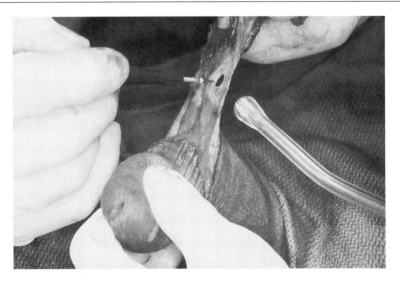

FIG. 9-10   The contact Nd:YAG scalpel is used to excise the foreskin during an adult circumcision. (Courtesy Dr. Frank Aledia.)

Partial Nephrectomy

The contact Nd:YAG laser is being used during partial nephrectomy procedures. The Nd:YAG probes and scalpels help excise the soft tissue very hemostatically to provide access to the kidney. The renal artery is identified and secured with a noncrushing vascular clamp. The branching vessels are isolated with contact Nd:YAG dissection and then ligated. The contact Nd:YAG laser energy helps provide precision and hemostasis throughout the procedure when the actual kidney tissue is excised. Thermal damage to the renal parenchyma is minimized because of the limited scattering associated with contact Nd:YAG technology.

REFERENCES

Gordon JO: TULIP: A less invasive approach to prostatectomy, *Clinical Laser Monthly*, p 121-123, Aug, 1993.

Tuttle JP: VLAP is quicker, less painful, and cheaper than TURP, *Clinical Laser Monthly*, p 187-189, Dec 1993.

SUGGESTED READINGS

Dretler SP: Laser photofragmentation of ureteral calculi, analysis of 75 cases, *J Endourol* 1(1):9, 1987.

Iammarino PJ: A nursing perspective on laser use in treating superficial bladder cancer, *AUAA J* p 7, April-June 1986.

Shumaker BP, Aledia FT, and Malloy TR: Urology (monograph), Philadelphia, May 1988, Surgical Laser Technologies, Inc.

Smith JA, editor: *The urologic clinics of North America*, Vol. 13, No. 3, Philadelphia, 1986, WB Saunders Co.

Stein BS: The use of lasers in urology, *AUAA J* p 4, April-June 1986.

10

GENERAL SURGERY AND ONCOLOGY LASER APPLICATIONS

The laser has been slow to gain acceptance in the field of general surgery because conventional methods offer accessibility and visibility, and the physician feels comfortable with traditional surgical tools that are easy to control during a procedure. Instrument development has advanced to meet the needs of the physician to incise or excise diseased tissue precisely and with fewer complications using minimally invasive techniques. Therefore, the general surgeon has not had a great desire to accept other tools, such as the laser.

Because the laser has not been as quickly accepted by general surgeons as it has by other specialists, its fate is still being determined. Unfortunately for general surgeons, the laser has allowed endoscopists, cardiologists, radiologists, and internal medicine specialists to perform the needed surgery from within organs or structures, thus eliminating the need for the general surgeon and incisional procedures.

During the late 1980s and early 1990s, laparoscopy was aggressively introduced to the general surgeon. Laparoscopic cholecystectomy became the preferred procedure over the open upper-abdominal method. Laser technology was the tool of choice for these beginning procedures since the physicians who developed this laparoscopic technique were also skilled in using the laser.

As laparoscopic cholecystectomy instruments and methods were refined, the value of the laser was questioned. Physicians were struggling to learn laparoscopy and laser technology at the same time. To become skilled with both the laparoscope and the laser was a tremendous challenge. Therefore, general surgeons began to use the tool they were already able to control: the electrosurgery unit (ESU). The laser began to be replaced as results showed that the ESU could also provide the cutting and coagulating needed during a laparoscopic cholecystectomy.

During this period, some general surgeons were trying to use the laser for every application. They were disappointed because they tried to do too much with the laser, or they did not use the most appropriate laser for a particular procedure. With the increased use of other tools, such as the ESU, the laser's popularity waned for general surgeons. Also, the physician could not justify the added patient charges for the laser and accessories.

Recently, laser technology has begun to spur the interest of general surgeons as new delivery systems and wavelengths are introduced that provide better results than those of conventional surgical methods. The laser offers precise cutting, coagulating, and vaporizing of tissue without undue trauma to the surrounding areas. There are also decreased complications and trauma to the patient. General surgeons are now attracted to the laser because of its hemostatic value in sealing small blood vessels. The tongue, scalp, neck, and other highly vascular areas tend to ooze with capillary bleeding when incised. When the laser has been used to treat these areas, surgeons appreciate its remarkable coagulative properties. The defocused CO_2 laser beam can seal blood vessels 0.5 mm in diameter and smaller, the argon laser seals vessels up to 1 mm in diameter, and the noncontact YAG beam coagulates bleeding vessels of up to 3 mm in diameter.

The laser is also valued for its hemostatic benefits in emergency situations with patients who have bleeding dyscrasias. Health care dollars are sometimes saved because laser intervention often allows earlier discharge from the hospital or may be performed on an outpatient basis. Because of these considerations, the laser is being increasingly accepted by general surgeons.

General surgeons have become skilled laparoscopists today, and many are beginning to attempt to meet the challenge of laser technology. As the laser's coagulation and precision capabilities during soft-tissue procedures (mastectomy, radical neck dissection) are realized, general surgeons are starting to use laser energy through the laparoscope. As hospitals restructure charge systems to lower the cost for laser usage, physicians are being enticed to use laser systems that were not being used. Residents are now being taught laser technology, so they too are becoming more familiar with it.

The rebirth of the laser is starting to evolve and will continue to grow with advances in delivery devices and wavelengths. Laser energy will continue to enhance endoscopy and laparoscopy because it can cut, coagulate, vaporize, ablate, and weld with great precision. Less bleeding, quicker recovery, and less damage to adjacent tissue are among the many proven characteristic benefits of laser technology. Some significant laser interventions are discussed in more detail in the following sections.

LASER PROCEDURES OF THE BREAST
Breast Biopsy and Treatment of Breast Abscess

A *breast biopsy* can be performed with the patient under local or general anesthesia. The area is infiltrated with lidocaine (Xylocaine) with epinephrine or a comparable solution. The epinephrine enhances the hemostatic effect of the laser. The breast is prepped with an antimicrobial solution and draped in the usual manner.

The incision line is a circumareolar or radial, depending upon the location of the lesion. The incision is made with a steel knife or with CO_2 laser energy in a focused beam of 25 to 30 W of superpulsed power (Figure 10-1). Traction is applied so that the plane of dissection can be easily identified. The power is increased to 30 to 50 W, depending upon the fat content of the breast, to raise a local flap. The specimen is resected, and the area is irrigated. If malignancy is expected, the wound may be "sterilized" by defocusing the CO_2 beam (spot size, 1.0 to 1.5 cm) and using 30 to 40 W of energy to desiccate the surface of the tissue. The smaller vessels are coagulated with defocused laser power of approximately 25 W; the larger ones are ligated with absorbable suture.

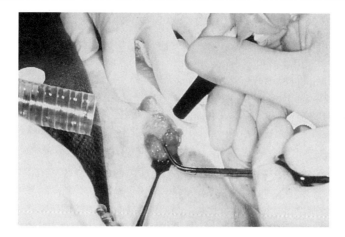

FIG. 10-1   A breast biopsy is performed using a CO_2 laser.

The contact Nd:YAG laser is also being used to excise a breast biopsy specimen. The contact scalpel or sculpted conical tip fiber precisely cuts the breast tissue very hemostatically with 8 to 15 W of energy.

The specimen is immediately delivered to the pathology department for examination. There is no difficulty in interpreting the disease of the breast specimen when the laser is used appropriately. Also, no change has been documented in being able to obtain accurate information on estrogen receptors on these specimens (Joffe, 1989, p. 26).

Whichever laser wavelength is used, the layers of breast tissue are sutured in the traditional manner if necessary, and the skin is approximated and subcutaneously, cosmetically closed. Because the laser seals the blood vessels and lymphatics effectively, a postoperative drain is not usually necessary. Steri-strips are applied directly to the incision line to help reinforce the closure. A thin layer of antibiotic ointment is applied to the surgical site. A nonadherent, bulky dressing is placed over the incision and obliquely taped so as to apply pressure. Postoperative bleeding and other complications are minimized because of the laser's sealing effects.

The patient may be instructed to use ice compresses on the surgical area to decrease the swelling postoperatively. Acetaminophen can be taken for discomfort. Usually breast biopsies performed with the laser result in less pain after the procedure than do biopsies performed with conventional methods. There may be less occurrence of seroma when the laser is used to excise breast tissue.

The dressing is removed on the first postoperative day; a light dressing may be reapplied to prevent clothing from irritating the surgical area. The steri-strips may begin to peel away but are not removed for 7 to 10 days. Nonabsorbable skin sutures, if used, are also removed after 7 to 10 days. When the dressing is removed on the first postoperative day, the patient can shower or bathe; the steri-strips will not wash off. The incision is gently dried and requires no other special care. The physician should be notified if redness, pain, or swelling occur at the surgical site.

A *breast abscess* can be treated with laser energy. The infected section of the breast is excised en bloc with approximately 60 W of CO_2 laser energy. Hemostasis is achieved, and the wound is irrigated with copious amounts of saline. The wound is sterilized by using a defocused CO_2 beam at 30 to 40 W to desiccate the surface tissue. The heat from the laser beam minimizes the possibility of recontamination and reinfection of the wound. The layers of tissue are closed over a closed-suction Silastic drain. A bulky dressing is applied, and postoperative antibiotics are prescribed. Home care of the wound is similar to that for a breast biopsy, but special attention is directed to the signs and symptoms of infection.

Mastectomy

The laser has proven to be a very valuable tool for the general surgeon performing mastectomy procedures. The CO_2 laser was the first wavelength used for this procedure.

When the CO_2 laser is used, a general anesthetic is administered and standard prepping and draping are performed. A skin incision is made with the CO_2 laser at approximately 25 W. The breast flaps are raised using 50 to 80 W of power in the continuous or superpulse mode. Steady traction is maintained to help define the plane of dissection. The laser handpiece is held to maintain the beam parallel to the flap for better control to prevent deeper penetration. Smaller blood vessels are coagulated with a defocused beam, and the larger vessels are ligated after being identified and isolated.

The breast is subsequently dissected laterally from the clavipectoral fascia. The axillary envelope is identified, and nodes can be excised using approximately 40 W of energy. Care must be taken to protect the underlying tissue from laser impact as the beam cuts through the target structures. A saline-soaked sponge or a titanium or quartz rod can be used as a backstop to prevent accidental injury from the beam. The surgical site is "painted" with a defocused CO_2 beam to decrease the chance of cancer recurrence from disseminated cancer cells.

General surgeons recently have turned their attention to contact Nd:YAG technology to perform mastectomies. Even though the CO_2 laser is useful for cutting and superficial coagulation, the contact Nd:YAG laser can cut, coagulate, and vaporize tissue with a controlled depth of thermal penetration. Some physicians have noted that the contact Nd:YAG delivery system is not as cumbersome as the articulated arm and handpiece of the CO_2 laser. Since the power density is localized at the tip of the contact scalpel or sculpted fiber, there is less scattering and damage to adjacent tissue. Therefore, there is a decreased need for backstops to protect the underlying tissue. Also, the contact Nd:YAG tip produces less plume than the CO_2 laser beam when striking tissue.

Contact Nd:YAG laser energy is delivered through scalpel tip with a diameter of 0.2 to 1.2 mm or a sculpted conical fiber of 1000 μm at 10 to 20 W to raise the flap. Initially, this procedure may take longer than the electrocautery technique, but as the skill level of the surgeon increases, less time is needed. The laser procedure is much more hemostatic, with less thermal damage to normal tissues (Figure 10-2). The lesion is excised easily as the smaller bleeders are coagulated and the larger ones are ligated. The axillary dissection is facilitated by the contact Nd:YAG's precision in not injuring the contiguous structures. The axillary vein is stripped by carefully dissecting the fatty tissue containing the lymph nodes. The CO_2 laser is harder to control in this area because the CO_2 beam could easily pop holes in the vein. The tactile sensation of contact laser technology minimizes this problem.

Whichever laser wavelength is used during the procedure, the wound is irrigated before closure; a small drain may be positioned to help decrease postoperative edema. If the field has remained dry throughout the procedure, the drain may not be needed. Drains are usually removed within 24 to 48 hours after the procedure. A bulky pressure

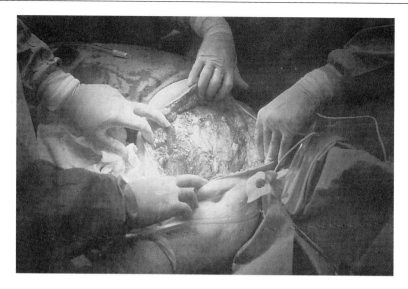

FIG. 10-2   The surgical site is very hemostatic after contact Nd:YAG laser technology is used to perform a mastectomy procedure. (Courtesy Dr. Thomas Vara.)

dressing is applied to minimize seroma formation and decrease postoperative discomfort and immobilization.

The laser is used for breast procedures for a variety of reasons. The laser's sealing effect provides a hemostatic surgical field and a decreased chance of spread of malignant cells to other areas of the body. Patients who are taking a blood-thinning agent, such as Coumadin, need not stop taking it because the laser provides such remarkable hemostasis. The breast flaps can be created with much precision, thus decreasing trauma to normal tissues. When an electrocautery device is used, there is always a chance of thermal damage to the flap. Also, the laser does not stimulate the underlying muscles and nerves, as electrocautery procedures do. There is also no chance of grounding pad burns or interference with the monitoring systems with laser technology. The laser dissection does not alter pathological examinations such as the estrogen receptor analysis. Infection is not a problem when the laser is used as it tends to sterilize the surgical site. Postoperatively, wound drainage may be decreased (because of the laser's sealing effects) to the point of possibly eliminating the need for drains. Patients reportedly recover more quickly and return to work earlier than with conventional methods.

Postoperatively, as contrasted to alternative methods, patients complain less of discomfort and are more willing to move earlier to facilitate the healing process. This may be due to the theorized sealing of nerve endings in the surgical area by the laser. Skin staples or sutures are left in place for 10 to 14 days. The patient is instructed to perform range-of-motion exercises regularly after the drains are removed. An in-bra prosthesis can be fitted after the swelling has subsided in approximately 4 to 6 weeks.

Recently, laser mastectomy has been performed as an outpatient procedure. Therefore, patient charges are much lower. However, not every patient can be sent home after this surgery. Patient-selection criteria for an outpatient laser mastectomy include having a home environment conducive to providing care for the patient, and having no comorbid complications. After a laser mastectomy procedure, the most intense pain occurs within 1 to 2 hours after the procedure, so the patient is usually retained in the postanesthesia care unit for 2 hours. When the electrosurgery unit is used for the mastectomy, patients have more postoperative pain and cannot be discharged on the day of surgery.

Because the patient's anxiety level may be high when an outpatient procedure is planned, a visiting nurse develops rapport with the patient before the procedure. The visiting nurse evaluates the patient at home after the procedure to make sure discharge instructions are being carefully followed.

LASER PROCEDURES OF THE NECK

The laser effectively cuts, coagulates, and vaporizes tissue during soft-tissue dissection of the head and neck area. This area is very vascular, and the hemostatic value and precision of the laser cannot be matched by that of other techniques. The CO_2 and contact Nd:YAG lasers are being used successfully during procedures such as parotidectomy, laryngectomy, radical neck dissection, and thyroidectomy. These procedures are similar in the following ways: The laser hemostatically seals the small blood vessels to provide a dry field so that delicate structures can be identified; it seals the lymphatics to decrease edema and the chance of malignant spread to other areas of the body; and it theoretically seals the nerve endings to reduce postoperative pain thus promoting quicker patient recovery. Radical neck dissection and thyroidectomy are discussed in detail as examples of laser intervention during soft-tissue surgery of the neck.

Radical Neck Dissection

General surgeons and ear, nose, and throat surgeons are performing radical neck dissections. The goal of this major procedure is to remove all of the tumor, metastatic lymph nodes, and nonvital structures on the involved side of the neck. All of the tissue under the skin is removed from the ramus of the jaw to the clavicle, from the midline to the angle of the jaw bone. Since metastasis occurs through lymph nodes and blood system, the sealing effect of the laser is extremely valuable.

A general anesthetic is administered and standard prepping and draping are performed. Usually a steel scalpel incision is made in the shape of a Y, H, or similar pattern. The CO_2 or contact Nd:YAG laser is used to dissect structures. Because contact Nd:YAG tips tend to offer great precision along with tactile sensation, they have become more commonly used for this procedure.

Skins flaps are retracted to expose the structures below. The surgeon identifies and isolates the muscles and vessels using the contact laser scalpel to carefully dissect the adjacent tissue. The surgeon precisely dissects selected muscle and vascular tissue while trying to preserve functionality of the area. Extreme care must be taken when directing the laser beam near the trachea because an accidental perforation could easily ignite the endotracheal tube. The lymph nodes are meticulously dissected along vessels and other structures. The contact Nd:YAG energy can easily be delivered to the hard-to-reach areas without any danger of extensive adjacent tissue or nerve damage.

After excision and repair of the appropriate structures are completed, the surgical field is examined for bleeding. Laser energy is directed to small oozing vessels for coagulation. The edges of the incision are approximated and closed in the traditional manner. A drain is positioned to provide adequate postoperative drainage to prevent excessive edema.

The patient is observed in the postanesthesia care unit for breathing difficulties caused by swelling in the tracheal area. Because of the laser's sealing effects during tissue dissection, edema is usually not a common complication. The surgical site is evaluated for bleeding at regular intervals after the procedure. The postoperative course for laser surgery is similar to that for conventional procedures, except for earlier removal of the drain and the possibility of less discomfort.

Laser Thyroidectomy

Thyroidectomy is often the treatment of choice for many thyroid conditions. Procedures can range from a simple excision of an adenoma to a subtotal or total thyroidectomy. Blunt and sharp dissection has been used to perform thyroid procedures. Prolonged surgical time and increased bleeding is associated with this technique. Electrocautery was increasingly used to help control bleeding, but problems of thermal and conductive injuries prevailed. Heat damage to normal tissue plus muscular contractions during the procedure limits the advantages of this tool. Recently, contact Nd:YAG technology has become popular. The contact tip provides clean dissection as smaller blood vessels are coagulated while cutting is done. Dissecting muscle fibers does not stimulate contractions because electrical energy is not used.

The patient is positioned with the neck slightly hyperextended. The surgical site is prepared in the traditional manner. The level of incision is marked approximately 2 cm over the midclavicular points. A skin incision about 6 to 7 cm long is made with a knife between the sternocleidomastoid muscles. The subcutaneous and platysma layers are excised with the contact tip or fiber using approximately 10 to 15 W of continuous Nd:YAG laser energy. Superior and inferior skin flaps are raised (Figure 10-3). Smaller blood vessels are coagulated with the laser energy; larger blood vessels are ligated. Fibrous structures and attachments are excised with the laser tip. The dryer surgical field enhances visibility, thus avoiding injury to the recurrent laryngeal nerve and parathyroid glands. Strap muscles are gently separated to expose the thyroid gland. The gland is palpated and assessed for disease (Figure 10-4).

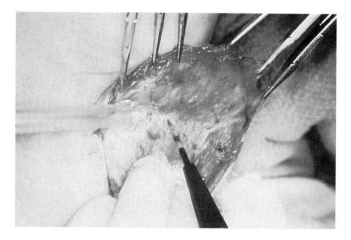

FIG. 10-3   A skin flap is raised using a contact Nd:YAG laser scalpel during a thyroidectomy.

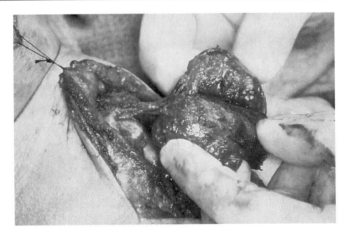

FIG. 10-4   The thyroid gland is exposed in a hemostatic surgical field.

In a total thyroidectomy, the superior pole of the gland is isolated, and the suspensory ligament is excised along with the lateral attachments. The superior thyroidal blood vessels are ligated. The parathyroid glands are identified, isolated, and protected. The lower portion of the thyroid is ligated and excised. The recurrent laryngeal nerve is identified at this level and preserved. The isthmus is transected, and larger blood vessels are ligated.

Complications associated with this procedure include injury to the recurrent laryngeal nerve, hypocalcemia, postoperative hematoma, or airway obstruction (Tyagi, 1993). These complications are minimized with the use of laser technology.

LASER PROCEDURES OF THE CHEST
Thoracoscopy to Treat Bullous Emphysema

With the introduction of the thoracoscope, general surgeons can access the chest cavity to perform a number of different procedures. Thus the patient recovers much faster because major surgery involving entry into the chest is avoided. Thoracoscopy to treat bullous emphysema is one of the newer techniques used to avoid major surgery.

Emphysema patients often have bullae that are abnormal air cysts located throughout their lungs. The bullae are formed from injured lung tissue that is located beyond the terminal bronchial trees. This injured lung tissue takes up space in the chest cavity but is not involved in the gas exchange during the respiratory cycle. Therefore, the breathing capacity of the patient is significantly reduced. The body tries to compensate for this deficit by increasing the size of the chest cavity by pushing the diaphragm down, creating a barrel-chest effect. But the chest cavity cannot expand indefinitely. Once the maximum size is reached, the patient experiences shortness of breath that continually worsens. Many patients become confined to wheelchairs and must receive oxygen continually. This condition, known as bullous emphysema, affects millions of chronic smokers or ex-smokers. In the past, few treatment options were available for these patients, but today contact Nd:YAG laser technology offers a new alternative treatment.

During the laser procedure, a general anesthetic is used with one lung ventilation. The patient is positioned with the affected lung up. The down-side lung is ventilated with 70%

to 100% oxygen. A rigid 10-mm thoracoscope is introduced into the chest cavity. A video monitoring system is used so that the entire surgical team can observe the procedure.

The main goal of this surgery is to shrink the bullae with the laser energy. The laser fiber is introduced to the surgical area through the thoracoscope. A large rounded probe is lightly held in contact with the bullae. Approximately 5 W of energy in a continuous mode gently heats the bullae, thus denaturing the protein. A white to yellow discoloration of the tissue results, and the bullae shrink. Normal saline is used to irrigate the laser site during the procedure to decrease the chance of vaporization or charring and to check for air leaks. If any bubbles are noted, then more laser energy is applied to the area. If an air leak persists, the bullous walls are oversewn by absorbable sutures. At the end of the surgery, chest tubes are inserted and connected to a drainage device (Wakabayashi, 1992).

This procedure shows promising results for patients with chronic bullous emphysema. Studies note that lung function can be improved from 21% to 86% after the procedure, and most patients no longer need oxygen.

Laser Bronchoscopy

The Nd:YAG laser delivered through a bronchoscope is beginning to gain recognition. Before the bronchoscopy, the patient's respiratory status must be carefully evaluated because respirations may be compromised during the procedure. The patient may be positioned with the healthy lung up so that adequate ventilation can be achieved. The procedure may be performed using a local or general anesthetic.

If a local anesthetic is used, the patient is given preoperative instructions that detail every step of the procedure. Intravenous sedation may be used to decrease the patient's anxiety. The back of the throat is sprayed with an analgesic to anesthetize the area for comfortable passage of the endoscope. Supplemental oxygen is delivered through a nasal cannula. Oxygen concentrations are kept below 25% to 30% at the surgical site. A flexible endoscope is passed into the bronchus, and a diagnostic bronchoscopy is performed. A biopsy or bronchial washings may be obtained through the flexible endoscope. The lesion is identified, and the supplemental oxygen is stopped. The area is quickly suctioned to decrease a high oxygen concentration that could support combustion. The noncontact or contact Nd:YAG laser is fired for a short time to impact the lesion. Any smoke is suctioned, and the supplemental oxygen is turned back on. The surgical site can be irrigated at this time. After the patient is adequately perfused, the process is begun again. The oxygen is stopped, the area is suctioned, the laser is activated, the plume is evacuated, the oxygen is turned back on, and the site is irrigated. This process continues until the surgery is complete.

When a rigid endoscope is used to treat bronchial lesions, a general anesthetic is needed. Special rigid bronchoscopes have been developed that provide a port for the anesthetic gases, laser fiber, and suction/irrigation tube. Larger specimens can be excised and removed through the larger lumen of the rigid bronchoscope. This bronchoscope can also be used to tamponade a bleeding vessel by applying direct pressure with the side of the endoscope. Sometimes a flexible bronchoscope is passed through a rigid bronchoscope to contact hard-to-reach areas. When performing laser surgery through a rigid bronchoscope, the surgeon need not pause to perfuse the patient because the anesthetic gases and oxygen are being delivered continually. The oxygen concentration must still be kept below 25% to 30%. (See Chapter 5 for a more detailed discussion of laser bronchoscopy.)

LASER PROCEDURES INVOLVING ABDOMINAL ORGANS

Different laser wavelengths are being used for a variety of procedures involving abdominal organs. Open procedures are being converted to laparoscopic techniques as minimally invasive applications are introduced. The anatomy is illustrated in Figure 10-5.

Liver

Because the liver is so vascular, laser applications are being refined to control intraoperative bleeding. CO_2 and noncontact Nd:YAG lasers have reportedly been used in liver applications but have not controlled bleeding or biliary spillage adequately. The noncontact Nd:YAG laser has also been combined with the ultrasonic dissector and finger blunt dissection for liver surgery. This technique decreases tissue damage and bleeding. New techniques and tools are being investigated for appropriateness in liver applications.

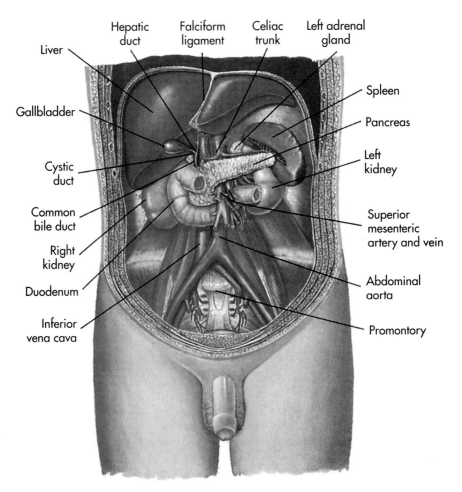

FIG. 10-5   Anatomy of the abdominal organs. (From Seidel HM et al: *Mosby's guide to physical examination,* ed 2, St. Louis, 1991, Mosby.)

Recently the contact Nd:YAG laser has proven to be very effective for liver procedures. Using this method, the surgeon can coagulate 80% to 85% of the blood vessels during a liver resection (Joffe, 1989, p. 83). The remaining larger blood vessels must be ligated or clipped. A new technique involves a disposable plastic "strapper" that is applied as a tourniquet to control the larger hepatic vessels. The liver section distal to the tourniquet is then hemostatically excised with the contact Nd:YAG laser device (Joffe, 1989, p. 83).

Hepatic resection is performed on patients with carcinoma, trauma, cysts, adenomas, hemangiomas, and other diseases. Before a liver resection, the patient's blood volume is assessed for adequacy, and any other associated conditions are controlled. Diagnostic examinations are performed, such as computed tomography, magnetic resonance imaging, hepatic angiography, and even laparoscopy. Adequate amounts of blood must be available for transfusion in case the patient loses a significant amount of blood during the procedure.

Different incision locations can be used depending on the site of the diseased area. The skin is incised with a scalpel or a laser scalpel at approximately 15 W of energy. Coaxial air or CO_2 gas is used to cool the laser tip and the connection to the fiber. The scalpel or probe is held in contact with the tissue using a light-touch technique. Traction and countertraction facilitate cutting and coagulation. Major blood vessels are ligated or clipped; smaller vessels, up to 3 mm, are coagulated by running the laser probe along the sides of the vessel to allow shrinkage and coagulation before transection. The involved part of the liver is hemostatically resected using the strapper technique previously mentioned. This method may take a little longer to perform, but when the procedure's hemostatic value is realized, this technique using the contact Nd:YAG laser becomes the preferred.

Postoperatively, the patient's blood volume is monitored for maintenance. Drains are placed, so the amount of drainage must be assessed. Copious drainage is usually expected, so the drains must be evaluated regularly to make sure they are patent. Delayed hemorrhage is usually not encountered when the noncontact Nd:YAG laser is used. If massive liver resection is performed, the patient should be treated postoperatively as if hepatic insuffiency existed, including administering albumin and vitamin K, hyperalimentation, and antibiotics.

Pancreas

Surgery of the pancreas is often difficult due to the anatomy and the blood supply to the pancreas. The CO_2 and Nd:YAG lasers have been explored for use during pancreatic procedures. The electrocautery, CO_2 laser, noncontact Nd:YAG, and contact Nd:YAG lasers were compared. The electrocautery, CO_2, and contact Nd:YAG laser were found to be superior to the noncontact Nd:YAG laser when the extent of thermal damage was evaluated (Joffe, 1989, p. 97).

Further studies note that the contact Nd:YAG laser can be used to precisely resect the pancreas while providing coagulation and preservation of surrounding tissues (Joffe, 1989, p. 98). More research is needed to explore innovative techniques such as endoscopic drainage of pancreatic cysts and other pancreatic resection procedures.

Spleen

The spleen consists of spongy material made of lymphatic tissue infiltrated with red blood cells. Because this organ is so fragile, it is difficult to treat. Historically, the spleen was removed after the hilar vessel was controlled. The current trend is to save the spleen if possible because it has been shown to contain highly selective immunological factors.

The Nd:YAG laser is used in the contact and noncontact mode to preserve as much of the normal spleen as possible while removing the traumatized or diseased area. Contact Nd:YAG laser energy offers precision; noncontact Nd:YAG technology provides deeper coagulation.

In a subtotal splenectomy, the hilar vessel is ligated, causing an ischemic demarcation line to appear. The noncontact Nd:YAG laser energy is used to vaporize the splenic capsule to a depth of 3 to 4 mm. The coagulated splenic sinusoidal and parenchymal tissue is suctioned while clips are placed on the skeletonized arteries. The procedure is continued until all of the spleen is resected. More research is needed on various techniques, delivery devices, and wavelengths to determine the value of the laser in procedures involving the spleen.

Intraabdominal Lesions

Laser energy can be directed through an endoscope to treat problems of the gastrointestinal tract (see Chapter 7, Gastroenterology and Colorectal Laser Applications). The laser is also occasionally used to treat conditions employing an intraabdominal approach, including open procedures and laparoscopy. The CO_2, contact Nd:YAG, and other lasers hemostatically excise lesions with minimal injury to adjacent tissue.

New methods and wavelengths are being explored to advance these types of procedures. A laser anastomosis system was recently introduced to provide precise laser welding of resected bowel. The laser bonds the structures of the bowel wall to form a strong anastomosis, so suturing is not needed. Welding glues are also being developed to assist with this procedure. Other similar applications are being explored as the effort to determine the true potential of the laser to facilitate and enhance surgical abdominal procedures continues.

Hernia

Hernia repair can be performed using the laser either through the laparoscope or during an open procedure. The benefits of laser technology are more pronounced during an open procedure. This type of hernia repair usually requires general anesthesia when an electrocautery device is used because of the discomfort associated with the flow of electrical current. An open hernia repair through a small incision can be performed using a local anesthetic if a laser is used. The electrocautery is not needed, so patient discomfort from electrical current is not a factor. Also noted is the laser's precision and hemostatic value, which allow vital structures to be easily identified.

Gallbladder

Cholecystectomies are performed on a regular basis to remove diseased gallbladders. Because an incision is made in the right upper quadrant, the patient is reluctant to move or breathe deeply after the procedure because of associated pain. This could complicate the recovery course if infection or a respiratory problem becomes evident.

The CO_2, contact Nd:YAG, argon, frequency doubled YAG, and other lasers have been used to excise the gallbladder during an open procedure. Because of the precision of the laser, adjacent tissue damage is minimized. Postoperative drains may be removed earlier because less drainage may result due to the laser's sealing effects. The recovery course is similar to that of conventional procedures except for reports of quicker recovery.

Today most gallbladder excisions are performed through the laparoscope using the electrocautery or laser. The incision in the large right upper quadrant is avoided because four smaller incisions are made to introduce the laparoscope and other instruments. The key to success is not the laser but the surgeon's skill in performing the laparoscopy. As general surgeons become more skilled and comfortable performing laparoscopic procedures, their use of the laser increases because of its precision and coagulation properties. This section discusses laparoscopic cholecystectomy using the laser.

Patient selection criteria must be followed strictly to ensure the success of the procedure. The patient must have documented stone formation or disease in the gallbladder and no evidence of extensive common bile duct disease. Previous abdominal surgery or trauma is not a contraindication to perform a laparoscopic cholecystectomy. A skilled laparoscopist may even attempt to perform a laparoscopic cholecystectomy when a patient has acute cholecystitis.

A general anesthetic is administered to the patient. A nasogastric tube and urinary catheter may be placed to decompress the stomach and bladder, respectively. This decreases the chance of organ perforation during the laparoscopic procedure.

The patient may or may not be placed in the Trendelenburg position (head down) to allow the organs to move toward the chest. A small umbilical incision is made and an insufflation needle inserted to fill the abdominal cavity with CO_2 gas. The needle is removed when the insufflation appears to be adequate. A trocar and sheath are inserted, and the trocar is removed to allow introduction of the laparoscope through the sheath. The light cord, video camera, suction, and insufflation hose are connected to the sheath or laparoscope.

The physician examines the pelvis and abdomen and identifies landmarks for reference. Other puncture sites are made at strategically placed positions to allow for the passage of other necessary instruments during the procedure. Figure 10-6 illustrates the traditional locations of the puncture sites. If the patient has a midline incision or other previous surgical incisions, the puncture sites are made elsewhere to avoid these areas (Figure 10-7).

The patient may then be placed in reverse Trendelenburg (feet down) to allow the transverse colon to move away from the surgical field. The gallbladder and other structures are identified. An intraoperative cholangiogram may be performed to determine the patient's specific anatomy. Forceps and laser energy are used to dissect any peritoneal attachments or adhesions from around the cystic duct or artery. The artery and duct are doubly ligated with two clips or sutures on the patient side and one on the gallbladder side. These structures can be divided with the laser energy (Figure 10-8).

The surgeon grasps the gallbladder to provide traction during its dissection from the liver bed with the laser energy (Figure 10-9). A long needle may be inserted into the gallbladder for decompression.

When multiple adhesions are present, or the gallbladder is difficult to excise from the liver bed, a technique involving partial resection of the gallbladder may be used. The anterior portion of the gallbladder is excised, leaving the posterior wall adhered to the liver bed. The laser is then used to vaporize the remaining posterior wall, and the area is irrigated so the surgeon can observe whether complete vaporization has occurred (Figure 10-10).

Depending on the technique used, the laparoscope may be moved from the larger umbilical port to another side port. The gallbladder is grasped and then gently pulled through the umbilical port sheath (Figure 10-11). If a large gallstone prevents removal of the gallbladder through the sheath, then the gallbladder can be pulled through the umbilical incision after the sheath is removed. The umbilical incision can also be extended to accommodate the removal of a large gallbladder or stones.

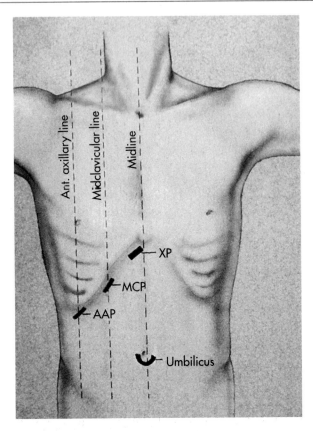

FIG. 10-6   Locations of traditional puncture sites for laparoscopic cholecystectomy. (Courtesy Dr. Jack Lomano.)

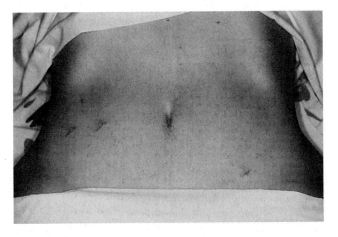

FIG. 10-7   Puncture sites are placed away from a midline incision for a laparoscopic cholecystectomy.

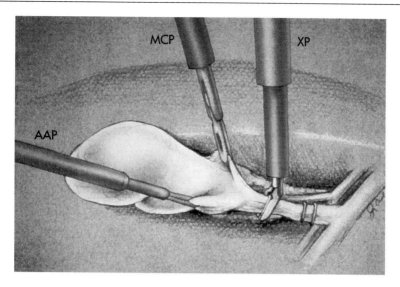

FIG. 10-8   The cystic artery and cystic duct are identified, clipped, and transected. (Courtesy Dr. Jack Lomano.)

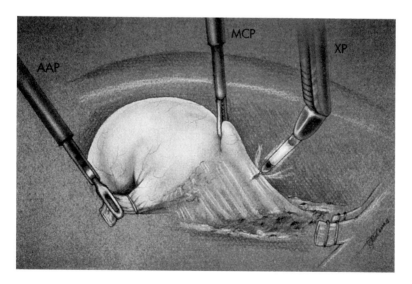

FIG. 10-9   The gallbladder is excised from the liver bed using laser energy. (Courtesy Dr. Jack Lomano.)

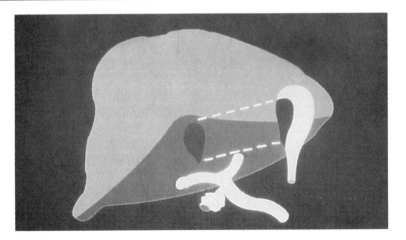

FIG. 10-10   Sometimes part of the gallbladder is left adhered to the liver bed. The remaining section is then vaporized with laser energy. (Courtesy Dr. Leonard Schultz.)

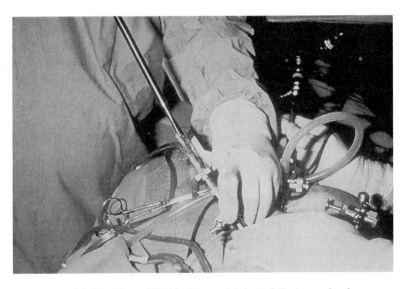

FIG. 10-11   The gallbladder is removed through the trocar sheath.

The liver bed is hemostatically coagulated with laser energy and then irrigated with a saline or an antibiotic solution. The surgical area is inspected for active bleeding and is coagulated if necessary.

At the end of the procedure, the abdomen is decompressed by gentle pressure to remove the insufflated gas. A suction may be attached to provide a closed system to eliminate any air contamination from the insufflation gas and tissue debris. A postoperative drain is not needed. All skin incisions are closed in the traditional manner.

Postoperatively, the patient may have shoulder pain, especially if any of the insufflation gas escapes into the preperitoneal space. This can be controlled with mild analgesics. Patients are usually discharged on the day of surgery or the next postoperative day. Most patients can return to unrestricted work within 1 to 3 days after the procedure.

The laser offers advantages over conventional methods when used to resect the gallbladder through the laparoscope. The laser provides great precision, thus adjacent tissue is not thermally injured. Capacitive coupling is not a concern, as it is with electrosurgery, and hemostasis is maintained. When the laser is used, most patients are discharged from the hospital and return to work quickly, with an uneventful postoperative course.

The main disadvantage associated with laser cholecystectomy is that the surgeon must not only become a skilled laparoscopist but also must understand and be in control of the laser energy. The potential complication of accidentally impacting the intestine with the laser energy must be avoided during the laparoscopic procedure. The surgeon must also understand that bleeding is harder to control through a laparoscope than in an open procedure.

As the general surgeon becomes an expert in laser endoscopy, fewer open procedures will be required to incise or excise internal diseased tissue. The laser will then become a more valuable tool and its true potential will be realized.

Biliary Stones

The flashlamp pulsed dye laser and the holmium laser are being used successfully to fragment biliary stones. An endoscope can be introduced into the biliary system via a percutaneous transhepatic approach. This can be done during the laparoscopic cholecystectomy procedure or during endoscopic retrograde cholangiopancreatography. The fiber is held in contact with the stone while short pulses of high-power laser energy are delivered to fragment the stone. Pure cholesterol or calcified stones are harder to fragment, but these can be reduced in size for mechanical removal with a stone basket.

PHOTODYNAMIC THERAPY

Cancer continues to kill thousands of people each year. The quest to eradicate cancer without harming healthy tissue remains a challenge to scientists, physicians, and nurses. A procedure called photodynamic therapy (PDT) shows great promise for eliminating cancer with minimal injury to adjacent cells.

In the 1920s, investigation of PDT began when researchers discovered that tumor cells produced a red-orange fluorescence when exposed to ultraviolet light (Joffe, 1989). This reaction is proposed to be caused by the endogenous porphyrins found in bacteria. An artificial porphyrin was then developed from the hemoglobin of cow's blood. The tumor's fluorescence was enhanced when it absorbed the porphyrin. Later studies showed that when the fluorescing tumor was exposed to light, it was destroyed by a reaction within the abnormal tissue (Joffe, 1989).

In 1978, Thomas Dougherty, PhD, and his associates at Roswell Park Memorial Institute in Buffalo, New York, began to further the investigation and development of this astounding therapy (Dougherty et al, 1978). The most effective combination of specific light and hematoporphyrin dye was explored to produce most impressive tumor death results. The U.S. Food and Drug Administration (FDA) has permitted clinical applications of this experimental procedure to selectively destroy cancerous tumors without harming healthy tissue. Different applications, such as bladder, bronchial, gastrointestinal, and dermatological, are being explored for approval by the FDA.

Two basic concepts characterize this procedure. One is that the dye is very light-sensitive and reacts when exposed to light energy. The other is that the dye stays concentrated in the tumor longer than it does in normal tissue. Neither the dye nor the light can be used alone. Only the appropriate combination of the light and the dye can produce successful results in destroying the tumor.

When a patient meets the strict patient selection criteria for this procedure, PDT can be performed. The expertise of a skilled physician is needed to calculate the appropriate dosages of dye and light and the exact time interval needed to allow the dye to clear from the normal cells. Most PDT procedures are currently performed on esophageal, bronchial, or urinary malignancies.

A specific amount of the special artificial dye is injected into the patient's vein. The dye rarely causes negative reactions for the patient. The dye is absorbed by all of the cells of the body, but leaves the normal cells within 1 to 2 days after injection. The abnormal, cancerous cells retain the dye longer. This obvious difference in concentrations within the body allows the dye to react in the tumor and not in the normal cells.

A red laser light, at approximately 630 nm, produced from a tunable dye laser system, is delivered to the tumor area by a laser fiber. The laser energy can be delivered to the tissue through external, endoscopic, interstitial, or retrobulbar exposure. The red wavelength is used because it penetrates tissue at a great depth to provide complete exposure to the beam.

When the laser energy reaches the tumor, which is filled with the light-sensitive dye, a definite reaction occurs. The light activates the dye, and a singlet oxygen (peroxide) is produced that causes tissue death of the tumor. Because the adjacent cells do not have a high concentration of the dye, they are relatively unaffected. The reaction inside the cell can be either mild or severe. A mild reaction produces swelling and inflammation; a severe reaction produces tissue death. This process is illustrated in Figures 10-12 to 10-16.

Researchers continue to investigate the most effective delivery systems, time lapse between injection and irradiation, dye composition, specific laser wavelength needed, and duration of light exposure.

The complications associated with PDT are minimal compared with those associated with chemotherapy or radiation therapy. The main side effect of PDT is that skin cells retain some of the dye. If the patient is exposed to sunlight, a reaction occurs in the skin cells, resulting in severe sunburn. Since sunlight contains the red light needed to activate the dye, swelling and redness of the skin result. Therefore, the patient must avoid sunlight for 6 weeks to 2 months after being injected with the dye. New dyes are being explored that minimize this complication.

With today's dye preparations, the patient is instructed to gradually increase sun exposure after 1 to 2 months after the procedure. This gradual increase should start with expo-

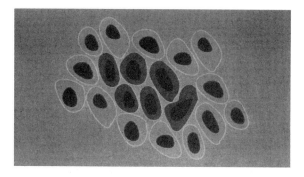

FIG. 10-12   The cancerous lesion is surrounded by normal tissue. (Courtesy Dr. Leonard Schultz.)

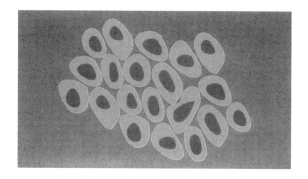

FIG. 10-13   A special light-sensitive dye is injected into the patient's veins and is absorbed by all the cells. (Courtesy Dr. Leonard Schultz.)

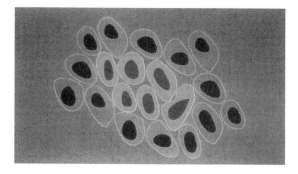

FIG. 10-14   After 1 to 2 days, only the malignant cells retain the special dye. (Courtesy Dr. Leonard Schultz.)

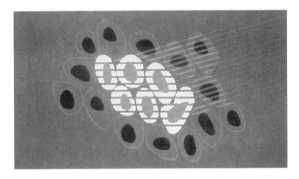

FIG. 10-15 The tumor is exposed to red laser light to activate the dye during photodynamic therapy. (Courtesy Dr. Leonard Schultz.)

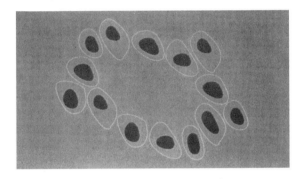

FIG. 10-16 Malignant cells are selectively destroyed. (Courtesy Dr. Leonard Schultz.)

sure to sunlight for 5 minutes, early or late in the day. If no reaction is evident, then a gradual increase in intensity and duration of sunlight exposure can be tried. The patient must carefully watch for any reactions to sunlight that may cause complications. Special sunblocks can be used that are more effective than sunscreens, which offer minimal protection. The patient is instructed to wear protective clothing while gradually increasing the time in the sun, to go outside only before sunrise and after sunset, and to beware of the intense sunlight that may shine through a window.

Detailed patient instructions are critical to the success of the PDT procedure and to minimize any reactions to the sun. Sample patient instructions are provided on page 258.

The success of PDT is being communicated throughout the world as researchers in various locations report remarkable results. Clinical applications are revealing that cancerous growths can be controlled and possibly completely eradicated.

Researchers are further refining the PDT procedure by exploring the use of other light-sensitive dyes and different laser wavelengths. They are perfecting laser delivery systems and documenting the exact amount of laser energy required to activate the dye.

Researchers are investigating clinical applications outside the United States and are noting responses to PDT in patients with premalignant conditions. For example, a special

---

Sample Patient Instructions: Photodynamic Therapy

Photodynamic therapy is a new treatment alternative that involves the injection of a light-sensitive dye that settles in cancerous tumors. Laser energy is used to activate the dye, and a reaction occurs that selectively destroys the tumor. The following instructions will help you understand the treatment and your role in this procedure.

BEFORE THE TREATMENT:
- An intravenous line will be started before the dye is injected.
- The light-sensitive dye will be injected into your vein through the intravenous line. The dye may feel cool during the injection. There have been very few reports of complications during this injection.
- The dye will be absorbed by all of the cells in the body but will remain only in the cancerous cells after 2 to 3 days. You may be discharged from the hospital after the injection and readmitted for the laser segment of the treatment. Light precautions must be followed after the injection of the dye (these are explained later).
- You will probably have other diagnostic tests, depending upon the extent of the cancer. Please ask questions about any of these tests.

DURING THE LASER TREATMENT:
- You will be taken to the operating room for your laser treatment 2 to 3 days after the injection. The type of anesthesia you will receive will be discussed with you.
- You will be protected from the bright lights in the surgery room during the treatment.
- The laser energy is delivered to the tissue through special fibers. The laser light causes the dye to react within the tumor to selectively destroy it. You may feel warmth in the area of the tumor, and you may have swelling at the site after the treatment. The length of the procedure depends upon the location and extent of the tumor.

AFTER THE TREATMENT:
- Hot or cold compresses may be ordered to help control swelling. A mild analgesic may be offered to relieve any discomfort.
- You should eat nourishing foods high in protein, vitamins, and minerals to help with the healing process. You should also drink plenty of fluids.
- Follow-up appointments will be scheduled so your physician can monitor your progress. You need to report any recurrence of symptoms, because early treatment has better results.
- Retreatment is possible with this therapy. The dye can be activated by the laser for a week after the injection. Repeated injections of the dye do not cause problems.

Continued

dye is being topically applied to the dysplastic cervix for absorption within an hour by the abnormal cells. The laser energy is delivered to activate the dye, and the response of the superficial cells is being studied. These trials are only in their preliminary stages, but oncology professionals eagerly await positive results.

Other studies are looking to PDT to help treat patients with severe pigmented vascular lesions. The injected dye is absorbed readily by the abnormal vessel growth, which is the

---

Sample Patient Instructions: Photodynamic Therapy—cont'd

SPECIAL LIGHT PRECAUTIONS:

- Special light precautions must be followed after the injection for 1 to 2 months because the skin cells retain some of the dye, and a severe sunburn can occur if light interacts with the dye.
- Window shades should be drawn during daylight hours. You can even sustain a sunburn during cloudy days. Regular hospital or home lighting will not activate the dye if you avoid windows with sunlight coming in.
- Artificial light of lower intensity does not cause sunburn, but the more intense light over a dentist's chair or at a beauty salon may cause some reactions.
- After going home, you can go outside, but go out very early in the morning or after sundown. If you must be outside during daylight hours, wear thick or dark protective clothing that covers as much of your skin as possible (long sleeves, hooded sweatshirt, gloves, hat, or scarf).
- Sunscreens with a high sun-protection rating offer minimal protection. Complete protection can be provided only by zinc oxide ointment.
- If you experience a mild sunburn, a lotion or soothing anesthetic preparation can be applied. If a severe reaction occurs, with blistering, your physician should be notified.

---

foundation of this condition. The laser light activates the dye, and the vessel growth is arrested, thus decreasing the severity of the problem. These studies are only preliminary, but results are encouraging.

PDT definitely has a bright future. The control of cancer and other conditions may lie just beyond the horizon and well within reach.

REFERENCES

Joffe SN, editor: *Lasers in general surgery,* Baltimore, 1989, Williams & Wilkins.

Dougherty TJ et al: Photoradiation therapy for the treatment of malignant tumors, *Cancer Res* 38:2628, 1978.

Tyagi NS: Contact tip YAG laser enhances safety of thyroidectomy, *Clinical Laser Monthly,* pp 7-9, Jan 1993.

Wakabayashi A: CO_2, Nd:YAG lasers make strides in treatment of bullous emphysema, *Clinical Laser Monthly,* pp 107-109, July 1992.

SUGGESTED READINGS

Ball KA: Photodynamic therapy of malignant tumors, *Today's OR Nurse* 9(6):9, June 1987.

Daly CJ, Gutierrez V, and Rader D: *General surgery (monograph),* Philadelphia, Oct 1987, Surgical Laser Technologies, Inc.

Lanzafame RJ: Breast surgery with the CO_2 laser cuts blood loss, enhances outcome, Laser practice report, *Clinical Laser Monthly* 3S, March 1986.

Lanzafame RJ: Cholecystectomy with lasers, *Laser Med Surg News Adv* p 31, December 1988.

McCaughan JS et al: Photodynamic therapy for esophageal tumors, *Arch Surg* 124, January 1989.

Meeker MH and Rothrock JC: *Alexander's care of the patient in surgery,* ed 10, St. Louis, 1995, Mosby.

Reddick EJ et al.: Laparoscopic laser cholecystectomy, *Laser Med Surgery News Adv* Feb:38, 1989.

11

CARDIOVASCULAR

LASER APPLICATIONS

New vascular laser applications are continually being introduced in the health care arena today. Research is noting the significance of using laser energy to perform angioplasty, vessel welding, and other vascular and cardiac procedures. Refinements in techniques coupled with new delivery systems and laser wavelengths are providing significant results to help determine the value of the laser. Various clinical applications in the cardiovascular specialty are addressed in this chapter.

ATHEROSCLEROSIS

Atherosclerosis continues to be a leading cause of morbidity and mortality in the United States, with 50% of all deaths attributed to this condition (Medi-tech Education Center, 1989). Atherosclerosis occurs when cholesterol, calcium, and other material accumulate along the inner walls of arteries. Eventually a plaque forms that interrupts blood flow.

Certain habits and lifestyles are contributing factors in the development of atherosclerosis. These include smoking, high serum cholesterol, high blood pressure, lack of exercise, family history of atherosclerosis, and diabetes.

Atherosclerosis can occur in any artery. Signs and symptoms of blood flow obstruction can occur at the occluded site or distal to the occlusion. The obstruction formation for peripheral artery occlusion is discussed as an example of this progressive process.

One of the first signs and symptoms of peripheral atherosclerosis is claudication. The patient notices pain in the legs, feet, and buttocks when exercising. Because muscles require more oxygenated blood during activity, pain is experienced when the blood flow is decreased. This discomfort may be relieved with rest.

As the condition progresses, pain caused by exercising is not relieved with rest and may be accompanied by changes in skin color and temperature. In cases left untreated, 8% of patients lose a limb within 5 years from the onset of these symptoms (Medi-tech Education Center, 1989).

As atherosclerosis continues and the blood supply decreases to a critical level, body tissues begin to die. Necrosis is an indication of severe atherosclerosis. Gangrene of the toes or feet may develop, and immediate surgical intervention is necessary to avoid amputation.

Early conservative treatment of atherosclerosis includes instructing the patient to stop smoking, decrease dietary intake of cholesterol and foods that increase blood pressure, and follow a regular exercise program. Patient-education booklets on atherosclerosis help increase awareness of and compliance with conservative treatment.

In the early stages of atherosclerosis, the patient may be given a prescription for a medication that enhances perfusion, e.g., pentoxifylline (Trental). The drug causes the membrane of the red blood cells to become more pliable, and thus increase their perfusion capability. Therefore, tissues receive oxygenation needed by the red blood cells.

PERIPHERAL LASER ANGIOPLASTY

Peripheral laser angioplasty is described in this section. Many of the details discussed apply to coronary artery laser angioplasty procedures described in the next section.

Diagnostic Testing

Diagnostic testing provides an arterial assessment of the severity of a patient's atherosclerosis. Noninvasive testing to note the ankle-brachial index may be performed. The ankle systolic pressure is divided by the brachial systolic pressure to determine the ankle-brachial index. Blood-pressure cuffs are positioned at various points on the leg for readings. A Doppler probe is used to accurately record the blood flow. The ankle systolic pressure and the brachial systolic pressure are compared. The following guidelines are used to assess the ankle-brachial index:

Ankle-brachial index

Normal	0.9-1.0
Mild disease	0.65-0.90
Moderate disease	0.45-0.65
Severe disease	0.45

Stress tests may also be performed to note tissue perfusion with exercise. If noninvasive testing is inconclusive or indicates the need for further studies, invasive testing is recommended.

Invasive testing is performed after the patient has been educated about the rationale for the diagnostic testing and procedure protocols for providing informed consent. An arteriogram is performed by injecting a special dye into the vessels. The exact location and extent of any arterial blockage is then identified. If atherosclerosis has progressed significantly to the point of compromising tissue perfusion, then surgical intervention is necessary.

Surgical Alternatives

Various surgical alternatives are available to the patient for the treatment of atherosclerosis. The goal of each procedure is to provide sufficient blood flow to perfuse the tissues.

Bypass surgery involves attaching a graft both above and below the blocked artery. This procedure involves major surgery, hospitalization, and a lengthy recovery.

Since major surgery can be associated with morbidity and mortality, the less invasive procedure of balloon angioplasty has become more common in treating peripheral atherosclerosis. Under fluoroscopic guidance, a deflated balloon is positioned across a lesion. A dilute solution of radiopaque contrast medium is used to inflate the balloon to allow visualization of the inflated balloon under fluoroscopy. As the balloon is distended, the dilating forces split and disrupt the plaque, opening fissures along the intimal (inner) layer of the artery. The medial (middle) layer of the artery is then split, and finally, after complete inflation, the adventitial (outer) layer is stretched beyond its ability to recoil. Thus, the arterial lumen is opened to the diameter of the balloon and reformed. Research has associated restenosis with fibrocellular filling in response to the controlled injury caused when the balloon stretches the artery.

Atherectomy is another procedure being investigated for treating atherosclerosis. A high-speed, rotating mechanical device is introduced into the artery, and the plaque is cut and removed. Problems with perforation, microembolism, and vessel-wall injury have been reported with this technique.

Laser angioplasty is another alternative introduced to complement balloon angioplasty. The initial problems noted with laser angioplasty were inadequate delivery systems, a high perforation rate, small recanalized lumen channels, and poor long-term patency.

Tremendous advances have helped to perfect the laser angioplasty procedure. Laser recanalization requires the introduction of a laser fiber into the occluded vessel to destroy the plaque. A balloon is then often used to make the channel larger to enhance blood flow (Figure 11-1).

Laser angioplasty is gaining popularity in the treatment of atherosclerosis. The goals of the procedure are as follows:

1. Increase the vessel lumen while promoting a smooth intimal layer in the artery.
2. Recanalize arteries that are difficult or impossible to treat with balloon angioplasty.
3. Decrease the incidence of restenosis.

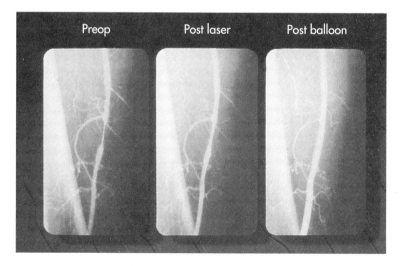

FIG. 11-1 Under fluoroscopic examination, the laser is used to create a lumen for blood to flow within a peripheral artery. Balloon angioplasty increases the size of the lumen.

History of Laser Angioplasty

The history of laser angioplasty began in 1963 when McGuff and Bushnell demonstrated that ruby laser energy could vaporize atherosclerotic plaque in cadaver vessels (McGuff and Bushnell, 1963). Almost 20 years later, Choy and his team reported the first transluminal laser angioplasty in canines (Choy et al, 1982). After artificially created thrombi were vaporized with laser energy, blood flow was restored. There was no evidence of debris formation and no postoperative thrombi, but there was a moderate degree of intimal necrosis.

Abela and his group studied the effects of different laser wavelengths on human atheromatous plaques and blood vessels; they investigated the CO_2, Nd:YAG, and argon laser energies. These researchers noted that the power and duration of exposure could be regulated to produce predictable degrees of arterial injury and that laser energy did, in fact, destroy atherosclerotic plaque (Abela et al, 1982).

Laser angioplasty continued to progress with the use of various methods and lasers to destroy arterial plaque. In 1985 Sanborn introduced the hot-tip method of vaporization of plaque. In 1986, Grundfest first used the excimer laser, while Lammer developed the contact Nd:YAG techniques for laser angioplasty. Also in 1986, Kramer introduced spectroscopy to assist with identifying plaque vs. vessel wall or blood. In 1988, Leon first used the dual diagnostic and therapeutic laser (Ball, 1990, p 173). Advances since this time have been steady; new wavelengths are being explored, and innovative delivery devices are being developed. The technique of laser angioplasty is continually being refined to establish a method that provides the best patient outcomes.

Patient Selection Criteria

Patient selection criteria for laser angioplasty have been developed over the years. Patients who qualify for the procedure can be characterized by the presence of the following conditions:

• Symptoms of atherosclerosis (such as claudication, pain during rest, or tissue necrosis)
• Obstruction of the iliac, femoral, popliteal, or tibial artery
• An artery occluded more than 85%
• An occluded arterial segment of less than 25 cm in length
• Patent distal vascular runoff
• No tortuous or bifurcated lesions
• No major medical or surgical conditions that would contraindicate the laser procedure

Preoperative Patient Education

Patient education is extremely important before laser angioplasty is performed. The nurse's role in preparing the patient for this procedure is highly significant. Education is paramount for decreasing the patient's fear of this new surgical alternative. Misconceptions and exaggerated fears that arise from laser technology's association with industrial and defense applications may be evident in discussions with the patient. Preoperative education must be explicit to help the patient totally understand the procedure and the anticipated results.

The physician is responsible for initiating patient education when the procedure is first recommended. As the patient reviews the information, questions may arise and be directed to the nurse. To address the patient's concerns, the nurse must understand the laser angioplasty procedure, comprehend the anticipated outcome of the surgery, and be aware of what the physician has already discussed with the patient.

The nurse should be able to empathize with the patient and offer emotional support. If the particular laser system to be used is still investigational, the patient must be informed about its status and sign a special consent form before the procedure can be conducted. The nurse should develop a rapport with the patient and encourage him or her to verbalize any negative or uncomfortable feelings. Intense perioperative education is vital, to convey what constitutes reasonable expectations and ensure patient compliance.

Intraoperative Procedures

Laser angioplasty techniques can be divided into three categories: thermal, photothermal, and photoablative.

Thermal laser angioplasty involves the use of argon or Nd:YAG laser energy to heat a biocompatible metal alloy probe tip attached to a fiberoptic waveguide. The tip is heated to a temperature of approximately 400° C (752° F). A thermographic image analysis illustrates that the most intense heat is generated at the tip of the metal end, and that lower temperatures are radiated by the periphery.

The thermal probe is introduced to the plaque. Using tactile pressure, the surgeon moves the hot tip through the obstruction to provide a small lumen for the blood to flow through. Advances have led to another type of probe, which permits part of the laser energy to escape from the middle of the probe, while most of the energy is used to heat the probe.

Research has shown that high temperatures inside the vessel can cause carbonization and necrosis of the vessel layers (Ginsburg et al, 1985). Another laser delivery system that has been introduced controls the temperature of the metal tip. By controlling the thermal output of the tip to maintain consistent thermal stability at lower temperatures, researchers are attempting to prove that a smoother, symmetrical lumen can be produced with less vessel damage or vascular spasm. A variety of tip sizes can be used to sequentially open the occluded artery.

Another thermal delivery system has a laser fiber positioned within a balloon to provide selective destruction and balloon dilatation concurrently. One balloon-laser angioplasty system allows the Nd:YAG laser energy to soften the plaque, which is then pushed against the vessel wall by the pressure exerted from a balloon. Researchers continue to refine balloon systems that are permanently coupled with laser technology.

A dual laser system has been introduced that has both therapeutic and diagnostic capabilities. The atheromatous plaque is identified by spectroscopic analysis performed by the laser fiber. The plaque is then evaluated by a computer diagnostic system. Based on this laser diagnostic information, therapeutic intervention is initiated with the laser fiber activated for selective ablation of the plaque. This spectroscopic detection system allows accurate discrimination between the plaque and the vessel wall, greatly decreasing the possibility of vessel-wall perforation (Leon, Lu, and Prevosti, 1988).

Photothermal laser angioplasty is the second classification of laser angioplasty techniques. This method involves a contact Nd:YAG probe that rapidly heats the plaque to the point of vaporization using a photo-optical effect. This selective plaque destruction allows for rapid cooling, thus decreasing arterial injury. Dr. Lammer in Graz, Austria, conducted studies to note specific postoperative vessel responses and successful long-term patency using this technique. Results showed that the contact Nd:YAG technique allows for an increased diameter of recanalized lumen, decreased scattering of the laser energy due to direct contact with the target tissue, and decreased vessel perforation because of the rounded configuration and precision of the contact probe (Lammer, Pilger, and Kleinert, 1988).

The photoablative laser angioplasty technique is the third method of removing atherosclerotic plaque with a laser. The excimer (excited dimer) laser uses different combinations of argon, xenon, and krypton with chloride or fluoride to generate laser energy at various wavelengths, most of which are in the ultraviolet range of 194 to 355 nm. The excimer laser provides high peaked power in pulsed nanoseconds that strips electrons from the nucleus. This action breaks bonds via shock waves or a photoablative effect. Selective destruction of plaque is achieved at lower temperatures, leaving a smooth vessel intima with no carbonization. A major concern about the use of the excimer laser is the possible mutagenic and carcinogenic effects of the ultraviolet wavelength's disruption of the DNA. Also, the gases used in this laser are highly toxic and pose a safety hazard that must be addressed. Research continues to determine whether the excimer laser's decreased thermal trauma to the vessel wall promotes decreased restenosis rates as compared with those resulting from thermal methods of laser angioplasty.

The holmium:YAG laser is being investigated for use during laser angioplasty because it, too, can produce a photoablative effect in breaking the bonds of the plaque. This laser does not involve a toxic gas and thus poses no additional safety hazards. Research with this wavelength continues.

Controversies exist today as to who will perform laser angioplasty procedures. Radiologists were the first physicians to become interested in this technique, followed by cardiologists. However, surgeons in the United States currently perform more laser angioplasties than do radiologists or cardiologists. This trend developed with the success of laser angioplasty, which has led to fewer bypass surgeries.

Another controversy concerns how and where the procedure should be performed. Radiologists and cardiologists tend to perform laser angioplasty percutaneously in the angiocatheterization laboratory or special radiology procedures room. Surgeons initially preferred to perform laser angioplasty using the open surgical approach, but the percutaneous approach is becoming more popular. Many surgeons prefer to perform laser angioplasty in the operating room environment, where problems or complications such as perforation can be immediately addressed. The setting for laser angioplasty usually depends on where the specialists perform most of their work. Radiologists and cardiologists feel more comfortable in the angio catheterization laboratory, whereas surgeons feel at ease in the operating room. Since angio catheterization laboratories and radiology suites are often the sites of numerous angiography and other special procedures, surgeons are having difficulty scheduling procedures in these areas. The hospital administration must be prepared to address these scheduling problems as the use of laser angioplasty increases.

Another dilemma is whether the surgeon should invite a radiologist to perform the balloon angioplasty part of the laser angioplasty procedure. If the radiologist is to assist with the procedure, then scheduling must be coordinated to ensure that the radiologist will be available. Some surgeons prefer to perform the entire procedure alone.

Laser programs will continue to be the focus of a battle over who should perform laser angioplasty and how and where the procedure should be performed. The hospital administration must solve these problems while trying to meet the needs of all the physicians who wish to use this less invasive surgical technique.

Various *imaging systems* can be used during laser angioplasty, including angioscopy, ultrasonic imaging, and fluoroscopy.

Angioscopy is performed using an ultrathin, flexible endoscope with multiple channels designed to conduct special instruments. Visual imagery fibers provide a direct view of the arterial lumen. During arterioscopy, a laser delivery system can be introduced to the plaque under direct visualization. A continuous flush of heparinized solution through the angioscope is required to displace the blood from the area being treated. Some limitations of the fiberoptic endoscope in laser angioplasty applications include the inability to enter small vessels or accommodate some of the larger laser delivery systems, and the need for a saline flush for visualization, which could lead to fluid overload.

Because delivering the laser energy through the endoscope is difficult due to size and guidance limitations, postlaser angioscopy is sometimes performed to evaluate the fluoroscopic laser angioplasty results. The arterioscope has been used to guide the delivery of an argon laser beam that glazes the inside wall of the artery to promote a smooth inner lining. As angioscopy is refined, the ability to directly visualize the effects of laser angioplasty during the procedure will help in the immediate determination of the actual vessel damage and procedure results.

Intravascular ultrasonic imaging is being perfected to provide an image of the inside lumen of the vessel for accurate diagnosis, precise plaque destruction, and reliable evaluation of the results. With this system, the physician evaluates a detailed, two-dimensional, cross-sectional view of the artery to accurately distinguish the plaque and the arterial wall. A tiny transducer at the end of a catheter is placed within the vessel to send and receive sound waves to distinguish the various tissue types. This system offers continual visualization of the laser destruction of the plaque.

The fluoroscopy unit is one of the more commonly used imaging systems today (Figure 11-2.) During laser angioplasty, the configuration of the operating room table must allow the portable, fluoroscopic C-arm to be positioned properly under the extremity with the occluded artery. When the procedure is performed in the operating room, difficulties are sometimes encountered in positioning the fluoroscopy unit appropriately because many surgical beds cannot accommodate this unit. When the procedure is performed in the radiology department or another area where the fluoroscopy equipment and the patient table are permanent, the visual images and manipulation capabilities of the fluoroscopy unit can be used much more advantageously.

Before the *laser angioplasty procedure,* an intravenous line is inserted for administration of medication and fluid to the patient during and after the procedure. Vital signs are continually monitored throughout the procedure. Frequent evaluation of the patient's hemodynamic status ensures early detection of most complications.

Anesthesia during laser angioplasty can be local, regional, or general depending upon the patient's condition and anticipated tolerance of the procedure. Because sudden movements can compromise the precise administration of the laser energy to the target tissue, sedation is often used. The patient may need to be strapped to the table to ensure immobility during the procedure. If the patient is to remain awake, preoperative education must prepare the patient for all aspects of the procedure, including the introduction of a large-bore catheter, the interaction of the laser energy, the fluoroscopic visualization, and any pain that may occur. Some patients have complained of a burning sensation in the leg during laser ablation of plaque in the femoral or popliteal areas.

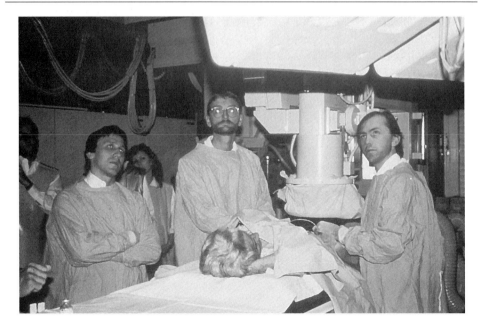

FIG. 11-2   Fluoroscopy is used to provide vascular imaging during a laser angioplasty procedure.

After the anesthetic is administered, the abdomen, groin, leg, and foot are prepped. The unaffected leg is prepped to the knee so that the physician can compare femoral pulses. Standard draping is performed to allow exposure of the area where the artery will be accessed. The back table setup includes instruments for a cutdown and the other equipment needed for the laser angioplasty.

A #7, #8, or #9 French sheath introducer set with a hemostasis valve and side ports is introduced into the femoral artery percutaneously. The cutdown method can be used to access the artery if needed. A heparinized, intravascular irrigant is administered through the arterial sheath via the side port for its antiembolism effects. A three-way stopcock on the side port of the sheath allows the introduction of the contrast medium and allows proximal pressure measurements to be made.

Baseline fluoroscopy of the involved segment is accomplished, landmarks are determined, and the fiber is introduced to the obstructed area. Depending upon the method of laser angioplasty used, the fiber may require calibration. This involves comparing the amount of energy that enters the fiber at the laser connection with the amount that exits the fiber. The laser is activated to recanalize the occluded artery. The position of the laser delivery system is checked periodically, and the recanalization is evaluated using small amounts of the contrast medium during fluoroscopy.

After successful recanalization, the artery lumen may be dilated even more by balloon angioplasty. If the diameter of the recanalized vessel is less than 50% of the diameter of the unaffected proximal vessel, then balloon angioplasty is performed to widen the channel (Grant Laser Center, 1987). The ultimate goal of laser angioplasty is to open the vessel without balloon angioplasty. Results will then reflect the true effects of the laser intervention as the sole method of opening occluded vessels. Until the laser delivery systems are improved to provide recanalization without balloon angioplasty, clinical data will not be as significant because they represent both technologies.

A final fluoroscopy is performed to note the results in terms of artery patency. The sheath and fiber are removed, and pressure is applied to the artery for at least 5 minutes if the angioplasty was performed percutaneously. If arteriotomy was performed, then the arterial access is closed.

As laser angioplasty technology progresses, the following advantages are being noted: The technique

- is minimally invasive,
- replaces major surgery,
- can be used on high-risk patients,
- can be performed with the patient under local or regional anesthesia,
- can shorten hospitalization,
- promotes cost efficiency, and
- is associated with potentially longer patency rates than other methods provide.

Some restrictions and limitations of laser angioplasty are being addressed as techniques are refined. Potential complications associated with laser angioplasty include vessel perforation, thrombus formation, vessel dissection, distal emboli production, and restenosis.

Studies indicate that the debris produced during laser angioplasty is very minimal and not large enough to cause distal occlusion (Case et al, 1985). The byproducts of laser angioplasty are primarily CO_2, H_2O, N_2, and short-chain organic molecules in various proportions. These byproducts are readily absorbed by the blood and probably produce no significant complications (Isner et al, 1983).

Postoperative Phase

The patient is evaluated in the postanesthesia room for hematoma, vessel perforation, and any other symptoms. The access point is assessed for signs of bleeding. An ice bag may be placed on the access site to decrease swelling. Color, temperature, and blanching of the affected leg are evaluated. The dorsal pedal and posterior tibial pulses are evaluated by palpation or by using a Doppler. A continuous heparin drip may be infused for 24 to 48 hours postoperatively to decrease the chance of embolism formation. Pain medication may be administered as needed. The patient is transported to the nursing unit when vital signs are stable and no other problems are noted.

An intravenous line may be maintained for 24 hours after the laser angioplasty to ensure adequate fluid intake. The patient is instructed to take 325 mg of aspirin orally every day for 3 to 6 months, unless contraindicated by other conditions, to decrease the chance of postoperative clot development. Walking at least three times a day is encouraged. The access site should be observed for signs of infection. The pulses and lower extremity perfusion are evaluated regularly until the patient is discharged. Just before discharge, arterial patency is evaluated with Doppler indexes and segmental pressures.

The patient is reevaluated at 1, 3, 6, and 12 months and then every year. Noninvasive Doppler studies are performed at each visit. Intense patient education to control smoking and cholesterol intake is conducted, and an exercise program is recommended. The patient usually undergoes repeat angiography in 6 months and 1 year or as symptoms warrant.

Laser angioplasty is still in its infancy. Intense research is leading to the use of different laser wavelengths and innovative methods to advance this special technology. Much work must still be done to develop the most effective laser wavelength, refine delivery systems, and compare the short- and long-term results of the various techniques. Technological development is accelerating as laser energy is being harnessed to ensure a bright future for peripheral angioplasty applications.

CORONARY ARTERY PROCEDURES

Laser Angioplasty

Coronary vascular laser therapy continues to excite health care professionals. Past outcomes of peripheral laser angioplasty spurred the development of procedures to perform coronary artery laser angioplasty. By introducing a small, very flexible laser fiber to the occlusion in the coronary artery, plaque can be selectively destroyed, thus eliminating the need for open-heart bypass surgery. The details discussed in the preceding section about peripheral artery laser angioplasty also apply to coronary artery laser angioplasty.

Indications that a patient needs coronary artery laser angioplasty include long lesions, aortoostial lesions, total occlusions, and saphenous vein grafts. Preliminary research has shown an overall success rate and a risk of major complications (including restenosis) comparable to those of balloon angioplasty (Litvack and Eigler, 1993).

Because perforation of a coronary artery could lead to devastating complications, laser angioplasty systems must be refined to provide high levels of precision. Researchers continue to develop systems that will distinguish the plaque, vessel wall, and blood. Chromophore-tagged monoclonal antibodies that selectively attach to plaque are being examined. This tagging technique enables the physician to distinguish the plaque and the vessel wall. When the plaque has been tagged, the therapeutic laser beam is absorbed only by the tagged areas. Thus the chance of damaging the surrounding arterial wall is virtually eliminated.

Research has shown that when intravenous tetracycline is administered, the excised diseased arteries are made to fluoresce. The outcome of ultraviolet laser ablation of these fluoresced areas has been compared to the outcome obtained with untreated atherosclerotic vessels (Murphy-Chutorian et al, 1985). Questions remain regarding the adequacy of this selective destruction of vascular plaque and the potential side effects associated with the procedure.

Coronary laser angioplasty is associated with many potential problems, including perforation, vascular spasm, cardiac arrhythmias, intimal dissection, and reocclusion.

Because coronary artery lumens can be very small and tortuous, the potential for laser perforation is more acute. Vascular spasms can occur from the heat produced during laser angioplasty, and cardiac arrhythmias may result from the introduction of the delivery device into the coronary system. Intimal dissection can occur if the vessel wall is damaged by the laser energy or from the follow-up balloon angioplasty to widen the lumen. Reocclusion may occur from thrombus formation or atherosclerotic plaque disruption.

Refinements in coronary artery laser angioplasty are needed to control plaque destruction, improve laser delivery and diagnostic systems, and prevent residual damage and reocclusion. Coronary artery laser angioplasty techniques will continue to generate much excitement because so many people have coronary artery disease.

Transmyocardial Revascularization

Dr. Mahmood Mirhoseini and his nurse, Mary Cayton, at St. Luke's Medical Center in Milwaukee, Wisconsin, are pioneering the use of transmyocardial revascularization (TMR), another procedure developed to treat clogged coronary arteries. This procedure is also being researched at other facilities, and the results are promising.

When the artery is occluded and perfusion of the heart muscle is inadequate, revascularization of the ischemic myocardium can be achieved by using the laser to drill small holes in the left ventricle. This allows blood to flow to the ischemic heart muscle from within the heart. As in a reptile's heart, channels in the myocardium cut by the laser allow blood from the ventricle to nourish the heart wall and possibly even restore damaged tissue.

Dr. Mirhoseini estimates that more than 300,000 people in the United States could be candidates for TMR. These are people with heart disease who cannot tolerate conventional treatments such as bypass surgery, balloon angioplasty, thrombolytic therapy, or medical management to control angina (*Clinical Laser Monthly,* October 1993). Typically, patients at high risk for surgery have problems with diabetes, diffuse disease or disease in areas not feasible for bypass surgery, early deterioration of previous bypass grafts, or a history of stroke.

TMR involves a CO_2 laser, set at 1000 W, that delivers a pulse in one twentieth of a second. This laser system was designed specifically for TMR. The surgery is usually performed through a small left thoracotomy incision but can also be performed during an open heart procedure (Figure 11-3). The laser fires computer-controlled shots between heartbeats into the left ventricle when it is full of blood. The blood in the chamber absorbs the energy, preventing it from continuing through the heart and possibly damaging other tissue. Approximately 10 to 25 channels about 1 mm wide are created. Epicardial bleeding from the laser impact is minimal and stops within a few minutes. The oxygen-rich blood from inside the heart then flows into the newly created channels, which become like new blood vessels, to perfuse the ischemic heart muscle. With an adequate blood supply, the progression of myocardial ischemia or angina can be slowed.

Evaluation of the channel lengths indicate that they remain patent for long periods. A thallium test showed perfusion still occurring through these channels in patients after 3 years (*Clinical Laser Monthly,* October 1993).

The normal hospital stay for patients undergoing TMR is less than 1 week vs. at least 16 days for open bypass surgery (*Clinical Laser Monthly,* October 1993). Therefore the

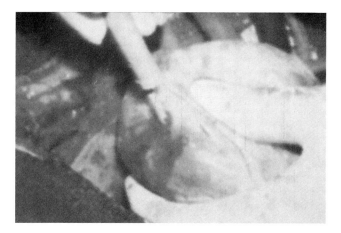

FIG. 11-3   The CO_2 laser energy creates channels in the heart muscle during transmyocardial revascularization.

financial savings associated with TMR is impressive. After discharge the patient is evaluated at 3, 6, 9, and 12 months and then annually.

Other researchers are investigating the use of a special contact Nd:YAG fiber or tip to perform TMR. More research is needed to determine the most appropriate delivery device and laser wavelength for this procedure.

Laser Thrombolysis

The holmium:YAG laser is being investigated for use during coronary artery laser angioplasty in revascularization during acute myocardial infarction (AMI) or heart attack. Recent studies show that only one third of AMI patients can take thrombolytic drugs that will dissolve clots (*Clinical Laser Monthly,* March 1993). Therefore, these patients might be treated with holmium laser angioplasty.

The excimer laser also has been researched for use in this application, but this laser needs more time to warm up (sometimes 20 to 40 minutes), which may not be practical for an emergency patient. When the holmium laser is used to provide thrombolysis, the thrombus and part of the arteriosclerotic plaque are destroyed. In comparison, balloon angioplasty merely displaces or moves the clot or plaque to one side. Even though balloon angioplasty has a success rate of approximately 93%, the residual blood clot restenoses in a significant number of patients (*Clinical Laser Monthly,* February 1992). Therefore, vaporization of the clot may produce more significant outcomes.

Opponents of the holmium laser procedure note that caution should be used in evaluating research techniques and results. They say that using the holmium laser to cut through an intravascular thrombus is like using a knife to cut through gelatin. Each time a cut is made, the gelatin collapses into the space created (*Clinical Laser Monthly,* February 1992).

VASCULAR WELDING AND INTRAVASCULAR SEALING
Laser Welding

Laser welding of vessels is attracting attention as an alternative to conventional suturing. The mechanism of laser welding is not fully understood. One theory is that welding occurs from the fusion of the collagen fibers (Figure 11-4).

Experiments were conducted to weld medium-size vessels (4 to 8 mm in diameter) using three different laser wavelengths. The CO_2 laser welds produced inadequate seals that could not withstand arterial pressure. The Nd:YAG laser welds were successful initially but failed after 20 to 40 minutes. The argon laser uniformly sealed the vessels only if they were accurately approximated. These successful arterial anastomoses tolerated 150 to 200 mm Hg of arterial pressure. Healing occurred almost completely within 4 to 7 weeks, with no evidence of pseudoaneurysms. The argon-welded vessels also produced less foreign-body response than did the sutured vessels (White et al, 1986).

Further research and refined techniques today show more promising results with different wavelengths. Arteriovenous fistulas are being successfully welded with argon laser energy. The strength of the anastomosis is remarkable because the laser energy causes the tissues to bond together to withstand the pressure of the blood flow.

Laser welding is being investigated for a variety of reasons:

- To eliminate the need to introduce foreign bodies (sutures) into the vessel,
- To decrease cross-clamping time,
- To decrease vessel trauma from excessive manipulation,

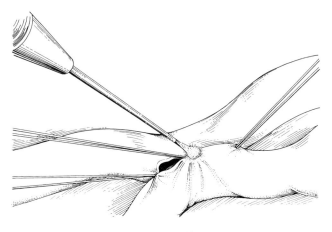

FIG. 11-4   Laser welding of vessels.

- To allow unrestricted vessel growth without the hindrance of suture material,
- To decrease any intimal damage of the vessel that may lead to platelet aggregation and thrombus formation, which can result from suturing, and
- To provide patency rates superior to those of conventionally sutured arteries.

With these goals in mind, laser wavelengths and delivery devices are being perfected to achieve these objectives. Also special glues are being developed for use as bonding pastes between the two ends of the structure being welded. Researchers are trying to determine whether certain glues provide stronger anastomotic bonds than others.

Intravascular Sealing

Laser intravascular sealing is another potential laser application for vascular procedures. A unique laser balloon angioplasty system has been investigated for improving the results of balloon angioplasty by also providing thermal sealing of the arterial dissections. Nd:YAG laser energy has been successfully used to seal separated intima-media layers of the arterial wall. This procedure helps maintain a patent and smooth lumen (Jenkins et al, 1988). Other researchers are trying to prove the benefits of laser glazing for the arterial lining after the lumen has been opened. This action has been theorized to promote a smooth arterial intima to decrease the chance of reocclusion from plaque buildup on a roughened, postsurgical vessel lining.

FUTURE CARDIOVASCULAR LASER APPLICATIONS

As laser vascular applications continue to advance, physicians and nurses must constantly be aware of changes and adapt to them. Laser use in cardiac and other vascular procedures offers an intellectual challenge and continues to be investigated and refined. Applications under study include the following:

- Myocardial laser vaporization for hypertrophic cardiomyopathy,
- Laser atrial septotomy for intractable left ventricular failure or congenital heart disease,

- Laser endarterectomy to mechanically remove atherosclerotic obstructions and diseased lumen,
- Laser valvuloplasty to destroy calcific valve deposits without the need for valve replacement, and
- Arrhythmia control through the destruction of conductive myocardial tissue with laser intervention.

Physicians and nurses should grasp the opportunity to participate in laser cardiovascular research and clinical applications because this area will expand rapidly over the next decade.

REFERENCES

Abela GS, Normann S, Cohen D et al: Effects of carbon dioxide, Nd:YAG, and argon laser radiation on coronary atheromatous plaques, *Am J Cardiol* 5:1998, 1982.

Ball K: *Lasers: the perioperative challenge,* St. Louis, 1990, Mosby.

Case RM, Choy DS, Dwyer EM et al: Absence of distal emboli during in vivo laser recanalization, *Lasers Surg Med* 5:281, 1985.

Choy DS, Stertzer S, Rotterdam HZ et al: Transluminal laser catheter angioplasty, *Am J Cardiol* 50:1206, 1982.

Ginsburg R, Wexler L, Mitchell RS et al: Percutaneous transluminal laser angioplasty for treatment of peripheral vascular disease, *Radiology* 156:619-624, 1985.

Grant Laser Center: *Laser angioplasty protocol with SLT Nd:YAG laser,* Columbus, OH, 1987, Grant Laser Center.

Holmium laser used to stop heart attack in progress, *Clinical Laser Monthly,* pp 17-19, Feb 1992.

Isner JM, Clark RH, Fortun RV et al: Preliminary analysis of photo-products emitted by laser therapy of atherosclerotic plaque (abstract), *Clin Res* 31:665A, 1983.

Jenkins RD, Sinclair IN, Anand RK et al: Laser balloon angioplasty: Effect of exposure duration on shear strength of welded layers of postmortem human aorta, *Lasers Surg Med* 8:392-396, 1988.

Lammer J, Pilger E, and Kleinert R: Laser angioplasty by sapphire contact probe. Experimental and clinical results, *J Intervent Radiol* p 3, 1988.

Laser coronary thrombolysis—A new treatment modality for revascularization in acute myocardial infarction (review), *Clinical Laser Monthly,* p 47, March 1993.

Laser technique shows promise as alternative to bypass surgery, *Clinical Laser Monthly,* pp 157-158, Oct 1993.

Leon MB, Lu DY, and Prevosti LG: Human arterial surface fluorescence: Atherosclerotic plaque identification and effects of laser atheroma ablation, *J Am Coll Cardiol* 12(1):94-102, July 1988.

Litvack F and Eigler N: Excimer angioplasty: Multicenter trials showing excellent results, *Clinical Laser Monthly,* pp 171-172, Nov 1993.

McGuff PE and Bushnell D: Studies of the surgical application of the laser, *Surg Forum* 14:143, 1963.

Medi-tech Education Center: Laser-assisted balloon angioplasty, *Fundamentals for nurses* (education booklet), Watertown, MA, 1989, Medi-tech/Boston Scientific Corp.

Use caution with laser angioplasty for heart attacks, *Clinical Laser Monthly,* p 21, Feb 1992.

Murphy-Chutorian D, Kosek J, Mok W et al: Selective absorption of ultraviolet laser energy by human atherosclerotic plaque treated with tetracycline, *Am J Cardiol* 55:1293-1297, 1985.

White RA, Abergel RP, Lyons R et al: Biological effects of laser welding on vascular healing, *Lasers Surg Med,* 6:137-141, 1986.

12

PODIATRY, ORTHOPEDIC, AND NEUROSURGERY LASER APPLICATIONS

The laser has rapidly gained acceptance in podiatry, orthopedics, and neurosurgery. The initial recognition of its value in these specialties was slower because the laser had not been an effective tool when used on bone. Because the water content of bone is low, laser energy (especially CO_2) could cause bone tissue to ignite and create necrosis. The fact that lasers were not effective for bone overshadowed their soft-tissue benefits.

The use of laser energy became more common when its hemostatic value for treating soft tissue was realized. Soft tissue could be excised or incised with minimal blood loss. Other benefits of the laser were soon discovered: it could seal nerve endings, thus reducing postoperative pain, and seal lymphatics, thus minimizing postoperative edema.

Other wavelengths were discovered that could be appropriately used on bony tissue. The holmium laser, for example, can be used in a fluid environment on cartilage and bone without charring this hard tissue. Delivery systems and surgical techniques were refined, and this laser has become an acceptable tool for many podiatric, orthopedic, and neuro-surgical applications.

PODIATRIC LASER APPLICATIONS

The CO_2 laser is the most commonly used laser in podiatry today. Many podiatrists have been so pleased with the benefits and the ease of using this sophisticated tool that they have purchased a CO_2 laser unit for their offices. Contact Nd:YAG, KTP, and holmium:YAG wavelengths are also used for podiatric procedures.

Podiatrists have used various methods for tissue excision, such as electrosurgery or curettage. In electrosurgery, the electrosurgical unit sparks tissue and achieves great depth of penetration as the layers are heated. This burning reaction destroys tissue in bulk; therefore, individual layers cannot be excised precisely. The curettage method removes tissue in chunks, which could result in destruction of healthy tissue. Unlike other modalities, the laser offers precision in performing tissue-destruction procedures. The laser destroys tissue layer by layer as nerve endings are sealed and smaller blood vessels are coagulated. The laser vaporizes diseased cells, which minimizes recurrence. The laser also heats the adjacent tissue to high temperatures, thus producing a sterilizing effect. Once the podiatrist or physician becomes skilled in using laser technology, the laser becomes the standard instrument for use in a variety of procedures.

Excision of Verrucae Plantaris

Approximately 7% to 10% of the general population has verrucae plantaris, or plantar warts (Borovoy, Klein, and Fuller, 1985). These warts, caused by the human papovavirus, are characterized by large vacuolated cells in the upper stratum and granular layer of the epidermis. The warts usually do not extend into the dermis; therefore, care must be taken to avoid penetrating the dermis during surgical removal.

Conventional treatment of verrucae includes topical chemicals, cryosurgery, electro-surgery, surgical curettage, and steel-knife excision. The results of these different treatments have been inconsistent because the warts tend to recur, cause pain, and form scars. The laser has been found to be a very effective alternative to these treatments.

The original use of the CO_2 laser in podiatry was for excision of verrucae. These lesions, which are usually on the bottom of the foot, are sometimes very resistant to conventional treatment because of their location in a weight-bearing area. Over the years, many variations of the excisional method have been developed, each with advantages and disadvantages. No single treatment regimen has produced consistent results. Usually podiatrists chose treatments that provided satisfactory results for the patient and used surgical techniques that they were most familiar with. For optimal outcome, a procedure should involve excising the lesion with minimal scarring, allow early return to ambulation, and result in a low chance of recurrence. Laser surgery became an acceptable modality that met these criteria in the treatment of plantar verrucae.

Laser excision of verrucae is performed on an outpatient basis or in the podiatrist's office. Usually 1% lidocaine with epinephrine is locally infiltrated; a field block is administered for more extensive disease (Figure 12-1). Epinephrine is used to help decrease intraoperative bleeding. The verrucae must not be injected directly, so as to minimize the iatrogenic spread of the virus. The foot is prepped and draped in the usual manner; the surgical area must be surrounded by wet towels to prevent laser ignition of dry combustibles.

The CO_2 laser is set at 8 to 20 W, depending upon the size and depth of the lesion. The wart is circumscribed at its periphery with continuous intermittent pulses of energy (Figure 12-2). The charred area ensures that any dormant virus, which may be located in the area around the lesion, is destroyed by the adjacent thermal effect of the laser energy. A dermal curette may be used at this time to remove the center core of the lesion for biopsy (Figure 12-3).

The remaining wart is then vaporized in the defocused mode using overlapping strokes in the horizontal, vertical, and oblique directions. Small bleeding vessels can be coagulated with direct, defocused laser energy. A wet sponge or curette is used to remove the charred tissue, and the depth of penetration is assessed. The lesion is sequentially ablated until the dermoepidermal junction is identified. The dermis is recognized by its characteristic tough consistency and pink, blood-oozing base. If the laser energy is delivered into the dermal layer, fat globules appear, and the chance of scarring is increased. Therefore, care must be taken not to penetrate too deeply into the dermal layer with the laser energy.

All the verrucae should be treated in one session. This decreases the chance of reinoculation of healthy tissue by lesions not yet treated.

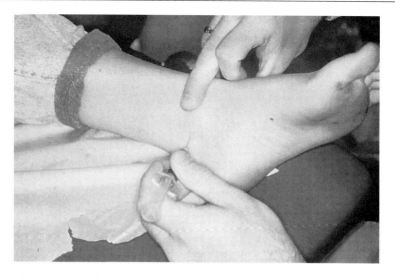

FIG. 12-1   A foot block is administered before laser excision of multiple plantar warts.

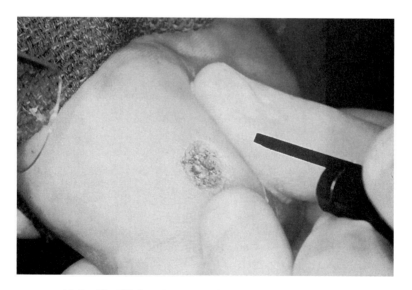

FIG. 12-2   The CO_2 laser beam vaporizes the plantar wart layer by layer.

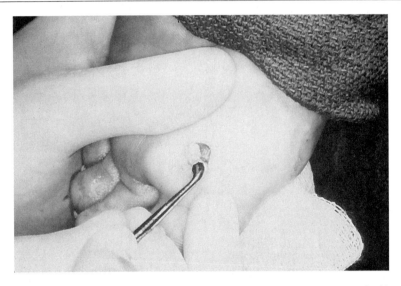

FIG. 12-3   A dermal curette is used to remove the center core of the plantar wart for biopsy.

After the surgery, an antibiotic ointment or topical antiseptic is applied (Figure 12-4). The surgical site is covered with a sterile bulky dressing. A special orthopedic shoe or slipper may be used if a regular shoe cannot be worn. The podiatrist may instruct the patient not to change the dressing until the area is evaluated 3 days after the procedure.

The patient is instructed to take acetaminophen for discomfort and to elevate the foot to reduce pain and swelling. An ice pack can be applied during the first few days to also help decrease swelling. The patient is usually instructed to apply the ice pack for 20-minutes, at 20-minute intervals.

The patient is also instructed to wash the foot in peroxide daily, apply the prescribed medication to the surgical site, keep the area covered with a sterile dressing, and not walk barefoot.

The patient is usually evaluated again in the physician's office 1 week after the procedure for observation of the healing process. Granulation tissue is expected to have filled in the surgical void. Healing usually is complete within 3 to 4 weeks.

Laser vaporization offers many advantages over conventional procedures to remove verrucae plantaris. The recurrence rate is decreased, scarring is minimized, and adjacent tissue necrosis, postoperative hemorrhage, and infection are greatly reduced. The laser stimulates the formation of granulation tissue to foster healing. Because of the theorized nerve-sealing effect by the laser energy, patients have less postoperative pain than with conventional methods and are able to walk on the affected foot with minimal discomfort.

Callus, Cyst, Corn, and Fissure Treatments

A *callus* is a thickening of the epidermal layer caused by chronic friction. In contrast with corns, calluses usually do not have a central core. This disorder frequently occurs on the sole of the foot, particularly under the metatarsal head, where pressure is constant. Some people may have a familial predisposition for development of calluses.

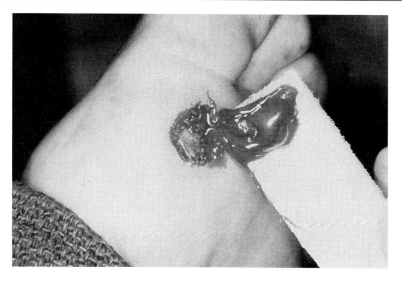

FIG. 12-4   A topical antibiotic ointment is applied after the plantar wart is vaporized with CO_2 laser energy.

The conservative treatment for calluses is to debride the area and fashion an orthotic insert to place in the shoe and redistribute the weight. Surgery involving bone reformation may be performed for an extensive problem.

Some podiatrists use laser energy to remove calluses. This treatment method is still controversial because sometimes the expense of using the laser cannot be justified. Before the laser procedure, the patient is injected with a local anesthetic below the callus. The CO_2 laser is set at 5 to 15 W of continuous or superpulse power to ablate the callus to the level of the subcutaneous dermis. The podiatrist sweeps the laser beam over the hypertrophied area and mechanically removes the char to note the depth of penetration. The laser energy continues to ablate the lesion until normal dermal tissue is identified. An antibiotic ointment is then applied, and a sterile bulky dressing is placed.

Postoperative instructions for the patient are similar to those for verrucae excision. Retreatment may be necessary if the callus reforms.

Porokeratosis is a hyperkeratotic lesion on the sole of the foot and is sometimes referred to as a plugged duct cyst. Some physicians believe that a porokeratotic lesion is initially caused by a verruca that disappears, leaving a depressed area. This disorder usually occurs at the pressure areas of the foot. The sweat glands deep within the dermis become dilated.

A local anesthetic is administered before the porokeratosis is removed. The CO_2 laser is used at approximately 10 W of continuous power to ablate the porokeratosis to the dermoepidermal junction. The physician then precisely vaporizes the lesion base by aiming the beam directly into the depression and applying the laser energy until a flash of white light appears, which indicates that the normal dermis has been entered. This technique ensures that the involved sweat duct and gland are also ablated. Postoperative care is the same as for verruca excision.

A *corn* is a thickening of the skin that is usually associated with pain caused by prominent underlying bone. Different types of corns include hard, soft, seed, and neurovascular corns; all can be ablated with CO_2 laser energy. The neurovascular corn, with a hemorrhagic vascular central core, responds very well to the CO_2 laser wavelength or to color-selective wavelengths. This type of corn appears on the sole of the foot or the bottom of the toe and resembles a human nail. It is characterized by longitudinal striations and is usually yellowish and hard.

A local anesthetic is administered before corn removal. The CO_2 laser energy is set at 6 to 10 W of continuous power, and the lesion is ablated easily. The epidermis is vaporized, and the charred tissue is removed with a wet sponge until the dermis is observed. The laser energy produces a sterilizing effect on the tissue, so there is less chance of postoperative infection. The nerve endings are sealed, so the patient does not have much discomfort after the procedure. Postoperative patient instructions are the same as for verrucae excision.

A *heel fissure* is caused by excessive callus formation on the heel (Figure 12-5). It is common in obese women and is most frequently found on the medial surface of the heel extending to the midarch. The condition is sometimes caused by dry skin, other systemic problems, or wearing open-backed shoes for extended periods. When the skin is rehydrated and any infection is eliminated, the healing process slowly begins. The CO_2 laser is used to reduce excessive callus and expose the epithelial surface to speed healing. The laser lightly vaporizes the fissure at 5 to 8 W. Usually no anesthetic is needed. The patient is instructed to keep the area clean and apply a thin layer of hydrating antibiotic ointment daily. For successful long-term results, the cause of the fissure or the contributing factor must be determined and then removed or altered. Retreatment may be necessary at a later date if recurrent callus formation prohibits complete healing.

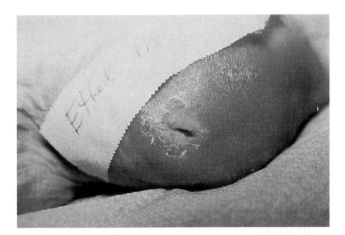

FIG. 12-5   A heel fissure is caused by excessive callus formation and can be treated with CO_2 laser energy. (Courtesy Dr. Jack Buchan, Jr.)

Nail Procedures

Deformities such as incurved, ingrown nails often cause discomfort and infection. The nail may be treated with conventional surgical or chemical methods. A portion of the nail or the entire nail may be removed (partial or total matrixectomy, respectively). This surgical excision may destroy the nail matrix (where the nail root produces the nail plate), preventing regrowth of the toenail. Postoperative pain and edema are associated with this procedure. Chemical methods require a longer treatment period that is marred by inconvenience, discomfort, possible infection, and prolonged drainage.

For the laser matrixectomy, the patient is given a digital nerve block. The affected area is prepped and draped in the traditional manner. A penrose drain is tightened around the base of the toe to provide a tourniquet effect to help control bleeding. A dry field is imperative for easy identification of the matrix. The nail is mechanically removed, and the matrix is exposed. The physician may use an operating microscope or optical loupes to enhance the image. The laser is set at 6 to 10 W of continuous power, and the matrix is precisely ablated. Nail-bed capillary bleeding is coagulated with a defocused beam. The matrix is lightly charred to ablate only the matrix tissue where nail growth is not desired. A wet cotton-tipped applicator is used to remove the char (Figure 12-6). Postoperative care requires changing the bandage daily and applying antibiotic ointment. Healing is complete within 2 to 3 weeks.

Fungus nail, or onychomycosis, is identified by characteristically thick, hypertrophic, deformed nails, usually with a yellowish discoloration (Figure 12-7). A fungus culture confirms the presence of infection. More than 60% of people over age 50 have this condition (Borovoy, Klein, and Fuller, 1992). Fungus nail may be painful and can lead to extensive infection and ulceration. The condition has been difficult to eradicate using standard methods, which involve mechanical debridement and topical antifungal medications.

The CO_2 laser is used effectively to treat this condition by vaporizing the fungal spores that cause the disease. The physician sets the laser at 6 to 9 W of power and sweeps the laser beam in a defocused mode over the infected toenail. This superficial brushing has a

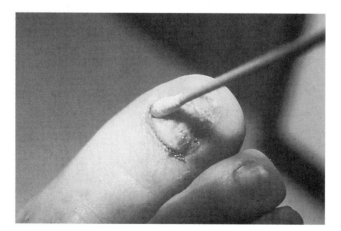

FIG. 12-6   A cotton-tipped applicator is used to remove the char during laser matrixectomy. (Courtesy Dr. Jack Buchan, Jr.)

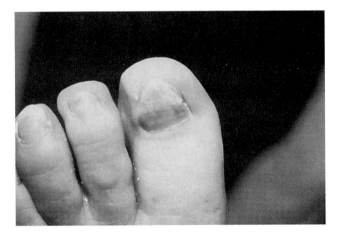

FIG. 12-7　Onychomycosis, or fungus nail, is a common condition in older people and can be treated with a CO_2 laser.

sterilizing effect on the area and shaves off the nail overgrowth. The matrix is preserved while the fungal infection is treated. An oral and a topical antifungal medication are prescribed until the nail returns to normal.

A waffling technique has also been introduced, in which the laser is used to cut small, interrupted holes (about 1 mm apart) in the toenail. Anesthesia is not necessary. The CO_2 laser is set at 8 to 10 W with pulse durations of 0.05 to 0.1 second and a 1-mm spot. The laser holes are cut through the fungus of the nail but do not penetrate the nail bed. Methyl alcohol can be used to remove the carbon eschar, making the fenestrations observable. An antifungal cream is applied directly to the nail and is easily absorbed by the nail plate through the holes, thus retarding fungal growth (Borovoy, Klein, and Fuller, 1992).

Postoperative patient instructions include cleansing the nail thoroughly with a brush and hydrogen peroxide before applying an antifungal cream twice daily. The patient is also instructed to debulk the nail weekly using disposable emery boards. The patient must understand that an emery board must not be reused because reinfection can result. The patient is seen monthly until healing is complete, usually in 12 to 18 months. The nail can be relased during this time if needed.

Laser treatment has become very common for treating fungus nail because of its successful results. Advantages of this method include shorter treatment time, less postoperative pain, preservation of the matrix, and subsequent healthy nail regrowth.

Subungual hematoma is being successfully treated with laser energy. The traumatized toe bleeds underneath the toenail, leading to pain and edema of the toe. This swelling can be relieved by firing the laser beam at right angles to the nail plate to form several holes, thus releasing the pressure under the nail (Figure 12-8). With the beam set at 10 W, no anesthesia is needed, and the physician can burn 5 to 6 holes in the affected nail plate. Spontaneous evacuation of the hematoma occurs, and the pain caused by the accumulated blood is relieved. The area is covered with ointment and bandaged for 2 to 3 days. When this procedure is performed within 24 hours of the accident, the nail usually does not fall off. Left untreated, the nail usually self-avulses.

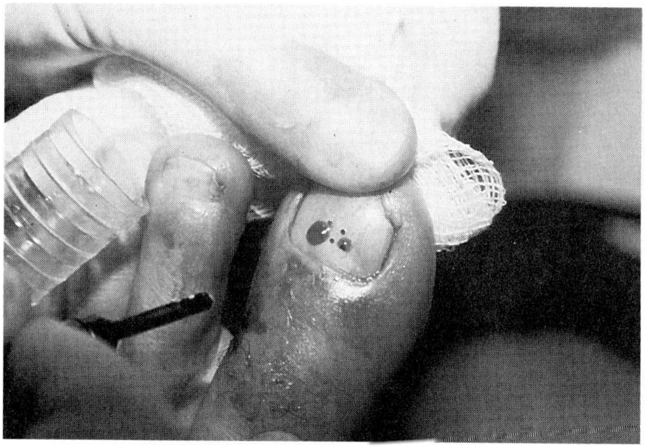

FIG. 12-8 Subungual hematoma can be treated by using the CO_2 laser to drill holes in the traumatized toenail to release the pressure under the nail. (Courtesy Dr. Jack Buchan, Jr.)

Neuroma, Cyst, and Other Soft-Tissue Excisions

Morton's neuroma, or interdigital neuroma, is a hyperplastic proliferation of the protective sheath of the common digital plantar nerve and is caused by a tumorous nodule or trauma formed by hyperplasia of the nerve cells. The most common nerve involved is the third digital nerve between the third and fourth toes. The condition is characterized by acute cramping or burning pain in the ball of the foot, with radiating pain into the third and fourth toes. Other symptoms include numbness and tingling of the toes. Sometimes removal of the shoe is needed to massage the foot for pain relief. Conservative methods using orthotics and special shoe padding are aimed at decreasing trauma to the nerve, but have limited success. Cortisone injections are also used to help decrease nerve inflammation. Surgical excision is sometimes necessary to remove the neuroma, but this method has been associated with stump neuroma symptoms.

The CO_2 or contact Nd:YAG laser can be used as an alternative treatment technique to excise the neuroma. A local anesthetic is administered, and an ankle tourniquet may be applied to decrease intraoperative bleeding. Because the laser provides great hemostasis, many podiatrists do not use a tourniquet or epinephrine, thus avoiding associated potential complications.

A dorsal incision between the third and fourth metatarsal heads is made with a steel knife or with the laser. The incision is deepened through the superficial fascia, and blunt dissection is used to access the interdigital space, cut the intermetatarsal ligament, and expose the neuroma. The neuroma is characterized by its white, glistening appearance. The podiatrist grasps the nerve, pulls it distally, and, using continuous power, vaporizes the neuroma base. The proximal portion of the neuroma recedes into the foot, and the distal portion of the neuroma is dissected and sent to the pathology department for examination (Figure 12-9). The incision is closed in the traditional manner, and a compression dressing is applied.

The patient walks in a special protective postoperative shoe and is reevaluated in 5 to 7 days for a dressing change and assessment of the surgical site. The sutures are removed in 1 week.

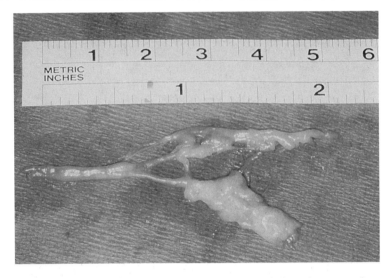

FIG. 12-9   A neuroma is excised from the foot and sent to the pathology department for examination. (Courtesy Dr. Jack Buchan, Jr.)

The advantages of the CO_2 laser for this procedure are less edema, less fibrosis or adhesion formation, and a reduced rate of recurrence of the condition. The laser energy seals the smaller blood vessels, making the surgical site more hemostatic so that delicate structures, such as nerves, can be seen and identified.

Ganglionic cysts can also be excised with laser energy. A ganglionic cyst is a synovial sac that contains synovial fluid and is lined with epithelium. These cysts can be found near any joint and are usually caused by mechanical pressure or trauma. The cyst can cause pain because of its size and location and tends to recur frequently.

The CO_2 laser can be used to excise the ganglionic cyst or vaporize the synovial villi to decrease recurrence. Physicians tend to prefer excision because a specimen can be sent to the pathology department for examination. When synovial villi vaporization is performed, the cyst is exposed and incised to drain the synovial fluid. The laser is then used to completely ablate the internal area of the sac. The incision is closed, and a compression dressing is applied. Postoperative care for this procedure is similar to that for neuroma excision.

Keloids and hypertrophic scars can be excised effectively with laser energy. A keloid is a hypertrophic scar that forms after surgery or trauma. This response is an abnormal intensification of the scar formation required for healing. This growth can easily be debrided with CO_2 laser energy. Recurrence is usually reduced when the laser is used, compared with recurrence rates when traditional excision with a steel knife is used.

The appropriateness of using the laser to treat *heel spurs* has prompted controversy because of the cost of using a laser system. The pain caused by this condition arises from chronic irritation or bursitis in the plantar fascia area. The CO_2, KTP, and Nd:YAG laser have been used to treat heel spurs. Advantages of using the laser include earlier pain-free walking, decreased pain (measured in terms of postoperative narcotics taken), reduced incidence of wound dehiscence, and decreased disability time (Kelly, 1993).

Laser debridement of ulcers has been very successful. Anesthesia is usually not necessary. Necrotic tissue within an ulcer is debrided with 10 W of continuous CO_2 laser power until bleeding is precipitated, marking the presence of healthy tissue (Figure 12-10). The laser energy has a sterilizing effect, thus removing infective tissue. This procedure is more successful in the absence of gross or bone infection.

The goals of laser debridement are to produce a sterilizing effect on the tissue to resolve the superficial infection and to cleanse the ulcer of necrotic tissue. Postoperative care involves close observation of the wound for 2 to 3 days. If no infection is present, a cast may be applied to enhance the healing process. The ulcer will heal within a few weeks if proper postoperative instructions are carefully followed (Figure 12-11).

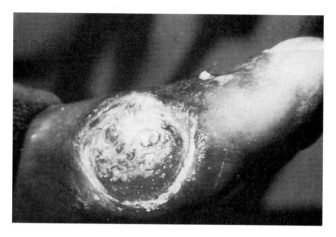

FIG. 12-10   A decubitus ulcer is treated with CO_2 laser energy, exposing normal healthy tissue. (Courtesy Dr. Jack Buchan, Jr.)

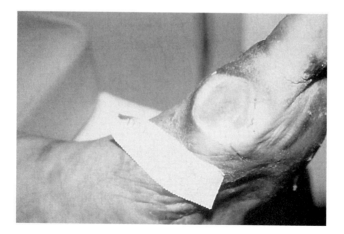

FIG. 12-11   An ulceration heals within a few weeks after laser debridement if postoperative instructions are followed closely. (Courtesy Dr. Jack Buchan, Jr.)

Studies are being conducted to explore the use of CO_2 laser energy for decubitus ulcers that involve bone exposure. The laser is used to excise and vaporize the necrotic tissue. A small (pinpoint) hole is drilled into the bone to tap into the haversian canal that provides the bone with an internal circulation system (Figure 12-12). By providing an artificial communication with the haversian canal, healing can take place more rapidly because this collateral circulation enhances perfusion to the area. Conclusive results have not been noted yet as to the effectiveness of this technique.

Cancerous tumors can be excised using different laser wavelengths. For example, a wide excision of a malignant melanoma on the side of the foot can be effectively performed with a CO_2 laser. The hemostasis achieved increases visibility and identification of delicate structures of the foot. The sealing effect of the laser energy decreases the chance of malignant cells spreading to other areas of the body (Figure 12-13).

ORTHOPEDIC LASER APPLICATIONS

Many orthopedic specialists are satisfied with their sophisticated drills, saws, rongeurs, and other hand tools; thus laser technology must offer significant improvements over these tools to be justified. To be accepted by orthopedists, laser energy must impact the bony structures without causing charring, and delivery devices must access hard-to-reach areas. The holmium laser recently has gained recognition as a versatile tool that meets these needs during orthopedic procedures.

Researchers are discovering other laser wavelengths and developing techniques and accessory instruments that are becoming attractive to orthopedic surgeons. Many clinical applications have already shown great promise and are being adopted. The laser has definitely become a more popular tool for the orthopedist during the past few years.

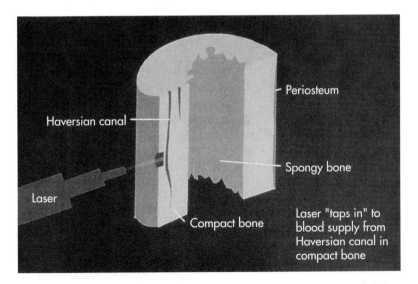

FIG. 12-12   The CO_2 laser beam drills a hole to tap into the haversian canal to assist with the healing process. (Courtesy Dr. Leonard Schultz.)

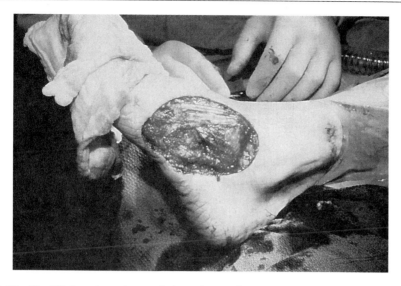

FIG. 12-13   The CO_2 laser is used to precisely excise a malignancy while providing a hemostatic surgical field.

Arthroscopic Procedures

Arthroscopy has become the standard method for diagnosing and treating joint conditions. Techniques have been simplified over the years, and instruments have been improved enough to use for surgery within the joint, making arthrotomy unnecessary.

The CO_2 laser was the first laser to gain acceptance for arthroscopy of the knee. During this procedure, the arthroscope is introduced into the knee joint in the traditional manner after a tourniquet is applied above the knee. The purposes of the tourniquet are to minimize bleeding during the procedure and decrease the chance of air-embolism formation. The disease is diagnosed, and the irrigation solution is removed. Because the CO_2 laser wavelength cannot be transmitted through fluids, a gas environment is necessary. The knee joint is insufflated with a gas, usually helium or CO_2. The laser is attached to the special arthroscopic waveguide with a coupling device (Figure 12-14), and low powers of CO_2 laser energy are directed to the diseased area. The smoke is evacuated immediately to provide adequate visualization.

The surgery is completed by totally lavaging the area. The key to the success of this arthroscopic procedure is to completely irrigate the surgical site to remove all of the charred tissue. If charred tissue remains in the joint, postoperative effusion in response to the necrotic tissue will occur. By irrigating the knee joint, the normal healing process can be initiated, and the chance of complications can be minimized.

Evaluations of the use of the CO_2 laser for chondroplasty and partial synovectomy have been favorable, but more research is needed to demonstrate this laser's full value. The CO_2 laser is also being used investigationally to vaporize cartilaginous and collagenous lesions of the shoulder joint. Because a tourniquet cannot be applied before the procedure, the chance of air-embolism formation is increased.

Contact Nd:YAG technology is also being used for arthroscopic procedures. Contact Nd:YAG energy can be delivered to tissue in a fluid environment. Therefore, a gas envi-

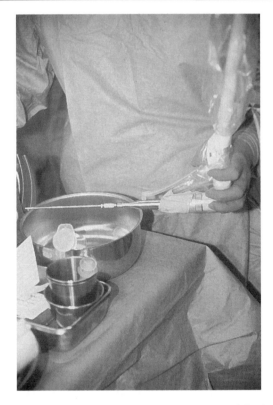

FIG. 12-14   The articulated arm of the CO_2 laser is attached to a special arthroscopic waveguide.

ronment is not necessary, and routine arthroscopy can be performed without removing the irrigant solution from the joint. The arthroscope laser delivery system consists of a quartz fiber surrounded by a ceramic jacket that delivers the Nd:YAG energy while being in contact with the joint structures (Figure 12-15). The depth of penetration of the beam is precisely controlled. Decreased adjacent tissue damage, accurate tissue ablation, and reduced postoperative complications are the advantages of contact Nd:YAG laser applications in arthroscopy.

The most commonly used laser for arthroscopic procedures today is the holmium:YAG laser. This laser's energy is delivered through the arthroscope or a second puncture site via a flexible fiber. This wavelength produces an air bubble that conducts the laser energy directly to the tissue, so the irrigating solution in the joint does not have to be removed before the laser is activated (Figure 12-16). The depth of penetration achieved with the holmium wavelength is shallow, which allows for precision by minimizing damage to normal tissue.

The holmium laser is gaining popularity for use in other joint procedures as well. Its wavelength is used to successfully treat a variety of conditions in the shoulder and ankle joints, for example (Figure 12-17). New and refined techniques are being introduced that continue to promote this laser's versatility.

Other wavelengths are being developed. For example, the erbium:YAG laser, with a wavelength of 2940 nm, holds promise for use in orthopedic procedures. This wavelength

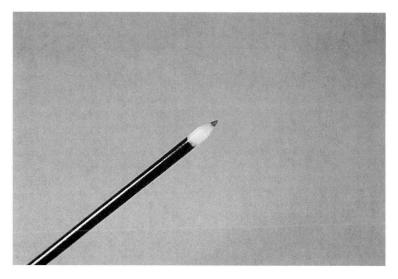

FIG. 12-15   The contact Nd:YAG delivery device consists of a quartz fiber surrounded by a ceramic jacket. (Courtesy Surgical Laser Technologies, Inc., Oaks, PA.)

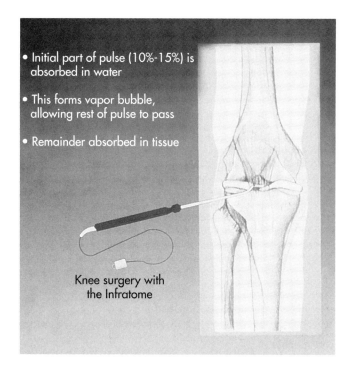

FIG. 12-16   The holmium laser beam is delivered to the tissue in an air bubble. (Courtesy Coherent, Inc., Palo Alto, CA.)

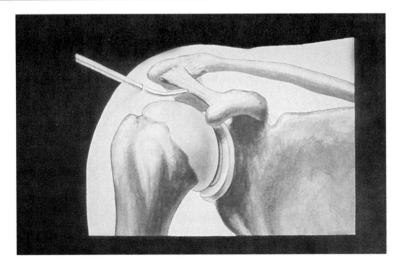

FIG. 12-17   The holmium laser is used successfully in the shoulder joint to treat a variety of conditions. (Courtesy Coherent, Inc., Palo Alto, CA.)

is highly absorbed by water and causes no heat damage to adjacent tissues. This characteristic is important when the erbium:YAG laser is used to cut or ablate bone or soft tissue. Modifications and refinements are being made that will enhance the delivery of this laser energy to tissue during orthopedic procedures.

Laser Discectomy

Traditional discectomy surgery involves prolonged recovery, high costs, and postoperative discomfort. Laser discectomy successfully combines the laser, which provides ultimate precision, with sophisticated imaging, such as computed tomography, magnetic resonance imaging, or endoscopy. Recovery is much quicker because the surgery is performed through a small incision or a percutaneous stick to ablate the center portion of the herniated disc, allowing it to slip away from the nerve to relieve pain.

The purpose of laser discectomy is to relieve leg pain, not back pain. Some surgeons state that low back pain may also be relieved as a result of treating the leg pain (*Clinical Laser Monthly,* April 1993).

Patient selection criteria include unilateral leg pain greater than back pain, positive straight-leg-raising test or crossover pain, weakness, reflex alteration, sensory changes, and a positive radiological examination showing a herniation at a location consistent with the clinical findings. Patients should not be considered for this procedure if there is evidence of severe degenerative disease, free fragments within the spinal canal, severe lateral recess stenosis, hypertrophy of the ligamentum flavum, or any other condition that would place the patient at high risk. A radiological examination is performed to aid in the proper diagnosis of the patient's condition.

Some manufacturers provide kits to simplify the surgical setup for laser discectomy. The kit includes the flexible trocar, cannulae, dilator, annular trephine, stylet, ruler, and marker (Figure 12-18).

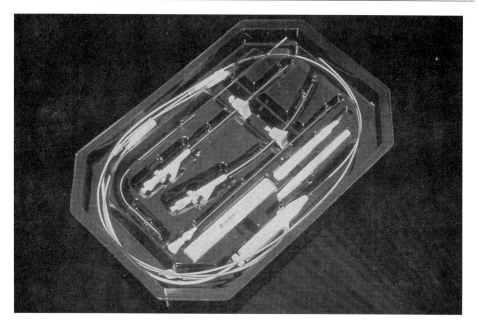

FIG. 12-18   Laser discectomy kits are available that contain the instruments needed to facilitate surgical set-up. (Courtesy Coherent, Inc., Palo Alto, CA.)

The KTP and holmium lasers have been used successfully for this procedure. Laser discectomy is performed with the patient under local anesthesia. Then the patient can let the surgeon know of any pain in a particular area so that nerve-root injury can be prevented. The percutaneous approach into the intervertebral space avoids direct injury to nerve roots, prevents further weakening of the annulus, reduces postoperative scarring, and does not complicate any future surgery.

Laser disc decompression can be achieved by several different methods. Using an advanced imaging system, the surgeon inserts the fiber into the herniated disc. After placing the fiber, the surgeon uses the laser to vaporize the nucleus of the disc; then the products of vaporization are sucked out. The heat produced at the end of the laser probe may result in thermal irritation of the nerve endings in the nerve root or annulus. Patients often complain of pain during the procedure; therefore, the procedure must be interrupted at intervals to allow the disc space and laser tip to cool.

One of the risks associated with this procedure is thermally induced neuropathy. This condition is minimized with use of the holmium laser, which penetrates only ½ mm the tissue, thus decreasing the hazard of damage to nerve roots.

Because of advancements in delivery devices, the laser probe can now be constantly cooled, allowing the procedure to progress without interruption and with minimal or no patient discomfort (Figure 12-19).

Spinal endoscopes are now available that provide direct visualization and guidance during laser discectomy. A flexible endoscope, approximately 1.7 mm in diameter, is introduced into the intervertebral disc space through a 2.8-mm cannula (Figure 12-20). The endoscope can be steered through the tissue, allowing the surgeon to identify landmarks and inspect the annulus and nucleus pulposus. Direct visualization allows for more con-

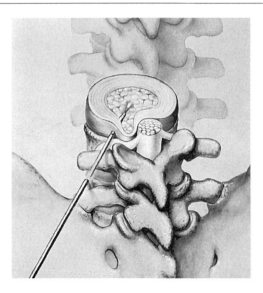

FIG. 12-19   The tip of the fiber is constantly cooled to decrease adjacent thermal injury during laser discectomy. (Courtesy Coherent, Inc., Palo Alto, CA.)

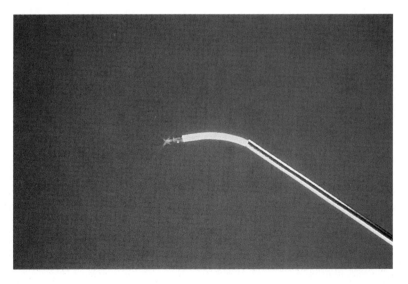

FIG. 12-20   A flexible, steerable spinal endoscope allows direct visualization during laser discectomy. (Courtesy Coherent, Inc., Palo Alto, CA.)

trol as the surgeon precisely ablates the nucleus, knowing exactly how much volume has been removed.

The endoscope and fiber are positioned posterior and lateral to the herniation, thus the decompression is direct and more effective (Figure 12-21). Because the holmium laser energy penetrates the tissue only $\frac{1}{2}$ mm, adjacent cells are not heated and nerve roots are preserved. Also, constant irrigation and suction help restrict any thermal conduction. The pulsed laser beam ablates the nucleus without mechanical trauma.

The skin incision usually does not require sutures. A sterile bandage is placed over the surgical site. Because laser discectomy is a minimally invasive procedure, the patient is discharged on the day of surgery, thus tremendously decreasing the cost of the procedure. A conservative postoperative physical therapy program with restricted activity is prescribed for a short period. Trunk stabilization and strengthening exercises should be performed. Continuing research and significant long-term results are encouraging orthopedic surgeons to learn the techniques of this procedure.

Laser Use for Soft Tissues

The laser has coincidentally proven to be very effective when used to cut soft tissue during orthopedic surgery. The laser energy seals blood vessels to provide hemostasis, seals lymphatics to decrease postoperative drainage, seals nerve endings to reduce postoperative pain, and sterilizes the tissue with high temperatures generated at the surgical site.

CO_2, contact Nd:YAG, KTP, holmium, and other laser wavelengths can be used to cut soft tissue during a total joint replacement, laminectomy, or other procedures that involve incision into the soft tissue to access the disease site. The laser, instead of the electrosurgery unit, is used as a dissecting tool. The laser precisely cuts and vaporizes adipose tissue, fascia, and muscle during the procedure. Bleeding vessels are treated with laser coagulation.

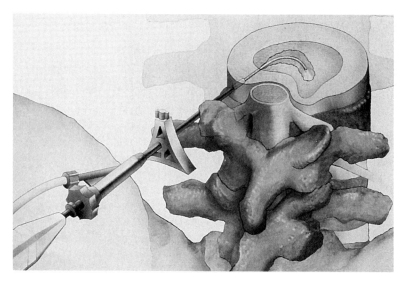

FIG. 12-21 The flexible endoscope bends the fiber around to directly impact the herniated disc from the posterior and lateral position. (Courtesy Coherent, Inc., Palo Alto, CA.)

When the laser is used to dissect soft tissue for lumbar laminectomies or total knee replacements, its advantages include earlier ambulation and return to full range of motion, less postoperative pain, less intraoperative blood loss, shorter hospitalization, and faster return to normal activities.

Vaporization of Polymethylmethacrylate

Joint replacement is performed to remove painful arthritic components and implant metal or plastic prostheses. Sometimes a bone cement called polymethylmethacrylate is used to stabilize the prosthesis. When it loosens, a revision arthroplasty may be needed to replace the old prosthesis.

The original prosthesis that is cemented in place must be extracted by the use of mechanical devices that may further traumatize or fracture the weakened bone. The CO_2 laser and other wavelengths impact the hardened cement to change its consistency for easy extraction.

Approximately 15 W of superpulsed CO_2 laser energy can be delivered directly to the bone cement. The old components are loosened and can be extracted easily. After the prosthesis is removed, the cement residue in the inner channels of the bone is treated with laser energy. The heat from the laser beam makes the cement more pliable, and the residue can be cleaned from inside the bone shaft.

Great care must be taken not to impact the cement with too much laser energy because the cement could ignite. The CO_2 laser must not be used on the bone because the bone will char and weaken. The plume and odor must be eliminated with a strong smoke evacuator. The gaseous byproducts of this plume consist of formaldehyde, hydrocarbons, carbon monoxide, and hydrocyanic acid. The CO_2 laser technique requires practice in the laboratory setting before expertise can be developed for clinical applications.

The advantage of this procedure is less chance of bone fracture during the extraction of the bone cement and old prostheses. Further research will refine this technique to decrease its risk of complications.

Laser Biostimulation

Laser biostimulation, or cold laser treatment, is attracting much attention around the world. This nonsurgical technique is used to decrease pain in joints or pain from past surgeries. A helium-neon laser light at approximately 630 nm is directed at a painful area or joint for a series of treatments. Some delivery devices contain a heat sensor in the tip. As the delivery device is moved over the painful area, the sensor detects increased heat, which indicates pain in that specific area. The laser is then activated for less than 30 seconds at that spot. The delivery device is moved to other areas where heat is sensed, and the laser is activated again. This process continues until multiple spots have been treated (Figure 12-22).

The physiological action of the laser on the tissue is not thoroughly understood, but theories have postulated that normal floating endorphins that decrease pain naturally are attracted to the area, and the pain is subsequently relieved. Other theories suggest that the quick relief of pain after the treatment results from pain gate blocking. When pain is decreased, the patient is more willing to perform postoperative exercises, which may release adhesions that could be causing the pain.

More research is being conducted in this area as biostimulation becomes less controversial. Subjective benefits must always be coupled with a proven physiological rationale

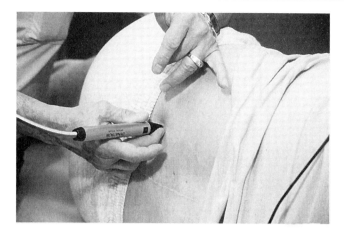

FIG. 12-22   Laser biostimulation decreases lower back pain resulting from adhesion formation after open laminectomy.

to support a scientific hypothesis. Methods are being devised to provide accountable and replicable physiological responses to this laser energy to prove its efficacy.

Reflex sympathetic dystrophy (RSD), also known as sympathetic maintained pain, is characterized by chronic pain in the arms and legs as a result of a minor injury, such as soft-tissue trauma or a fracture. Approximately 6 million Americans suffer from RSD. This condition affects the part of the nervous system that controls heart-rate, blood pressure, and other vital functions. Traditional treatment involves injecting a pain medication into the neck nerve plexus once or twice a week for 12 weeks. Side effects of this treatment can include nausea, vomiting, and severe headaches (*Clinical Laser Monthly,* May 1993).

Laser treatment for RSD involves delivering the helium-neon beam, at 632.8 nm, to the nerve plexus in the neck at 10 to 15 mW over a 1-cm exposure area. This area is aimed to decrease arm pain. The laser energy is delivered to the lower back for patients with leg pain. Total exposure time per treatment ranges from 30 to 240 seconds, depending upon the patient's response. Treatment is administered one to two times per week for a total of 15 treatments. The patient senses faint tingling or a vibration during the procedure. The key to this RSD therapy is early treatment and aggressive physical therapy to prevent deterioration, useless limbs, and chronic pain (*Clinical Laser Monthly,* May 1993).

Other investigations of this wavelength show that it encourages RNA synthesis and growth. Because scar tissue prevents regrowth of nerve cells, this property is extremely important in decreasing pain (*Clinical Laser Monthly,* May 1993).

A new laser has become available in the United States to treat repetitive stress injury (RSI). This laser, with a wavelength of 830 nm, is a hand-held, low-energy infrared laser whose beam penetrates up to 5 cm into the tissue. It has been known to affect nerve function, decrease inflammation, and increase blood flow. Thus it reduces pain and swelling in tendons and tissues.

This laser was first used successfully in Asia and Europe to treat inflammation and RSI. It has been particularly useful for treating carpal tunnel syndrome, which is a common form of RSI. This laser is not approved by the FDA in the United States, but its results are very promising.

During one study of the treatment of carpal tunnel syndrome, volunteers from 10 major automobile manufacturing sites participated. Employees with carpel tunnel syndrome were treated in a double-blind study. Half received physical therapy and laser treatment; the other half received physical therapy and a nonfunctioning laser treatment. During the actual laser treatments, the delivery device was held over the inflamed area for approximately 33 seconds for a duty cycle totaling 99 seconds per treatment. Patients were treated three times a week for 5 weeks. Further comparisons noted that the laser group generally felt better faster and returned to work more quickly than those treated with the conventional carpal tunnel surgical procedure (*Clinical Laser Monthly,* September 1993).

NEUROSURGICAL LASER APPLICATIONS

The CO_2 laser was the first wavelength used to treat tumors of the brain. Other wavelengths were then introduced to the neurosurgical arena, such as the noncontact and contact Nd:YAG, frequency doubled YAG, holmium, and argon lasers. Refinements in technique and instruments continue to increase the benefits of using the laser for neurosurgical applications.

Laser Procedures of the Brain

Many different wavelengths are effective for excising brain lesions because they can be used to precisely ablate and excise tumors with minimal tissue damage to adjacent healthy structures. Traditional surgical procedures require much tissue manipulation during tumor excision, causing a rush of fluid into the area to help with the healing process. This normal response leads to fluid accumulation within the brain after surgery, causing cerebral edema. The patient may remain comatose if the pressure of the swelling persists during the healing process.

When the laser is used to excise a brain tumor, less tissue manipulation is involved, and therefore less trauma occurs. The small blood vessels are coagulated and tissues are sealed, helping to decrease postoperative edema. The reduction in cerebral edema also allows patients to become alert more quickly.

Brain tumors are classified into three distinct categories. Lateral sphenoid tumors are frequently globular with involvement of the dura, bone, and orbit. Middle third tumors are usually globular and may extend to the internal carotid artery. These tumors may be attached to the large sphenoid bone at the base of the skull. Medial tumors can wrap around the internal carotid or middle cerebral arteries. These lesions may extend into the optic foramen or the cavernous sinus.

Diagnostic testing is performed before laser surgery to determine the position and extent of the tumor and the extent of adjacent tissue destroyed by the tumor. The patient is prepared for the craniotomy in the traditional manner. The surgeon makes the skin incision with a steel knife and uses the laser to detach the muscles from the skull. The bone is removed with high-speed drills and perforators. The surgeon coagulates bleeding vessels of the dura mater and uses scissors to enter the dura mater.

Brain retractors that will be positioned close to the laser-tissue impact site should be dulled or ebonized to prevent direct reflection. Also, wet sponges may be used to cover shiny instruments to decrease reflection of the laser beam.

The tissue is manipulated as little as possible, and the tumor is identified. The laser may be coupled with a microscope at this point to enhance the image of the tissue for accuracy. When the vessels of the tumor are coagulated, the tumor may begin to shrink. The tumor is carefully and precisely debulked and excised by laser power at appropriate wattages, depending upon the size and consistency of the tumor. Vessels are recognized and coagulated or ligated as the tumor is removed. After removal, the tumor base is vaporized to destroy as many of the abnormal cells as possible.

The laser has proven to be an extremely useful tool for excising these various lesions. The advantages of using the laser are controlled hemostasis, an improved view of the operative field because of decreased bleeding, less trauma to adjacent healthy tissues (decreasing the chance of postoperative seizure disorders), and more thorough removal of the tumor.

Acoustical neuroma removal is safer and easier when the laser is used compared with other surgical tools. This lesion is a basal skull tumor that can enlarge to become an intracranial tumor. The cochlear and facial nerves are initially affected by this growth. The blood supply to the brain stem may then become involved as the tumor spreads. Traditionally, the tumor has been approached from the posterior fossa. However, a high incidence of neurological deficit and disfigurement from the resection is associated with this approach.

The CO_2 laser is being used in a translabyrinthine approach. This procedure allows direct entry to the tumor through penetration of the base of the skull, where the tumor originates. The tumor is identified and precisely removed with the laser energy without extensive manipulation or damage to healthy structures.

The contact Nd:YAG laser is becoming more commonly used for brain tumor excisions. The advantages of this application include greater precision because tactile sensation is restored for the physician, shallow depth of penetration, minimal plume production, no carbonization of the edges, hemostasis, distinct control of the dissecting plane, minimal thermal damage, accessibility of deeper tumor tissue, and sterilization effects.

The argon and frequency doubled YAG lasers have been found extremely useful in removing smaller vascular lesions of the brain. Because of their color selectivity, only the pigmentation in the tumor absorbs the energy, leaving the adjacent tissue unharmed. Hemostasis is sometimes improved when these wavelengths are used. These laser beams can also be conducted through cerebrospinal fluid if necessary. Laser welding of vessels is being researched for use in the treatment of microvascular anastomoses during intracranial bypass surgery.

Laser Procedures of the Spinal Cord

The laser is valued for its precision in removing tumors from the spinal cord area. Complete anesthesia is critical to ensure that the patient does not inadvertently move during the delicate excision of the tumor from the spinal cord. Because the laser beam is so precise, the surgeon can now shave a tumor away from the vital cardiovascular and cardiorespiratory centers of the brain stem. The surgeon and anesthesiologist must work closely as a team to ensure that the patient remains totally still during this phase of the procedure. The surgical site is frequently irrigated to decrease thermal buildup that may conduct heat to adjacent normal tissue.

Research is being conducted to develop new techniques, wavelengths, and delivery systems to treat delicate spinal cord problems. Contact Nd:YAG technology provides the tactile sensation for the surgeon, fostering precision for the removal of tumors of the spinal cord. Spinal endoscopes are now available to assist with this delicate surgery by providing direct visualization.

Stereotactic Endoscopic Laser Surgery of the Brain

Guided imaging in stereotactic surgery, coupled with the sophistication of the laser and the endoscope, is revolutionizing neurosurgery. Stereotactic techniques enable the surgeon to precisely determine the location of a specific lesion or structure in the brain.

Stereotactic laser endoscopy has many advantages over conventional craniotomy. It provides for the determination of the exact location of the lesion. The vessels and major motor areas of the brain are avoided as the tumor is accessed. The procedure requires shorter hospitalization and may be performed using a local anesthetic or intravenous sedation. The surgical wound is merely a bur hole made to access the operative area; the postoperative course is usually only 2 days. Operating time is reduced significantly, and complications such as bleeding and infection are minimized.

In the radiology department, the stereotactic device is positioned on the patient's head. The fixation pins are stabilized on locally anesthetized areas on the head. Computed tomography (CT) is performed, and the patient is then taken to the operating room with the hardware in place.

The physician enters the information from the CT scan into a computer to calculate the exact location of the lesion. After the coordinates are determined, the patient is carefully transferred to the surgery table. A local anesthetic is administered so the patient can respond to questions throughout the procedure. The surgical area is infiltrated with an anesthetic. A small incision is made, and the periosteum is elevated. A craniotome is used to make the bur hole, and the dura mater is entered. An aiming bow is attached to the stereotactic frame, and the flexible or rigid endoscope is positioned within the holder. The aiming bow acts as the guiding system for the endoscope. Biopsy specimens or cultures are taken as needed as the endoscope is introduced into the brain.

The patient is reminded that the moistened eye pads protect the eyes during laser surgery. Everyone in the surgery room dons protective eyewear in preparation for the procedure. The laser fiber is introduced through the endoscope port. The tumor is vaporized with contact or noncontact Nd:YAG laser energy or another wavelength. Any tissue impacted by the laser is irrigated and evacuated; the tumor is mechanically removed. At the end of the procedure, the stereotactic apparatus is removed, and the incisions are closed in the traditional manner. The patient's vital signs and neurological status are evaluated in the postanesthesia care unit for about 1 hour after the procedure.

The advantages of using the stereotactic laser endoscopy procedure for tumor removal include intraoperative coagulation of blood vessels, direct visualization through a small incision, access to deeper brain tumors without alteration of the structures or damage to adjacent tissues, easy vaporization and aspiration during the procedure, minimal postoperative swelling and cerebral edema, shorter hospitalization, and cost savings. As neurosurgeons become more experienced in performing this procedure, other procedures that can be performed through an endoscope are being introduced. The potential for performing major cranial procedures through the endoscope is within reach in today's health care environment.

REFERENCES

Borovoy M, Klein JT, and Fuller TA: Carbon dioxide laser methodology for ablation of plantar verrucae, *J Foot Surg* 24(6):431, 1985.

Borovoy M and Tracy M: Noninvasive CO_2 laser fenestration improves treatment of onychomyocosis, *Clinical Laser Monthly*, pp 123-124, Aug 1992.

Kelly PF: KTP laser application enhances recovery from heel spur surgery, *Clinical Laser Monthly*, pp 55-56, April 1993.

Low-energy laser shines light on stress injury treatment, *Clinical Laser Monthly*, pp 143-144, Sept 1993.

Non-thermal laser could spell relief for chronic pain, *Clinical Laser Monthly*, pp 76-77, May 1993.

Orthopedic surgeons discover new method for treating leg pain, *Clinical Laser Monthly*, pp 59-60, April 1993.

SUGGESTED READINGS

Bieglio C and de Bisschop G: Physical treatment for radicular pain with low power laser stimulation, *Laser Med Surg News Adv* 6(4):122, August 1988.

Frykberg RG, editor: *Clinics in podiatric medicine and surgery*, Vol. 4, No. 4, Philadelphia, Oct 1987, Saunders.

Jain KK: CO_2 laser provides safe, complete excision of difficult brain tumors, *Clinical Laser Monthly* 3(1):1S, Jan 1987.

Koch F and Poisson C: Targeting cerebral tumors, combining image-guided stereotactic endoscopy with laser therapy, *AORN J* 49(3):741, March 1989.

Owens PA and Emmons WF: Lumbar laminectomy patients recover faster with laser procedure, *Clinical Laser Monthly* 6(7):3S, July 1988.

Sherk HH: Arthroplastic revision in joints less traumatic than regular surgery, *Clinical Laser Monthly* 6(1):1S, Jan 1988.

Winckelbach JK: Use of the Nd:YAG laser in the excision of Morton's neuroma, *Clinical Laser Monthly*, pp 103-104, July 1993.

Wright G: Laser matrixectomy in the toes, foot and ankle, *Clinical Laser Monthly* 9(5):246, April 1989.

13

LASER TECHNOLOGY
AND ANIMALS

New technology, including laser technology, often involves animals during the evolution and advancement phases. Animal research assists in product development and justifies proposed outcomes of procedures before human studies are permitted. Appropriate animal use has fostered the introduction of new applications, delivery devices, and wavelengths throughout the years. Then, after a laser technique has been established and accepted for human use, it can be used in veterinary medicine to benefit animals.

This chapter discusses laser research and applications at these two opposite ends of the progression and use of laser technology. The first section discusses the evolution of animal research and the development of animal research protocols for a laser program. Administrators are often given the responsibility to expand a laser program to include animal use in laser courses and research. Careful planning and observance of specific government regulations ensure successful completion of this task.

The second section describes some examples of laser applications in animal surgery. Opportunities are evolving for health care providers experienced and skilled in laser applications as this technology gains popularity in veterinary medicine. For example, a competent clinical laser nurse experienced with laparoscopy may be a valuable assistant during a laser laparoscopic procedure on a race horse. This section illustrates some unique and beneficial laser applications performed on animals.

ANIMAL USE IN LASER RESEARCH
History of Animal Use in Research

The use of animals in research has been debated since early times, and valuable information has resulted. In 1628 William Harvey wrote *On the Motion of the Heart and Blood* and began more extensive research on the newly discovered circulatory system. The cardiovascular systems of animals were studied, and scientists were able to introduce new theories about the human anatomy. These significant findings partially justified the use of animals in research. Immunology pioneers began to use animals to study the effects of vaccines and the routes of infective diseases. Medical science has advanced tremendously over the years because animals were used for investigations.

During early times human dissection was unacceptable, so human anatomy could not be adequately studied. Cadavers were dissected but were difficult to obtain. In 1832 a law was passed in England to legalize the sale of cadavers for dissection and to stop the practice of body snatching from cemeteries. With the quest for more knowledge about anatomy, scientists began to dissect animals because obtaining human cadavers continued to be controversial, and bodies were not readily available. Animal research was then justified because cadaver dissection was unpopular and considered unethical.

In 1831 Marshall Hall proposed five principles to govern animal research (Zurlo, Rudacille, and Goldberg, 1994):

1. An experiment should never be performed if the results can be obtained through observation.
2. No research should be performed without a clearly defined and obtainable objective.
3. Scientists should thoroughly study the works of predecessors and peers to avoid needless repetition of an experiment.
4. Experiments that are justified should be performed causing the least possible suffering for the animals.
5. Every study should be performed using methods that provide the clearest possible results and decrease the need for repetition.

In 1959, the publication of *The Principles of Humane Experimental Technique*, by W.M.S. Russell and Rex Burch, marked the beginnings of an organized movement to alleviate inappropriate use of animals in medical research. The three R's—replacement, reduction, and refinement—became the approach to animal use in investigational studies. Powerful antivivisectionist lobbies began to oppose any and all use of animals in research and became involved with a significant animal protection movement.

Today, many concerned people do not object to the humane use of animals for the prevention and treatment of disease, but many of them question using animals for product development and routine safety testing. Animals continue to be used for safety testing of cosmetics, shampoos, soaps, and medicines. A dilemma exists as to what criteria should be employed in determining whether an animal should be used for medical or scientific research.

The first law designed to govern the use of animals for research, the Cruelty to Animals Act, was enacted in Great Britain in 1876. In the United States, the Animal Welfare Act was passed in 1966 and has been revised many times since. This law sets standards for the transportation and husbandry of laboratory animals, excluding rats, mice, and birds.

In 1985, an amendment to the Animal Welfare Act established the need for facilities to form institutional animal care and use committees (IACUCs) to review all protocols for studies or research involving warm-blooded animals. Each approved facility performing research with animals must form an IACUC consisting of at least five members. One member must be a doctor of veterinary medicine, who will oversee the activities involving animals at the institution. Other members must include at least one practicing scientist, one person whose primary concerns are not medical or scientific (attorney, minister, etc.), and one person who is not connected to the facility except for membership on this committee. The IACUC members must annually evaluate procedures using animals and inspect facilities. They must review the policies and procedures of the facility, including the choice of animals for a particular activity, numbers of animals to be used, and degree of pain and discomfort the animals may experience. They must also determine whether the scientist has considered the use of replacement, refinement, and reduction alternatives to whole animals in conducting the research. The IACUC usually is highly respected within the facility. Because public demand for accountability is increasing, this peer-review system has become very popular and effective.

Animal Research Protocols

Many hospitals, especially those in academic settings, apply to the United States Department of Agriculture (USDA) for approval to become a site for animal research. The USDA sends the facility a packet of information about the application process.

A facility may conduct research with or without providing housing for the animals. If housing the animals is necessary, then USDA investigators must conduct a more extensive review. A facility must be prepared to house and care for animals if survival research is conducted. If a facility wants to use animals for research without providing housing, then less stringent rules are applied. This type of research is usually involved with animal euthanasia after experiments are completed. A doctor of veterinary medicine is always involved with these procedures.

Some laser courses use warm-blooded animals to assist in demonstrating a particular laser technique or illustrate laser impact with a certain wavelength. Cutting, coagulating, and vaporizing can easily be demonstrated on live tissue. Dogs, rabbits, and cats have been used in the past as animal models in laser courses for physicians, but these animals are usually categorized as pets. Lately, pigs and goats have become more acceptable animal models.

When a facility seeks approval for animal research without housing, many internal policies must be developed. The facility must form an animal care and use committee, delegate responsibility to the committee members, file documents and reports, acquire animals, and develop a public relations policy. Samples of these policies are provided on the next pages to assist laser program administrators when they develop an animal research program. Those involved must carefully review current regulations and guidelines when they develop these policies to ensure applicability and appropriateness.

LASER APPLICATIONS IN VETERINARY MEDICINE

Laser applications in veterinary medicine have become more common over the past few years as procedures that have proven to be beneficial in human medicine are modified for use in veterinary medicine. The CO_2 and Nd:YAG lasers appear to be the most preferred wavelengths used today. Opportunities for laser team members involved with human surgery have been extended, and they can now use their knowledge and skill to assist with laser procedures in animals. Laser technology to benefit animals is becoming more widely accepted as laser education and laser systems become more available to the veterinarian.

Veterinarians are attending laser courses designed for human medicine even though there are some differences between the practices. Animal medicine requires unique skills. First, veterinarians must be able to diagnose conditions, illnesses, and injuries from objective symptoms since animals cannot communicate subjectively. Veterinarians must also be able to treat a variety of animal species and thoroughly understand each animal's distinctive characteristics. Veterinarians must serve as the general practitioners of animal health and many times must also practice as the surgeon, internist, radiologist, and pathologist. Sometimes veterinarians must practice in less sophisticated settings than those used for humans, with limited instruments and diagnostic equipment.

Formal laser education provides information and hands-on experience to enhance the skill level of the veterinarian to foster safe and appropriate use of the laser. High-quality standards must be maintained, and laser safety must be enforced. Inappropriate use of laser energy must be discouraged because complications and negative results will hinder the progress of laser technology as used to benefit animals.

New technology, such as laser technology, is usually not readily available for use in veterinary medicine. Many hospitals have formed collaborative and mutual relationships with veterinarians practicing at zoos, marine parks, and animal sporting arenas such as race tracks, or in private practice. The laser then can be loaned to a veterinarian when an animal's condition warrants laser intervention. Animal hospitals providing equestrian services have purchased lasers because funds are more readily available for treatment of

---

Sample Policy
Animal Care and Use Committee
Membership

Purpose:

To provide consistency with the Department of Agriculture's animal welfare guidelines for membership on the Animal Care and Use Committee.

Policy:

1. The Committee shall consist of at least five persons: Chairman, attending veterinarian, investigator scientist/physicians, and an outside member who is not affiliated in any way with the hospital other than as a member of the Committee.
2. The outside member is to provide general representation of the community for the proper care and treatment of animals at the facility. The outside member cannot be a member of the family of anyone connected with the hospital and cannot be a former employee or member of the staff, or a supplier or vendor to the hospital.
3. All Committee members should possess sufficient ability to assess animal care, treatment, and practices.
4. If the Committee consists of more than five members, not more than three members shall be from the same administrative unit of the hospital.
5. The members of the Committee are to be appointed by the president of the hospital and/or the director of medical education.
6. The Medical Education Department will maintain an up-to-date list of Committee members, indicating the name, degree, position, qualifications, address(es), and telephone number(s) of each member. A copy of this list is to be sent to the attending veterinarian.

Sample Policy
Animal Care and Use Committee
Responsibilities

Purpose:

To provide consistency with the Department of Agriculture's animal welfare guidelines for responsibilities of the Animal Care and Use Committee.

Policy:

I. A quorum shall be required for all formal actions of the Committee, including inspections. A quorum is defined as a majority of the Committee members.

II. The Committee shall inspect all animal study areas at least semiannually, with no more than 6 months between inspections.

    A. A report will be filed with the Department of Agriculture and a copy maintained in the Medical Education Department.

    B. A report shall include but should not be limited to the following:

        1. Date of inspection

        2. Signature of the Committee members

        3. Reports of any violations or deficiencies of the regulations or standards

        4. Any deviations from the approved research protocols that adversely affect the animals

        5. Any other information or concerns of the Committee regarding the status or conditions of the animals or the facility

        6. Any corrections made by the facility

    C. If deficiencies are noted by the Committee, the Committee will notify the administrative representative of the facility in written form. If the deficiencies are not corrected within 30 days, the Committee shall notify the Department of Agriculture.

III. The Committee shall evaluate all protocols for proposed animal use in research and training.

    A. All protocols involving the animals will be kept on file in the Medical Education Department and will be available for inspection by the Department of Agriculture and the Animal Care and Use Committee.

    B. The Committee shall approve the protocols if they

        1. Ensure that animal pain, distress, and functional or sensory impairment are minimized.

        2. Ensure that all survival surgery is performed using aseptic technique.

        3. Ensure that adequate veterinary care is planned for and provided.

        4. Ensure that the type and number of animals are appropriate and necessary as an essential part of the protocol.

        5. Ensure that the appropriate use of anesthetics, analgesics, tranquilizers, or euthanasia is used in accordance with the Department of Agriculture protocol.

        6. Ensure that provisions for transportation to accredited facilities are made for animals involved with survival research.

IV. All other responsibilities are in accordance with the USDA's written protocol on file in the Medical Education Department.

Sample Policy
Animal Care and Use Committee
Documentation and Report Filing

Purpose:

To provide consistency with the Department of Agriculture's animal welfare guidelines for documentation and report filing from the investigational facility (name of hospital).

Policy: The Medical Education Department will keep on file the following reports:

1. A copy of reports of the USDA inspection of the facility.
2. The sales record that accompanies the animal from the vendor.
3. The acquisition/disposal form, which should include
   a. Acquisition date
   b. Animal type and number
   c. Place of acquisition
   d. Description of the animal (color, type)
   e. Sex of the animal
   f. Method and date of disposal
4. A copy of the annual report that the facility submits to the USDA.
5. A copy of the veterinarian's program of care, representing the initiation of the contract with the veterinarian and refiled every three years thereafter.

Sample Policy
Animal Care and Use Committee
Acquisition

Purpose:

To provide consistency with the Department of Agriculture's animal welfare guidelines for the acquisition of animals.

Policy:

1. Animals will be procured only from a reputable and USDA-approved dealer.
2. The animals will be transported to the veterinarian's facility one day before or on the morning of the day the animals are needed for the investigational or educational purposes.
3. The veterinarian will prepare and transport the animals to the research laboratory site at the hospital.
4. A copy of the sales receipt from the vendor will accompany the animals and will be kept in the Medical Education Department.
5. The animals will be removed by the veterinarian for proper housing or euthanized before removal. The animals will be properly disposed of by the veterinarian.

Sample Policy
Animal Care and Use Committee
Public Relations Policy

Purpose:

To provide consistency of format whenever action is required to explain or justify the use of animals for investigational or educational purposes at (name of hospital).

Policy:

1. Whenever a statement is required in answer to a demand for an explanation of the rationale for using animals for investigation or education at (name of hospital), the director of public relations or his or her designate will be immediately notified.
2. No statement will be made by any other member of (name of hospital) or staff physician.
3. The following statement will be read to the public or media regarding the use of animals at (name of hospital) for investigational or educational purposes:

    (Name of hospital)'s policy regarding the use of animals for medical research is consistent with that of other leading health care research centers in the country. (Name of hospital) follows strict guidelines for the care of animals as established and monitored by the U.S. Department of Agriculture and the Animal Welfare Act. (Name of hospital) meets all standards established by the National Institutes of Health governing experimentation, including quarters, space, cleanliness, comfort specifications, and the use of anesthetics for potentially painful experiments. We believe the use of animals for medical research is both necessary and appropriate.
4. No member of the public will be granted entrance to observe the use of animals unless accompanied by a police officer or other law enforcement officer of a legally constituted law enforcement agency with general law enforcement authority (not an agency whose duties are limited to enforcement of local animal regulations). If the purpose of the visit is to search for a particular animal, the law enforcement officer will furnish the facility with a written description of the missing animal and the name and address of its owner before making such a search. No entrance will be granted to antivivisectionists wishing to conduct a general inspection.

Sample Form
Animal Care and Use Committee
Inspection

Date ——————————————— Inspection area ———————————————

Please evaluate the following areas:

1. Animal pain, distress, and functional or sensory impairment are minimized.

Yes ————— No—————

2. Adequate veterinary care is planned for and provided.

Yes ————— No—————

3. The types and numbers of animals are appropriate and necessary for the research protocol or laser conference.

Yes ————— No—————

4. Anesthetics, analgesics, tranquilizers, and/or euthanasia are used in accordance with the Department of Agriculture protocol.

Yes ————— No—————

5. Violations or deficiencies noted:

6. Concerns regarding the status or condition of the animals or the facility:

Signature ———————————————————————————————

horses. Veterinarians have also procured laser systems that are outdated for human surgery or systems that have been reconditioned but are still safe and operational. These units cost considerably less than newer units.

Laser technology in veterinary medicine has evolved as specific advantages have been documented, such as hemostasis when the laser seals small blood vessels, the sterilizing effect of laser energy, sealing of lymphatics, shorter surgery time, less post-operative edema, decreased inflammation and pain, and rapid healing with less scar formation.

When a laser is to be used on an animal, appropriate assessment and planning must be completed before the procedure is performed because the animal's response cannot always be anticipated. Normal vital-sign ranges, anesthesia required, positioning and other intraoperative practices, instruments, the animal's response to the surgery, and postoperative recovery course must be appraised. Careful follow-up after the procedure is mandatory since some animals may need assistance during this period.

Different laser wavelengths have been used for surgery on large and small animals. Some of the uses for veterinary laser surgery are listed below (Crane, 1986).

- Management of malignant or benign cutaneous lesions by vaporization of abnormal tissue.
- Endoscopic laser vaporization or fulguration of malignant or benign tumors in body cavities or tubular structures, including the nasal cavity, sinuses, lower portions of the respiratory tract, gastrointestinal tract, and abdominal structures.
- Control of hemorrhage from excisions or incisions into parenchymal organs or other tissue.
- Excision or ablation of infected cutaneous wounds, ulcers, sinuses, and fistulae.
- Precision microdissection of laryngeal tissue, brain tissue, and other delicate structures when postoperative edema is undesirable.

Animals manifest a very high rate of benign and malignant lesions, thus the use of photodynamic therapy (PDT) is increasing. This less invasive technique to selectively destroy abnormally growing cells is a valuable alternative to more invasive excisional surgery. Primary and collaborative studies of veterinary and human treatments in PDT research are opening new avenues of treatment for dysplastic lesions.

Laser Surgery on an Elephant

Laser technology is being used successfully for excisional procedures on animals, resulting in less surgery time and better control of intraoperative bleeding. The CO_2 laser was used at the San Francisco zoo to vaporize a papilloma virus lesion about the size of a small orange from the foot of a 7-foot-tall elephant weighing over 6700 lb. The elephant was first weighed on a portable truck scale since the proper dose of anesthetic was dependent on the exact weight of the animal. A sedative was injected into a vessel in the elephant's ear, and an oxygen tube was inserted into her trunk. A podiatrist used a CO_2 laser to excise the lesion, which was later diagnosed as benign. Intraoperative bleeding was minimal. The elephant recovered very quickly and returned to her normal diet of 100 lb of rolled oats, carrots, and oranges. The operative foot appeared not to cause any significant postoperative discomfort.

Laser Surgery on Horses

Contact Nd:YAG laser technology is being performed through the endoscope to treat upper airway obstructions in horses. The goals of this surgery are to reduce the morbidity associated with conventional surgery, promote outpatient surgery for standing horses and for those placed under general anesthesia for a short period, provide precise excision, promote improved hemostasis, shorten the period of recovery and convalescence, and improve overall outcome (Tulleners, 1989).

Most of these procedures are performed through the endoscope on standing horses on an outpatient basis. With customized instruments, a variety of upper-airway conditions can be treated using contact Nd:YAG laser technology, including the excision of cysts, polyps, pyogranulomas, abscesses, ethmoid hematomas, and tracheal ulcers, and the correction of epiglottic entrapment.

Before the laser surgery can be performed, a thorough assessment must be completed, including palpation and inspection of the head and neck and auscultation of the heart and lungs. Horses may manifest symptoms of exercise intolerance, abnormal respiratory noise, coughing, dysphagia, epistaxis, or weight loss.

A flexible fiberoptic endoscope, 1 mm in diameter, is used to diagnose and treat the disease. The endoscope is usually inserted through the right nasal passage. The horse is sedated, standing, and restrained so that accidental injury will not occur. A radiological examination may be needed to help the veterinarian diagnose the disease. Topical anesthesia helps decrease the discomfort of the endoscope. The horse's eyes may be covered for protection; however, as long as the laser energy is confined inside the horse's body, it may be advisable not to use eye protection because it usually causes the horse to become disoriented. Every person in the room wears eye protection. Smoke-evacuation equipment may be needed because small amounts of plume are generated during laser vaporization.

After the procedure, the horse is not allowed food or water for 2 hours. The pharynx is sprayed twice daily with a special pharyngeal spray to reduce inflammation. Exercise is limited depending upon the area and extent of the surgical procedure. Usually an endoscopic reexamination is scheduled 1 week after the procedure to verify healing effects and determine when the horse can return to exercise.

Laser surgery has become a very attractive alternative to many traditional techniques used to perform upper-airway surgery in horses. Because most procedures can be performed on an outpatient basis with the horse standing, the need for general anesthesia is eliminated and other risks are minimized. The expense of an inpatient hospital stay and round-trip shipping fees are decreased or eliminated. Postoperative care can be provided by the owner or trainer. Therefore, time away from exercising and training is minimized.

Laser Surgery on a Dolphin

The first laser procedure on a dolphin was performed in 1993 at Sea World in Ohio to treat perioral and intraoral squamous cell carcinoma (Figures 13-1 and 13-2). In 1991, before laser surgery was considered, the growing lesion was treated with cryosurgery to freeze the dysplastic tissue. This therapy was not successful in arresting the cancerous growth; therefore, other alternatives had to be considered. The marine-animal veterinar-

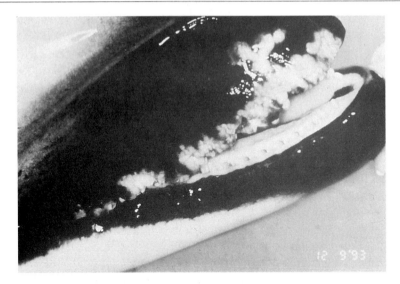

FIG. 13-1   Slow-growing squamous cell carcinoma invades the outer portions of a dolphin's mouth. (Courtesy Sea World, Inc., Orlando, FL.)

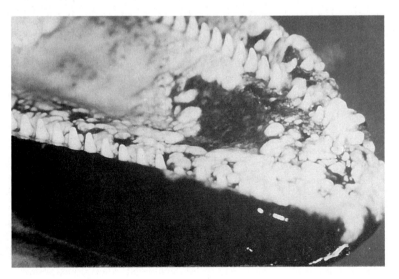

FIG. 13-2   The cancerous lesion extends to the upper palate, resulting in necrotic and friable intraoral tissue. (Courtesy Sea World, Inc., Orlando, FL.)

ian had recently attended a comprehensive laser training program and realized that contact Nd:YAG technology would be very appropriate for treating this dolphin's condition. Two consulting laser-credentialed surgeons and a perioperative laser nurse specialist (the author) assisted with the procedure. Private companies donated a laser and smoke evacuator for use during the procedure.

The dolphin was approximately 16 years old, which is middle-aged for this animal, and weighed 300 lb. No other conditions were present that would complicate the procedure. The dolphin's routine blood analyses indicated that no abnormalities were present. The surgery was planned, and the surgical team, including the trainers, were educated about laser-tissue interaction and safety measures.

On the morning of the surgery, the dolphin was sedated and placed on a foam pad (Figures 13-3 and 13-4). The laser and smoke evacuator were wheeled into position (Figure 13-5).

The trainers stabilized the dolphin and kept her skin wet with a constant flow of water. They also helped assess her pulse, respirations, temperature, and other responses during the procedure. The dolphin's vital signs all stayed within normal limits throughout the procedure (temperature, 98° to 99° F; pulse range, 90 to 120 beats per minute; respirations, 8 to 12 every 5 minutes).

The dolphin's eyes were protected from the laser beam with a towel, and a mouth gag was used to help her keep her mouth open. Xylocaine solution was applied to the lesion surfaces on the upper palate. Everyone involved with the procedure wore protective eye wear. The LED (light-emitting diode) readout on the laser display board was difficult to see because the procedure was performed outdoors. Shading the control panel made the readout easier to see.

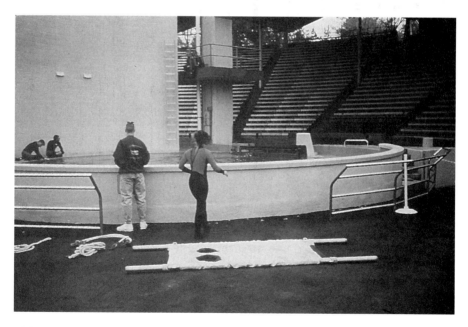

FIG. 13-3   A special stretcher that is contoured to the dolphin's body is used to safely move the dolphin to the surgical bed.

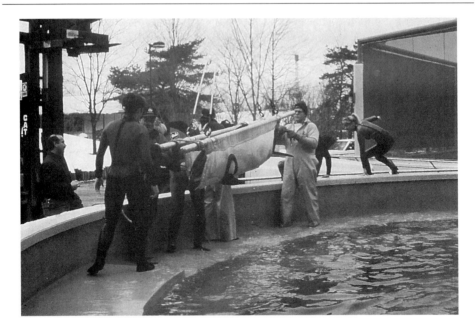

FIG. 13-4   The dolphin is gently lifted from the water for the laser procedure.

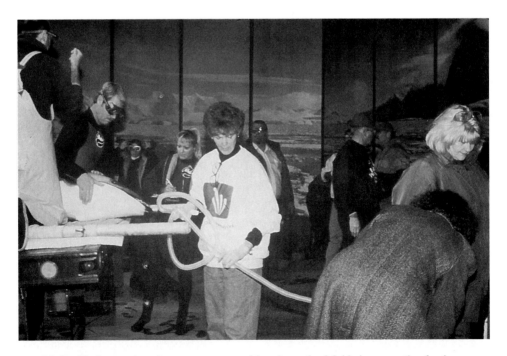

FIG. 13-5   The laser and smoke evacuator are positioned near the dolphin in preparation for the surgery while the team monitors and cares for the patient.

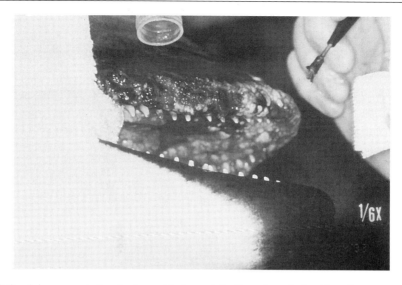

FIG. 13-6   A large rounded probe is used to hemostatically and precisely ablate the cancerous lesion using Nd:YAG laser energy. (Courtesy Sea World, Inc., Orlando, FL.)

A large (10-mm diameter) rounded probe attached to a general surgery handpiece was used to ablate the cancerous tissue (Figure 13-6). A slow saline drip helped to irrigate the surgical site. The probe was kept clean by wiping the tip when tissue debris accumulated on the surface. A biopsy was not needed because several biopsies had been taken on previous dates to diagnose the disease. The mouth, lip, and palate of a dolphin are highly vascular, but the surgical field remained extremely hemostatic throughout the procedure because the laser energy sealed the smaller blood vessels.

The dolphin was very compliant and remained still during the procedure. When the cancerous tumors had been ablated on the outer surfaces of the mouth and on the upper palate, the surgical site was inspected to make sure that the lesion had been vaporized to the level of normal tissue. The mouth gag was removed, and the dolphin was transported back to the salt-water pool, which is always maintained at 55° F. The stretcher was gently placed in the water, and the dolphin easily swam away.

The dolphin was closely assessed throughout the remainder of the day and was given fish to eat after 1 hour. She was reunited with her two dolphin companions and appeared to have no pain or discomfort.

The surgical site was evaluated daily. Healing on the outer surface was remarkable, and cosmetic results were satisfactory. The upper palate also healed rapidly and without complications. The results of this laser procedure were that the tumor spread was arrested, cosmetic and tissue integrity were maintained, and no intraoperative or postoperative difficulties were encountered. Therefore, laser surgery proved to be highly beneficial in eradicating disease and preserving the health of this dolphin.

REFERENCES

Crane SW: State of the art message: Lasers in veterinary surgery, *Lasers Surg Med* 6:427-428, 1986.

Tulleners EP: Transendoscopic contact YAG laser correction of upper airway obstructions in the horse, American Association of Equine Practitioners, 35th annual convention proceedings, Dec 1989, Boston.

Zurlo J, Rudacille D, and Goldberg AM: *Animals and alternatives in testing,* New York, p 37, 1994, Mary Ann Liebert, Inc. Publishers.

SUGGESTED READINGS

Charlton C and Tulleners E: Transendoscopic contact neodymium:yttrium aluminum garnet laser excision of tracheal lesions in two horses, JAVMA 199(2):241-243, July 15, 1991.

Tulleners E: Transendoscopic contact neodymium:yttrium aluminum garnet laser correction of epiglottic entrapment in standing horses, JAVMA 196(12):1971-1980, July 15, 1990.

Tate LP, Little ED, and Bishop BJ: Experimental and clinical evaluation of Nd:YAG ablation of the laryngeal ventricle and laryngoplasty in horses with left laryngeal hemiplegia, *J Clin Laser Med Surg* 2(3):139-144, 1993.

ADMINISTRATIVE ASPECTS OF A LASER PROGRAM

Today's competitive world of health care opportunities is characterized by the use of laser technology as an alternative or adjunct to conventional procedures. In addition, this amazing tool has opened the way for the development of other procedures, which would not have been possible otherwise. Because of the growing popularity of laser technology, the administration of a laser program requires the dedicated efforts of many people, including administrators, physicians, nurses, and laser team members.

As the benefits of laser technology are realized, physicians are welcoming the laser as a valuable tool in their surgical armamentarium. The media continue to promote this innovative and exciting technology by educating patients about its many benefits.

This part addresses the key elements of initiating, managing, promoting, and expanding a laser program in the areas of administration, financial management, legalities, marketing, and education. Critical factors that are vital to maintaining a comprehensive and successful laser program are explained in detail.

14

FORMING THE
INFRASTRUCTURE OF
A LASER PROGRAM

As the popularity and success of laser technology in health care continue to grow, more laser programs are being initiated. Developing and maintaining a comprehensive laser program require careful and intense planning. Ensuring the program's success requires the development of a firm infrastructure that provides a strong foundation for growth. Forming a laser committee, preparing a business plan, formulating a physician credentialing policy, providing appropriate staffing, addressing ethical issues, and properly expanding laser services are all vital elements in laser program development and maintenance. Each of these components is discussed in detail in the following sections.

LASER COMMITTEE

The first step in developing a laser program is to form a laser committee. For beginning programs, this group initially can be an ad hoc unit of the existing surgical committee. As the program expands, the Laser Committee usually becomes an independent committee of the hospital. The structure and responsibilities of the Laser Committee must be understood as initial meetings are planned.

Structure

Membership on the Laser Committee should include but is not limited to the following:

Representative from administration
Physicians representing different subspecialties
Laser safety officer
Laser team member(s)
Operating room director
Librarian
Hospital risk manager
Public relations and marketing representative

317

Others can be invited to serve on the Laser Committee as needed. Departments involved with the laser program, such as the endoscopy laboratory or the radiology department, may also participate on the committee. The committee must also acknowledge the presence of ophthalmic lasers in an outpatient clinic and include this staff in laser program decisions.

At least one official physician representative from each of the specialty departments should serve on the committee. The committee can communicate through these representatives to the various departments as needed. Departments represented could include neurosurgery/orthopedics, general surgery, gynecology, urology, ophthalmology, otolaryngology, dermatology/plastic surgery, oncology, radiology, and pathology. Usually subspecialties such as colorectal or vascular are part of the general surgery department.

The Laser Committee may choose to appoint a medical director of the laser program. If the program advances to the point of becoming a separate department, regulations require that a medical director oversee the activities of the department (Joint Commission on Accreditation of Healthcare Organizations, 1988). This person should work closely with the administration and the laser nursing director/manager.

Meetings should be held on a regular basis, usually once per month. More active laser programs may have a subcommittee that meets on a weekly basis. The meetings should be open to anyone who is interested or involved in the laser program. This will encourage participation by more people.

The *mission* of the Laser Committee is to provide guidance for the laser program so that patient care will be enhanced by laser technology. The direction and success of the laser program are largely dependent upon the coordinated and progressive activities of the committee.

Responsibilities

Strategic planning is one of the major responsibilities of the Laser Committee. The committee members should stay current with the ever-changing world of laser technology and make decisions that will benefit patients and promote the strengths of the program.

One of the most vital responsibilities of the Laser Committee is to formulate written safety policies and procedures. Guidelines must be set so that patient care and laser safety can be ensured and remain consistent within the laser program. Various reference sources for information on laser safety are provided on pages 319-320.

The policies and procedures developed at each facility must be openly communicated to the health care team involved in laser procedures. The Laser Committee must be notified if any infractions occur regarding laser safety and must be aware of any problems that may arise as safety parameters are enforced. Incidents in which safety has been compromised should be documented and reported to the Laser Committee. The committee should react appropriately to guarantee that laser safety guidelines are being implemented and followed.

Safety policies and procedures should address eye and fire hazards, medical surveillance, and other aspects of laser safety. All policies and procedures should be reviewed annually for appropriateness. A safety procedure should never be so specific that it cannot be followed. Policies and procedures are general guidelines for practice and should reflect the standard of care of the institution.

Communications and networking is another responsibility of the Laser Committee. Advances and trends in laser utilization should be announced regularly at the committee meetings. Open discussion should be fostered to promote innovative ideas and support

Laser Safety Reference Sources

Agency for Health Care Policy and Research
Executive Office Center, Suite 501
2101 E. Jefferson Street
Rockville, MD 20852
(301) 594-1433

American National Standards Institute
11 West 42nd Street, 13th floor
New York, NY 10036
(202) 639-4090

American Nurses Association
600 Maryland Avenue SW, Suite 100 West
Washington DC 20024-2571
(202) 651-7000

American Society for Lasers in Medicine and Surgery
2404 Stewart Square
Wausau, WI 54401
(715) 845-9283

Association for the Advancement of Medical Instrumentation
3330 Washington Boulevard, Suite 400
Arlington, VA 22201
(703) 525-4890

Association of Operating Room Nurses
2170 S. Parker Road
Denver, CO 80231
(303) 755-6300 or 1-800-755-AORN
FAX (303) 750-2927

Center for Devices and Radiological Health
Food and Drug Administration
5600 Fishers Lane
Rockville, MD 20857
(301) 443-6143

Joint Commission on Accreditation of Healthcare Organizations
One Renaissance Boulevard
Oakbrook Terrace, IL 60181
(708) 916-5600

Laser Institute of America (publishes ANSI standards)
12424 Research Parkway, Suite 125
Orlando, FL 32826
(407) 380-1553

Occupational Safety and Health Administration
Bureau of National Affairs
1231 25th Street NW
Washington DC 20037
(202) 452-4200

Continued.

Laser Safety Reference Sources—cont'd

PUBLICATIONS

Standards and Recommended Practices (published annually)
Association of Operating Room Nurses
2170 South Parker Road
Denver, CO 80231
(303) 755-6300 or 1-800-755-AORN
FAX (303) 750-2927

Advanced Technology in Surgical Care
(formerly Clinical Laser Monthly) (Published monthly)
American Health Consultants, Inc.
3525 Piedmont Road NE
Building 6, Suite 400
Atlanta, GA 30305
(404) 262-7436 or (800) 688-2421

Journal of Clinical Laser Medicine and Surgery (monthly)
Mary Ann Liebert, Inc.
1651 Third Avenue
New York, NY 10128
(212) 289-2300

Lasers in Surgery and Medicine (monthly)
Wiley-Liss, Inc.
605 Third Avenue
New York, NY 10158-0012
(212) 850-8800

Minimally Invasive Surgical Nursing
(formerly Laser Nursing) (quarterly)
Mary Ann Liebert, Inc.
1651 Third Avenue
New York, NY 10128
(212) 289-2300

Medical Laser Report (monthly)
Penn Well Publishing Company
Advanced Technology Group
10 Tara Boulevard
5th Floor
Nashua, NH 03062-2801
(603) 891-9177

Medical Laser Buyer's Guide (annually)
Circulation Department
10 Tara Boulevard
5th Floor
Nashua, NH 03062-2801
(603) 891-9177

for the laser program. Minutes from the meetings should be recorded and distributed to each member. The performance, enthusiasm, and ambition of the committee members will directly influence the activity of the laser program and its destiny.

BUSINESS PLAN DEVELOPMENT

One of the first projects of the Laser Committee should be to develop a business plan that will guide the activities of the laser program. Whether one laser or a dozen lasers are involved, a comprehensive business plan will determine which steps to take to foster steady growth.

The business plan consists of at least five sections. A sample outline of a comprehensive business plan is provided on page 322.

The first section is the *executive summary,* which provides a brief, concise overview of the entire plan and highlights the mission of the program. The wording should be precise and forceful since this is the most carefully read part of the business plan. Many times this is the only section that will be completely read by administration, physicians, and staff members. The rest of the text is reviewed only if more detail is desired.

The second section consists of an *external assessment* of laser services. A historical perspective traces the evolution of laser technology in health care. A description of any regulatory issues notes limitations and rules imposed on laser technology. Demographics detail the characteristics of the community served, and an assessment is made of the community's need for laser surgery. A study of the geographical competition and market share of patients is performed to determine what other forces may negatively affect the laser program.

The third part of the business plan is an *internal assessment.* A careful look at the existing laser program reveals a good deal of valuable information. The structure of the laser program and the persons involved is illustrated on an organizational chart. Technical support is described, noting how service and preventive maintenance for the lasers are to be accomplished. The current laser program is detailed by noting the types of lasers, surgery volume, laser utilization by specialties, and patient demographics. Economic considerations such as costs, charges, and reimbursements are discussed. Fiscal needs are ascertained through budget development for the laser program to determine the financial commitment required. Current marketing projects are assessed and evaluated. Finally, a SWOT analysis is performed to list the strengths, weaknesses, opportunities, and threats of the laser program so that strategic goals can be set.

The next section outlines the *short-term, intermediate, and long-term goals* that are set. Goals are the desired targets expressed as statements beginning with the word "to" followed by an action verb. For example, a goal can be "to increase laser volume by 10% within one year."

Short-term goals can be achieved within 1 year; intermediate goals are achievable within 2 to 5 years, and long-term goals are usually attainable after 5 years. Laser technology is so dynamic that stating long-term goals is very difficult, thus these goals are often quite broad in scope.

Goals can involve financial performance, laser volume, medical staff development, program development and expansion, laser and other equipment acquisition and replacement, laser education and research, quality improvement, and marketing.

The *action plan* follows the section on goals and describes in detail how each goal can be achieved. For example, the goal "to increase volume" can be accompanied by an action plan to monitor monthly laser usage, conduct a survey to assess physicians' needs for

Sample Business Plan Outline

I. Executive summary
   A. Description of laser program
   B. Mission
   C. Historical trends and market analysis summary
   D. Summary of SWOT (strengths, weaknesses, opportunities, and threats) analysis
   E. Major strategic goals
II. External assessment
   A. Historical evolution of lasers
   B. Regulatory issues
   C. Demographics
   D. Community needs
   E. Competition
III. Internal assessment
   A. Description of existing laser program
   B. Organizational structure and staffing
   C. Technical support
   D. Current laser systems
   E. Laser volume trends
   F. Laser use per specialty
   G. Laser patient demographics
   H. Costs, charges, reimbursements
   I. Marketing
   J. SWOT analysis
IV. Strategic goals
   A. Short-term goals (less than 1 year)
      1. Financial performance/volume
      2. Medical staff development
      3. Program development
      4. Laser system and accessory acquisition/replacement
      5. Laser education and research
      6. Quality improvement
      7. Marketing
   B. Intermediate goals (1 to 5 years)
   C. Long-term goals (more than 5 years)
V. Action plan
VI. Evaluation process

laser systems, explore validity of laser charges, or identify a key physician in each specialty who will promote the advantages of laser technology.

The business plan's final section describes the *evaluation process*. Since goals should never be set in cement, a process needs to be defined that will provide for continual evaluation of the action plan. This allows for changing activities as needed to promote and enhance growth and maintenance.

The business plan must be developed, implemented, and evaluated by everyone involved with the laser program. This fosters ownership in the success of the laser program. In many failed laser programs, administration was not involved in this process, so ownership was limited. Dedication is encouraged when the entire team has a voice in deciding how the laser program should function and grow.

PHYSICIAN CREDENTIALING

Because the Laser Committee is responsible for formulating safety policies and procedures, laser credentialing usually falls into this category. The specific laser credentialing protocol is determined by the hospital governing board. Currently, there are no federally or state controlled regulations to mandate laser credentialing but there are guidelines to assist with the development of credentialing policies. The American National Standards Institute (ANSI) standard Z136.3 recommends that a physician attend a course that covers basic laser physics, laser-tissue interaction, and clinical application. The course should also include a hands-on segment so the physician can actually use the laser in a laboratory setting. The course should be at least 8 to 10 hours, including the hands-on experience (ANSI, 1988). Many hospitals require a 14- to 16-hour laser training program.

Because laser technology is sometimes introduced in medical school, special consideration should be given to physicians who obtained laser didactical and clinical experience during their medical education process. A letter from the college educators stating the laser experience and education may substitute for attendance at a laser conference. Many ophthalmologists qualify for this special consideration.

After the physician attends a laser workshop, the Laser Committee may be called upon to review the coursework. Comments are given to the main credentialing body of the hospital. Temporary laser privileges usually are granted so that the physician can be preceptored. The precepting physician, who is already credentialed to use a particular wavelength, monitors another physician during one or more laser procedures. The preceptor then provides written documentation of the other physician's safe and appropriate use of that particular wavelength. The number of preceptorships required to become credentialed is determined by the hospital's credentialing body with advice from the Laser Committee. After the physician completes the preceptorship(s), his or her laser credentialing request usually is approved or denied by the hospital executive committee or board of trustees.

Hospital credentialing protocols usually require the physician to become credentialed for each laser wavelength. When programs are initiated and no one is credentialed to use the laser, the preceptorship requirement may be altered or eliminated on the recommendation of the Laser Committee. A sample physician credentialing policy is provided on page 324.

The Laser Committee should address the need for residents to become credentialed in using the laser. Some facilities require the resident to attend a laser conference or view laser videos that specifically address laser safety and application before assisting with a laser procedure (Ball, 1986). The resident should meet with a laser team member or the laser safety officer to review the operation of the specific laser that will be used. The resident must be allowed time to practice with the laser system in a laboratory setting. A sample resident certification policy and procedure is provided on page 325.

An annual credentialing review is important to document physician laser utilization. Some facilities review the actual number of laser procedures that individual physicians perform each year. This process is simplified by entering laser statistics into a computer

Sample Physician Credentialing Policy and Procedure

Purpose:

To establish a written policy, for physicians who wish to use lasers within the hospital complex, requiring the physician to obtain the necessary training and experience in the safe and appropriate use of lasers.

Procedure:

1. STAFF PRIVILEGES: The physician seeking laser credentials must have staff privileges at the hospital.
2. LASER COURSEWORK: The physician must send a copy of the certificate of attendance at a laser course with hands-on laboratory training to the Medical Staff Office. The certificate should state the types of lasers involved and the number of contact hours given. (Ideally, a course brochure should be attached.) The physician must have attended a course(s) with at least 14 hours of lecture and hands-on experience. Courses with less than 14 hours will be considered individually by the Laser Committee.

   Special considerations will be made by the Laser Committee for physicians who received laser coursework and experience in their medical-school training. Appropriate documentation must be submitted to verify this experience.
3. LASER COMMITTEE REVIEW: A copy of the certificate of attendance or documentation of the laser education is sent to the laser safety officer. The laser coursework or education program is reviewed by the Laser Committee for appropriateness.
4. TEMPORARY LASER PRIVILEGES: The Medical Staff Office contacts the specialty department chairperson to award temporary laser privileges to the applicant. The applicant is notified of these privileges. If temporary privileges are not awarded by the specialty department chairperson, then the applicant must wait until the credentialing privileges are approved at the next specialty department meeting.
5. PRECEPTORSHIP(S): The physician seeking laser credentials must contact a physician already credentialed for that particular wavelength to act as preceptor during a laser procedure(s). The precepting physician observes the laser procedure and documents the safe and appropriate use of the laser by completing a preceptor form. The laser team member delivers the completed form to the laser safety officer. The physician must be preceptored according to the laser wavelength—the usual requirement is one preceptorship for external procedures and two preceptorships for endoscopic or microscopic procedures. The Laser Committee determines preceptorship requirements.
6. REVIEW-AND-APPROVAL PROCESS: The laser safety officer submits the copy of the laser preceptor form(s) to the Medical Staff Office for filing in the physician's folder. The folder is maintained at the dedicated facility. The physician's credentials are processed through the Specialty Department Committee, Credentials Committee, and Medical Executive Committee for approval.
7. AWARDING OF LASER PRIVILEGES: The physician receives written confirmation of the laser credentials approval; a copy is kept in the physician's file in the Medical Staff Office. Physician credentialing status is maintained in a credentialing book by the laser safety officer for all areas using the laser.
8. INVESTIGATIONAL LASER PRIVILEGES: To use a laser that is not approved by the FDA for a specific procedure, laser-credentialed physicians must provide the Institutional Review Board (IRB) of the hospital with the patient-selection criteria, procedure protocol, and special consent for the procedure. The IRB reviews the request and grants approval to perform the procedure if all specified criteria have been met. The IRB routinely monitors the status of each investigational protocol to allow the continuation of the investigation.

monthly. If the number is unusually low (sometimes set at fewer than three laser procedures per year), then the physician is contacted to discuss how he or she is staying current
with this ever-changing technology. Since laser use requires skill, a physician who has
not used the laser for a long time may need a refresher course. Sometimes this annual credentialing review also offers the Laser Committee the opportunity to determine why a
physician is using the laser more frequently at another hospital. A sample of an annual
credentialing review procedure is on page 326.

STAFFING: THE LASER TEAM

Another critical element in laser program development is staffing. According to ANSI
standard Z136.3, the laser safety officer is the individual with the "authority and responsibility to monitor and enforce the control of laser hazards, and to effect the knowledgeable

---

Sample Resident Certification Policy and Procedure

Purpose:

To establish a written policy, for residents who wish to assist with laser procedures or use
lasers within the hospital complex, requiring the resident to obtain the necessary training and
experience in the safe and appropriate use of lasers.

Procedure:

1. LASER COURSEWORK: The resident must attend a course that offers at least 14 hours
   of classroom lecture and hands-on experience. Topics should include laser biophysics,
   laser-tissue interaction, safety, and clinical application. A copy of the certificate of attendance must be sent to the Medical Staff Office and should include the types of lasers involved and the number of contact hours given. A video session specifically approved by
   the Laser Committee may be substituted for the laser didactic session. After completion of
   the video session, the resident makes an appointment with the laser safety officer or a designated laser team member to review specific lasers. The resident will practice with the
   laser(s) and become familiar with the operation. Documentation of this experience is sent
   to the Medical Staff Office.
2. LASER COMMITTEE: The Medical Staff Office sends a copy of the laser coursework/
   experience to the Laser Committee for review. The Laser Committee recommends approval or disapproval to the resident's specialty department.
3. SPECIALTY DEPARTMENT: The coursework/experience information is sent to the chairman of the specialty department for review. The resident is given privileges to assist or perform laser surgery by the specialty department.
4. PRECEPTORSHIP: The resident must work under the direction of an attending physician already credentialed to use the laser.
5. CERTIFICATION LIST: Documentation of the resident's laser privileges is maintained
   by the Medical Staff Office. A list of residents, their specialties, and the laser wavelengths
   they are authorized to use is also maintained and is communicated to the laser team members by the laser safety officer.
6. PERMANENT LASER CREDENTIALING: After residency training is completed and
   permanent laser credentialing is desired, the resident contacts the Medical Staff Office.
   The Medical Staff Office directs the laser coursework/experience to the Laser Committee,
   the resident's specialty department, the Credentialing Committee, and the Medical Executive Committee.

Sample Annual Credentialing Review Policy

Purpose:

To provide a means to review physician laser utilization and monitor laser credentialing status on an annual basis.

Procedure:

1. A laser subcommittee consisting of the laser safety officer, administrative representative, and the chairperson of the Laser Committee will review physician laser utilization every year.
2. Using computer printout statistics for the previous year, each credentialed physician's laser utilization will be noted.
3. Physicians with fewer than three laser procedures in a 1-year period will be designated "low users."
4. The laser safety officer will contact each physician to determine the reason for the low laser utilization and report to the laser subcommittee.
5. The laser subcommittee will report to the Laser Committee the results of the utilization analysis.
6. The Laser Committee will review the analysis and recommend corrective measures to increase utilization and to help physicians who are low users to remain proficient in safe and appropriate laser use.
7. An operating room or laser center room, staffed with a laser team member, can be made available if needed for the low users to review and practice laser applications with various wavelengths.

evaluation and control of laser hazards" (ANSI, 1988). Each facility should designate one laser safety office to supervise laser safety. Laser team members work directly with the laser safety officer in providing a safe laser environment.

Laser team members are given the responsibility and authority to turn off the laser system during a procedure if the hospital's safety policies and procedures are not being followed. Therefore, the written safety policies must be current, and the laser team members must understand them completely. The Laser Committee should support the laser team's decisions and actions while enforcing the facility's laser standards. This provides a safe environment for the patient and surgical team and minimizes the potential for litigation.

The backbone of a progressive laser program is the laser team, whose members often determine the success of the program through their dedication and enthusiasm (Figure 14-1). The skill level and expertise required to perform the duties of a laser team member sometimes bring extra financial compensation for the added responsibilities involved.

The *responsibilities* of the laser team members are significant in determining the success of a laser program. Some of these responsibilities include the following:

- Operating the laser
- Ensuring that laser safety measures are being followed
- Performing minor trouble-shooting on the laser
- Providing preventive maintenance on the laser

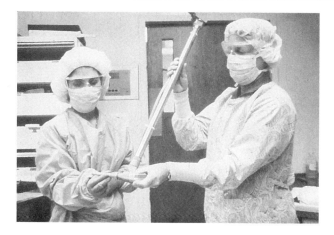

FIG. 14-1   A laser team member helps the scrub nurse connect the CO_2 laser handpiece to the articulated arm.

- Documenting laser service and preventive maintenance
- Documenting laser utilization on the patient chart and on the laser log
- Taking inventory of and maintaining laser supplies and equipment
- Attending Laser Committee meetings
- Assisting with patient education
- Assisting with physician credentialing criteria

The laser team members are known as the laser resource persons for this dynamic technology. Because of the rapid expansion and advances involved, the team must remain current in laser technology. This requires them to attend continuing education laser conferences and read up-to-date laser publications. Sometimes laser team members learn about a new development and encourage a physician to become involved with it. Thus the laser program continues to grow.

The *education* of the laser safety officer and laser team requires them to attain a special skill level to properly perform all of their assigned duties. Initially, they should attend a laser training program to learn about the technology. This program should include lectures on laser biophysics, laser-tissue interaction, laser units and delivery systems, accessory equipment, safety, developing and maintaining a laser program, clinical applications, and future laser procedures that are currently investigational. The laser team members are generalists who must understand how the laser is used clinically in all of the specialty areas. Unlike physicians, who focus on their own specialties, the laser team must be able to provide support for laser procedures in various areas of medicine (Figure 14-2).

Health care professionals in different *positions* can become laser team members. When a laser program is initiated, a perioperative nurse usually is the one assigned to function as the laser safety officer. The nurse not only performs the basic duties of the laser safety officer, but also develops and implements the laser perioperative patient education program.

The laser nurse is vital in helping the patient understand the laser procedure before it is performed. The nurse reinforces what the physician has already described to the patient.

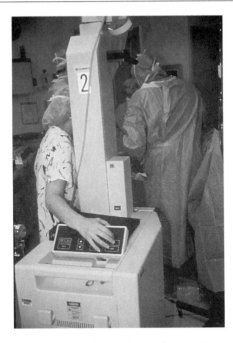

FIG. 14-2 The laser team member constantly monitors safety practices and is ready to put the laser quickly on standby if necessary.

When a patient is told that surgery is needed, the patient often is very anxious about this unknown. When a patient is told that laser surgery is needed, then two unknowns exist, and the patient may become even more anxious. Therefore, some time should be provided for the nurse to spend with the patient before the procedure.

Because the laser is being used increasingly with procedures that require local anesthesia, thorough preoperative teaching helps ensure patient compliance during the procedure. The patient should know what to anticipate during the surgery, what sounds may be heard, what odors may be produced, why eye protection is needed, and any other expectations of the procedure. Discussing all of these concerns usually helps patients become more relaxed during the procedure.

The laser nurse is also involved in providing discharge instructions to the patient. Postoperative visits to the inpatient are often well received and help assess the patient's special needs and expectations after the surgery. Because many laser procedures are performed on an outpatient basis, written discharge instructions are needed. Preprinted discharge instructions often are completed by the physician and discussed with the patient. Usually the patient signs to affirm that the instructions were given; a copy of the instructions is given to the patient, and another copy is kept with the chart. The laser nurse should go over the postoperative discharge instructions with the patient, allowing plenty of time for questions.

The laser nurse has often been placed in the compromising position of having to circulate during the procedure as well as operate the laser. Being accountable for two roles tremendously increases the responsibility required of the laser nurse. Thus, the potential for injury to the patient, physician, and staff members is greater. In the traditional operating room environment, the standard of care in laser technology requires that a laser team member operate the laser while a perioperative nurse circulates during the procedure. This ensures that the patient receives quality care and that a safe environment is promoted. If the circulating duties are minimal and the patient is healthy, maybe only one nurse is needed to circulate and operate the laser. Specific situations must be addressed, with the focus on providing the safest environment for the patient.

Industry has addressed staffing limitations by producing a remote control that can be placed in a sterile sleeve. This remote can then be regulated by the surgical team at the sterile field. The laser should always be in the standby mode even if the scrub nurse, technician, physician, or assistant is controlling the laser.

Another staff member who may be part of the laser team or function as the laser safety officer is the surgical technician. A scrub technician who has attended a laser course and met the requirements of the hospital usually qualifies to become a laser team member and is often called the laser safety technician. This person ensures laser safety, participates during the laser procedure, and assists the nurse with other tasks pertaining to the laser procedure.

As laser use increases and more laser systems are acquired, a biomedical laser technician may also be a laser team member and may function as the laser safety officer. The position of biomedical laser technician requires biomedical or laser/optic training. The main responsibility of this technician is to provide preventive maintenance on the lasers, troubleshoot as needed, and provide service that the technician is qualified to perform. The biomedical laser technician can be an employee of the maintenance department or be part of the surgical staff.

The biomedical laser technician must document all service and preventive maintenance for accreditation requirements. A central file that contains the appropriate service documentation is vital to trace the service history of a laser unit. This information can be recorded on computer for easy storage and retrieval. Lasers are extremely expensive, and regular preventive maintenance will decrease system failure and allow optimal laser performance. When a laser is purchased, the vendor sometimes will agree to train the biomedical laser technician to properly maintain and service the laser.

If a laser program does not have a biomedical laser technician, the hospital can purchase service contracts for preventive maintenance and service on the laser when its warranty expires. As the number of laser systems in a program increases, the need for a biomedical laser technician may prove to be more economically justifiable.

The position of laser director may be added as the laser program expands. This person may also be the laser safety officer. The laser director is usually a registered nurse who has management and operating room experience and thus understands the patient care required. If the laser director is not expected to oversee patient care, the position may be filled by an experienced manager who is not a nurse. The laser director assesses, plans, coordinates, and directs all activities of the laser program. Sometimes the laser program may become a separate department that offers laser support throughout the hospital (e.g., in operating rooms, angiocatheterization and gastrointestinal laboratories, outpatient clinics). Since the laser director is dedicated strictly to the expansion of the laser program, steady growth is usually realized. In today's economic crunch of health care services, the laser director may be expected to assume other management roles, such as director of the endoscopy laboratory.

Sample job descriptions for the laser team members are provided below and on pages 331-332.

A laser team member must be available for emergency laser procedures. As emergency laser cases increase and laser support is required, an availability call schedule should be implemented. The Laser Committee needs to address how to handle the laser cases that will be performed at off-shift times. This protocol must be discussed with the laser team members so that arrangements can be made to accommodate this need. As the use of laser technology becomes more common, using the laser during emergency situations will also increase. Some hospitals make sure that the evening and night surgical staff members have attended a laser training program and can function as a laser team member.

**Sample Job Description
Position: Laser Director**

Summary of responsibilities:

Under the general direction of the vice president of nursing, directs, organizes, and coordinates all activities of the laser program. Functions as facilitator of nursing practice for quality patient care and administratively for services provided on an inpatient and outpatient basis.

Typical responsibilities:
1. Hires, supervises, and evaluates the staff of the laser program.
2. Assesses and evaluates the quality of care delivered and determines action to be taken in correlation to patient acuity, staffing patterns, and staff development needs. Maintains, evaluates, and reports quality assurance indicators.
3. Coordinates the activities of the laser program within the operating room and other hospital departments.
4. Collaborates with medical staff to meet the needs of the physician, patient, and hospital.
5. Develops annual operating and capital budgets for the laser program, ensuring budget adherence following implementation.
6. Identifies learning needs of patient, family, physicians, and staff. Plans, develops, coordinates, implements, and evaluates teaching tools for individual and group health education and support. Oversees physician laser credentialing process.
7. Initiates research methodology to advance patient care, cost containment, and human resources. Monitors reimbursement issues.
8. Makes presentations on the use of lasers in the health care arena for professional and community audiences. Works closely with public relations and marketing departments to promote the laser program.
9. Initiates and recommends policies and procedures necessary to achieve the objectives of the laser program.
10. Serves on the Laser Committee and presents monthly administrative reports.
11. Reviews, reports, and evaluates laser statistics to note trends and recommend action to enhance the laser program.
12. Assists with laser procedures as needed.
13. May serve as the laser safety officer.

Sample Job Description
Position: Laser Nurse

Summary of responsibilities:

According to prescribed policies and procedures and under the general supervision of the director of the laser program, participates in the planning and implementation of nursing care plans for laser patients. Develops and implements laser inservices and continuing education programs for the operating room and laser team. Assists and encourages proper and safe use of the laser using guidelines and appropriate equipment. Assumes responsibility for laser operation and documentation during laser procedures.

Typical responsibilities:

1. Participates in the planning and implementation of nursing care plans for laser patients.
2. Visits laser patients preoperatively and postoperatively to alleviate fear and evaluate patient's concerns.
3. Makes follow-up phone calls to outpatients who have had laser surgery.
4. Develops and implements inservices and continuing education programs for the operating room and laser staff.
5. Oversees daily scheduling of patients in the laser program.
6. Participates in investigatory research projects.
7. Assumes responsibility for laser operation and documentation during laser procedures.
8. Assists and promotes safe and appropriate use of the laser following written guidelines.
9. Maintains the laser logs and records for all laser procedures.
10. Provides a relaxed atmosphere when the laser is being used.
11. Prepares and maintains laser equipment and attachments for use.
12. Functions as the laser resource person to physicians and staff members.
13. Remains current in the field of laser medicine and surgery.
14. May serve as the laser safety officer.

Documentation is a vital responsibility of the laser team. Laser use should be recorded on the patient's chart according to the protocols of the hospital. Abbreviations should comply with the hospital's accepted listing. For example, if "w" is used to designate "watts," then this abbreviation must be approved by the hospital before it can be documented on the chart. This reduces the chance of confusion with other meanings, such as "w" for "west." Complete and accurate documentation will help avoid potential medical and legal problems.

Usually the laser power, duration, and other parameters are documented along with the use of smoke evacuation equipment and other safety measures. This may be documented on the intraoperative surgical record or on a hospital-approved laser log form. This information can also be transcribed onto a computer program that can produce periodic reports on laser use trends. The Laser Committee can study these trends to determine the most favorable direction for the program to follow. A sample laser log is provided on page 333.

Sample Job Description
Position: Laser Safety Technician

Summary of responsibilities:

According to prescribed policies and procedures and under the general supervision of the director of the laser program or the laser nurse, assumes responsibility in the daily clinical operation and documentation of lasers, and assists with and oversees the proper safe use of lasers using protocols and equipment guidelines.

Typical responsibilities:

1. Assists with the setup of laser equipment for each procedure.
2. Monitors and ensures safe laser use for each procedure.
3. Documents laser use on the operative record and on the laser log.
4. Assists with inservices and continuing education programs for physicians, nurses, and the community.
5. Assists in maintaining preventive maintenance and service records on the lasers.
6. Remains current in the field of laser medicine and surgery.
7. Reports problems or concerns involving the safe use of the laser.
8. Acts as a resource person for laser technology in health care.
9. May serve as the laser safety officer.

Sample Job Description
Position: Biomedical Laser Technician

Summary of responsibilities:

According to prescribed policies and procedures and under the general supervision of the director of the laser program or the laser nurse, assumes responsibility for operating, maintaining, and repairing the laser and related equipment.

Typical responsibilities:

1. Operates, maintains, and repairs the lasers and related equipment. Contacts service representatives as needed.
2. Performs preventive maintenance checks on all lasers. Records service and preventive maintenance on lasers.
3. Evaluates equipment and systems and makes recommendations for upgrades or changes.
4. Participates in the development of laser procedures and related systems.
5. Assumes responsibility for laser operation and documentation during procedures. Monitors laser safety.
6. Develops and implements inservices and continuing education programs for physicians, nurses, and the community.
7. Remains current in the field of laser medicine and surgery.
8. Participates in investigational and research projects both technical and clinical.
9. Functions as laser resource person for physicians and staff members.
10. May serve as the laser safety officer.

Sample Laser Log

Date _____   Total charges _____

Patient name _____

Hospital number _____   Zip code _____

Sex _____ Patient status: In _____ Out _____ Patient age _____

Anesthesia _____   Insurance _____

Physician _____   Referring _____

Procedure _____

Laser _____

Power _____   Duration _____

Total energy _____   Spot size _____

Total laser time _____

Delivery system _____

Smoke evacuation   Yes _____ No _____

Laser team member _____

Comments _____

_____

_____

ETHICS

Hippocratic ethics provides the foundation of moral values in medicine, such as the duty to refrain from harming the patient and keeping patient information confidential (Maley and Epstein, 1993, p. 3). High technology, such as laser technology, has introduced a new arena of ethical concerns that must be addressed.

Hospitals today usually have ethics committees to provide education, formulate policies, and advise health care professionals on dilemmas that cause confusion and debate. There is no consensus currently on the exact role an ethics committee should take, but the committee usually does not solve ethical issues or provide legal guidance. It merely helps the practitioner work through a problem by noting the risks and benefits of or alternatives to specific treatments or care to help provide an acceptable ethical solution.

Many laser-related ethical dilemmas can confront physicians, laser team members, risk managers, aand administrators. For example, a physician knows that a specific laser application will provide quicker recovery for the patient, but the insurance company will not reimburse for the procedure. It will reimburse for the traditional nonlaser, more invasive technique, however. This ethical problem must be handled carefully to allow the patient to participate in the decision-making process concerning the care to be delivered.

Laser research opens yet another new world of ethical concerns. The most common problem in research ethics occurs when the patient has a false impression that the treatment outcome will be much better than what should realistically be anticipated. For example, a patient receiving photodymanic therapy for a bronchial tumor must know the realistic expectations of the risks involved and the predicted outcome.

Some physicians have tried to elevate laser technology to being the panacea for all surgeries. They profess that the laser can be used for more procedures and with better results than can conventional procedures. This unrealistic expectation of laser technology produces an ethical problem because of the expense incurred during laser procedures that could be performed without the laser at less cost. Any technology, including laser technology, has limitations. There has to be a fine balance between when physicians use the laser safely and appropriately and when creativity and innovation provide new techniques to benefit patient care.

The acquisition of laser technology can present an ethical problem when physicians help finance the purchase of a laser system or the construction of a center that provides laser services. This can present a conflict of interest because these physicians may tend to use the laser or the center more than they otherwise would. When physicians are within a large group of investors, this conflict usually is less evident.

Hospitals and physicians need to be alert to problems associated with always having to provide the latest technology. For example, if an expensive laser system is purchased to provide the latest technology, the need to get the most use out of the system becomes paramount. The focus often shifts from patient-driven to technology-driven. This situation presents an ethical concern.

The concept of managed care has begun to create some turmoil in today's health care environment. Managed care encourages providers to work within limited reimbursements, therefore all costs must be controlled. Incentives affecting participating physicians encourage less use of more expensive technology even though it may positively affect patient outcomes. Hospitals and physicians must understand that they should not rely on decisions of the gatekeepers concerning new technology but should base their use of a technology on proven clinical studies.

The science of bioethics has become an exciting and interesting field as health care professionals struggle to make appropriate decisions to benefit patients. Just as technology continues to advance, the system of ethics continues to evolve to form a complementary dyad.

Expanding Laser Services

The results of the research conducted to prepare a business plan will determine the type of laser program that is needed. The three most common types are integrated, semifreestanding, and freestanding laser programs.

In the integrated laser program, the most common type of program, laser services are consolidated in the operating room environment. A laser is purchased and is placed in the surgical area, where it is available to physicians credentialed in laser use. An endoscopy suite or outpatient clinic may also obtain a laser.

As the need for lasers increases and more laser systems are procured, the laser program may require expansion, which could involve building or renovating an area solely for laser applications.

The semifreestanding laser program offers laser services in the surgical suite and in a dedicated laser center facility. Grant Laser Center in Columbus, Ohio, was one of the nation's first laser programs to offer an ambulatory local anesthesia laser center as a semifreestanding laser program within the medical center complex. This center is equipped with six treatment rooms designed for laser procedures requiring local anesthesia. If general anesthesia is required, the procedure is performed in the operating room. This type of program has proven to be financially successful and very convenient for the patient and physician.

Laser centers are now being complemented with other local anesthesia services. For example, laser-surgi centers offer local anesthesia applications with and without the laser. The nonlaser procedures may be breast biopsies, hernia repairs, plastic surgery procedures, and other surgeries that do not always involve laser technology. By moving the less invasive procedures that require local or no anesthesia to a laser-surgi center, the operating room can be used for the more major procedures. In a less threatening local anesthesia surgery center, which has an office-type setting, patients feel more comfortable and secure about undergoing procedures.

The freestanding laser program is designed for performing local and/or general anesthesia laser procedures and is separate from a medical center or hospital complex. Beckman Laser Institute in Irvine, California, is an excellent example of this type of program. Policies and procedures must be formulated to develop the protocol necessary for transportation if a patient requires hospitalization after laser surgery.

Freestanding laser facilities are being expanded to incorporate nonlaser procedures that can be performed on an outpatient basis. Advances in flexible and rigid endoscopy are allowing more procedures to be moved from the hospital operating room to less invasive settings.

When considering the planning and building of a semifreestanding or freestanding surgical facility, many factors must be addressed, including the physical plant and layout, patient flow, scheduling, furniture, and patient privacy. As the focus of health care changes from hospital environments to alternate settings, the increased development of ambulatory surgery centers tend to encourage these trends.

A successful laser-surgi center is usually located on the first floor of a building to provide easy access for patients. Free parking or valet parking usually is provided, thus promoting patient-focused services.

A number of concerns must be addressed as the architectural design is drawn. Nurses must be involved with this process to ensure that the needs of patient care will be met (Figure 14-3). Special water and electrical hookups must be considered as the layout of the center is planned. The placement of each laser within a treatment area must be determined so that the appropriate room size can be agreed upon. Doors and rooms must be large enough to accommodate wheelchairs since some of the laser-surgery center patients may be older and less mobile. A laser should be positioned within the treatment room so that the beam is fired away from the entrance. A laser may be located in one room, while its fibers may be directed through a window into another room. For example, a tunable

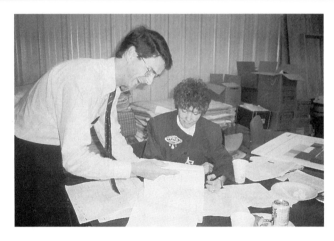

FIG. 14-3   The nurse must be involved with the architectural design and plan development for a laser center.

dye laser can be connected to a slit lamp for ophthalmic applications in one room, while the fiber is directed through a port into an adjacent room where a treatment table is placed for dermatology applications (Figure 14-4). Windows can be planned for the laser rooms, but they must be covered with drapery or other window covering that will stop or absorb the laser beam.

The exhaust system must provide adequate air movement and exchange to prevent air stagnation and possible infection. If plume-producing lasers or electrosurgical units will be used, a centralized smoke evacuation system may be designed.

A small recovery area needs to be planned so that patients can rest immediately after a procedure, if necessary. For example, a cold compress often is applied to the operative eye after laser surgery. The patient can comfortably recline in a chair in this type of room (Figure 14-5). Significant others usually are encouraged to stay with the patient in the recovery area.

Other rooms need to be carefully designed. The waiting room must be large enough to accommodate patients and their families or friends. A television and reading materials help decrease dissatisfaction and restlessness if waiting is prolonged. The nurses station must be large enough to accommodate files and a computer for documentation and patient information. Storage areas must be large enough to provide space for the laser equipment, accessories, instruments, and surgical supplies. (Surgical environments rarely have enough storage space.) The soiled and clean rooms should include containers for regulated medical waste, an autoclave or other sterilizing equipment, sinks for manually cleaning instruments and supplies, proper ventilation for glutaraldehyde chemical soaks, a hopper, linen bags, and a storage area.

The flow of patients must be planned so that proper areas can be arranged to provide privacy and comfort during the registration process and patient education (Figure 14-6). The patient must be assessed before the procedure is performed. Thus, a place must be designated where the nurse can meet with the patient to have the consent form signed, vital signs taken, and overall patient appraisal conducted (Figure 14-7). The patient should

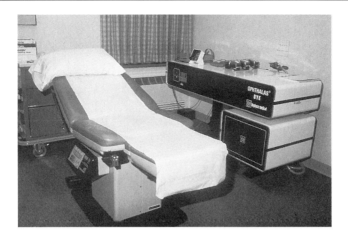

FIG. 14-4   The laser fiber can be passed through a window behind this laser to connect to the ophthalmology slit lamp in the next room.

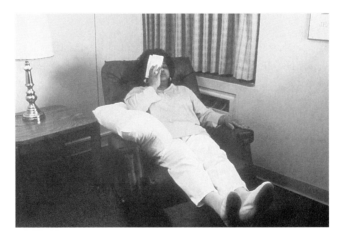

FIG. 14-5   The patient comfortably reclines in the recovery area while applying a cold pack after ophthalmic laser surgery.

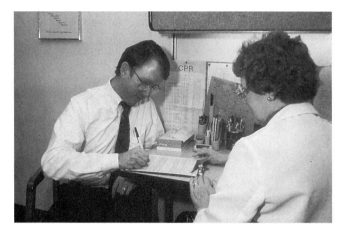

FIG. 14-6   Privacy is maintained as the procedure is discussed and the patient signs the surgical consent form.

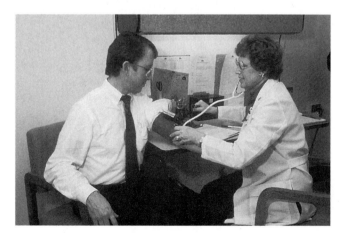

FIG. 14-7   The patient's vital signs are taken before the surgical procedure to determine baseline levels.

be shown the laser, and any questions should be answered before the procedure (Figure 14-8). The patient may be accompanied by a support person, such as a family member or significant other, who should be allowed to participate in as much of the surgical experience as possible. Sometimes a support person is allowed to stay with the patient during and after the procedure (Figure 14-9). Thorough preoperative education will ensure that everyone involved understands safety measures, such as the reason to wear eye protection during a laser procedure.

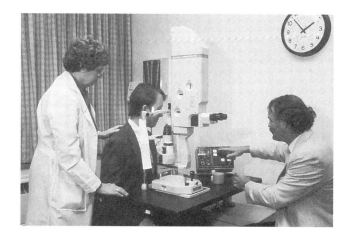

FIG. 14-8   The patient is shown the laser, and any questions are answered.

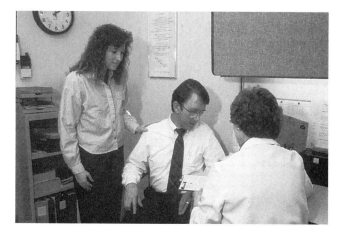

FIG. 14-9   A support person is present when the discharge instructions are discussed.

Postoperative education is of great importance since the patient will be recovering at home. Compliance with discharge instructions is directly related to postoperative complications and outcomes of the procedure. Written discharge instructions must outline in simple terms what is needed during the postoperative phase. The patient must be encouraged to participate fully. For example, a patient who has had hypertrophied nasal tissue (from rhinophyma) excised with the CO_2 laser must be allowed to see the surgical site before a dressing is applied. This will help the patient realize the extent of the surgery and enforce the need for following the discharge instructions closely.

A follow-up postoperative phone call to the patient will encourage compliance with the instructions for home care (Figure 14-10).

The decor and furniture of the laser-surgi center must provide a feeling of warmth and comfort. Hallways and some of the procedure areas, such as ophthalmic rooms, usually are carpeted to convey a relaxed atmosphere. Paintings and wall hangings are used as accents or to provide diversion. For example, a picture hung above a gynecology treatment table will provide a distraction for the patient during the procedure. Rocker-recliners can foster patient comfort during the immediate postoperative period.

Lighting can be provided through overhead or accessory surgical lights, but the room lighting should be adjustable so it can be muted to provide a relaxed setting. Physicians often request that the lights be dimmed during procedures involving a slit lamp or microscope.

Other rooms can be included in the planning of an outpatient laser-surgi center. A conference room or staff lounge provides an area for the surgery team to relax and participate in continuing education. A research laboratory can be used to conduct investigational studies to promote new techniques or validate nursing practices.

If a press conference or news release is planned, these areas can be used to greet the media representatives. Appropriate decorating and furnishing can provide an ambiance of sophistication that will showcase and represent the laser program in a positive manner.

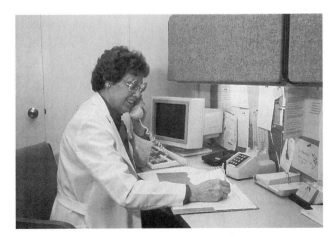

FIG. 14-10   A follow-up phone call to the patient helps ensure compliance with discharge instructions for home care.

Participating in planning the design and style of a laser-surgi center can be a stimulating challenge for the perioperative nurse, can foster creativity, and can promote innovation. The nurse must remember that all decisions regarding the new facility must revolve around patient needs and not the desires of physicians or enthusiasm for the technology.

REFERENCES

American National Standards Institute, Inc.: American National Standard for the safe use of lasers in health care facilities, ANSI Z136.3, Toledo, OH, 1988, Laser Institute of America.

Ball K: Developing a laser program, *Today's OR Nurse* 8(8):16, 1986.

Joint Commission on Accreditation of Healthcare Organizations: *Accreditation manual for hospitals,* Chicago, 1988, JCAHO.

Maley RA and Epstein AL: *High technology in health care, risk management perspectives,* Chicago, 1993, American Hospital Association.

SUGGESTED READINGS

Absten GT and Joffe SN: *Lasers in medicine: An introductory guide,* London, 1985, Chapman & Hall Ltd.

Allard D: Defining performance expectations for laser nurses and technicians, *Clinical Laser Monthly,* pp 12-15, Jan 1993.

Ball KA, guest editor: Seminars in perioperative nursing, *Lasers* 1(2):79-82, April 1992, WB Saunders Co.

Computerized log streamlines laser center administration, *Clinical Laser Monthly,* pp 85-91, June 1993.

Jones WV: Mapping your organization's future: Developing a multiyear business plan, *Minimally Invasive Surgical Nursing,* 7(4):145-150, Winter 1993.

Laser specialists will find key role as public educators, *Clinical Laser Monthly,* pp 145-148, Oct 1993.

Pfister JI, Kneedler JA, and Purcell SK: *The nursing spectrum of lasers,* Denver, 1988, Education Design, Inc.

A sampling of LSO job descriptions, *Laser Nursing* 5(2):44-46, Summer 1991.

15

FINANCES OF A
LASER PROGRAM

L aser technology can be a financial risk if appropriate planning is not incorporated into the laser program. This chapter discusses the process of laser procurement, cost-charge-reimbursement issues, cost containment, and maintaining adequate utilization of laser systems.

PROCUREMENT OF LASER SYSTEMS

The first step in procuring a laser system is determining the degree of interest and the level of enthusiasm the facility has for this technology. Often a physician may attend a training seminar and become inspired by the multiple applications of the laser. This physician then requests that the hospital administration purchase a laser system. Or, hospital administrators may read or hear about the success of laser technology and try to generate physician interest in this new treatment modality that tends to attract patients. Sometimes a perioperative nurse or a laser team member may attend a conference and learn about the benefits of a particular laser system or procedure. This information is then shared with the physicians. Whatever initiates the original excitement, enthusiasm must be fostered, and the physicians must voice a genuine interest in the laser.

Laser technology continues to blossom because of technological advances, but this progression sometimes increases the price of laser systems. Lasers cost from $15,000 to $150,000 or more. Some facilities are not financially able or willing to risk producing the cash needed to buy a laser system. Therefore, budget manipulation is mandatory because procuring these capital expenditures becomes essential to maintain current technology. Creative procurement methods allow the facility to take advantage of this rather costly technology. Laser procurement should be a well-coordinated process involving justification, evaluation, and acquisition (Ball, 1991).

Justification

The Laser Committee must design a *feasibility study* to help justify the procurement of a laser system. This study is conducted by surveying physicians to determine their interest level. The survey should note the anticipated physician laser utilization, case mix, potential revenue, and return on investment. The information obtained from the physicians can be validated through data tallied by the Medical Records Department. For example, if a facility is interested in purchasing a laser lithotripsy unit, urologists and general surgeons should be surveyed. An estimate that a urologist will perform at least 10 procedures per month using the lithotripsy laser can be verified by noting the number of patients with ureteral stones that the physician has admitted. This type of investigation helps ascertain physician interest.

The determination of whether to evaluate laser systems is made from the survey results. If the Laser Committee decides that there is not enough interest or that the laser purchase would not be an economically sound investment, then the committee will continue to monitor the laser market for evaluation at a later date.

Evaluation

The second step in the procurement process is conducting an evaluation of laser systems from several vendors. This evaluation is arranged when the Laser Committee determines that there is enough interest to justify procurement of a laser. Arrangements are made to bring in specific laser systems for evaluation. A memo should be sent to each physician who will be involved with the evaluation, stating the dates, times, and other conditions of the evaluation. The laser team is also notified of the evaluation. It is very important to make sure that all of the physicians and laser team members are involved in the evaluation process to ensure that everyone has a voice in the decision.

Transportation, setup, and preparation can be very costly for the vendor that provides a laser for evaluation. Therefore, to help control these expenses, the vendor appreciates a well-planned, well-orchestrated evaluation program. Communication must be adequate to inform all those involved of the evaluation period so that continuity can be maintained. Some hospitals have one laser at a time demonstrated for evaluation; others prefer to have all of the lasers demonstrated at the same time for comparison.

As the physicians and laser team members review the lasers being evaluated, written comments should be made. The Laser Committee should meet in an open session to discuss the evaluation so that all opinions can be heard. The decision about which laser unit to procure is usually the product of the combined preference of the physician, administration, and laser team.

The *deciding factors* for laser procurement are based on a number of considerations. The length of time before delivery can be expected is critical because facilities want the most current and advanced laser systems. Many times a facility has to wait to procure a newer, more advanced laser because manufacturing is behind schedule. The Laser Committee should note how long it will take to receive the laser after the purchase order is given.

Another deciding factor is the warranty and maintenance of the laser. Many questions should be asked of the manufacturer because service is just as critical as the laser system itself. Some sample questions are:

- What does the warranty cover and for how long?
- When the warranty has expired, what different service contracts can be purchased, and how much does each one cost?

- How much will service cost if a service contract is not purchased?
- Where will the service representative be coming from, and who is responsible for the travel expenses?
- What is the response time for service when the laser fails?
- If the laser cannot be repaired in the field and must be sent back to the manufacturer, will a replacement laser be provided? At what cost, if any?
- What similar facilities have used your service?
- Is a service manual provided along with the operating manual for the laser at no extra cost?
- Are training programs available for a biomedical laser technician? At what cost?
- Is the cost of training the hospital biomedical technician included in the purchase price?

Other questions that must be answered during a laser evaluation involve ancillary expenses. The cost of laser accessories must be considered for budgeting purposes. For example, the cost of a smoke evacuator and related supplies (filters, tubing) must be determined when a CO_2 laser is purchased. The cost of laser fibers and contact tips must be understood so that no surprises occur after the laser has arrived.

The expense of continuing education must be addressed during the evaluation of the various lasers. After the initial inservices, there may be additional charges if the hospital wants the vendor to continually educate the staff members or physicians. Laser vendors are usually good resources for current information on laser workshops for laser safety officers and physicians.

Those laser procedures that have been approved by the Food and Drug Administration (FDA) must be communicated during the evaluation period. The Federal Food, Drug, and Cosmetic Act granted the FDA authority to regulate drugs, cosmetics, and foods. The Medical Device Amendments granted additional power to the FDA in 1976 to regulate medical devices. According to this amendment, there are four ways in which companies may sell medical devices such as lasers:

1. Devices sold before 1976 are grandfathered and can continue to be sold without additional requirements.

Devices sold after 1976 must receive clearance by the FDA in the following ways:

2. The medical device is considered substantially equivalent to the pre-1976 and existing devices; the process involved is called 510(k).
3. The medical device has been proven clinically to be safe and effective; the process involved is called premarket approval or PMA.
4. The medical device can be sold on a limited basis under a special exemption called an investigational device exemption, or IDE, to gather the clinical data needed to submit a 510(k) or PMA.

The vendor should submit a list of procedures that have been approved by the FDA for use with a particular laser system. Just because one laser has received approval does not mean that all companies with a laser that uses a similar wavelength automatically have received approval.

If the Laser Committee wishes to procure a laser that is currently being investigated and has an IDE, then an investigational agreement must be made. The vendor has to enlist the aid of the principal investigators for the laser and document this for the FDA. The hospital Investigational Review Board (IRB) must approve the investigational protocol that will be used within the facility. The principal investigator and coinvestigators sign a contract as to the intent of the study. The written protocol must be followed, including patient selection criteria, procedure protocol, documentation and report filing, and evaluation. The vendor gathers the documentation for the laser procedures as the investigatory work is completed and summarizes the findings for the FDA. If the FDA notes any discrepancies, the investigation is altered and then may continue with the required changes incorporated. If the clinical data prove that the laser is safe and effective for that particular patient procedure, the FDA approves the system to be sold under the 510(k) or PMA status.

If a hospital wants to use a laser that is still investigational for a particular procedure, this can be done without the hospital becoming involved as an investigator. The hospital IRB must approve the procedure's patient selection criteria, protocol, and anticipated outcome. Documentation of the procedure is not reportable by the vendor because the hospital is not listed as an investigatory site.

Ideally, when an investigatory procedure is performed with a particular laser, the hospital should be involved as an approved investigational site. This helps ensure proper compliance with the protocol and continuity of the study. The danger of having a patient sustain injury during a procedure outside of the specified investigational protocol could potentially compromise the FDA evaluation and approval process.

During any investigational study of a laser system, it is imperative that the patient realize that the laser is still experimental for that particular procedure. The patient signs a special consent form noting that the physician has discussed with the patient the investigational status of the laser.

After the Laser Committee has determined the specifics of each laser system, the evaluation period for laser procurement is completed. The Laser Committee should obtain written comments from all persons involved in making the decision. This documents responses and offers a fair and comprehensive process for appropriate laser selection.

Acquisition

When the Laser Committee has justified the need for a laser and has determined which laser to procure, the accounting department begins the third step of laser procurement: acquisition. The accounting department has financial expertise, and knows the hospital's fiscal stability and can determine the most economical method to procure a laser system. Different procurement methods should be reviewed and compared to note the most beneficial and cost-effective arrangement for the health care facility. Creative financing has become attractive to hospitals when they try to determine how to obtain an expensive laser unit. No longer is outright purchase the only method of acquiring costly equipment.

Various laser procurement methods are available, primarily ownership methods, leasing agreements, and limited partnerships. Knowing the advantages and disadvantages of each method aids in the process of deciding which is most desirable. Whichever method is used, the facility must realize the amount of cash needed initially, the succeeding cash commitments required, the impact of the net present value concept, the life expectancy of the laser, and the actual cash spent compared with the income received from laser use.

The *outright purchase* or ownership method of laser procurement has been commonly used historically because it offers immediate possession. Many facilities enjoy the prestige associated with ownership and equate their worth with the amount of equipment they own. With the ownership procurement method, a tangible asset is immediately realized, and the money used to purchase the system is spent. Therefore, costs for the laser purchase do not appear on the operating expense reports, and there is no need for planned monthly budgeting for cash expenditures for a laser.

The main disadvantage of the ownership method of procurement is the loss of investment monies. Thus this immediate cash expenditure limits the facility's cash flow. Also, it is difficult to gauge income without actually entering a laser expense on the ledger or in the financial operating report on a monthly basis. If the money spent on the laser were instead put in a money market fund, the value of the interest earned would have to be considered as potential income. Because of the time value of money, the value of a dollar held today is more than the worth of the dollar tomorrow. Therefore, savings of cash today increase the value of the cash on hand because the net present value of the dollar is higher today than it will be in the future.

If cash is not readily available for investment in a laser system, the facility could opt to borrow the money required to procure the laser. When lending money for laser procurement, the financial institution will want to examine the credit worthiness of the health care facility requesting the loan. All reasonable options for obtaining the funds must be considered. The possibility that a member of the hospital's board of directors is on the board of a local bank should not be overlooked when preferential treatment is needed. Some states float bonds and make available monies needed to buy expensive medical equipment at lower interest rates. Whatever source is used to borrow the money to buy a laser, interest rates must be compared to determine the best method of procuring the equipment.

Another way to obtain ownership is through donations. Money from fund-raising events and charitable donations can help defray the cost of an expensive laser system. Because laser technology is new and is a viable alternative to conventional surgery, community organizations and individuals are eager to donate money to help make the most current health care technology available.

Leasing arrangements are the second major laser procurement method. With laser technology changing so rapidly, the prestige of ownership is not as attractive. Leasing structures involve monthly payments with an option to buy at the end of the contract. At the end of a 5-year contract, a hospital may determine that the leased laser is outdated and thus the buyout option is not desirable. Therefore, the hospital assumes less risk in dealing with this ever-changing technology. Lasers should never be leased for more than 5 years because laser technology is constantly advancing. Usually a 3-year leasing agreement is most appropriate.

The leasing procurement method also leaves potential investment money untapped so that investments can be made to compensate for the interest expense of the lease. Because leasing reduces capital requirements, more funds are available to procure more than one type of laser system, and the lasers can generate revenue while the lease is being paid off. Leasing agreements assist in cash budgeting because the monthly cost of the laser appears on the operating expense report. True profitability and income are more accurately analyzed and compared as the expense is measured against the revenue generated each month.

The disadvantage of the leasing method is that the cost of the lease must be budgeted because this is a regular financial commitment that will affect cash flow. If the cash income is low for the month, the hospital may have to borrow to finance the cash expenditure.

The two most commonly used sources of laser leasing funds are the manufacturer/distributor and the third-party financier. Manufacturer/distributors have recently become more interested in expanding sales by offering leasing options. However, sometimes third-party financiers can quote lower leasing terms because lending money for expensive equipment is their business. A financier who specializes in the health care laser market probably could offer the lowest leasing rates. When a hospital wishes to borrow money for a laser lease, its creditworthiness is not as important as the value of the equipment. Therefore, facilities with lower credit ratings may find obtaining a lease easier than borrowing the cash for a laser purchase.

Some manufacturer/distributors offer a lease-per-use program in which the lessee (the one who leases the equipment) pays a certain amount for each procedure performed with the laser. This allows a hospital and those involved to evaluate a laser system by using it before deciding whether to purchase or lease. Facilities just entering the laser arena find this method valuable because it requires no immediate financial commitment. The lease-per-use method is most desirable for use over short-term periods because payments can become very expensive as the laser caseload continues to increase. Also, if payment is required for a minimum number of laser uses each month, this option can become financially undesirable if laser use is below the minimum.

Sometimes companies form a contractual agreement with the facility that lowers the purchase price if the laser is leased by the month. For example, a hospital may lease a laser for 6 months. At the end of this period, the hospital decides to purchase the laser. Part of the monthly leasing payments are used to lower the cost of the laser according to the prearranged agreement.

Leases usually include an option to buy at the end of the specified leasing period. The three most significant types of buyout plans are the $1.00 buyout, the one-extra-payment buyout, and the fair-market buyout. Buyout plans that offer the laser for $1.00 or one extra payment usually require a higher monthly payment. The true lease or fair-market-value buyout allows a lower monthly payment, with the buyout fee being the fair market value of the laser (sometimes quoted at 10% of the original cost of the laser). The true lease is the type of lease needed to qualify for medical equipment Medicare reimbursement. New federal regulations eliminate this type of reimbursement.

Facilities often opt not to buy the laser at the end of the lease and thus are better off having the lease with the lowest monthly payments. The disadvantage of a true lease is that the buyout cost is often overlooked during budgeting, and when money is needed at the end of the period, other arrangements must be made to finance this cost.

If the leasing method of procurement is chosen, the accounting department must thoroughly review the contract. Terminology must be defined simply. For instance, "guaranteed renewal protection" really means that the return option is not effective until after a specified renewal period. "Purchase protection" really protects the lessor (the leasing company) because this wording actually means that the lessee must either purchase the laser or renew the lease. No option to return the laser is offered.

The accounting department should be thoroughly cognizant of the terms specified in a leasing contract. The following questions should be answered:

- Who is responsible for the insurance and shipping of the laser if it is to be returned?
- What condition does the laser have to be in when returned?

- Is the lease automatically renewed for a specified monthly payment and period of time if the lessor is not notified by a certain date of the intention to return the laser?
- Does the hospital have to update the laser to current technology standards if it returns the laser?

All of these questions are critical for those deciding whether to sign the leasing contract. Many hospitals have been stuck with outdated and nonfunctional equipment because they overlooked the small print on a leasing contract.

It is important to be on guard against the deadly "4 Rs" sometimes included in the return-policy section of the lease: return ripoff, resale racket, restocking scheme, and restoration (Anderson and McCoy, 1984). The return ripoff mandates that the facility pay for the privilege of returning the laser. If a laser is to be returned, a reasonable destination and the individual responsible for shipping should be determined at the initiation of the lease. The contract should be studied carefully to determine whether advance notice must be given before the laser is returned. Sometimes, if advance notice is not given, the laser lease is automatically renewed for a specified period of time.

In the resale racket, the hospital must assume the risk of low laser resale value. Beware of the contract stating that if the lessor cannot sell the laser for the fair market value, the lessee must make up the financial difference. The restocking scheme forces the hospital to pay an additional amount to have the lessor accept the laser into their stock. The restoration clause is a subtle statement that requires the laser to be returned "like new," in "upgraded" condition, or meeting "current specifications." The contract should read that the laser is in "as is" condition or has been "subjected to normal wear and tear."

The accounting department should be acutely aware of the terms and specifications of a laser leasing contract. A few flowery and ambiguous words can turn a financially beneficial method of procurement into a nightmare.

Laser rentals, another type of leasing, has developed during the past few years. Renting a laser has become a common method to ensure that a facility can offer the most advanced technology (Figure 15-1). Laser rental companies purchase a variety of laser systems. They hire nurses and technicians who have attended laser training programs and can be categorized as laser team members. When a hospital, clinic, or physician's office needs this technology, the company delivers the laser, guarantees its proper functioning, furnishes the laser fibers and/or other accessory devices, and provides a laser team member to operate the laser and ensure that laser safety practices are being followed. Written policies should be in place to determine how the rental equipment and the nonemployee function within the facility's surgical environment. Often the circulating nurse or an extra employee of the facility is present to complete the laser documentation form.

Laser rental agreements can be made for each procedure or by the day. The facility must make sure that the appropriate installation needs are met before the laser is brought in for use. This laser rental system has been widely accepted as an innovative method to provide the technology, control costs, and evaluate systems to provide justification for purchase.

Limited partnership is the third major laser procurement method. Physicians (individuals or groups) may opt to form a limited partnership to purchase or lease a laser system when a hospital is unwilling or financially unable to procure a system. Then a lease-per-use schedule can be established, with the hospital paying a specified amount each time the laser is used. A monthly installment plan that does not reflect laser utilization may

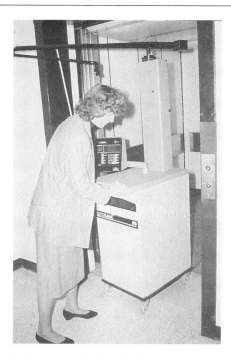

FIG. 15-1   A rental laser is wheeled into the hospital in preparation for a scheduled laser procedure.

also be implemented. A certificate of need is not required when a limited partnership buys a laser. The net worth of the partnership increases as revenue is generated as a result of this purchase. Physicians are more motivated to use the laser and will encourage other physicians to use it, thus increasing utilization of the system. Physicians are discouraged from buying lasers for their offices because with the limited partnership they share the wealth from the laser revenue while the hospital assumes the responsibility for staffing and operation of the laser.

A laser system can be an important, depreciable piece of equipment to a limited partnership. Because tax laws may be altered or adjusted each year, the benefits of tax write-offs must be reviewed for cost-effectiveness. Changes in the financial advantages of limited partnerships appear to be decreasing the popularity of this arrangement.

Each of the three major laser procurement methods should be evaluated thoroughly for advantages and disadvantages. Creative financing is vital for health care organizations as they develop comprehensive laser programs that include a variety of laser systems. Since the cost of lasers can be prohibitive, careful consideration and strategic planning must be used to ensure the financial viability of the facility and its laser program. The high cost of current technology demands that medical and surgical managers become more involved in the managerial accounting in today's ever-changing health care environment.

To successfully compete in today's laser marketplace, hospitals must optimize any financial investment. Usually a combination of laser procurement methods offers the most financially sound arrangement for providing the latest laser technology. Appropriate laser system procurement can help facilities meet their medical equipment needs in the future, help preserve financial viability, and ultimately enhance the quality of health care services provided.

When the laser has been ordered, plans should be made to provide the appropriate water or electrical hookups. Changes should be made immediately so that the physical plant is ready when the laser is delivered. Many hospitals do not plan appropriately for the special laser requirements; thus, when the laser is delivered, it sits unused as the warranty period elapses. This poor planning causes the hospital to lose potential revenue and allows the laser program to stagnate.

LASER ECONOMICS

The three most important elements in measuring the economical status of a laser program are costs, charges, and reimbursements. Charges and reimbursements should be more than the costs of performing laser procedures if a program is to remain financially viable. These three factors must be monitored and controlled on a continual basis.

Costs

The actual cost of the laser procedure must be determined before charges can be set and the adequacy of reimbursement can be assessed. As with any surgical procedure, the direct and indirect expenses must be noted.

The direct cost of the laser system can be estimated by dividing the purchase price of the laser by the total number of anticipated usages. This amount is then divided by 5 since laser systems are depreciated over a 5-year period. This formula is as follows:

$$\text{Cost per procedure} =$$
$$(\text{Cost of laser/Anticipated number of uses per year})/5$$

For example, an $80,000 laser with an estimated use of 50 procedures per year divided by a 5-year life expectancy determines a laser cost of $320 per procedure. With increased usage to 200 procedures per year with this same laser, an $80 cost can be calculated. Therefore, the impact of increased laser volume directly affects the cost per procedure of the system.

Other costs must be determined for a laser procedure, including laser service and preventive maintenance, laser fibers, smoke-evacuation supplies, drapes, and instruments. Staffing expenses must also be determined. Indirect costs such as marketing, physical plant overhead, and administrative expenses must be determined to portray a true analysis of actual costs. This information is then used to determine the appropriate amount for either a procedure or laser charge.

Charges

When a laser program is initiated, a method to charge for laser services must be developed. Charges in the operating room should be consistent with other department charges. For example, if a CO_2 laser is used in an outpatient clinic and in the surgery suite, then the CO_2 laser charges should be compatible.

There are three ways to develop a laser charge: A charge per laser use, a charge per time interval, or a charge that is incorporated in the procedure charge.

The laser charge per use is determined by noting the various direct and indirect costs of the laser and laser supplies. One predetermined laser charge is then assessed each time the laser is used without consideration of the length of time per use.

The laser charge per time interval sets an equitable fee schedule that charges for laser use in time increments. This type of charge addresses complaints about having the same charge for the laser whether it is used for 5 minutes or 2 hours.

The laser charge may also become a hidden part of the procedure charge. The procedure charge, whether the laser is used or not, includes the charge for the laser system itself. Most facilities issue an extra charge for smoke-evacuation supplies, fibers, or contact tips. These different charges should be based on the actual cost of the supply or equipment. This type of charge system encourages physicians to use laser technology since an added charge for the laser unit is not an extra expense.

A debate as to whether there should be a standby charge for laser use has heated the marketplace. Some hospitals feel that a charge should be submitted if the laser is scheduled and not used. There is a hospital expenditure for staff time to set up the laser system and time involved with waiting to see if the laser will be used. Others state that the laser charge should be bundled into the operating-room service charge and an extra fee should not be assessed. This dilemma presents an ethical issue in determining whether a patient should be charged for the laser if it is not used. But the cost has to be incurred by someone. So the debate will continue as hospitals struggle with this concern (*Clinical Laser Monthly*, July 1993).

Reimbursement

The amount of reimbursement for a laser procedure is a constant concern for hospital administrators, physicians, and laser team members. Since laser technology can be a rather expensive venture, the return on investment is paramount. In today's environment of managed care, reimbursement is usually not equal to the amount of the charge. Therefore, actual costs must be determined to appropriately illustrate the profitability of a laser program. The cost to perform the procedure, the charges, and the reimbursement rate are valuable information for those involved in a laser program.

Physician reimbursement is based on the Current Procedural Technology (CPT) codes. If a physician has difficulty receiving reimbursement for a particular procedure, then the third-party carrier should be contacted directly to determine the reason. Many times the third-party carrier does not understand the laser application.

The physician should charge an amount equal to that of a procedure done without the laser. For example, a laser conization of the cervix should not warrant a tremendous increase in charges compared with a conization of the cervix with a knife. The laser, in this example, is merely a tool for the physician. In comparison, the physician charge for an endometrial ablation may be similar to that for a vaginal hysterectomy because the procedure is performed as an alternative to a hysterectomy. If there are no CPT codes for a specific procedure, the physician should submit a letter of explanation of the rationale and description of the laser procedure, a copy of the operative record, and the amount of the charge. If there are complications associated with the procedure, then the physician must code the procedure accordingly and note the complication, such as advanced scarring at the surgical site or a cardiac condition that had to be monitored.

Reimbursement is a complicated process because each carrier uses different criteria for payment. Surgeries are subject to interpretation by the carriers, and the amount of reimbursement may differ depending upon the geographical location of the patient. Payors are interested in the surgery performed and the patient's outcome, not the technology used.

Currently research is being conducted to determine whether a code modifier can be used for laser procedures to establish a reasonable rate of reimbursement. These codes are being developed through surveys sent to physicians in every specialty. The criteria being compared for different procedures will be used to determine one relative value scale. These criteria involve risk to the physician, risk to the patient, skills required, time required, and severity of the illness (*Clinical Laser Monthly,* Sept 1993).

Physicians today are reimbursed by Medicare using a resource-based relative-value scale (RBRVS) system. Medicare continues to control payments by monitoring the relative value unit (RVU) of specific CPT codes. An RVU is divided into three components: work, overhead, and malpractice costs (*Clinical Laser Monthly,* April 1993).

A controversial issue that has risen in recent years is limited physician reimbursement for procedures that can be performed in the physician's office. This impacts the RVU component of overhead costs. Medicare payment structures are making a "site-of-service differential," meaning that there may be a 50% reduction in the overhead payment segment of the cost of the physician's services if the procedure is performed in a hospital's surgery or outpatient department instead of the physician's office. For example, an ophthalmologist can expect less reimbursement for physician services when a posterior capsulotomy is performed in a hospital laser center as opposed to the physician's office. The rationale behind this decision is that Medicare can also expect to pay the hospital a facility fee for the procedure. The site-of-service differential is still being refined to provide equitable reimbursement while controlling health care expenditures.

This type of reimbursement payment system will encourage physicians to purchase lasers for their offices. Instead of one laser being positioned in a laser center for five physicians to use, now each physician may feel pressured into purchasing a laser for his or her office. This is not the best utilization of laser technology.

If a physician purchases a laser system for the office, then financial considerations must be made to determine the initial cost of the laser, accessories and medications needed for the procedure, service and preventive maintenance, and staffing costs. A careful calculation of these amounts will assist in determining whether purchasing a laser system can be justified.

Facility reimbursement can be divided into inpatient and outpatient reimbursements. Facility reimbursement for an inpatient procedure is often predetermined, as with the Medicare diagnosis-related group (DRG). A DRG is based on the patient's discharge diagnosis. Each DRG allows for a specified amount of reimbursement no matter how long the patient is hospitalized, what tools are used to perform the procedure, or what the different charges total. If the patient can be discharged earlier, then the costs are less for the hospital and a profit is realized. If the patient requires a longer hospitalization, the hospital does not receive more money unless special conditions are met. When the laser is used during surgical procedures, often the patient recovers more quickly and can be discharged earlier. This helps to control costs and make the DRG system profitable.

When the DRG system was initiated, its purpose was to increase the number of outpatient procedures and control or decrease the amount of inpatient costs. The use of laser technology is consistent with those goals. When the laser is used during a surgical procedure, many of the benefits of laser technology, such as the sealing of blood vessels to decrease the amount of blood loss, help the patient recover more quickly. Since the laser can be used through the endoscope, many procedures that normally require an external incision to access an organ can be performed through an endoscope. Therefore, laser technology has helped to control health care dollars.

When the prospective payment system for inpatients was implemented, the government compiled a list of procedures that could be performed on an outpatient basis. This list is known as the ambulatory surgery center (ASC) list. The procedures listed must be performed on an outpatient basis now, or special circumstances must be documented that justify the patient's admission as an inpatient.

There is currently a prospective payment system that addresses the amount of reimbursement for outpatient procedures for Medicare patients. This system is still being refined. The different ASC procedures are placed into different groups and reimbursement is made according to the groups. Other third-party carriers are also implementing this type of reimbursement system.

Bundling of charges is beginning to occur in the health care environment today. For example, the physician's charge and the facility fee are reimbursed with one amount. Usually the facility receives the payment and then sends the physician the amount of payment for his or her professional services. This type of reimbursement mandates that everyone involved with the procedure practice as cost-effectively as possible.

Laser program officials must constantly be aware of reimbursement changes. The payor mix of the patients should be determined to note the various anticipated reimbursement amounts. Cost-containment measures are critical in controlling costs when reimbursement amounts are low. The cost of various supplies should be studied compared with the actual reimbursement for them to justify their expense. Laser fibers can be very expensive if reimbursement does not cover the cost of using a new fiber every time. Cost-containment measures may call for a hospital policy of reprocessing the fibers to get more use out of each one.

In today's world of uncertainty with regard to reimbursement for expensive supplies and equipment, a laser program must constantly monitor costs vs. reimbursement. An astute laser committee will report changes in reimbursement on a regular basis. With constant vigilance regarding the financial impact of laser technology, a laser program can continue to be economically successful. For example, local-anesthesia laser centers have proven financially successful for many institutions. Patients do not have to pay for the added overhead of a general-anesthesia surgical suite for a local-anesthesia laser procedure. The laser center concept allows the procedure to be performed in a mini-operating-room environment that is more cost-effective because of lower overhead. These types of programs will begin to develop as reimbursement limitations influence health care arenas.

COST CONTAINMENT

Cost containment can be the key to maintaining a cost-efficient laser program. Cost containment requires the constant effort of everyone involved in the laser program, including laser team members, operating room staff, department directors, and physicians. An awareness of the expense of various items or pieces of equipment coupled with the knowledge of the actual reimbursement encourages the laser team to manage costs through creative strategies.

Strategic planning is a critical element in helping to control costs. Intense coordination of laser system evaluations ensures that the appropriate laser is procured. Preventive maintenance costs should be reviewed before a laser is purchased. Many times a laser company will charge extraordinary fees to service a laser if a service contract is not purchased after the warranty has expired. Sometimes a facility will have to pay the travel expenses of a service technician coming from across the country when a service call is needed. Costs can be decreased if the facility determines that the service technician is located nearby to avoid excess travel expenses.

Resource management for cost containment can prove very beneficial. Sometimes a laser team member can be scheduled to work on flextime with the surgical schedule followed very closely, noting the times that laser services are required. If a procedure is not booked until 9:00 AM, the laser team member can begin work at 8:30 AM to increase staff utilization. Special attention is paid to avoiding conflicts in the scheduling of the available laser equipment. This in turn increases laser-system utilization and staff productivity.

Computerization has had an impact on the use of laser technology in health care. Computers can be used to promote cost-efficiency by documenting laser inventory, laser utilization, service, and preventive maintenance schedules. Computers can analyze statistical data, and trends can be noted that will influence the laser program and help maintain cost-efficiency (Figure 15-2).

Computerization can point out the highly profitable procedures so that a marketing program can be developed to increase the visibility of these procedures. Computers can also be used to determine which physicians are generating the most revenue for the laser program so that their special needs can be specifically addressed.

Special laser supplies and equipment can be very costly. "Cheaper is not always better" is a guideline that should be followed. Less expensive items can often lead to safety concerns that will increase liability and hazards during the laser procedure.

There are many suggestions for maintaining cost-efficiency when obtaining the necessary supplies and equipment for a laser procedure. Instruments should be selectively anodized or ebonized to decrease reflectivity. Not every instrument used during the laser procedure needs to be nonreflective. Only those instruments that will be used in the immediate laser-tissue impact area need to be treated. Existing instruments can be sent to have the nonreflective surface applied so that special instruments do not always have to be purchased.

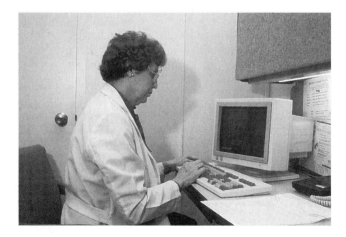

FIG. 15-2   Laser procedures are entered into a computer program that will analyze information to determine trends in the laser program.

Quartz rods that are individually packaged can be used again after appropriate cleaning and sterilization. Glass rods should never be used as backstops even though they are less expensive because the heat generated by the laser energy will cause them to shatter.

Lasers can often be shared between departments to promote increased utilization and cost-efficiency. For example, the gastrointestinal laboratory may be able to use the same Nd:YAG laser system as the operating room if special attention is given to scheduling. Most lasers can be easily transported from one area to another.

Care must be taken to protect endoscopes from laser damage. Backscatter from an Nd:YAG laser beam can destroy the end of an endoscope. The laser fiber must extend past the end of the endoscope, and the physician must observe the fiber tip in the surgical field before the laser is activated. Video monitoring of the procedure helps to ensure the proper positioning of the fiber before the laser is activated because the laser team member also can note the fiber location.

The end of a bare laser fiber is sharp and can tear the inside lumen of the biopsy channel of a flexible endoscope. The end of the fiber can be protected by introducing the fiber into medical-grade tubing with the tip recessed inside the tubing. Then the whole unit is passed through the biopsy channel. Once the fiber tip inside the tubing is through the end of the endoscope, the tubing is withdrawn to expose the fiber tip. This helps protect the inside lumen of the endoscope.

Many Nd:YAG fibers can be repolished for use in more than one procedure. Research has led to disposable fibers. Some facilities have been forced to reprocess these fibers because of reimbursement limitations. Sterilizing cases are commercially available that can contain the clean fibers for gas sterilization if the fibers are to be used again (Figure 15-3). This action helps decrease the cost of each fiber use, but the facility must understand that liability is assumed when it reprocesses a single-use item.

Laser protective eyewear can be very expensive. Care must be taken not to scratch the lens surface. CO_2 glasses can be stored in lengths of stockinette for protection. It is best to shop around for the best prices on laser eyewear, but to make sure that the eyewear meets ANSI regulations for appropriateness and safety (specific wavelength and optical density).

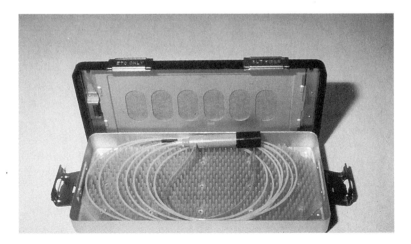

FIG. 15-3   A laser fiber is reprocessed and placed in a protective container for gas sterilization.

Special laser endotracheal tubes are being manufactured to decrease the chance of airway explosion during upper airway procedures. Wattage and power-density limitations associated with the use of the laser endotracheal tube must be noted. To control costs, some facilities use red rubber endotracheal tubes wrapped in reflective foil tape. Each batch of foil tape should be test-fired to note how it reacts to laser impact. This practice may control expenses but also will increase the liability to the facility and physician.

Changing the smoke-evacuation filters as required will increase the efficiency of the smoke-evacuation system. Filters that contain coconut-based charcoal are more effective in removing odors than the less expensive, wood-based charcoal ones. Some smoke evacuators are equipped with a light that appears when the suction decreases, indicating that the filter needs changing.

Contact tips used during Nd:YAG procedures can be very costly if not cared for appropriately. Special storage units are available that can be autoclaved and placed within the sterile field to help keep track of these small tips. Making sure that the physician is skilled in using the tips helps tremendously in avoiding tip fracture or damage. Lateral stress must be avoided so that the longer contact scalpels are not broken. The side ports that deliver the coolant to the contact tip must be kept patent to allow the purge to flow to prevent the tip from becoming thermally damaged. The contact tips can be soaked in hydrogen peroxide before the cleaning process to loosen any adhering tissue. If time is taken to care for these tips appropriately, their life expectancy can be tremendously increased and money will be saved.

The costs of special CO_2 laser gas or the laser purge gases from different vendors should be compared. Sometimes specialty gas companies can supply these gases at a lower cost than that of the laser manufacturer. The proper concentrations of CO_2 laser gas must be obtained to ensure adequate functioning of the laser. If specific concentration requirements for the CO_2, nitrogen, and helium are not met, the laser will not operate properly.

Custom packs tend to help control costs by minimizing waste. Turn-around time between cases is decreased because the setup time for custom packs is less. Custom packs not only save time, but also save storage space and simplify inventory maintenance (Figure 15-4). Sterile custom packs are available, but can also be purchased clean for those endoscopy procedures that do not require a sterile setup. This helps control costs significantly.

Cost containment need not be an overwhelming task, but it does take commitment and initiative. With effort and planning, laser programs can be very cost-effective in a world of everchanging and demanding technology.

Maintaining Adequate Laser Utilization

One of the most critical challenges today is to get the most use out of new technology. Laser technology has been confronted with other advances, such as endoscopy, that also mandate skill and experience. The use of lasers in some specialties has gone from no use, to much use, to limited use. The question now is, How can we get physicians to use lasers when they are appropriate? A number of considerations can be explored to increase laser use:

Laser charges: To increase utilization, the first area that should be examined is the amount of the laser charge. The charge for the laser system must not be prohibitive. Sometimes hospitals have completely paid for a laser system, but the charge continues to increase each year. Many physicians who would like to use the laser complain that the patient's laser charge is too high, so they use other tools instead.

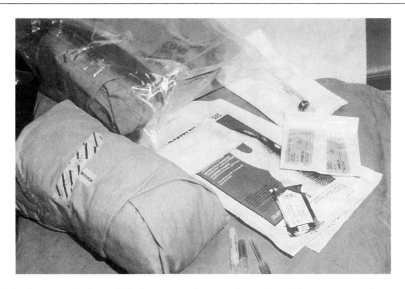

FIG. 15-4   Items regularly used for laser procedures can be packaged in a custom pack to control the cost of maintaining a large inventory.

Supply charges: Charges for laser fibers, contact tips, smoke-evacuation accessories, special endotracheal tubes, and other supplies must be monitored to ensure that charges are appropriate. Some of these charges may be incorporated into the bundled procedure charge.

Physician credentialing: A facility's written laser credentialing policy should not deter physicians from participating. For example, a policy that requires 10 preceptorships before credentialing can be granted for a particular wavelength is inappropriate and unnecessary. Written policies on credentialing must provide a safe surgical environment with skilled practitioners but must not discourage physicians from wanting to use the laser. Sometimes an elite "old boys club" is promoted by requiring too many preceptored procedures as only a few physicians are allowed to use the laser.

Multispecialty laser systems: Laser units that can be used by a variety of specialties will often increase utilization. A tunable dye laser can be used by ophthalmologists and dermatologists; a holmium laser can be used by otorhinolaryngologists, orthopedists, and neurosurgeons; and a CO_2 laser can be used by podiatrists, gynecologists, urologists, plastic surgeons, otorhinolaryngologists, and a host of others. If a laser system can only be used for one specialty, then careful justification of actual caseload must be determined to ensure the return on investment.

Laser team: An astute and eager laser team is often the stimulus needed to encourage laser utilization. When a physician realizes that a talented laser team member is providing support for a procedure, then the physician may be more willing to use this technology.

Laser literature: A member of the laser team or the laser safety officer should constantly monitor laser articles. Often a monthly literature search is conducted by the hospital library to note any new laser developments. Articles can be copied and sent to the appropriate physicians to help them remain current with laser technology.

Continuing education: Ongoing education is paramount to a successful laser program. Laser utilization can be increased by providing new knowledge and skills to the physicians and team members. Keeping physicians informed about the results of different procedures may increase their interest in using a laser system.

Ongoing physician training laboratories: Periodic training sessions can be arranged for physicians to practice with specific laser systems. When a physician feels secure about a laser system and can control its energy, then he or she will be more apt to use the laser clinically.

Communication about the laser program: The Laser Committee should send regular reports to the various specialty departments regarding the laser program. New equipment, accessories, and laser systems should be communicated so that physicians understand the status and availability of this technology.

Laser newsletter: A periodic (monthly, quarterly) laser newsletter can be published by the Laser Committee that communicates advances in laser technology, reviews written safety policies, and provides an ongoing assessment of the program and market.

Administrative support: Administrative support for a laser program is vital to maintaining an active laser department. If the hospital administration does not value the program, then money will not be designated to upgrade or maintain laser technology.

Marketing: The Laser Committee and laser team members should actively challenge negative press or inaccurate information about laser technology. A consistent marketing plan will promote laser technology and increase interest. Encouraging all of the physicians who use the laser to participate in a marketing plan will create a positive atmosphere for support. (More information about laser marketing is detailed in Chapter 17.)

REFERENCES

Anderson R and McCoy J: *Anatomy of a lease,* South Barrington, IL, 1984, Leasing Associates of Barrington.

Ball KA: Procuring a laser system, *AORN J* 54(5): 1049-1055, Nov 1991.

For laser services not rendered: Where's the bottom line?, *Clinical Laser Monthly,* pp 100-102, July 1993.

Laser payments cut under RBRVS; site of service penalties imposed, *Clinical Laser Monthly,* pp 62-64, April 1993.

New code modifier for lasers?, *Clinical Laser Monthly,* p 133, Sept 1993.

SUGGESTED READINGS

Apfelberg DB, editor: *Evaluation and installation of surgical laser systems,* New York, 1987, Springer-Verlag.

Ball KA: The impact of reimbursement requirements on local anesthesia laser surgery, *Laser Nursing* 5(2):67-68, Summer 1991.

Ball KA, guest editor: Seminars in perioperative nursing, *Lasers,* 1(2):61-66, April 1992, WB Saunders Co.

Bundling laser fees with OR charges draws physicians, *Clinical Laser Monthly,* pp 118-125, Aug 1993.

Buying a new laser? Training and maintenance are key factors, *Clinical Laser Monthly,* pp 177-179, Nov 1993.

Collins T: Acquiring a new laser, *Minimally Invasive Surgical Nursing* 7(2):57-59, Summer 1993.

Laser personnel build solid case for IRB approval, *Clinical Laser Monthly,* pp 159-164, Oct 1993.

Maley RA and Epstein AL: *High technology in health care, risk management perspectives,* Chicago, 1993, American Hospital Association.

Morrison DM: Capital equipment for endoscopic and laparoscopic surgery, *Minimally Invasive Surgical Nursing* 7(1):24-25, Spring 1993.

Per-case rental could solve scheduling, financing problems, *Clinical Laser Monthly,* pp 14-16, Jan 1994.

16

LEGAL ASPECTS OF
LASER SURGERY

A s laser technology continues to grow, so does the number and variety of legal pitfalls that accompany it. New laser procedures involving specialties from neurosurgery to podiatry are being introduced as clinical investigations continue to enhance the technology. As the potential of the laser is discovered, increased patient benefits are realized. The standard of care is changing because the laser provides less invasive surgery, less hospitalization, and quicker recovery. Because of the dynamic nature of laser technology, many legal problems may arise within a laser program. Legalities regarding laser program administration, patient consent and education, and physician liability must be addressed.

LASER PROGRAM ADMINISTRATION
Standards of Care

Standards of care exist for laser technology today. Every laser program, no matter how small, should have a laser committee or a laser subcommittee of the surgical committee to develop standards of care. A standard is a written value statement that defines a level of performance established by expert consensus (Allard, 1993). The American National Standards Institute (ANSI) developed the standard Z136.3 to address laser safety in health care environments. This standard is meant to be used as a guideline for facilities in developing safety policies and procedures.

The Laser Committee should participate in total quality management for the laser program and formulate policies and procedures for the safety of the patient, physician, and staff. Written guidelines should be established and communicated before the laser is used within the facility. If a hospital does not have any written policies, then a patient may be able to sue based on another facility's standards. The patient may also be able to sue the hospital for failure to act reasonably by not initially adopting protective standards (Schwartz and Zaslow, 1985a).

Trends in the health care environment indicate that the national standard of care is becoming accepted as standard practice (Schwartz and Liberator, 1985b). This movement toward national standards is beginning to negate geographic distinction as hospitals using similar lasers are being held liable for the national standard of care regardless of location.

Therefore, the smaller rural hospital with only one CO_2 laser is expected to provide the same standard of care as a large teaching hospital with 20 laser systems.

One national standard of care that has developed in laser technology requires that a laser team member be available whenever a laser is used. This person is responsible for ensuring that the laser safety standards written in the hospital's guidelines are being followed. The laser team member is also held liable for understanding laser safety and procedures. For example, a laser team member who knowingly repairs a laser fiber incorrectly is legally responsible for potential injury to the patient. If the laser team member turns on air to purge the Nd:YAG fiber during an endometrial ablation and the patient suffers from an air embolism, the laser team member can be implicated. Because of the Respondeat Superior standard, the employer is also responsible for the employee's actions because the employee acted within the scope of the employment conditions (Schwartz and Zaslow, 1985b).

A second circulating nurse is recommended because the laser must be put in the standby mode when not being used. The circulating nurse should not be expected to assume the responsibility for laser operation and assistance along with performing circulating duties. For example, if the circulating nurse is too busy to place the laser in standby and the laser is inadvertently activated, causing the drapes to catch on fire, the hospital would be liable for not providing another circulating nurse or a laser team member to operate the laser (because this is the national standard of care). The laser should always be respected as a potentially hazardous piece of equipment, and safety measures must be strictly enforced.

Documentation

Documentation helps minimize liability at a later date. Documenting the laser wavelength, power, pulse duration, tissue type involved, and various safety measures followed (e.g., special endotracheal tube, smoke evacuation in place) provides an adequate report of the laser use. Documentation of laser parameters should be made on the patient's chart on the operative record. Many facilities also opt to complete a laser log to generalize laser utilization so that trends can be noted. If the laser use is only documented on the laser log, the log must be approved by the hospital as a permanent part of the patient's record (Ball, 1987). Complete laser documentation is invaluable to help recall actions taken if testimony is needed during a lawsuit.

Proper documentation of laser-related accidents is mandatory. Even the most insignificant incidents should be reported in written form because even minor injuries could result in complications. Documentation should always be factual and objective and should not place blame on anyone. Each state has different rules regarding the discoverability and confidentiality of incident reports.

Reports of infractions of laser safety or incidents of injury to patients should be presented to the Laser Committee for review. The risk manager of the hospital should also be actively involved in promoting laser safety. Sensitivity to laser incidents can help in enforcing laser safety guidelines. Appropriate changes can be made when deficiencies are pointed out tactfully.

Defective laser equipment should be immediately removed from service. The hospital should have policies that address malfunctioning lasers that include the following:

- Monitoring process for identifying product hazards
- Method for handling product recalls

- Procedure for removing defective laser equipment from service for evaluation or repair
- Procedure for reporting laser equipment that has been involved with a patient injury or death
- Method for reporting equipment failure that could have caused injury to patients, staff members, physicians, or visitors

Investigation into a device failure should be conducted by experienced technical personnel. Persons without appropriate knowledge and skill should not be allowed to examine the device. Any products used during a procedure in which the patient was injured must be removed from service until the reason for the failure is determined. The following process is recommended when a device fails:

1. Complete an incident report immediately.
2. Remove the equipment from service immediately.
3. Document the event completely and carefully.
4. Preserve the equipment so that an investigation can be completed.

On November 28, 1990, the Safe Medical Device Act (SMDA) became law, expanding the authority of the Food and Drug Administration (FDA) to regulate medical devices. This ruling requires reporting to the FDA any serious illness, serious injury, or death caused by a medical device in hospitals, nursing homes, ambulatory surgery sites, outpatient treatment and diagnostic facilities, and sites of home health care providers. Unfortunately, this law does not regulate physicians' offices and therefore is very inconsistent because many procedures are performed in physicians' offices. Reporting must take place within 10 days after determining that the device caused the problem. Reportable illnesses or injuries include those that:

- Are life threatening
- Result in permanent impairment of a body function or permanent damage to a body structure
- Necessitate medical or surgical intervention to preclude permanent impairment to a body function or permanent damage to a body structure (Maley and Epstein, 1993, p. 34)

Hospitals usually delegate the responsibility of reporting adverse events to the risk manager. A summary of reported events must be made every July and January. The risk manager must understand the reporting process completely.

In June 1993 a new FDA program was implemented, called MEDWatch. This is a voluntary system that encourages reporting of adverse events caused by products regulated by the FDA. The simplified form does not require identification of the patient but does require information relevant to the device failure and the patient's condition.

The FDA recommends that a facility develop a device report decision-making team to determine what should and should not be reported. A decision flow chart should be designed so that an investigating FDA agent can easily note how decisions were made. The FDA suggests that copies of reports to the FDA and to the device manufacturer be kept for at least 2 years.

Documentation of electrical equipment service and preventive maintenance is required by the Joint Commission for the Accreditation of Healthcare Organizations (JCAHO).

Since the laser is a piece of electrical equipment, it must be maintained according to these standards. A written policy or job description should define who is responsible for preventive maintenance and service. A centralized file containing this information not only helps document the service or maintenance, but also notes trends in equipment care. A maintenance log decreases the liability of the hospital by showing that the laser is maintained in good working order. The maintenance log also traces the status of any ongoing problems so that they can be identified and solved. Computerized service and maintenance records help with storage, quick retrieval, and determining trends. The service history of a laser can be easily traced from a computerized log to note when replacement is necessary.

Environmental Controls

Environmental controls are needed to provide a safe environment for employees. Since laser technology can be damaging to eyes, many facilities have incorporated eye examinations for staff members into the laser program. A baseline eye examination is performed initially; another is required after any laser ophthalmological incident. When the staff member terminates employment with the hospital, another eye examination is performed to document optical health to decrease the possibility of future litigation or challenge litigation if appropriate. These examinations do not ensure safe laser practices.

Physician Credentialing

Physician credentialing is another legal aspect in the administration of a laser program. Laser conferences offer certification of attendance at a laser conference but normally do not credential the physician as a safe laser user. Therefore, every hospital must develop a physician credentialing policy to regulate laser use within the confines of their own health care facility. Most laser credentialing policies require attendance at a hands-on laser course and completing a preceptorship to become credentialed in laser use.

A facility's policy should not state that if a physician is credentialed at another area hospital, then laser privileges are granted at their own facility. This places the facility in a compromising position if the laser coursework needs to be presented during a lawsuit and is located elsewhere.

Copies of the physician's laser course and preceptorship should be kept on file in the Medical Staff Office. The JCAHO may inspect the files to note if this information is available or if a written hospital policy requires its presence. Many times a credentialing log book is kept in the surgical department or laser area to trace the credentialing status of each physician. As the number of physicians using the laser continues to grow, a credentialing log book is vital for quick reference. This log must be kept current to provide accurate information and must be shared regularly with the laser team.

Maintaining privileges today to perform particular procedures, such as infertility surgery, often require that a minimum number of procedures be performed each year to maintain credentialing. For many hospitals, performing a certain number of laser procedures is required to continue laser credentialing. This policy has caused much dismay and concern for physicians who only perform a few laser surgeries each year. Hospitals are developing these types of policies to decrease potential liability, to provide a safe environment for the patient, and to ensure that a high skill level is maintained by the physician. Providing a program of continuing education and preceptoring will help sustain the physician's competence and proficiency.

Physicians already credentialed in laser use often question the liability involved when they function as a preceptor for another physician. Some reports have noted that if the preceptoring physician does not charge the patient for his or her role during the procedure, the preceptoring physician is not liable. Other reports indicate that the preceptoring physician is liable for any laser-related patient injury during the preceptorship. Government regulations and previous court rulings must be studied to arrive at an answer to this legal liability dilemma.

Total Quality Management

Total quality management of a laser program can be tedious but results note that patient safety is guaranteed, injuries are minimized, and lawsuits are decreased. Three key elements in assisting with quality management are education, networking, and personnel support (*Clinical Laser Monthly*, January 1994). Education includes continual offerings to enhance the knowledge and skills of physicians and laser team members. Innovative patient education helps patients gain a thorough understanding of the laser procedure. Networking fosters the sharing of information by physicians and laser team members. Learning from others assists in noting procedural techniques, adverse reactions, safety considerations, and a host of other laser technology concerns. Providing personnel support helps build a strong infrastructure to implement the goals of the laser program. By providing an environment that continually strengthens the experience of the laser team, maximum support can be offered during each laser procedure. All of these factors help provide strong bonds that will advance a laser program to a level of excellence.

Outcome analysis provides information to a laser program so that constant changes can be made to continuously improve laser services. Today's health care environment must be accountable for surgical results and must provide continuous quality improvement (CQI) to obtain better patient outcomes. CQI is based on the theory that quality can be improved on a continual basis. Everyone must participate in this activity to make it work. The process involves collecting data, involving everyone in identifying problems and solutions, and implementing changes as needed.

Facilities focused on proving value and improving quality are the ones who will survive in the current competitive health care arena. Analyzing outcomes requires that every patient be monitored so that CQI can be achieved. This takes time, effort, and money to conduct adequately, and the research must be honest. Even the negative events or results must be exposed. A mere sampling is not enough for a comprehensive quality assurance program. Computerization has facilitated the task of documenting and examining information to detect trends. Databases are being developed that can make outcome analysis affordable and meaningful.

PATIENT CONSENT AND EDUCATION
Patient Consent

Patient consent has presented another legal quandary. Patient informed consent should address the various laser procedure risks and benefits. Patients must also be made aware of the alternatives to laser surgical intervention so they can make an educated choice between laser or conventional surgery. The consent form should communicate that the physician may have to proceed with conventional surgery if unforeseen conditions arise, such as laser system failure, or if laser use is later deemed inappropriate for the patient condition noted. Patients often regard laser surgery as a panacea and are extremely disappointed if the laser was not used during the procedure.

Written consent merely verifies that the physician has discussed the procedure with the patient. Too often, more emphasis is placed on whether the consent form is signed than whether the patient fully understands the impending laser procedure. There is a major difference between signing the written consent form and giving an educated informed consent for the procedure. Patients should never be asked to sign a consent form after a sedative or an anesthetic has been administered. Emergency treatment that saves the life of a patient does not require consent unless it is known in advance that the patient did not want emergency treatment (Maley and Epstein, 1993, p. 32).

The informed consent procedure begins in the physician's office when the decision to perform the procedure has been made. At this time, the physician should discuss the procedure with the patient and explain that the laser may or will be used. The patient's knowledge and anxiety level should be assessed to determine proper understanding of the procedure. The nurse helps to restate and reinforce what the physician discusses with the patient. The written consent form can be signed at this time or on the day of the surgery, when the patient's level of understanding about the procedure is again determined. If more patient education is required to provide informed consent, the physician or nurse can again discuss the procedure with the patient. Procedure-specific written materials or video tapes can enhance this education process.

In completing the written consent form, many physicians prefer to document that the laser may or will be used during the procedure to provide as much information to the patient as possible. Some physicians prefer not to note the specific laser type because more than one laser wavelength may be used during the same procedure.

Proper informed consent about laser surgery is very important because this new technology is often misinterpreted by patients as being the miracle cure that the media often describes. For example, a patient may expect a complete lightening of a port-wine stain, when in reality the laser may only produce a 70% lightening. Laser technology has in some instances produced extraordinary results, but each patient must thoroughly understand the anticipated outcome of a particular procedure so that expectations are realistic. Emphasis must be placed on open and truthful communication with the patient to build rapport. The best assurance is showing the patient a caring attitude and ensuring that the patient truly understands the laser surgical application. Caring health care professionals tend to stay out of the courtroom.

If a patient refuses to sign a consent for the laser procedure, this should be documented on the patient's chart. The hospital risk manager should be notified, especially if refusing the laser procedure could compromise the patient's well-being.

Patient Education

Patient education is imperative in laser intervention, and clear communication is critical during a laser procedure. The patient must understand the intraoperative instructions and the rationale for the action. For example, a patient undergoing a local-anesthesia surgical procedure must realize the need to remain still while the laser is being activated. The nurse is instrumental in supporting the patient during this period. If the patient moves during a crucial time and injury occurs, the patient may think that suing for neglect is appropriate. In reality, the patient may be held liable for contributory neglect if instructions were given as to the necessity of remaining still during the procedure.

Immobility during laser surgery is critical during delicate procedures when precision is vital. Anesthesiologists are becoming more cognizant of their responsibility to provide total muscle relaxation during laser surgery in which any patient movement could cause injury during laser activation. Negligence on the anesthesiologist's part could easily become a debatable issue (Cerullo and Koht, 1983).

According to JCAHO requirements, ambulatory surgery patients should receive written postoperative instructions (JCAHO, 1988). Special discharge instruction forms can be designed for each laser procedure specialty, such as endoscopy, gynecology, dermatology, ophthalmology, and podiatry. Frequently, the patient is asked to sign the form, which indicates that the postoperative instructions were discussed with the patient. Ideally, one copy of the form remains as a permanent record on the chart, and the patient receives the other copy. Liability is minimized when the patient understands the rationale and action needed during the postoperative phase of the laser procedure. The purposes of the written postoperative discharge instructions are to:

- Ensure continuity and consistency in perioperative care
- Reinforce the postoperative care instructions that were discussed with the patient
- Provide legal documentation indicating that the patient received written postoperative discharge instructions
- Provide contact information for the patient should any complications arise after discharge (the hospital and/or physician's emergency phone numbers)

PHYSICIAN LIABILITY

Physician liability has become an issue because laser technology is relatively new. Currently, malpractice insurance rates are not increased when the physician uses the laser for surgical procedures. The physician must possess a basic knowledge of laser physics, laser-tissue interaction, safety, and appropriate application before becoming credentialed. The physician should know how to assemble the laser equipment before a surgical procedure. If a malfunction occurs, the physician should be able to determine where the problem exists. And even though the laser team member is expected to perform a preoperative laser safety and performance check, the physician is ultimately responsible for this action (Schwartz, 1983). For example, the laser team member tests the alignment of the CO_2 beam with the aiming beam before the laser procedure. If the physician does not realize that the beams are out of alignment and causes injury to the patient, litigation could occur. The physician could be held liable for not assuming the responsibility for checking such a critical factor as beam alignment, and the laser team member could be held liable for not communicating that the laser beam was out of alignment.

The need for laser intervention continues to cause debate among some physicians. Since the technology is still in its infancy, application disagreements between doctors can occur. What one physician considers to be the standard of care, another physician may deem negligent (Schwartz, 1985). For example, a gynecologist who uses 35 W of CO_2 laser power to ablate the cervix may be considered negligent by a physician who uses 10 W. Expert witnesses sometimes have opposite opinions on laser application because the technology's standards are still being developed.

A physician who purchases a laser for office use must understand the liability implications when the laser is used by another physician. If the laser functions properly, and the owner cannot prove that the borrowing physician has deviated from the standard of care, the owner of the laser could be held liable for a patient injury. The owner of the laser could also be held negligent for not screening the borrowing physician's laser expertise level. Sometimes a physician who owns a laser system may offer the laser to another physician only after an indemnification agreement has been signed by the borrowing physician releasing the owner from liability (Schwartz and Liberator, 1985a).

After a laser is procured, an innovative physician or biomedical laser technician may decide to alter the laser to enhance its efficiency or power. Modifying the internal components of the laser could change the unit from FDA approved to experimental. Any alteration shifts liability from the manufacturer to whoever made the changes on the laser (Murphy, 1984). Any alteration or modification of the laser unit should be scrutinized for possible liability changes.

Laser technology has developed and expanded quickly over the past decade. This ever-changing field will continue to grow at an astonishing pace as long as ideas and interest flourish. There are legal ramifications to this whirlwind of activities. Today's standard of care may be changed with tomorrow's developments. Until laser applications become more stable and permanent, legal pitfalls will be present. Health care facilities must carefully develop their laser programs so that the potential for risk and liability is minimized. Unplanned and inconsistent laser programs are destined for failure; a single negligence suit that results from poor preparation can cause the downfall of the entire laser program.

REFERENCES

Allard D: Defining performance expectations for laser nurses and technicians, *Clinical Laser Monthly*, pp 12-15, Jan 1993.

Ball K: Legal aspects of laser surgery, *Today's OR Nurse* 9(2):23 Feb 1987.

Cerullo L and Koht A: Anesthesiologic considerations in laser neurosurgery, *Lasers Surg Med* 3:38, 1983.

Joint Commission on Accreditation of Healthcare Organizations: Accreditation Manual for Hospitals, Chicago, 1988, JCAHO.

Maley RA and Epstein AL: High technology in health care, risk management perspectives, Chicago, 1993, American Hospital Association.

Murphy E: Legal implication of OR laser use, *Today's OR Nurse* 6(6):32, 1984.

Risk management and quality assurance are keys to low injury rate, *Clinical Laser Monthly*, p 5, Jan 1994.

Schwartz D, editor: Expert legal comments on 13 clinical laser dilemmas, *Companion publication to Clinical Laser Monthly*, p 7, 1983.

Schwartz D: Uniform protocols keep laser programs out of the courtroom, *Clinical Laser Monthly* 3(11):125, 1985.

Schwartz D and Liberator J: Legal question. *Clinical Laser Monthly* 3(4):47, 1985a.

Schwartz D and Liberator J: Legal question. *Clinical Laser Monthly* 3(10):117, 1985b.

Schwartz D and Zaslow J: Legal question. *Clinical Laser Monthly* 3(1):5, 1985a.

Schwartz D and Zaslow J: Legal question. *Clinical Laser Monthly* 3(6):71, 1985b.

SUGGESTED READINGS

Ball KA, guest editor: Seminars in perioperative nursing, *Lasers* Vol. 1, No. 2, April 1992, WB Saunders Co.

Laser programs embracing quality improvement process, *Clinical Laser Monthly*, pp 97-100, July 1993.

Outcomes analysis: Proving value and improving quality, *Clinical Laser Monthly*, pp 165-168, Nov 1993.

17

MARKETING A
LASER PROGRAM

Because laser technology is constantly evolving, marketing efforts are needed to communicate the success of laser surgery. A current definition of marketing is "the analysis, planning, implementation, and control of carefully formulated programs designed to bring about voluntary exchanges of values with target markets for the purpose of achieving organizational objectives" (Kotler, 1979).

Historically, hospitals have marketed according to internal facility needs, promoting services designed to affect the consumer. This traditional marketing is being replaced with marketing efforts geared toward satisfying patient needs and being responsive to changing needs as mandated by the patient.

Health care marketing is now being scrutinized carefully by hospital administrators because of intense competition. Since laser technology is experiencing tremendous growth, competition is becoming exceedingly acute in the laser arena. Physicians and administrators are realizing the need to educate the community and the referring physicians on the benefits derived from the laser.

After meticulous planning, a laser program is developed to meet a variety of patient needs. Many programs deteriorate when they fail to follow through with a marketing plan to initiate or increase laser utilization. Therefore, the "dusty laser syndrome" occurs as large amounts of money are dedicated to pay for laser units, supplies, and specialized staffing, but because of the lack of marketing, the lasers are not used (Ball, 1987). The physicians become upset because there are no patients to use the laser on, the administrators are disappointed because the physicians are not using the expensive laser equipment, and the laser team is disgusted because they are not using their special laser training. The missing link is marketing to promote the laser to the community.

DEVELOPING A MARKETING PLAN

Marketing is the combination of art and science to satisfy patient needs and wants through an exchange process. A marketing plan is dynamic and should be able to be altered as patient needs change.

Developing a marketing plan is very similar to developing a business plan but not quite as involved. The components are basically the same, but the wording focuses on marketing issues.

External and Internal Assessment

An *external assessment* must be made to analyze the laser market for health care applications. This analysis documents laser technology in general and notes trends over the years. This foundation will provide information significant in recognizing the overall direction of lasers in medicine and surgery. Libraries, workshops, and visits to other laser facilities can offer references for the development and expansion of laser programs. Information on trends can be derived from studying articles about laser technology in professional journals. Over 11.5 million surgical procedures are performed each year; of these, an estimated 40% could utilize laser technology (Swergold, Chevitz, and Sinsabaugh, Inc., 1987). Therefore, laser technology continues to grow as new procedures and wavelengths are developed.

The external environment must be explored to note consumer needs and the competition's marketing efforts. Discovering what the consumer wants and how other hospitals are promoting their laser programs can be vital in charting the direction of a marketing plan. Questions must be answered, such as:

Are other hospitals offering more specialized and skilled laser team members to support the program?
Are the laser services at another facility more convenient and personalized?
What laser equipment and supplies are being used at other hospitals?
What marketing efforts are being made to promote other laser programs in the area?
How many laser procedures are being performed at other facilities?
What physicians are performing laser procedures at other facilities?
How does the administration financially support a laser program?
What does the patient understand about laser technology?
What are the patient's needs when laser surgery is performed?
What are the patient's expectations of laser surgery?

An *internal assessment* must also be made to note the strengths and weaknesses of existing resources within the hospital. Performing a thorough self-examination can help in determining the status of a laser program and planning for the future. Resources must be identified and questions asked, such as:

How many laser procedures are currently being performed?
What do the physicians already know about laser technology and how can they help promote the laser program?
Which physicians are credentialed in laser use, and are they using the laser at other hospitals?
Which laser specialty areas or procedures are most profitable for the hospital?
What monies have been budgeted for marketing the laser program?
What type of marketing and advertising plans have been successful for the hospital in the past?

What internal capabilities of the hospital can provide marketing efforts (e.g., writing the script for a television commercial, providing camera-ready art for newspaper ads, surveying and evaluating a marketing program's success)?

Which personnel can be used to assist in marketing a laser program?

How much interest and enthusiasm is there for the laser program?

What do the various hospital departments know about the laser program?

In what direction is the laser program headed with the existing laser technology at the hospital? Are newer laser systems needed before marketing can be implemented to offer the most current technology?

How much administrative support can be expected?

What do patients like about the existing laser services?

Can the marketing plan address the concerns of the patients, physicians, and laser team members?

After a comprehensive study has been externally and internally conducted and reviewed, a determination of where the laser program can fit into the arena of local competition can be made. Opportunities for the laser program can be highlighted, and threats to the viability and growth of the program can be noted.

Establishing the Focus of the Marketing Plan

Defining the *objectives* is the next step in developing a comprehensive marketing plan. Objectives must be measurable so that they can be appropriately evaluated to note what was accomplished. Objectives should be specific, attainable, and documented in writing. They should begin with "to" followed by an action verb. For example, the following short-term objectives could be developed for a laser program for achievement within 1 year:

- To increase laser utilization by 15% over that of the previous year
- To expand the number of physicians credentialed to use the laser by 10%
- To plan and conduct four physician laser conferences
- To plan and conduct three training programs for laser team members
- To implement a preoperative laser education program for inpatients
- To develop a patient education brochure that explains local-anesthesia laser surgery
- To present laser technology to 10 community organizations
- To conduct laser inservice presentations for five other departments within the hospital
- To arrange for a training program with hands-on laser experience for the new residents each July

A laser marketing program should be geared toward educating patients and physicians about laser technology, and be sensitive to meeting their needs in providing this service. Open communication among everyone involved in the marketing plan is paramount. This ensures continuity, in that everyone is participating to achieve the same goals to enhance the program while meeting the needs of consumers. When everyone is involved, ownership of the program is felt, and dedication is fostered. For example, when laser team members are asked to become involved in developing a marketing plan, their motivation to participate in the implementation is heightened.

Identifying the *target audience* is the next phase in developing a marketing plan. The patient is usually the primary target because patient-focused care is the critical element in the competition and survival of hospitals today. The patient target can be determined by studying the geographics (location or zip code delineations), demographics (age, income, race, education, sex, family status, occupation, etc.), and psychographics (lifestyles and attitudes) of the potential groups. Traditionally, the female is the health care decision maker of the family, so many laser marketing programs are often targeted toward women over age 30. Secondary targets could be the potential laser-using physicians or the referring physicians. When the primary and secondary targets have been identified, all marketing efforts should consistently be geared toward them.

Determining the *position* of the laser program involves defining distinctive characteristics. The laser program's uniqueness should be determined so that patients and physicians will be attracted to the laser services. Concluding where the laser program currently stands and where those involved would like the laser program to be, can help in making decisions regarding the marketing niche to be filled or an exceptional characteristic that is needed to draw attention to the program. Creativity is extremely helpful in conveying the uniqueness of the program. Being recognized for a specific characteristic allows the program to be easily identified.

Budgetary commitment must be resolved before a marketing plan is implemented. If there are financial limitations, the marketing plan must be altered to accommodate them. An ongoing review of monies spent during the marketing plan's implementation should be conducted so that the plan can proceed with no surprise expenditures that could hinder the progress of the program. The value of the marketing plan must be scrutinized for its long-term and overall success. A return on investment cannot necessarily be realized immediately from the direct efforts of marketing.

IMPLEMENTING A MARKETING PLAN

Implementation of the marketing plan is the next step in the marketing process. Open communication should be maintained during this phase so that everyone involved with the plan is acutely aware of the various marketing projects and schedules. For example, the laser team must be prepared to answer questions and make physician referrals after a television commercial about the laser program has been shown.

When implementing a marketing plan, everyone involved should carefully study each objective to make sure achievement can be maximized. For example, the objective "to increase the number of credentialed physicians" can be achieved through a variety of approaches. Physicians in multispecialties can be inspired to use laser technology by presenting information about clinical applications and patient outcomes. Networking can be valuable when physicians encourage their colleagues to use the laser. Often a practice laboratory helps physicians become more skilled so they feel more secure about using the laser clinically.

Increased laser utilization can also be promoted when the names of physicians who use the laser are given to the referring physicians. Letters sent to referring physicians can help educate them about the laser services available, clinical techniques, and expected outcomes when a laser is used.

Open communication with physicians about the laser program will increase interest. A one-page description of the laser program or new laser advances can be handed out at medical staff meetings to promote interest. A periodic newsletter sent to referring and specialty physicians can highlight laser procedures or new developments so that the laser program is constantly being recognized. Potential laser users can be identified and personally contacted to help them find the appropriate laser training program. Presentations at professional meetings can provide testimonials from physicians about their experiences with laser technology.

Marketing can be achieved through advertising, personal selling, sales promotion, and publicity. A combination of these different methods is usually necessary to promote the laser program in the most cost-effective manner.

Advertising

If money is available for advertising, information about a laser program can easily reach its target audience. The best way to impact the prospective target must be determined within budget constraints. The advertising campaign should strive to get the most promotion for the least money. A look at the competition and where others are in the advertising marketplace will help to guide advertising efforts.

Those involved should not make promises to the consumer through advertising. Liability may become an issue if the advertising states that the laser is the answer to all problems. Qualifying words such as "the laser *may be* an alternative to conventional surgery" or "the laser *may be* used for a particular procedure" are preferable.

An advertising campaign should also present the possible benefits of laser surgery to the public and should not focus on the laser program itself. Consumers want to hear or read how the laser will benefit them. Simple words and phrases are easily retained by the consumer who may be attracted. The advertisement should draw attention and interest and arouse a desire for action. It also should promote commitment from the laser program to address the needs of the patient.

If the hospital does not have an active marketing or public relations department, an outside agency may be used to assist with the advertisement of the laser program. The steps involved in selecting and working with an outside advertising agency are as follows (Roman and Maas, 1976):

1. Determine what is to be expected from the advertising agency.
2. Survey agencies that appear to have experience in health care advertising, have a professional and knowledgeable staff, have a philosophy about advertising objectives similar to the laser program, and are the appropriate size to provide the needed services.
3. Interview the selected agencies and discuss the budgetary limitations and objectives of the campaign. The agency should provide a work sample and a list of references. These references should be checked for client satisfaction.
4. Determine which agency will best meet the advertising needs of the laser program. Honestly discuss the money available for advertising. Discuss the planning and implementation phase of the campaign and the degree of desired involvement in the advertising decisions.
5. After the contract has been signed, continue to be involved with the campaign. If an idea or an ad is not appropriate, tell the agency immediately so that the needed changes can be made.

6. Be consistent with deadlines, and always review any advertisements.
7. Set up informal work sessions with the advertising agency to discuss and foster creative advertising.
8. If you are not satisfied with the agency's representative and products, ask that a new person be assigned to the account. Don't immediately change agencies.
9. Monitor the expenditures of the agency to ensure appropriate use of the marketing budget.

Determining which type of media will be the most successful often is difficult when marketing a laser program. Statistics have shown that consumers obtain most information about a health care product or service from print media, such as newspapers. Television advertising and physician referrals are also important in supplying information to the consumer. The patient can also receive details about a laser program from hospital employees and friends.

All ads should have similar components: Purpose, target, uniqueness, response mechanism, tone, and synergism. Each ad must have a purpose. The target audience needs to be identified and reached. The consumer should be able to readily determine the uniqueness of the service or product through the innovative message that is communicated. In response to the ad, the consumer should be called to action. For example, the phone number for laser information should be highlighted so the consumer will easily be able to contact the facility. The tone of the ad should promote a personality or attitude that attracts the consumer. Synergism or consistency should prevail, through the use of similar colors, themes, layout, or typefaces in advertising materials so all ads can immediately be identified with a particular laser program.

Reach and frequency must be addressed to achieve the expected results of the advertising campaign. Reach is the number of people the ad is intended to affect during each event, or the coverage per run. Frequency is the number of times that the ad must be shown to affect the total number or percentage of the audience desired. For example, an ad must usually be run six times in print for a target audience to realize the message that is being conveyed (Dubuque, 1988).

A laser advertising campaign is usually most effective when a media mixture is used to reach the client. A variety of media avenues are available for advertising a laser program, including newspaper, radio, television, outdoor advertising, or direct mail. Each of these approaches have specific characteristics that should be studied to determine the most advantageous ways to promote a laser program.

The *newspaper* is the backbone of advertising, with a market area penetration of 60%. Usually persons aged 35 to 64 with higher income and more education than average read the newspaper most often. This audience can easily understand a rather complicated specialty such as laser surgery. The newspaper is often read during leisure time because it is readily available in the home, and Sunday is the most significant newspaper reading day for leisure readers. Friday's edition is usually read by younger people, while Saturday's newspaper is more often read by the elderly. The Wednesday edition is read widely by females because this midweek newspaper is usually full of shopping coupons. The morning newspapers are often read by business people (Dubuque, 1988).

The newspaper can be retained by the reader for future reference so that a response can be made to the ad. Because the newspaper ad can be read over and over, a complicated advertisement scheme can be used. Usually the simpler ads are read first, though.

The headline of the ad should capture the reader's attention because it is read twice as often as the body of the ad. The target audience is frequently attracted to the advertisement by its pictorial appeal. If people are pictured in the ad, warmth and caring can be conveyed through touch. The type in the ad should be large enough so that the consumer can easily read the print without exertion. Serif print (letters with feet) is easier to read than sans serif print (letters without feet) (Dubuque, 1988).

A newspaper advertising campaign can be very effective if the same location and position on the page is used every time the ad is run. If several different ads are to be used during a campaign, an identifiable trait in each ad should create immediate awareness to link the ad to a specific laser program.

Radio offers a quick, opportunistic approach as a good supplemental medium for reinforcing advertisements in the newspaper or on television. The same announcer should be used for every radio advertisement to promote consistency and decrease confusion since the radio only offers audio imagery. The radio is listened to by the upper-middle and upper classes while driving to and from work between the hours of 7:00 and 9:00 AM and 4:00 and 6:00 PM (Dubuque, 1988). Most listeners will alternate between two favorite radio stations, so the most popular radio stations need to be determined for an area.

The laser program phone number should be readily identifiable and repeated so that the audience can retain the information. The initial wording must immediately grab the audience's attention and the product or service should be mentioned frequently. The words should be kept simple so that the audience can easily listen and appreciate the message.

A memorable sound should be heard during the radio ad that readily reminds the listener about the laser program if heard again. A distinguishing sound or piece of music that is different from the normal sounds of the radio station should be used to grab the listener's attention. For example, if you are advertising on a country radio station, country background music should be avoided.

Some laser programs have found that the radio is not the appropriate medium for advertising laser surgery. Because the laser beam consists of light and light is visual, radio cannot easily convey the concept of laser surgery. Often monies that were used for radio advertising have been shifted to newspaper or television ads to provide the visual component.

Television commercials have high penetration into the target audience with a basic buy achieving 85% to 90% market penetration (Dubuque, 1988). Television advertising is expensive because the commercial must first be produced and then time must be bought to show the commercial. Television is an excellent medium for promoting a new product or service. Statistics show that NBC is viewed the most frequently across the United States, whereas ABC appeals to a younger audience, and CBS appeals to older groups (Dubuque, 1988). Advertising on cable television during reruns of popular shows is an excellent way to reach select audiences. Television advertising is skewed towards the less educated and lower income consumers.

A television ad should capture the viewer's attention within the first 5 seconds (Dubuque, 1988). The commercial must be simple, with a key identifiable characteristic that is carried throughout the ad. The name of the laser program should appear frequently, and the call for action or the phone number should also be displayed.

The tone of the commercial should match the product or service being promoted. Therefore, laser surgery should be complemented by high-technology music and visuals. Testimonials from patients often establish credibility for the advertisement. Animation can be used selectively to help reinforce the message of the ad. A laser program with caring health care professionals can easily be portrayed in a television commercial. An ad with a nurse holding a patient's hand during the laser procedure conveys the warmth and security that the audience is sensitive to.

A television ad must be repeated to reach the expected target. The process of buying time can be done through an experienced agent who understands the system and can get the most advertisement for the amount of money budgeted.

Outdoor advertising has been used lately by health care facilities. Outdoor advertising, such as that on billboards, has a higher reach than television and a higher frequency than radio (Dubuque, 1988). This type of advertising can be very cost-effective and should be used as a supplemental medium. Statistics show that the cost of reaching 1,000 people with outdoor advertising is 10 to 30 times less than that of other media, such as newspaper, television, and radio (Dubuque, 1988).

Outdoor advertising usually obtains the best results if the community already has been introduced to the product or service being advertised. If a laser program is already recognized within a geographical area, then outdoor advertising could be very effective. The billboard illustrates services or products as larger than life, so simplicity must be the rule. Since many people drive by a billboard quickly, the message must be short and to the point. A characteristic theme should make the ad immediately identifiable as representing the laser program.

Direct mail is another advertising medium that can be very cost-effective. Since mailing lists are readily available, a specific target can be easily reached. The elderly tend to read direct mail more often than the young do. Complicated messages are easily conveyed in direct mail since space is not a problem. The envelope or the opening words must attract the reader so that the entire ad will be read. The reader should be inspired to respond to the ad immediately, and the response mechanism must be easily performed. For example, a direct mailing could request the reader to place the "Yes" sticker on the return request for more information on laser surgery. Advertising efforts using the direct mail method are usually more successful if a personalized letter can be included.

Whenever advertising promotes a telephone number to call for further information, there must be a voice to respond at the other end of the telephone line. If the laser program has specific hours of operation, then an answering machine should be purchased to take messages when calls are received during the off-shift hours. Messages and requests should be acknowledged promptly to maintain interest and generate business.

When a patient asks about the possibility of a laser being used for a certain medical condition, a nonphysician should not respond; instead, the patient should be referred to a physician who uses the laser. If the laser is not appropriate for a particular condition or surgery, the physician should be the one to relay this information to the patient. If contact between the physician and the patient has been established and the physician has determined that the laser is not appropriate for a particular procedure, a patient-physician relationship has been developed. The patient may then use the physician's services for other conditions.

Personal Selling

If budgetary limitations are placed on a marketing plan, less expensive and more creative ways to market the laser program must be instituted. Personal selling has tremendous impact in increasing the visibility of the laser program.

Speaking engagements on laser technology scheduled by the program director, physicians, or laser team members can help increase the recognition of the program tremendously. Kiwanis clubs, Rotary organizations, Lions clubs, or church groups who meet on a regular basis are usually interested in inviting speakers to talk about the latest advances in health care. A slide presentation can appropriately and simply illustrate laser technology from a description of what a laser is to the various clinical applications. Most community organizations request speakers to present a 30- to 45-minute program. The slide show can be enhanced by the distribution of a brochure or pamphlet that describes the laser services. The telephone number of the laser program should be readily available so that anyone who wants to request more information can call at a later date.

Physicians or nurses involved with the laser program can also volunteer to speak at professional organizations on their experiences with laser technology. Testimonials or success stories help validate the program and encourage other physicians to use laser services.

Laser team members can help deliver the message about the laser program within the hospital by giving presentations to other departments. This promotes enthusiasm for the laser services among hospital employees and expands the program's marketing. Internal marketing is a very effective strategy to promote a laser program.

Increased laser volume can be achieved in a number of ways through personal selling. The laser team can encourage physicians to use the laser services by sending relevant articles to different specialists to stimulate them to review and possibly become involved with a new laser procedure. Many articles published by health care professionals discuss laser procedures and the merits of laser technology. The hospital should subscribe to laser journals. Sharing these articles and publications with physicians will show them that the laser team is interested in expanding the laser program by helping with new procedures. A physician feels more secure with the laser after realizing that this support from the laser team is available.

The head of laser services should keep in constant contact with the Medical Staff Office. When a potential laser user is granted staff privileges at the hospital, a personalized letter, followed by a phone call introducing the laser program, is valuable and appreciated. A description of the laser services and available laser systems and instrumentation will help encourage the physician to become credentialed in laser use.

A hands-on laboratory or practice laser session is always helpful to new physicians who need to increase their skill and feeling of control with the laser. When a laser team member takes the time to devote attention to support or help the physician understand the intricacies of a specific laser system, the physician will be more apt to use the laser.

The annual credentialing review procedure documenting physician laser use can be beneficial in determining trends in laser use. Physicians who do not use laser technology much can be asked why this is so. Many times the personal contact is enough to encourage the physician to use a hospital's laser services more. Physicians enjoy the personalized treatment that this type of marketing allows, and they often transfer to a hospital that offers this type of caring attitude and concern.

Physicians who are active laser users can encourage other specialists to use the laser by elaborating on their experiences with the technology. Often one physician's experiences with a particular wavelength can be communicated effectively to a physician in another specialty who may be able to use the same wavelength, thus leading to increased laser volume. For example, a gynecologist can discuss with a podiatrist the technique and results of CO_2 laser vaporization of condyloma. The podiatrist may then be encouraged to try the laser on plantar warts.

Sales Promotion

Sales promotion is another method used to market a laser program. A promotional event can often lead to media coverage that could increase the visibility of the laser program. For example, a hospital could offer to supply a laser to the veterinarian of a zoo to perform laser surgery on an animal. A specialist from the hospital could be made available to help with the procedure. Plantar warts can be easily vaporized with a CO_2 laser. A monkey with endometriosis could benefit from a laparoscopy using a laser to vaporize the endometrial implants. Media attention to these unusual events would focus on the collaboration between the zoo and the hospital's laser program, thus the hospital would also enjoy recognition.

Another way to market laser services is to participate in planned promotional events. Sometimes community organizations plan athletic challenges for participation by large corporations and hospitals. Laser program t-shirts or other identifiable costumes (such as running inside a mock laser box with the name of the laser program clearly displayed; see Figure 17-1) will attract attention to the laser program. Creativity and innovation cause people to become intrigued and interested in what is being promoted.

Another promotional event that will attract media attention is using a laser to cut the ribbon at a grand opening. For example, the ribbon can be cut with a CO_2 laser to open a new local-anesthesia laser center. At the 1993 Association of Operating Room Nurses (AORN) conference, the ribbon at the entrance to the vast display floor of surgical products was cut by the president of AORN and the chairman of the Exhibitor's Advisory Committee (Figure

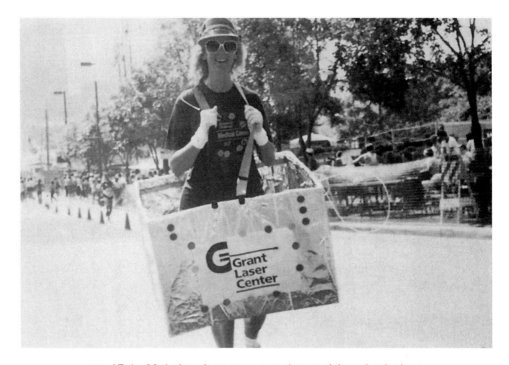

FIG. 17-1   Marketing a laser program requires creativity and enthusiasm.

17-2). This signified the arrival of new beginnings and technology in the surgical arena as the display floor was officially opened. When a laser is used to cut a ribbon, safety precautions must be followed to prevent accidental injury or ignition of the ribbon.

Publicity

Newsworthy information on laser surgery can be used to publicize and market the laser program. When a unique laser procedure is scheduled, the hospital's public relations department should notify the media. Usually the media are eager to report on new surgical techniques or procedures that will benefit patients. With this news type of coverage, a third party (the newscaster) appears to be testifying on behalf of the new advancement. The audience views this as support for the technology, and interest is then generated.

New laser procedures such as percutaneous discectomy, stapedectomy, treatment for snoring, thoracoscopic treatment for emphysema, or welding could be publicized, especially if the procedure is being performed for the first time in a specific geographical area. A hospital must make sure that the physician feels secure about performing the procedure before the media are notified. A procedure usually is performed several times before the media are invited to videotape and generate a story for the news show. The media must be given accurate and simple information so that the laser will not be misrepresented to the public. The laser must be promoted as a tool that the physician uses during a procedure. The laser must not be described as a panacea. Sometimes the media sensationalize a new development and do not represent the technology accurately.

A *booth display* on laser information can promote a laser program (Figure 17-3). A portable display booth that allows informational graphics and pictures to be changed easily can be taken to health fairs, career days, and other relevant events or meetings to pro-

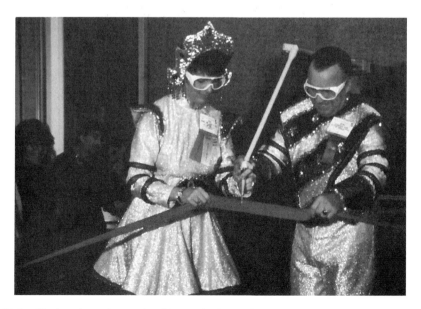

FIG. 17-2 The laser is used to cut the ribbon to the display floor at the annual Association of Operating Room Nurses conference.

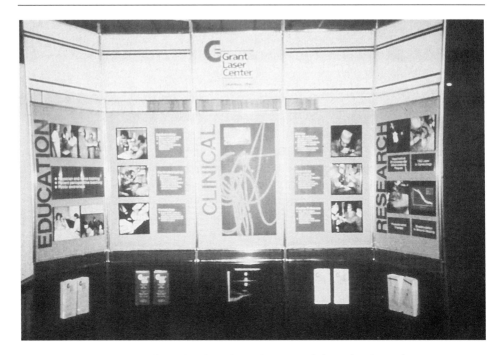

FIG. 17-3   A portable display booth can be used to present information about a laser program.

mote the laser program. This type of booth can also be displayed at professional meetings to increase awareness and use of laser services. A videotape showing various laser applications can also be presented to attract people to the booth. The public relations department can use a list of area health fairs, career days, and physician or nurse conferences to develop a schedule for booth displays.

Informational brochures can be used to increase awareness about the laser program (Figure 17-4). A promotional brochure should have attractive visuals to hold the reader's attention. Simple descriptions of laser biophysics and clinical laser applications will help potential patients and physicians understand laser technology and its impact on health care. When an individual or group requests information about the laser program, this marketing brochure can be sent.

Patient education brochures can be designed regarding laser use for individual specialties or procedures. Usually the computer or informational services department of a hospital can design these brochures at lower costs. For example, a patient education brochure on laser angioplasty could include the following:

- What is atherosclerosis?
- Signs and symptoms of atherosclerosis.
- Testing for atherosclerosis.
- Treatment alternatives for atherosclerosis.
- Laser angioplasty (from hospitalization to discharge).
- Recovery course and home care.

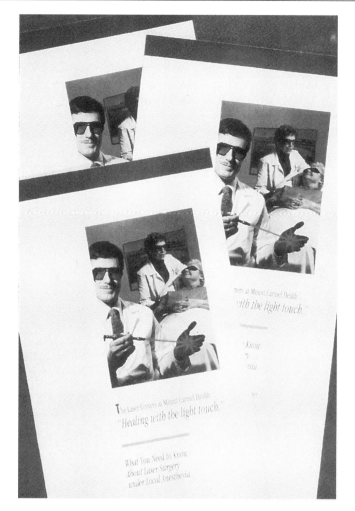

FIG. 17-4   Laser brochures can be used to describe laser services or educate patients about laser procedures and the laser program.

Patient brochures should be available in specialists' offices. A central phone number should be highlighted on the brochure to give the patient easy access to further information. Brochures can also be available to interested persons in the audience when a physician or nurse speaks to a community group about laser technology. When a patient calls the laser program office about a specific concern, an appropriate brochure can be sent to the patient to provide information on a specific laser procedure.

Patient brochures can also complement video programs that can be shown within the hospital's private network system on patient televisions. Also, audio programs have been designed for use over the telephone. The patient can access these programs by dialing a special number and then selecting from different short informational presentations. Programs for selection might include the history of laser technology, how a laser works, preparation for a specific laser procedure, different clinical applications, or benefits of laser technology.

Business cards should be made for the laser team members to help publicize the laser program (Figure 17-5). Because the laser team members are usually actively involved in implementing the marketing plan, they must be given a vehicle for providing information about laser surgery to anyone who requests it. Laser technology is dynamic and exciting, thus people have a strong desire to learn more about it. A business card gives the recipient ready access to a telephone number and the name of a person who can be contacted later for more information.

Publicizing the laser program can also be achieved by giving laser program t-shirts to patients or to attendees at laser courses and conferences (Figure 17-6). Any time the name of the laser program can be displayed, the opportunity should be seized. For example, a laser course manual should have the name of the program written on the binding so it can be seen when placed on a bookshelf. Creative ideas can be explored to provide the most appropriate publicity ventures.

EVALUATING A MARKETING PLAN

The success of a laser marketing program often depends on the strength and continuity of the evaluation phase. Evaluation of marketing activities should be documented to determine the effectiveness of each marketing project or method. The marketing plan should be flexible and changeable as continual evaluation notes strengths and weaknesses.

One of the greatest indicators of laser program success is patient satisfaction. If a patient is pleased with the services of the laser program, then that patient will tell friends

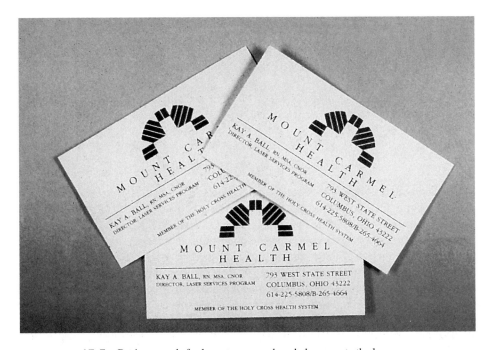

FIG. 17-5   Business cards for laser team members help promote the laser program.

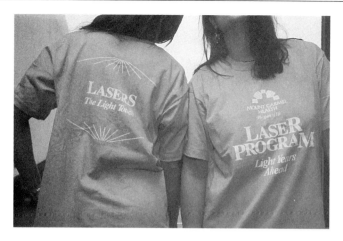

FIG. 17-6   Laser-program t-shirts can be given to attendees at laser courses and conferences.

and family members about the laser experience, thus patient referrals are made. A caring attitude must be conveyed in all laser program marketing to encourage and invite patients to use the laser services. Patients are attracted to facilities whose staff members go beyond the call of duty to ensure patient comfort and satisfaction.

Thorough perioperative education is an effective marketing tool and is critical in helping the patient truly understand laser surgery. When good rapport is developed with the physician and nurse, the patient feels much more secure about the procedure and the anticipated results. Postoperative visits by the nurse to inpatients or phone calls by the nurse to outpatients help foster the caring environment that promotes patient satisfaction. Patients who have a positive laser surgery experience will readily communicate this to others.

Evaluation of a laser program's marketing plan can be accomplished in a written annual report, which provides a powerful vehicle for promoting the laser program. It gives the laser program participants a way to boast about the successes and achievements experienced during the year.

An annual report should include an overview of the laser program, including volume, patient characteristics, laser-credentialed physicians, comparisons of laser-wavelength use, and trends in laser technology or use. Program activities should be highlighted, including networking, new laser acquisitions, laser presentations, staff development, and marketing projects. The annual report also includes a list of the achieved goals that were set the previous year. Finally, the report should summarize the goals for the next year.

An annual report is valuable for noting trends within the laser program so that marketing can be redesigned to address any changes. For example, if a trend is noted that one specific geographical area is not using the hospital's laser services, then intense marketing can be focused on this target area during the next year. Constructive and worthwhile information can be gathered from a well-produced, comprehensive annual report.

Marketing requires the intense efforts of many people. Designing a comprehensive marketing plan, implementing the plan, and evaluating the results can ensure that the laser program will expand and be enhanced through its increased visibility.

REFERENCES

Ball K: Laser marketing, *Today's OR Nurse* 9(4):126, April 1987.

Dubuque S: Lecture on advertising a laser program, Clinical Laser Management Postconference, Aug 27, 1988, New York City.

Kotler P: *Marketing for Nonprofit Organizations,* New Jersey, 1979, Prentice Hall.

Roman K, Maas J: *How to Advertise,* New York, 1976, St. Martin's Press.

Swergold, Chevitz, and Sinsabaugh, Inc.: Experts predict strong laser market over next five years, *Clinical Laser Monthly* 5(1):1, 1987.

SUGGESTED READINGS

Ball KA, guest editor: Seminars in perioperative nursing, *Lasers,* Vol. 1, No. 2, April 1992, WB Saunders Co.

Hartwig P: Where have all the lasers gone? *Minimally Invasive Surgical Nursing* 7(4):151-152, Winter 1993.

Mackety C: Developing marketing strategies for laser programs, *Minimally Invasive Surgical Nursing* 5(2):56-58, Summer 1991.

Proven strategies for increasing laser utilization, *Clinical Laser Monthly* 11(8):113-132, Aug 1993.

18

LASER EDUCATION

Since laser technology is forever changing, fostering and expanding the education component of a laser program is extremely valuable. Laser education focuses on three audiences: patients, the community, and health care professionals.

PERIOPERATIVE PATIENT EDUCATION

Perioperative patient education is one of the most critical segments of laser education for a laser program. Educating the patient about laser technology can be a challenging responsibility for the nurse. During the past 10 years, nursing researchers have studied the effectiveness of structured patient education. They have noted that preoperative patient education has been successful in "decreasing patient anxiety, altering unfavorable attitudes, influencing postoperative recovery, and promoting satisfaction with care" (Rothrock, 1989).

The perioperative patient education program must be sensitive to patient needs and not be a packaged program that is given to all patients before the laser intervention. The patient-centered care concept helps staff approach the patient in a holistic way to focus on what the individual patient needs and not what the nurse believes the patient wishes to know.

Many obstacles discourage nurses from engaging in patient education. Nurses are being required to discuss more complex information, such as laser technology, with the patients in a shorter period. Many times the procedure is performed on an outpatient basis, giving the nurse even less time to interact with the patient. Sometimes perioperative nurses must struggle to find the time during a busy surgery schedule to discuss an impending laser procedure with an inpatient (Figure 18-1). Inpatients needing laser education are often sicker and less interested in participating in laser education. Because of these limitations, the nurse must regard every encounter with the patient as an opportunity for education.

Initiating Laser Education

Preoperative patient education begins in the physician's office or during a physician referral visit in the hospital. Physicians and nurses have learned that they must develop a rapport with a patient before education about a laser surgical procedure can be intro-

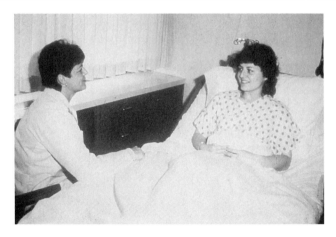

FIG. 18-1   A perioperative nurse visits an inpatient to discuss the laser procedure that will be performed the next day.

duced. Touching the patient's hand or patting a shoulder can be powerful in conveying the message of caring. The nurse becomes very effectual in assuring the patient or restating what the physician has discussed with the patient. The physician is responsible for supplying the details of the procedure, including alternative treatments, risks, and anticipated outcomes. What the physician and nurse tell the patient about the laser procedure must be consistent. Information from the two health care professionals should not conflict, or the patient's anxiety level will rise.

The nurse should feel comfortable about discussing the laser procedure with the patient (Figure 18-2). If the nurse is unsure about the technology, the patient will sense this uneasiness and become more anxious.

Preoperative patient education is valuable and beneficial to the patient, family, nurse, and hospital (Table 18-1) (Woodward, 1983).

The goal of preoperative teaching is for the patient to receive the information and then comply with what has been taught (Woodward, 1983). Nurses can easily evaluate the effectiveness of the preoperative teaching by noting the patient's conformity to the instructions. For example, a patient under local anesthesia undergoing CO_2 laser vaporization of a plantar wart was instructed preoperatively as to the rationale for remaining completely still during the procedure. The patient's verbal response during the procedure, "Don't worry, I'll make sure I hold very still," indicated that the patient was complying with the instructions. Patients are motivated to follow the preoperative directions when they realize it is in their best interest to do so.

Preoperative information is given to the patient for three reasons:

1. To increase the patient's understanding of the procedure.
2. To develop rapport with the patient so that confidence is encouraged.
3. To satisfy legal criteria to document that the patient received preoperative education about the procedure.

The preoperative education program should promote rapport between the physician or nurse and the patient. Providing an environment that is conducive to allowing the patient

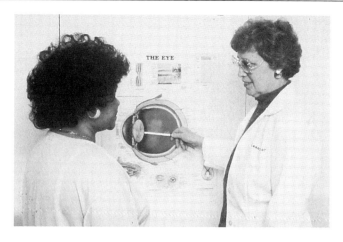

FIG. 18-2   An experienced clinical laser nurse discusses an ophthalmic laser procedure with a patient.

TABLE 18-1

Benefits of Preoperative Patient Education

Who Benefits	Benefit Derived
Patient	• Quicker return to activities of daily living • Postoperative complications decreased • Self-esteem increased, anxiety decreased • Intraoperative and postoperative pain reduced • Hospitalization costs decreased
Family	• Less anxiety • Increased feeling of support to the patient, thus increasing self-esteem
Nurse	• Increased patient compliance with care needs • Less stress since the patient is less anxious • More time devoted to holistic patient care instead of focusing on anxiety of the patient
Hospital	• Decreased liability • Economic benefits • Decreased recovery time for the patient • Increased bed turnover when the patient is discharged earlier • Enhanced public relations • Compliance with JCAHO requirements

Modified from Woodward S: Preoperative patient education seminar, Resource Applications, Inc., Denver, 1981.

to ventilate feelings and concerns helps to decrease patient anxiety. This approach to patient education provides open and effective discussion.

Assessment

The patient should be initially assessed to determine his or her desire to learn about the laser procedure. Skeptical patients receiving information about a procedure can react either with less concern or more fear. Research has shown that patients favor being given information about their surgical procedures (Rothrock, 1989). Shimko (1981) noted that anxiety actually increased after preoperative education was given to patients who already had a high anxiety level. The rationale to support this finding is that for patients with high preexisting levels of anxiety, preoperative information merely augments the apprehension. Also, if the patient was denying the anxiety before the instruction, then the reality of having to face the surgical procedure removed the denial coping mechanism, thus increasing stress.

The patient must be instructed on what to expect from the laser intervention. If the patient is encouraged to relax during preoperative education, more information will be retained. The procedure should be explained, along with reasonable expectations and activities that will occur preoperatively, intraoperatively, and postoperatively. If the procedure is described carefully, noting the sensory experience to be expected during the intervention and discussing the postoperative phase, the patient can more easily form a mental image of the impending event. The patient then can control responses such as pain, ambulation, and recovery more appropriately.

Assessing patients and providing preoperative education requires privacy. A comfortable room and a relaxed environment will help decrease the patient's stress level. Usually a family member or significant other is available to offer support. The nurse and physician must direct education not only to the patient but to the support person(s) as well.

Planning

Planning involves determining which teaching method to use. Often there is a tendency for one to teach as one was taught, or pedagogically. The pedagogical method is based on a concept of teacher-student interaction as conducted in a formal, authoritarian environment. Learning needs are determined by the teacher and directed by the curriculum. This type of patient education method was used initially, when health care professionals began to design education programs for the patient.

A more effective method is andragogy, which focuses on the adult-adult relationship. The patient, physician, and nurse determine what needs to be discussed in a more informal, supportive environment. This type of individualized patient education method has proven to be much more effective in helping the patient during the perioperative experience.

Many methods can be employed for patient education to enhance the learning process. Teaching aids that stimulate more than one sense are more effective in helping the patient retain information. Discussing the laser procedure with a patient is helpful, but showing the patient a picture of the laser or the surgery at the same time is much more effective.

Tape-recorded messages for the patient are available, but since they offer only auditory stimulation, other methods are more successful. Some physicians and nurses draw pictures to help the patient understand the laser procedure. Teaching programs that use slides with taped information have been successful in ensuring patient compliance (Abrams, 1982).

Pamphlets and booklets about specific procedures have also proven extremely effective in enhancing patient understanding of a procedure. Studies were conducted to determine the effectiveness of using booklets for patient education. Results noted that patient understanding and compliance was fostered, anxiety was decreased, coping behaviors were improved, and nursing time needed to teach specific behaviors was decreased (Rothrock, 1989).

When a study was conducted on the effectiveness of sending educational pamphlets or booklets to the patient before surgery, it was revealed that patients appreciated the information and that preoperative anxiety decreased (Rice and Johnson, 1984). This study indicates that patients desire as much information as possible before their procedure so that they may more appropriately participate in their treatment and recovery.

An illustrated preoperative patient education manual can help the patient understand the impending procedure. For example, an ophthalmic laser teaching manual can be designed for use in a local-anesthesia laser center or a physician's office. The manual can include a variety of pictures to educate the patient and thus relieve anxiety. Illustrations that can be used include a picture of the laser and how the patient is positioned at the slit lamp, the method used to administer preoperative eyedrops, the placement of a contact lens on the eye, how the beam is emitted, and applying a cold pack to the eye after the procedure. By experiencing the procedure first in pictures, the patient will have more realistic expectations, and apprehension and tension will be minimized.

Some facilities have videotapes on specific procedures for the patient to view during the preoperative education process. A strong advantage of this method is that the actual preoperative education that was presented can accurately be documented and retrieved if litigation occurs.

Teaching aids have proven to be very helpful in enhancing a preoperative education program. A teaching aid should never be used in place of personal contact, however. The aid must be only a secondary tool for ensuring patient understanding of the procedure. When the personal touch is removed from the education process, rapport with the patient is not fostered, and a patient-centered education program is not provided.

The patient's support system must never be overlooked. Family and friends can be a powerful tool for helping the patient during this sometimes stressful intervention. The support system should always be included in the patient education process from the time of initial contact with the patient to the postoperative phone call. By fostering and encouraging the involvement of the support persons, the patient is made to feel less alone, resulting in added strength and understanding (Figure 18-3).

When an experimental laser procedure is performed, the patient must be aware of the procedure protocol, anticipated results, risks, complications, and alternatives. The patient should also be informed of the costs that may be incurred because some insurance carriers will not reimburse a physician or hospital for an investigational procedure and the patient must assume full financial responsibility. The patient must sign a special consent form after reviewing it with the nurse or physician. The patient must thoroughly understand that the procedure is experimental and results may be questionable (Figure 18-4).

Implementation

During the implementation phase of patient education, the nurse should provide a positive environment that is relaxing and conducive to learning. The following guidelines

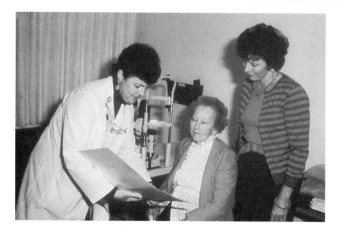

FIG. 18-3   Support persons should be invited to be present when the laser procedure is discussed with the patient.

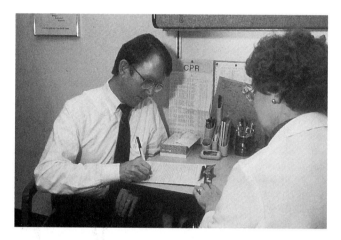

FIG. 18-4   Before an investigational laser procedure is performed, the patient must sign a special consent form stating that the patient understands the risks, alternatives, and experimental nature of the procedure.

will help decrease patient anxiety about the laser procedure during the preoperative discussion phase:

- Provide privacy for open discussion of the procedure and include family members or other support person(s).
- Sit near the patient and indicate that there is no hurry to complete this education discussion. Rapport is more easily developed when physical distance from the patient is reduced.
- Use therapeutic touch (such as holding a hand or patting a shoulder) and eye contact to communicate a caring attitude.

- Assess the patient's existing knowledge of the procedure and the surgical course so that a patient-centered perioperative education program can be implemented.
- Encourage questions from the patient and support persons to show that the patient's input and response to the laser education is valued.
- Provide simple and honest explanations of the laser procedure as the patient expresses a desire to learn.
- Listen to and observe the patient for any nonverbal negative communication.
- Document patient education and observations of the patient's reactions to the preoperative education discussion.

Patients may have many questions if laser technology is unfamiliar to them. Some patients still equate lasers with futuristic notions such as star wars technology and need more time than others to process the information that is provided. Some patients fear that the laser beam will blast through the surgical site, the way a laser gun would fire. Sensationalism about laser technology must be minimized, and realistic explanations about laser surgery must be conveyed.

Patients sometimes ask questions about the following:

- How the laser energy is generated
- Risks and safety of the laser
- Pain during and after the procedure
- Effectiveness of the laser being used
- Alternatives to laser surgery
- Postoperative care
- Cost of the procedure

Patients also question the expertise and skill level of the physician who will perform the laser procedure. Many physicians have their laser course certificate framed and hung on the wall in their office to validate the specialized education and training they received. Nurses should be prepared to respond to questions concerning the specialized education required to promote the safe and appropriate use of the laser.

Preoperative patient education should include a simple explanation of the type of laser used. Many patients want to know the differences among the various lasers and what determines which one will be used. A brief description of how the laser energy interacts with tissue will help dispel any previously formed unrealistic or impractical impressions. The following uncomplicated explanations can be offered to the patient:

- The laser energy is hot (for most lasers) and will burn the abnormal cells in a very controlled and precise manner.
- The laser can destroy diseased cells while leaving the normal cells virtually unharmed.
- The laser energy can seal small blood vessels, so less bleeding usually occurs during the procedure than during conventional procedures.
- Surgery time is sometimes decreased when the laser is used.
- The laser may seal nerve endings, so sometimes less pain is experienced after surgery.
- Laser energy can destroy bacteria, so there may be less chance of infection after a laser procedure.

- Safety glasses or goggles are worn by everyone in the surgery room to protect their eyes from the laser energy. The patient's eyes are always protected, too.
- A patient's pregnancy is not compromised when the laser is used because the radiation is nonionizing and will not affect the embryo/fetus.

Sometimes it is difficult to address pain during and after the laser procedure because everyone has a different pain threshold. Just mentioning the possibility of decreased pain is often enough to help the patient control intraoperative or postoperative discomfort.

Gynecology patients undergoing cervical ablation must understand the difference between pain and cramping. The laser procedure may produce cramping from prostaglandin release when the uterus is manipulated and the cervix is ablated. This release physiologically causes the uterus to cramp. By anticipating this sensation, the patient is better able to handle the discomfort during the procedure. Sometimes a patient can be instructed to focus on a picture hung on the ceiling to provide diversion.

Cosmetic results from laser surgery should be discussed in detail with the patient preoperatively so that anticipated results will be realistic. For example, a patient may expect a complete lightening of a port-wine stain when only partial lightening can be achieved. Before-and-after pictures of other patients often help promote realistic expectations. A mirror should be readily available in the laser treatment room so the patient can look at the immediate results of a laser dermatology procedure. This will help the patient more fully understand the postoperative care needed to achieve the expected outcome.

Patients often ask about scarring after a laser procedure. Research has shown that less scarring occurs when the laser is used than when electrocautery is used. Electrocautery heats the tissue to over $1000°$ C, whereas the laser heats the tissue only to approximately $100°$ C. Therefore, there is minimal thermal damage when the laser is used (Lobraico, 1984).

The anesthetic to be administered should be discussed with the patient before the procedure. If a patient is to remain awake, then thorough preoperative preparation is needed for patient compliance. The patient must be educated as to what to anticipate during the procedure. The sounds, odors, and discomforts should be discussed so the patient's mental image of the procedure can be as accurate as possible before the procedure. Since patients are afraid of the unknown, every effort must be made to help the patient understand as much information as possible (based on what they want to hear) during the preoperative education process.

Evaluation

The nurse or physician must constantly evaluate the patient's response to the education process. If too much information is given at one time, the patient will not absorb the facts. If the patient appears to be overloaded with information, then a secondary tool such as a videotape or a pamphlet can be given to the patient to use at home. Time must be allowed for questions and concerns that arise immediately after the operation. The procedure and postoperative instructions should be reviewed again with the patient.

During the education process, the patient can be expected to progress through four stages of adjustment as the patient realizes the significance of the impending surgical intervention: impact, regression, acknowledgment, and reconstruction (Lee, 1970). These phases are characterized as follows:

Impact: The patient feels a sense of helplessness, including fear, anxiety, and loss of control.

Regression: As the patient is forced to address the situation, regression may occur in dealing with the reality of the situation. The patient may show anger at the situation and may appear unwilling to learn about the procedure.

During these first two phases, the nurse can be effective in helping the patient to progress into the next stages. When the patient is ready, the nurse can help the patient understand the procedure by answering questions honestly and simply. The patient should be encouraged to share openly any feelings about the procedure.

Acknowledgment: The patient begins to acknowledge the need to undergo the procedure and expresses a desire to learn more about the procedure so as to feel more in control of the situation.

Reconstruction: This is the most positive phase of the education process, as the patient is now ready to plan for the recovery period because of a new feeling of self-worth. Positive reinforcement is needed during this time to ensure that the patient will remain in this phase.

These four phases are not clearly delineated because the duration of each one is variable. The time the patient spends in each phase is directly related to the patient's coping mechanisms and support system (Fox, 1986). The nurse needs to be cognizant of these phases so that various patient responses can be anticipated and addressed.

After the patient appears to understand the information provided through the perioperative education, he or she must sign the surgical consent form to document informed consent. "Consent" means permission to touch an individual. If a person is touched without approval, "battery" may be cited as a charge. "Informed consent" means permission to perform a procedure after the procedure, risks, complications, and alternatives have been discussed with the patient who gave permission. If the patient has been apprised of all of the procedural information and has signed the form, then informed consent can truly be documented. Ideally, the physician should be the person who requests the patient's signature on the consent form, but this task is often delegated to the nurse. This procedure is acceptable as long as the physician has thoroughly discussed the procedure with the patient.

State, local, and facility regulations must be followed regarding who has the authority to sign a consent form. State regulations usually require that the individual be over 18 years of age. An emancipated minor may also sign a consent form. A minor who qualifies to be emancipated usually is a minor who lives away from home and is responsible for himself or herself, is married, or has been or is pregnant.

The person who signs the consent form must be of sound mind, or else another person who is responsible for the patient must sign. If the patient is able to sign, then his or her signature should be obtained. Often the spouse of a patient having laser eye surgery will want to sign because the patient has difficulty seeing. The physician can document the receipt of informed consent in his or her notes if the patient is unable to sign. A patient who signs with an "X" should have two witnesses also sign the form.

Whether to include the word "laser" on the consent form is controversial. In providing as much information to the patient as possible, there is a trend toward specifying laser intervention by noting it in the procedure description. For example, instead of stating "laparoscopy with removal of endometrial implants," the consent form will state "laparoscopy with CO_2 laser vaporization of endometrial implants."

When patient education is addressed, one of the final questions a patient may ask is, "Would you undergo the laser procedure?" or "Would you recommend this procedure to one of your family members?" By personalizing the experience, the patient is asking about the physician's or nurse's feeling of comfort, security, and trust in the procedure. If the answer is "Yes," it must be honest so that the patient can maintain confidence.

The patient education process continues throughout the surgical experience. For example, during a local-anesthesia laser procedure, the patient is once again reminded of some of the highlighted patient education instructions. The patient is supported throughout the procedure because words of encouragement help promote patient compliance and comfort.

Postoperative observation will determine whether the patient is following or using the educational information that was given regarding the patient's role in the recovery phase. Many times the patient will have to be reminded about the postoperative care because anxiety during the laser procedure may obscure any recollection of previous instructions given (Figure 18-5).

Written discharge instructions are reminders for patients of the care needed at home. This educational tool is required by the Joint Commission on Accreditation of Healthcare Organizations (JCAHO) for all ambulatory patients. The physician and nurse will discuss the discharge instructions, and a written copy of the instructions will be given to the patient. Ideally, the patient should sign the instruction sheet, and a copy should be retained on the chart to document that the instructions were given.

Written discharge instructions can be individually developed for each specialty area. The physician can complete the form by noting which areas apply to each patient. Sample discharge instructions are provided on pages 394 and 395.

The physician or nurse should visit the inpatient postoperatively to reinforce the patient education process. The expectations of the surgery can be reviewed to note any patient needs that were not addressed. Changes in laser education programs are based on patient suggestions.

The nurse should make a postoperative phone call to all patients having laser surgery to follow up on the care that was given, the patient's response, and compliance with discharge instructions (Figure 18-6). Because of today's nursing shortage and time constraints, only ambulatory patients are usually called to follow up on their care. Many patients go back to work very quickly, so phone contact is limited. The nurse should tell the patient to expect a postoperative phone call. The patient, in turn, should tell the nurse whether he or she should call the patient at work. The patient may not wish to be called at work, especially if the laser procedure was relatively minor or confidential (such as vaporization of condyloma).

The education process is documented throughout the perioperative phase. Documentation validates the physician and nursing measures employed to help the patient understand the laser procedure and patient care required. If litigation occurs, the physician and nurse can recall the education process easily with accurate and complete documentation.

Perioperative patient education is a dynamic process. The nurse must be aware of technological changes that will help enhance the patient's understanding of the procedure. Advances in audiovisual capabilities are resulting in highly effective and sophisticated

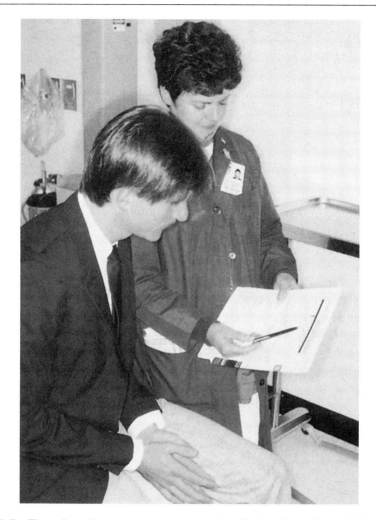

FIG. 18-5   The perioperative nurse reviews postoperative discharge instructions with the patient.

patient education programs on laser technology, and computerized teaching programs are being designed and implemented for this purpose.

COMMUNITY EDUCATION

Since laser technology has received a lot of media coverage in the past decade, interest in laser advances has blossomed. Community organizations seek health care professionals to present talks on current laser technology. No matter what the focus of the organization is, health care is a common denominator that always attracts attention.

The hospital's public relations department can be valuable in providing contacts to community organizations. Its speaker's bureau, with names of speakers on laser technology, can be shared with the public to promote interest.

Sample Discharge Instructions:
Laser Gastroscopy

The following instructions will help you care for yourself, or be cared for, upon your return home today. These guidelines are for the immediate postsurgery period.

Medications	_____ Resume own medications.
	_____
	_____
Activity	_____ Resume normal activities in_____
	_____ Return to work/school on_____
Diet	_____ Nothing by mouth for 4 hours, then fluids and light diet today, resume regular diet tomorrow.
	_____ Special diet as follows: _____
	_____
Anesthesia precautions	_____ Do not operate a vehicle (car, bicycle, motorcycle), machinery, or power tools; make any important decisions; or drink alcoholic beverages for 24 hours.
Expectations of surgery	_____ Mild abdominal bloating or gas.
	_____ Throat irritation.
	_____
Call your doctor for additional instructions	_____ Temperature above 100° F.
	_____ Persistent or heavy breathing.
	_____
	_____
	_____
	_____
Emergency phone numbers	_____
	_____

I have received and understand the above instructions:

_____
(Patient, Parent, or Guardian)   Date

Sample Discharge Instructions:
Laser Dermatology

The following instructions will help you care for yourself, or be cared for, upon your return home today. These guidelines are for the immediate postsurgery period.

Medications   _____ Resume own medications.

_____

_____

Activity   _____ Resume normal activities in_____

           _____ Return to work/school on_____

Wound care   _____ Apply _____
to the lesion(s) and apply sterile gauze pad over the
lesion(s). Wash hands before touching the dressing.
Do not touch the surgical area.

           _____ Do not remove dressing.

           _____ Remove dressing on (date)_____

_____

Anesthesia   _____ Do not operate a vehicle (car, bicycle, motorcycle),
precautions   machinery, or power tools; make any important decisions; or drink alcoholic beverages for 24 hours.

Expectations   _____ Drainage from lesion(s).
of surgery
           _____ Minimal pain.

           _____ Mild burning sensation at operative site.

_____

Call your   _____ Temperature above 100° F.
doctor for
           _____ Persistent or heavy bleeding or drainage.

           _____ Redness, swelling, or pus at operative site.

           _____ Severe pain at operative site.

Additional   _____
instructions
_____

_____

_____

Emergency   _____
phone numbers
_____

I have received and understand the above instructions:

_____

(Patient, Parent, or Guardian)   Date

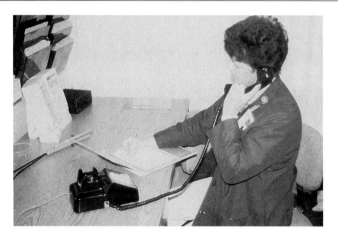

FIG. 18-6   With a postoperative phone call, the perioperative nurse evaluates patient compliance with the discharge instructions.

Slide Presentation

A slide presentation that focuses on educating the community about laser technology in health care can be very valuable. To promote laser use in health care, a general overview of different specialties can be presented to provide a generic summary. The following presentation format can be used:

1. Brief history of laser technology
2. Simple description of laser biophysics, systems, and safety
3. Benefits of laser surgical intervention
4. Major clinical applications in each specialty area (progress from neurosurgery to podiatry)
5. Future laser applications and research
6. Question and answer period

A 30- to 45-minute presentation can provide an appropriate synopsis of laser technology in health care. The presenter should be prepared for questions regarding the costs of laser application, various conditions that warrant laser use, and method of referring patients to particular physicians. Sometimes names of physicians are requested for immediate referrals. Printed materials distributed during the presentation can serve as valuable marketing tools and should include the phone number to call for further information.

Nurses, physicians, and hospital administrators can represent the laser program by providing information on laser advances and benefits. A physician specialist should remember to promote other specialty areas when delivering a presentation on his or her own area of expertise.

A slide show can also be valuable in providing inservice presentations about the laser program to various departments within a hospital. Employees of a hospital should recognize and understand the laser program in case they are asked for information by potential patients or other interested persons. Other departments should be able to offer patients a phone number to call and have their questions appropriately and promptly addressed.

Laser technology offers a fascinating career opportunity to individuals who enjoy challenges. Schools often request speakers for career days to inform students about opportunities in highly technological fields. The following career choices in laser technology can be promoted: physicians who use the laser in specialty practices, perioperative nurses, biomedical technologists, surgical technologists, and researchers involved with advances in laser technology. The opportunities are endless as this technology continues to expand into other arenas.

Students enjoy researching, reviewing, and reporting laser technology because the field is stimulating and ever-changing. Packets of information about laser technology and the hospital's laser program can be sent to interested students. A list of laser resources and references can help the student complete a report or explore laser opportunities.

Booth Display

A booth display can be developed to help educate the community about laser advances for health care. A portable booth can be taken to health fairs to illustrate how laser technology has affected the medical and surgical arena. Someone should always be available at the booth to answer questions or refer patients to physicians who use laser technology. Showing a videotape on laser applications will often attract people to the booth.

Informational Brochures

Informational brochures on specific laser procedures are beneficial in helping the community understand laser applications. Terminology should be kept simple and illustrations should be readily understood. Laser procedures that tend to be popular can be highlighted in these informational brochures. Laser procedures such as dermatology procedures, angioplasty, endoscopy, ophthalmic applications, and podiatric procedures can easily be illustrated. These brochures may be distributed through physicians' offices or at laser presentations.

By increasing community awareness through presentations, booth displays, and informational brochures, laser use in health care can be promoted. A laser program will expand as marketing efforts to educate the public attract patients. Increasing the visibility and understanding of the laser services offered will help promote the availability of laser technology. As the community becomes more aware of the potential of the laser, perioperative patient education will be widely accepted because the public will have a foundation of laser knowledge.

HEALTH CARE PROFESSIONAL EDUCATION

The health care professional can be educated about laser technology through performance appraisals, conferences, preceptorships, journals, videotapes, inservice presentations, videoteleconferencing, computerized learning programs, mentors, didactical sessions, and others. Some of these methods are discussed in detail in this section.

Performance Appraisals

Standards are being developed by which to judge competencies and levels of practice. Standards are written value statements that describe the responsibilities for which practitioners of the nursing profession are accountable. Standards also reflect the priorities of the profession and provide direction for professional nursing practice and a framework for evaluation of this practice.

The Nursing/Allied Health Division of the American Society for Laser Medicine and Surgery adopted "Standards of Perioperative Clinical Practice in Laser Medicine and Surgery" in 1994. These standards, which are divided into "Standards of Care" and "Standards of Professional Performance," are presented in the Appendix. The details of each section are described as follows:

Standards of Care	Standards of Professional Performance
Assessment	Quality of care
Diagnosis	Performance appraisal
Outcome identification	Education
Planning	Collegiality
Implementation	Ethics
Evaluation	Collaboration
	Research
	Resource utilization

Guidelines or recommended practices are specific to a clinical condition or situation (e.g., the need for eye protection during laser surgery) and assist the laser team by describing recommended courses of action for these clinical situations. Guidelines are based on the foundation of practice that accepted standards address.

Many hospital training programs are developing performance appraisals based on competencies that evolved from national standards, guidelines, and recommended practices. For example, a competency description may require that the laser team member participate in ongoing educational activities related to laser medicine and surgery. During the team member's annual review, the achievement of this competency is noted.

A checklist of various expectations can be developed to measure the laser team member's skill level and maintenance of expertise (Figure 18-7). The checklist can also be used as an orientation tool for novice laser team members to specify performance expectations, validate progress, and identify future learning needs (Allard, 1993).

The need for national certification of laser knowledge and skill is being debated today. Proponents state that physicians and laser team members should be required to take written and verbal tests to evaluate their laser knowledge and experience. This type of system would be directly or indirectly affiliated with a recognized professional organization to increase its legitimacy. Opponents of national certification state that the laser is merely a surgical tool, similar to the electrosurgical unit, and users need not become certified in its use. Opponents also state that if national certification were ever required, laser technology would stagnate because most physicians would be irritated by this requirement and would not want to be bothered by another regulating body.

Developing a Laser Conference

As a laser program expands, the desire to provide education for health care professionals may develop. The commitment of a core group of individuals in the laser program is instrumental in initiating the first laser conference. A physician must be involved in developing a physician laser conference, whereas a nurse must be involved in developing a laser nursing conference so that appropriate information is communicated. Too often a nurse will attend a physician training program and will be disappointed because nursing considerations were not presented. In contrast, nursing conferences focus specifically on the nurse's role during laser intervention.

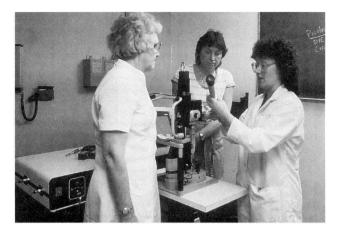

FIG. 18-7   Laser team members demonstrate how the laser fiber is connected to the slit lamp during an annual performance appraisal.

Obtaining *hospital commitment and permission* is the first step in developing a laser conference. Financial details must be reviewed in case the conference does not attract registrants and fails. Holding the first conference is usually a risky and expensive venture for the hospital, so there should be appropriate consideration of the economical impact. Once a budget has been determined, the conference plans can then be pursued.

A *conference coordinator* is appointed as the key individual to coordinate the educational offering. This person must be granted the time, authority, and resources to plan the laser conference. Coordinating a successful laser conference requires a great deal of time, energy, creativity, and dedication. A planning committee can be formed. If nursing contact hours are to be given, then the planning committee must include a nurse with a bachelor's degree in nursing. If the course is targeted toward licensed practical nurses (LPNs), then an LPN must serve on the planning committee.

The *target audience* must be determined so that the marketing and promotional efforts for the course can be planned. If the target audience is only gynecologists within one state, then mailing labels for those physicians should be obtained. If the course is geared toward nurses in a five-state area, then labels for nurses or operating room directors can be ordered.

Written objectives must be developed that are consistent with the course content. The objectives must be measurable, appropriate for the level of the registrants and course content, and realistic and attainable. Objectives should use verbs that can be measured, such as: list, describe, outline, name, demonstrate, and summarize. Examples of laser course objectives can be presented as follows:

At the end of the session, the registrant will be able to:

1. List three characteristics of laser light.
2. Describe four laser-tissue interactions.
3. State laser safety principles and actions.
4. List five elements in developing a laser program.
5. Describe the perioperative role during laser procedures.

6. Outline various laser applications for the different specialties.
7. Summarize laser investigation that is being conducted.
8. Demonstrate the safe and appropriate use of the laser in the laboratory.

The *course format,* including a detailed description of the content and times for topic presentation, must be determined. There usually is a didactic or theoretic component, as well as hands-on clinical experience. Most laser conferences last 1 to 3 days, depending upon the course content.

Speakers need to be contacted and asked to participate. Presentation topics must be clearly delineated so that duplication of information is avoided. Honorariums and expenses should be discussed with the speaker before a contract is signed.

The speaker's teaching methods should vary during the laser conference. A valuable method to convey a message is to deliver a slide presentation and then provide a videotape of the actual laser procedure. The registrants can quickly relate to the procedure when they observe the laser-tissue interaction and see the protocol presented.

The most powerful tool in laser education is made possible through videoteleconferencing. The audience can remain in the conference room while the audio and video signals are transmitted from the surgery suite during an actual procedure. The audience can actively participate in the surgery by asking questions of the surgical team while the procedure is described. This unique learning experience offers the best alternative to hands-on participation.

Continuing education units should be offered to provide the health care professional with documentation of an educational experience. The course should be approved for continuing education depending upon the type of health care professionals who attend. A laser nursing course should offer continuing education units, called contact hours, from an accredited approval body. Usually 50 minutes of course work equals one contact hour. A laser conference for physicians should offer continuing medical education (CME) units or other recognized approval units. Usually 60 minutes of course work equals one CME unit (Figure 18-8). Lunches and breaks are not included in the calculation of continuing education units.

A laser course should receive approval from an accrediting body to give the course credibility. Many times registrants are more apt to attend a course that has been approved because continuing education is required by many states and certification programs. A certificate is then awarded to document the registrant's attendance. Ideally, the certificate should include the name of the course, the laser wavelengths involved, and the number of credits or hours granted.

A *brochure* can be printed after the plans for the laser conference have been finalized. A layout that will feature a logo or other distinguishing characteristic should be included on each conference brochure to promote a recognizable identity for the laser program. Laser conferences can be marketed through professional journals or direct mailings of brochures.

The *didactical session* may cover the following topics:

• Laser history
• Laser physics
• Laser-tissue interaction
• Laser types and delivery systems

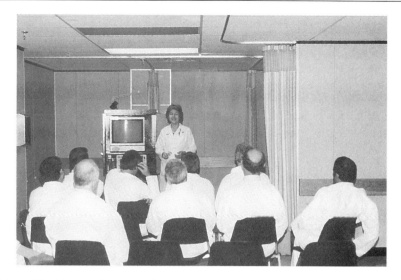

FIG. 18-8   Physicians receive continuing medical education credits for attending a laser conference.

- Special instruments and accessories
- Laser safety
- Developing a laser program
- Benefits of laser surgery
- Clinical laser applications
- Perioperative considerations
- Future of laser technology in health care
- Review of laboratory exercises

The schedule of the course content should flow from one area to another. For example, laser biophysics should be the initial presentation, with laser safety following. The time for each speaker should be fairly allotted so that one topic does not overshadow another. Time limitations must be followed closely. The speaker must be told that a presentation may be interrupted if it runs over the set time to maintain the schedule and continuity with the rest of the program. A speaker who continues beyond the specified time limit can be very disturbing to the audience. A discussion period should be provided so that the registrants can ask questions of the speakers. An introduction, breaks, and lunch must also be included in the schedule.

Appropriate audiovisual equipment must be available for the speakers, including a slide projector, a videotape player (usually ½ inch), an overhead projector, or a chart board, as requested. Empty carousels will be needed for slide presentations. An extra room with a slide projector and videotape player close to the conference room should be available for speakers to organize and practice their presentations. A microphone should be used according to the conference room size. Some speakers like to use a lavaliere microphone so they can walk around the room or into the audience. If the conference is large, floor microphones in the audience will be needed for questions and comments. The speakers must remember to repeat questions or make sure the inquiry is heard, especially if the session is being taped. Speakers usually request a laser pointer since the conference is on laser technology. A laser pointer can also be used to demonstrate the characteristics of a laser beam.

The conference registrants should receive a manual with detailed information about laser technology. The front and spine of the manual should include the name of the laser program or other sponsor of the conference. This provides continual recognition for the laser program after the manual is placed on an office bookshelf. An address and phone number also should be printed somewhere on the manual. Usually three-ring notebooks are used for laser manuals because more information can be added at a later date. Pockets on the inside of the notebook can hold brochures. The manual can include articles on laser biophysics, safety, development of a laser program, various clinical laser applications, and laser research results. If an article is copied from a publication, written permission must be granted before copies are made. Speakers should be asked to contribute articles for the manual. An outline of a speech helps the learner follow the flow of the presentation. Registrants will not have to take as many notes if the printed articles also highlight the presented information. Notepads and pens should be available at the conference.

A *laboratory experience* should have a limited number of participants at each station (Figure 18-9). Registrants get the most valuable and satisfying experience at stations with fewer than six students. Laboratory exercises should be written so that the instructors and participants can refer to them for guidance. This also helps to provide consistency between similar laboratory stations to ensure that the same information is being presented.

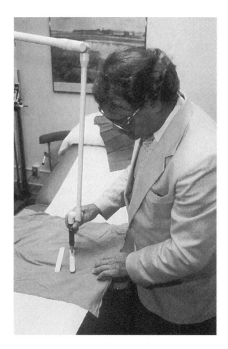

FIG. 18-9   Hands-on laboratory experience allows the physician to practice with different laser wavelengths.

During the hands-on laboratory experience, a variety of exercises can be used. After a brief discussion of the laser system and delivery devices, the laser wavelength character- istics are demonstrated (Figure 18-10). Depth of penetration, color selectivity, reflectivity, and transmission are demonstrated. Each participant must be given adequate time to prac- tice with the laser system. Some laboratory exercises are provided on pages 404-405.

Inanimate objects can be used to demonstrate the various laser wavelengths. The depth of penetration of the CO_2 laser can be demonstrated by impacting a piece of plexiglass using different power settings (Figure 18-11). Power density can be illustrated easily on a pork chop or an orange by varying the spot size, wattage, and duration of exposure. Color selectivity of the argon or yellow light lasers can be demonstrated by implanting small bits of dark liver on a light pork chop or by using the laser to pop a red balloon that is in- flated inside a white balloon (Figure 18-12). These wavelengths will react with the red or

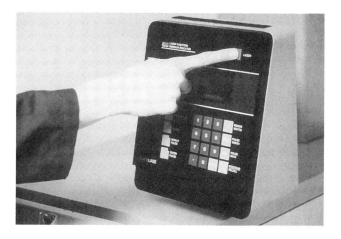

FIG. 18-10   The laser control panel is reviewed in detail with laser course registrants.

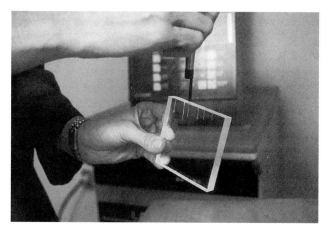

FIG. 18-11   The depth of penetration of the CO_2 laser beam is demonstrated by firing the laser into a piece of plexiglass at different power settings.

Laser Laboratory Exercises

The following format will be used to demonstrate the various laser systems and wavelength characteristics.

I. Introduction to the laser system
  A. Control panel
  B. Installation requirements
  C. Aiming systems
  D. Delivery systems—Demonstrate the various delivery systems that conduct the laser energy to the tissue.
      CO_2:
          Articulated arm
          Coupler with CO_2 laparoscope
          Waveguide through operating port of laparoscope
          Micromanipulator to connect to microscope
      Nd:YAG:
          Bare fiber (noncontact)
          Catheter fiber (noncontact)
          Contact tip (contact)
          Sculpted fiber (contact)
      Argon or KTP:
          Fiber (may be connected to handpiece)
          Connected to microscope
          Connected to automatic scanner
      Holmium:
          Fiber (may be connected to handpiece)
II. Characteristics of various laser wavelengths
  A. Power density and depth of penetration
     Tissue response to laser energy depends upon three parameters:
     1. Power (wattage)
     2. Duration of exposure
     3. Spot size (or beam diameter)
     Deliver the laser energy to a piece of chicken or liver using a variety of settings. The extent of tissue interaction can be changed by varying these three parameters. Each parameter can be noted by varying one while keeping the other two constant. Use a scalpel to cut through the lasered areas to note the depth of penetration of the laser energy.
         Depth of penetration:
             CO_2:   0.1 to 0.2 mm
             Nd:YAG: Less than 1.0 mm (contact)
             Nd:YAG: 2 to 6 mm (noncontact)
             Argon or KTP: 0.5 to 2 mm
             Holmium: 0.4 to 0.6 mm

Laser Laboratory Exercises—cont'd

II. Characteristics of various laser wavelengths—cont'd
B. Transmission of laser beam
Place a piece of liver in a bowl of water. Direct the laser beam through the fluid to the tissue to demonstrate whether the beam can be transmitted through fluid.
Effect of water:

CO_2:	Absorbed by water
Nd:YAG:	Transmitted through water
Argon:	Transmitted through water
KTP:	Transmitted through water
Holmium:	Transmitted a short distance through a vapor bubble

C. Color selectivity
Sweep the laser beam across a tongue blade with different colors on the blade. If the beam is color-selective, it will be highly absorbed by certain colors, such as red or black. This characteristic can also be demonstrated by placing implants of darker liver on a light-colored pork chop or chicken meat. Or a red balloon can be inserted into a white balloon. Both balloons are inflated and the laser beam is fired onto the balloons. The beams that are highly absorbed by red pigmentation will cause the inner balloon to burst, while the outer white balloon stays intact.
D. Reflectivity
Cause the laser beam to be reflected off the surface of a shiny instrument to impact a styrofoam cup. This is best demonstrated with the CO_2 laser. The Nd:YAG or KTP beams will be more readily absorbed if a black or red spot, respectively, is drawn on the cup. Compare the reflectivity of the laser beam with a shiny instrument, an ebonized surface, and an anodized surface.

---

darkened colors while leaving white or light-colored structures unharmed. Writing on an egg yolk (without breaking it) using an Nd:YAG contact scalpel mimics the speed and precision that is needed for this delivery system. Fresh placenta is a good model for demonstrating laser laparoscopy and endometrial ablation procedures. A cow's tongue will react similarly to cervical tissue during an Nd:YAG laser conization.

Sometimes live animals are used to demonstrate the living-tissue response to the different laser wavelengths. When animals are used, strict enforcement of U.S. Department of Agriculture regulations must be followed. Only animals procured through approved vendors for research may be used. A qualified veterinarian must be in attendance to anesthetize and control the animals. State and federal regulations should be determined when live animals are used. Usually research dogs or cats are not used for laser demonstrations today; rats, rabbits, pigs, and goats are more acceptable models. If a basic laser course is being taught, a live-animal laboratory is not necessary.

Vendor participation is helpful if laser equipment and supplies are to be brought in for the conference. A letter documenting the equipment or supply needs, delivery address, set-up time, and disassembly information should be sent to the vendor. A verbal or written

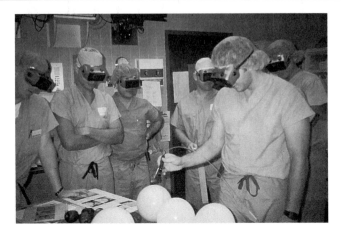

FIG. 18-12   Color selectivity is demonstrated by firing an argon beam through a white balloon to burst a red balloon that is inflated inside the white one.

commitment must be received from the vendor to reconfirm the agreement to assist with the conference. The role of the vendor should be discussed before the conference so that the vendor is prepared to teach or be available at a laboratory station.

If special electrical or water requirements are needed to operate a specific laser, details of these specifications must be addressed before the conference. Any equipment or supplies must be set up in advance. The laboratory station must be functional before the registrants enter the area.

An *evaluation* of the laser conference by the participants should include rating the speakers, content, objectives met, and laboratory experience. The evaluation will document participant satisfaction with the strengths of the course. Any weaknesses described can be addressed so that changes can be made if the course is offered again.

Evaluations should be summarized and reviewed by the persons involved with coordinating the conference. A written report of the conference should be prepared and submitted to the laser committee. Expenses vs. revenue should be noted to provide a financial report and determine profits or losses. The hospital administration should receive a detailed outline of the conference achievements, strengths, and weaknesses. A summary of the laser course will help justify offering another conference in the future.

Preceptorships

Attendance at a laser course is usually only the first step in laser credentialing. Today many physicians are required to have a laser-credentialed physician observe them performing one or more procedures before laser privileges for a particular wavelength are granted. The physician seeking laser credentials may have to arrange for his or her own preceptor. Sometimes the laser team members will assist with this process.

The number of required preceptored procedures is determined by the hospital credentialing committee and is often advised by the Laser Committee. If the number of required procedures is high, a physician may become discouraged and use other tools. The required number of preceptored procedures should be realistic and should not become an obstacle. Safety of the patient and the laser team must be considered when the ideal number of mandated preceptored cases is determined.

Some hospitals require that physicians perform a certain number of procedures each year to maintain credentials. The JCAHO is also exploring the need to have this requirement, which is justified as follows: If a physician has not performed a particular procedure or used a certain tool, then the skill level drops and the patient's safety is threatened. For example, if a physician has not used a CO_2 laser for a year, can his or her skill level still be guaranteed? This is also a quality control issue that hospitals are investigating so that potential litigation can be decreased.

If a physician is already credentialed to use the laser at another hospital and his or her laser activities can be documented, the credentialing committee may decide to forego the preceptorship requirement. This decision should be documented in the physician's file in the Medical Staff Office.

Sometimes a physician seeking to qualify for or maintain laser credentials has difficulty finding a preceptor for a procedure. This may be due to scheduling conflicts or the fact that some physicians may not want to encourage others to use the laser if this means a potential loss of patients. Some physicians enjoy having the market share without the threat of competition. So the dilemma is that a physician wants to become laser-credentialed but there is no one who will preceptor a procedure. This is the time that videoteleconferencing may help. By transmitting the audio and visual images over telephone lines, a credentialed physician may preceptor another physician from afar. This remote preceptorship is becoming an acceptable alternative to having a preceptor at the surgical site. The resolution and detail of the visual image is so well defined that distortion is not a concern. The ½-second delay in transmission is insignificant in the health care arena. This technology eliminates the problem of scheduling conflicts or inability to find a preceptor within a hospital. Videoteleconferencing of preceptorships for initial credentialing and for maintaining privileges is an exciting alternative to promote quality and skilled health care services.

After observing the procedure and noting the safe and appropriate use of the laser, the preceptor signs a written form. If the credentialing policy does not require a specific number of preceptored procedures, the preceptor may be the one who decides whether more procedures should be observed before credentialing is granted. Any documentation of preceptorships should be kept in the file of the physician who is seeking laser credentials. When the preceptorship requirement for a laser wavelength has been fulfilled, the physician is allowed to use that wavelength without supervision.

Laser education of the professional can be a rewarding experience for everyone involved. Being recognized as a premiere site for laser education helps promote leadership in the area of laser technology. Physicians and patients are attracted to laser programs of excellence that are known for being pacesetters of innovative practice in highly technological fields such as laser surgery.

REFERENCES

Abrams L: Resistance behaviors and teaching media for children in day surgery, *AORN J* 35:244, Feb 1982.

Allard D: Defining performance expectations for laser nurses and technicians, *Clinical Laser Monthly,* pp 12-15, Jan 1993.

Fox V: Patient Teaching, *AORN J,* 44(2):1234, Aug 1986.

Lee J: Emotional reactions to trauma. *Nurs Clin Am* 5:1577, Dec 1970.

Lobraico R: Unique concerns in patient education. Clinical lasers: Expert strategies for practical and profitable management, p 272, Atlanta, 1984, American Health Consultants.

Rice VH and Johnson JE: Preadmission self-instruction booklets, postadmission exercise performance, and teaching time, *Nursing Research* 33:147-151, May/June 1984.

Rothrock JC: Perioperative nursing research, *AORN J* 49(2):1614, Feb 1989.

Shimko C: The effect of preoperative instruction on state anxiety, *J Neurosurg Nurs* 13:318, Dec 1981.

Woodward S: Preoperative patient education seminar, Denver, Oct 21, 1983, Resource Applications, Inc.

SUGGESTED READINGS

Ball KA, guest editor: Seminars in perioperative nursing, *Lasers,* Vol. 1, No. 2, April 1992, WB Saunders Co.

Developing an ideal laser education and training program, *Clinical Laser Monthly,* pp 52-54, April 1993.

Owens P: Perioperative laser nurse's role in patient education, *Laser Nursing* 4(1):7-9, Spring 1990.

Pfister JI, Kneedler JA, and Purcell SK: *The nursing spectrum of lasers,* Denver, 1988, Education Design, Inc.

Rogalla C: Laser education program during nurse orientation, *Laser Nursing* 6(4):129-134, Winter 1992.

Tougher training standards, enforcement on the horizon, *Clinical Laser Monthly,* pp 65-68, May 1993.

Winning combination: Education, Employees and Enthusiasm, *Clinical Laser Monthly,* pp 127-129, Aug 1993.

STANDARDS OF PERIOPERATIVE CLINICAL PRACTICE IN LASER MEDICINE AND SURGERY*

S tandards are authoritative statements that describe the responsibilities of practitioners of a profession. Nursing standards reflect the values and priorities of the profession and provide direction for professional nursing practice and a framework for evaluation of this practice.

The American Nurses Association (ANA), in collaboration with numerous specialty nursing organizations and groups, developed a master model called "Standards of Clinical Nursing Practice" and published it in 1991. In 1992, the Association of Operating Room Nurses (AORN) published the "Standards of perioperative clinical practice" and "Standards of perioperative professional performance" using the ANA model. In 1994, the Nursing/Allied Health Division of the American Society for Lasers in Medicine and Surgery developed the "Standards of Perioperative Clinical Practice in Laser Medicine and Surgery," using these two publications as models.

The American Society for Lasers in Medicine and Surgery is a dynamic professional association dedicated to the exploration and application of laser technology in medicine and surgery. The goal is to ensure the highest quality of patient care during laser treatment. It is the responsibility of the Nursing/Allied Health Division of the society to formulate standards for reference to be used by clinical nurses and allied health care providers to assist in the establishment of safe, effective laser services in hospitals and other health care settings.

*Adapted from the Association of Operating Room Nurses: *AORN Standards and Recommended Practices for Perioperative Nurses,* Denver, 1993, The Association.

"Standards of Perioperative Clinical Practice in Laser Medicine and Surgery" includes Standards of Care and Standards of Professional Performance, as follows:

Standards of Care	Standards of Professional Performance
Assessment	Quality of care
Diagnosis	Performance appraisal
Outcome identification	Education
Planning	Collegiality
Implementation	Ethics
Evaluation	Collaboration
	Research
	Resource utilization

STANDARDS OF CARE

Standard I: Assessment

The perioperative nurse collects patient health data.

Criteria

1. The priority of data collection is determined by the patient's immediate condition or needs and the relationship to the proposed laser intervention. Pertinent data include but are not limited to
   - current medical diagnoses and therapies
   - physical status and physiological responses
   - psychosocial status of the patient
   - cultural, spiritual, and lifestyle information
   - individual understanding, perceptions, and expectations of the laser surgery or treatment
   - previous responses to illness; hospitalization; and surgical, therapeutic, or diagnostic procedures
   - results of diagnostic studies
2. Pertinent data are collected using appropriate assessment techniques.
3. Data collection involves the patient, significant others, and health care providers when appropriate. It may be accomplished through diverse means, such as interview, review of records, assessment, and/or consultation.
4. Data collection is systematic and ongoing.
5. Relevant data are documented in a retrievable form.

Standard II: Diagnosis

The perioperative nurse analyzes the assessment data in determining diagnoses.

Interpretive statement: Nursing diagnoses are concise statements about actual, or high risk for, health problems or clinical conditions that are amenable to nursing intervention. Diagnoses result from analysis and interpretation of data about the patient's problems, needs, and health status.

Criteria

1. Diagnoses are derived from the assessment data.

2. Diagnoses are validated with the patient, significant others, and health care providers when possible.
3. Diagnoses are documented in a manner that facilitates the determination of expected outcomes and plan of care.

Standard III: Outcome Identification

The perioperative nurse identifies expected outcomes unique to the patient.

Criteria

1. Outcomes are derived from the diagnoses and are formulated with the patient, significant others, and health care providers when possible.
2. The patient's present and potential physical capabilities and behavior patterns are congruent with the expected outcomes from the laser surgery or treatment.
3. Outcomes are attainable with consideration of the patient's capabilities and material resources.
4. Outcomes are documented as measurable goals and include a time estimate for attainment.
5. Outcomes are prioritized.
6. Outcomes provide direction for continuity of care.

Standard IV: Planning

The perioperative nurse develops a plan of care that prescribes interventions to attain expected outcomes.

Criteria

1. The plan of care reflects current nursing practice in laser technology.
2. The plan of care is individualized to the patient's condition and needs.
3. The plan of care is developed with the patient, significant others, and health care providers when appropriate.
4. The plan of care specifies nursing diagnoses and a logical sequence of interventions needed to achieve the outcomes.
5. The plan of care provides for continuity of care.
6. The plan of care is documented and communicated to the appropriate people.

Standard V: Implementation

The perioperative nurse implements the interventions identified in the plan of care.

Criteria

1. Interventions are consistent with the established plan of care.
2. Implementation of the plan of care is an ongoing process and based on the patient's response.
3. Interventions reflect the rights and desires of the patient and significant others.
4. Interventions are implemented in a safe and appropriate manner.
5. Interventions may be assigned or delegated as appropriate.
6. Interventions are documented and communicated as appropriate to promote continuity of care.

Standard VI: Evaluation

The perioperative nurse evaluates the patient's progress toward attainment of outcomes.

Criteria

1. Evaluation of the effectiveness of interventions is systematic and ongoing.
2. The patient's responses to interventions are documented and retrievable.
3. The effectiveness of interventions are evaluated in relation to outcomes.
4. Ongoing assessment data are used to revise diagnoses, outcomes, and the plan of care as needed.
5. Revisions in diagnoses, outcomes, and the plan of care are documented.
6. The patient, significant others, and health care providers are involved in the evaluation process when appropriate.

STANDARDS OF PROFESSIONAL PERFORMANCE
Standard I: Quality of Care

The perioperative nurse systematically evaluates the quality and appropriateness of nursing practice in laser medicine and surgery.

Criteria

1. The perioperative nurse participates in quality-of-care activities appropriate to the individual's position, education, and practice environment. Such activities may include
   - identifying and assigning responsibility for monitoring and evaluation activities
   - delineating the scope of patient care activities or services
   - identifying aspects of care
   - developing quality indicators for each identified aspect of care
   - establishing thresholds for evaluation of the quality indicators
   - collecting data related to the aspects of care and indicators
   - evaluating care based on the cumulative data collected
   - taking actions to improve care or services
   - assessing the effectiveness of the action(s) taken and documenting the outcomes
   - communicating data throughout the organization
2. Knowledge gained via the quality assessment and improvement process is used to initiate change in perioperative nursing practice in laser medicine and surgery.

Standard II: Performance Appraisal

The perioperative nurse evaluates his or her practice in the context of professional practice standards and relevant statutes and regulations.

Interpretive statement: Performance appraisal is a process that includes defining and evaluating professional practice behaviors.

Criteria

The perioperative nurse
   - identifies the behaviors that support the level of performance desired within the role(s) of perioperative nursing practice in laser medicine and surgery

- assesses perioperative practice behaviors in laser medicine and surgery on a regular basis and seeks constructive feedback
- identifies areas for personal and professional development
- takes action to achieve goals identified during performance appraisal
- periodically monitors and evaluates the progress of goal achievement
- participates in peer review when appropriate

Standard III: Education

The perioperative nurse acquires and maintains current knowledge in nursing practice in laser medicine and surgery.

Criteria

The perioperative nurse
- participates in ongoing educational activities related to clinical knowledge and professional issues of laser medicine and surgery,
- has primary responsibility for seeking experiences to maintain clinical skills in laser medicine and surgery
- identifies learning needs based on performance behaviors and seeks knowledge and skills appropriate for practice in laser medicine and surgery

Standard IV: Collegiality

The perioperative nurse contributes to the professional growth of peers, colleagues, and others.

Criteria

The perioperative nurse
- shares knowledge and skills about laser medicine and surgery with colleagues and others through inservice sessions, seminars, preceptoring, mentoring, role-modeling, publishing, consulting, problem solving, and other methods
- provides peers with constructive feedback regarding lasers in medicine and surgery
- contributes to a positive environment conducive to education of novice perioperative practitioners
- acts as a role model for perioperative nursing competencies and correct implementation of policies, procedures, and protocols

Standard V: Ethics

The perioperative nurse's decisions and actions on behalf of patients are determined in an ethical manner.

Criteria

1. The perioperative nurse acts as a patient advocate and is guided by the ANA's *Code for Nurses.*
2. Patient confidentiality is maintained.
3. Perioperative care is delivered in a nonjudgmental and nondiscriminatory manner that is sensitive to cultural, racial, and ethnic diversity.
4. Care is delivered in a manner that preserves and protects patient autonomy, dignity, and rights.

5. The perioperative nurse uses available resources to help formulate ethical decisions.

Standard VI: Collaboration

The perioperative nurse collaborates with the patient, significant others, health care providers, and others in providing care.

Criteria

The perioperative nurse
- communicates pertinent information relative to perioperative care involving laser technology
- consults with health care providers and others
- makes referrals, including provisions for continuity of care, as needed

Standard VII: Research

The perioperative nurse uses research findings in laser medicine and surgery practice.

Criteria

1. The perioperative nurse uses interventions substantiated by research as appropriate to the individual's position, education, and surgical setting.
2. The perioperative nurse participates in laser medicine and surgery research through involvement in one or more of the following activities:
   - identifying clinical problems
   - participating in data collection
   - sharing research activities with others
   - conducting research
   - reading and critiquing research for application in surgical practice
   - participating on a research committee
   - using knowledge gained through research findings to initiate change

Standard VIII: Resource Utilization

The perioperative nurse considers factors related to safety, effectiveness, efficiency, environmental concerns, and cost in planning and delivering patient care in laser medicine and surgery.

Criteria

The perioperative nurse
- evaluates factors related to safety, effectiveness, efficiency, environmental concerns, and cost when two or more practice options would result in the same expected outcome
- assigns tasks or delegates care based on the needs of the patient and the knowledge and skill of the provider selected
- assists the patient or significant others in identifying appropriate services available to address perioperative patient needs involving laser medicine and surgery

GLOSSARY

ablative surgery Vaporization or removal of tissue.

absorption Action of the tissue in taking up the laser energy, causing a reaction within the tissue.

accessible radiation Radiation that the human eye or skin may be exposed to during laser procedures.

active medium Substance within the laser head that is energized to produce photons and laser energy.

amplitude Half of the height of the wave from the top of one peak to the bottom of the next; measures the power of the wave.

average power Total amount of laser energy delivered divided by the duration of the laser exposure.

aversion response Movement by the eyelid or head to avoid a noxious stimulus or bright light. This can occur within 0.25 seconds, including the blink reflex.

coagulation Heating the tissue to a temperature below the level at which vaporization effects occur, approximately at 60° to 65° C. Often used to stop bleeding.

coherence State in which all the waves of the laser beam are in phase with each other in both time and space.

collimation State in which all the waves are parallel to each other with low convergence or divergence.

continuous mode (CW) Constant delivery of the laser beam without pulses.

controlled area Area that requires control and supervision for protection from laser hazards.

cooling system System of circulating water or air to keep the laser head from overheating.

delivery system Method used to deliver the light energy from the laser system to the target area.

diffuse reflection Change in the spatial distribution of the laser beam in many different directions (scattering) after it impacts a surface.

divergence Increase in the diameter of the beam as the beam gets farther from the exit aperture of the laser.

electromagnetic spectrum Continuum that graphs the various frequencies and wavelengths of different atomic systems.

energy Capacity to do work. Total energy (joules) = watts × time.

excited state State of an atom that has an electron orbiting in a higher shell, causing a high-energy state.

feedback mechanism System of mirrors in the laser head that promotes population inversion by amplifying the light energy.

fluence Amount of energy delivered to the tissue, determined by watts $\times$ time divided by the spot size (in cm^2).

focal length Distance between the lens and the focal point (point at which the beam is most intense).

focal point Exact point at which the laser beam has converged and is most intense.

free-flowing tube Tube with which laser gas is pulled from an external source and is excited to produce laser energy. The byproducts are discharged from the laser system.

frequency Number of wave peaks that pass a given point per second, inversely related to wavelength.

gas laser Laser system that uses gas as the active medium.

Gaussian curve Cross-section of radiant power density.

ground state State of an atom at a very low energy level.

helium-neon laser Device often used to provide the aiming beam for invisible laser wavelengths, 632 nm.

hertz (Hz) Frequency measurement of a wave in cycles per second.

infrared radiation Electromagnetic radiation with a wavelength in the range of 750 nm to 1 mm.

ionizing radiation Electromagnetic radiation that could be hazardous with continual tissue exposure because it may disrupt cellular DNA.

joule (J) Unit of energy. 1 J $=$ 1 watt $\times$ 1 second.

laser Device that produces an intense and directional beam of light. Acronym for light amplification by the stimulated emission of radiation.

laser chamber Resonating cavity that has two reflective mirrors at each end of the chamber and contains the active medium.

laser safety officer Physician, nurse, or technician who has the authority and responsibility to monitor and enforce the control of laser hazards during laser procedures. Usually one person is assigned the role of laser safety officer in a hospital.

maximum permissible exposure Radiation level a person may be exposed to without hazardous effects to the skin or eye.

micromanipulator Device that attaches to the microscope or colposcope to control the direction of the laser beam.

monochromatic Composed of photons of one color or wavelength.

nominal hazard zone Space near the laser-tissue impact area where direct, scattered, or reflected radiation exceeds the applicable maximum permissible exposure. Special eye and skin precautions must be enforced.

optical cavity See laser chamber.

output coupler Partially reflective mirror that allows a portion of the laser energy to escape from the laser chamber.

photon Light energy given off by an excited atom.

population inversion State in which the number of excited atoms in a laser medium exceeds the number of atoms not excited.

power Rate at which energy is transferred, received, or emitted; measured in units of watts (joules per second).

power density Irradiance or amount of power delivered to a specific area; measured in watts divided by the spot size (cm^2).

protective housing Protective enclosure that surrounds the laser components.

pumping Process of supplying energy to the laser head to activate the medium.

reflectance Ratio of the total reflected energy to the total energy that impacts the reflective substance.

scattering Process in which a light beam is distributed in many different paths after striking a surface.

sealed tube Sealed gas tube that contains a special catalyst for reorganizing and regenerating the gas to produce more lasing action.

specular reflection Mirrorlike direct reflection of the laser beam that occurs when the angle of the reflection is equal to the angle of the oncoming light.

spontaneous emission Release of a photon of absorbed energy from an excited atom.

stimulated emission Release of photon energy from an atom already in the excited state after being struck by a photon of equal energy.

TEM Transverse electromagnetic mode; determines the precision of the laser beam from the power distribution over the spot area.

transmission Passage of energy through a medium.

ultraviolet radiation Electromagnetic radiation with shorter wavelengths than those of the visible wavelengths; usually 100 to 400 nm.

vacuum pump Device that provides the force to pull the laser gas into the laser head.

vaporization Conversion of a solid or a liquid into a vapor; usually occurs in tissue at 100° C.

velocity Rate of speed at which a wave travels, which is approximately 186,300 miles per second.

visible radiation Electromagnetic radiation detectable by the human eye, in wavelengths of 400 to 750 nm.

watt (W) Unit of power; 1 W = 1 joule per second.

wavelength Distance between two successive peaks on a wave, usually measured in millimeters, micrometers, nanometers, or angstroms; determines the color of the light.

INDEX

A

Abdominal organs, laser procedures involving, 248-255
  anatomy and, 248
  biliary stones and, 255
  gallbladder and, 250-255
  hernia and, 250
  intraabdominal lesions and, 250
  liver and, 248-249
  pancreas and, 249
  spleen and, 249-250
Ablation, endometrial, 214-220
Abrasive tattoo, removal of, 179
Abscess, 198
  breast, 240-242
Absorption, laser-tissue interaction and, 15-19
Accidental tattoo, removal of, 179
Acetic acid
  cervical conization and, 202
  condylomata acuminata and, 235
Acknowledgement, laser education and, 391
Acoustical neuroma, 297
ACS; *see* Ambulatory surgery center
Actinic cheilitis, 177-178
Action plan, business plan development and, 321-322
Active medium of lasers, 30-31
Adenoma of soft palate, 153
Adhesiolysis, 220
Adhesions, 213, 214, 220
Administrative aspects of laser program, 315-408
Administrative support for laser program, 358
Advertising in marketing of laser program, 371-374
Airway, laser safety in, 141, 145
Airway explosion, fire safety and, 82-86

Alexandrite laser, 179
  Q-switched, 159, 181
Allergic rhinitis, laser surgery for, 136-137
Ambulatory surgery center (ASC), 353
Amenorrhea, 214
American National Standards Institute (ANSI), 58, 359-360
American Nurses Association (ANA), 409
American Society for Laser Medicine and Surgery (ASLMS), 59
American Society for Lasers in Medicine and Surgery, 409
American Urologic Association Symptom Index, 232
Amplitude, 6
ANA; *see* American Nurses Association
Ancillary components of lasers, 31-32
Andragogy, laser education and, 386
Anesthesia
  condylomata acuminata and, 236
  peripheral laser angioplasty and, 267
Angiomas, spider, 170-171
Angioplasty, laser; *see* Laser angioplasty
Angioscopy, 267
Animal care and use committee
  acquisition, 305
  documentation and report filing, 305
  inspection, 307
  membership, 303
  public relations policy, 305
  responsibilities, 306
Animal use in laser research, 300-302
Animal Welfare Act, 301
Animals, laser technology and; *see* Veterinary medicine, laser technology and

Ankle-brachial index, 202
ANSI; *see* American National Standards Institute
ANSI standards, 59, 62, 323, 325, 359-360
AORN; *see* Association of Operating Room Nurses
Aphthous ulcers, 154
Apnea, sleep, 152
Architectural design for laser-surgical center, 335-341
ArF; *see* Argon fluoride
ArF excimer laser; *see* Argon fluoride excimer laser
Argon fluoride (ArF), 55
Argon fluoride (ArF) excimer laser, 126
Argon laser, 15, 52-53, 61
    absorption of, 19
    adhesions and, 220
    allergic rhinitis and, 136
    arteriovenous malformations and, 193
    bladder tumors and, 225, 226
    brain procedures and, 297
    cervical vaporization and, 203
    characteristics of, 52-53
    closed-angle glaucoma and, 120
    condyloma acuminata and, 206
    control panel of, 32
    delivery systems of, 53
    dental applications and, 154
    depth of penetration of, 33
    dermatology and, 157, 159-160
    ectopic pregnancy and, 213
    endometriosis and, 210
    fibroids and, 221
    gallbladder applications and, 250
    green-only, 159
    hemorrhoids and, 196
    laparoscopy and, 208
    laser angioplasty and, 264, 265
    laser microlaryngoscopy and, 145
    laser tonsillectomy and, 150
    nasal conditions and, 137
    neurosurgical applications and, 296
    oculoplastic surgeries and, 130
    retinal conditions and, 112-113
    sealing of blood vessels by, 240
    spider veins of legs and, 171
    tattoo removal and, 179
    trichiasis and, 126
    urology applications and, 224
Argon laser trabeculotomy, open-angle glaucoma and, 119
Arterioscopy, 267
Arteriovenous malformations, 193
Arthroscopic procedures, 287-290
Arthrotomy, 287
Articulated arm, CO_2 laser and, 35
Asherman's syndrome, 214

ASLMS; *see* American Society for Laser Medicine and Surgery
Assessment
    external and internal, in marketing of laser program, 368-369
    of laser services, business plan development and, 321
    in perioperative patient education, 386
    in Standards of Care, 410
Association of Operating Room Nurses (AORN), 60, 376, 409
Atherosclerosis, 261-262
Atomic physics, basic, 7-8
Atoms, 8
Audience, target, in marketing of laser program, 370

B

Background diabetic retinopathy, 109-110
Backscattering of laser beam, 15
Backstops, safety and, 88
Bare fiber, fiberoptics and, 45
Baseline eye examination, 74-75
Battery, consent and, 391
Beckman Laser Institute, 335
Biannual credentialing review policy, 326
Bilateral prostatic hypertrophy (BPH), 231-234
Biomedical laser technician, 329, 332
Biophysics, laser; *see* Laser biophysics
Biopsy, breast, 240-242
Biostimulation, laser, 293-296
Bipolar electrosurgery unit, 21, 22
Bipolar scissors, 21
Bladder tumors, 224-229
Bleeding lesions, GI, photocoagulation of, 191-193
Blepharoplasty, laser, 182-184
Bloodborne pathogens, surgical smoke and, 98
Blooming effect, CO_2 beam and, 208
Booth display
    in community education, 397
    in marketing of laser program, 377-378
BPH; *see* Bilateral prostatic hypertrophy
Brain
    laser procedures of, 296-297
    stereotactic endoscopic laser surgery of, 298
Brain tumors, 296-297
Breast, laser procedures of, 240-244
Breast abscess, treatment of, 240-242
Breast biopsy, 240-242
Brochures
    informational, in marketing of laser program, 378-380
    laser conference and, 400
Bronchoscopy, laser; *see* Laser bronchoscopy
Budgetary commitment in marketing of laser program, 370

Bullous emphysema, thoracoscopy to treat, 246-247
Bundling of charges, facility reimbursement and, 353
Business cards in marketing of laser program, 380
Business plan development, 321-323

C

Café-au-lait macules, 169
Calculi, ureteral, 230-231
Callus, 278-279
Capacitive coupling, 21-23, 24
Capsule contraction syndrome, 126
Capsulotomy, posterior, 124-126
Carbon dioxide (CO_2) laser, 6, 32-39, 61, 94, 340
  adhesiolysis and, 220
  adhesions and, 214
  allergic rhinitis and, 136
  arthroscopic procedures and, 287-288
  bone tissue and, 275
  brain procedures and, 297
  breast abscess and, 240-242
  calluses and, 279, 280
  cavernous hemangioma and, 168
  cervical disease and, 202, 203
  characteristics of, 32-34
  condylomata acuminata and, 206
  corns and, 280
  decorative tattoo removal and, 179, 180
  decubitus ulcer and, 285
  delivery system of, 35-39
  dental applications and, 154
  dental cavities and, 155
  depth of penetration of, 33
  dermabrasion and, 174
  dermatology and, 157
  ectopic pregnancy and, 213
  excitation source of, 30
  fibroids and, 222
  fungus nail and, 281-282
  gallbladder procedures and, 250
  gingival overgrowth and, 155
  gynecology applications and, 200
  heel spurs and, 284
  hemorrhoids and, 196
  intraabdominal lesions and, 250
  laparoscopic applications and, 206-207
  laser angioplasty and, 264
  laser bronchoscopy and, 147-148
  laser microlaryngoscopy and, 145
  laser tonsillectomy and, 150-151
  laser turbinectomy and, 137
  laser welding and, 272
  laser-assisted uvula palatoplasty and, 152
  liver applications of, 248
  malignant melanoma and, 286
  mastectomies and, 242
  Morton's neuroma and, 283
  mucoceles and, 153

Carbon dioxide (CO_2) laser—cont'd
  neurosurgical applications of, 296-297
  oculoplastic surgeries and, 129-130
  operational modalities of, 39, 40-41
  pancreatic procedures and, 249
  pilonidal cysts and, 198
  podiatric laser applications and, 275
  port-wine stain and, 166
  radical neck dissection and, 244
  repair of pierced ear and, 184-185
  safety checklist for, 65
  sealing of blood vessels by, 240
  skin incisions and, 172
  soft tissues and, 293
  spider veins of legs and, 171
  subungual hematoma and, 283
  superpulse, facial chemical peel and, 178
  telangiectasia and, 169
  transmyocardial revascularization and, 271
  tubal reanastomosis and, 221, 222
  types of, 34-35
  ultrapulse, 178
  urethral strictures and, 229
  urology applications and, 224
  vaginal conditions and, 204
  vaporization of polymethylmethacrylate and, 294
  verrucae plantaris and, 276-278
  veterinary medicine applications and, 302
  vulvar conditions and, 205
  waffling technique and, 282
Carcinoma
  excision of, laser microlaryngoscopy and, 139
  penile, 237
  in situ, 201
  squamous cell, in dolphin, laser surgery for, 309-313
Cardiovascular laser applications, 261-274
  coronary artery procedures and; *see* Coronary
    artery procedures
  future, 273-274
  peripheral laser angioplasty and; *see* Laser angio-
    plasty, peripheral
  vascular welding and intravascular sealing and,
    272-273
Cardiovascular laser applications atherosclerosis and,
  261-262
Caries, dental, detection of, 155
Carpal tunnel syndrome, 295-296
Catheter fiber, fiberoptics and, 43
Cavernous hemangiomas, 168
Cavities, dental, detection of, 155
Cayton, Mary, 270
CDRH; *see* Center for Devices and Radiological
  Health
Center for Devices and Radiological Health (CDRH),
  58-59
Centralized smoke evacuation systems, 102
Cervical conditions, 200-204

Cervical conization, 202-203, 204
Cervical intraepithelial neoplasia (CIN), 200-203
Cervix
  erosion of, 200
  vaporization of, 202
Charges for laser services, 350-351
Cheilitis, actinic, 177-178
Chemical effects of lasers, 19
Chest, laser procedures of, 246-247
Cholecystectomy, 250-255
Choroid
  anatomy of eye and, 110
  malignant melanoma of, 129-130
Choroidal neovascularization, 112
Chronic cystitis, 235
Ciliary body, anatomy of eye and, 110
CIN; see Cervical intraepithelial neoplasia
Circumcision, 237, 238
Cladding of fiberoptics, 43
Classes I to IV lasers, 61
Claudication, atherosclerosis and, 261
Closed-angle glaucoma, 120-121
CME; see Continuing medical education
Coagulation of lasers, 34
Coherent laser light, 10
Collaboration in Standards of Professional Performance, 414
Collegiality in Standards of Professional Performance, 413
Collimated laser light, 9-10
Colon polyps, 194, 195
Colorectal laser procedures; see Gastroenterology and colorectal laser procedures
Colorectal tumors, 194-195
Colors, laser, 29
Communication
  about laser program, 358
  laser committee and, 318-321
Community education; see Laser education, community
Computed tomography (CT), stereotactic endoscopic laser surgery of brain and, 298
Computerization, cost-efficiency and, 354
Condyloma acuminata vaporization, 94, 206
Condylomata acuminata, 235-236
Cones, anatomy of eye and, 110
Conference coordinator, laser conference and, 399
Consent, informed, 363-364, 391
Console of lasers, 31
Contact Nd:YAG laser, 47-50
  adhesiolysis and, 220
  arthroscopic procedures and, 287-288
  bilateral prostatic hypertrophy and, 234
  bladder tumors and, 225, 227
  brain tumor excisions and, 297
  brain tumors and, 298
  breast biopsy and, 241
  cervical procedures and, 202, 203

Contact Nd:YAG laser—cont'd
  chronic cystitis and, 234, 235
  circumcision and, 237
  colorectal tumors and, 195
  delivery device for, 289
  dermatology and, 158
  ectopic pregnancy and, 213
  endometriosis and, 210
  fibroids and, 213, 222
  hemorrhoids and, 196, 197
  intraabdominal lesions and, 250
  laparoscopic presacral neurectomy and, 212
  laser microlaryngoscopy and, 145
  laser surgery on horses and, 309
  laser thyroidectomy and, 245
  laser tonsillectomy and, 150-151
  laser-assisted uvula palatoplasty and, 152
  liver procedures and, 249
  mastectomy and, 242
  Morton's neuroma and, 283
  nasolacrimal duct surgery and, 138
  neurosurgical applications of, 295
  oculoplastic surgery and, 129
  ovarian procedures and, 212
  partial nephrectomy and, 238
  pilonidal cysts and, 198-199
  podiatric laser applications and, 275
  radical neck dissection and, 244
  soft tissues and, 293
  spinal cord procedures and, 297
  urethral strictures and, 229
Contact tips of lasers, 47-48, 49, 356
Contact YAG laser, spider veins of legs and, 171
Continuing education, 357-358
Continuing education units, laser conference and, 400
Continuing medical education (CME) units, laser conference and, 400
Continuous quality improvement (CQI), 363
Continuous wave (CW) mode, 13, 40-41, 61
Contraceptives, oral, endometriosis and, 210
Control panel of lasers, 32, 64
Controlled treatment area, laser safety and, 76-78
Cooling system of lasers, 32
Copper vapor laser, 55-56
Core of fiberoptics, 43
Cornea, anatomy of, 126
Corneal reprofiling, 126
Corns
  neurovascular, 280
  podiatric laser applications and, 278-280
Coronary artery procedures, 270-272
  laser angioplasty, 270
  laser thrombolysis, 272
  transmyocardial revascularization, 271-272
Cosmetic tattoo, removal of, 179
Cosmic rays, 7

Cost containment, laser program and, 353-356
Costs of laser procedure, 350
CO₂ laser; *see* Carbon dioxide laser
Coumadin, 243
Course format, laser conference and, 400
CPT codes; *see* Current Procedural Technology codes
CQI; *see* Continuous quality improvement
Cramping, pain and, 390
Credentialing, physician, 323-325, 357, 362-363
Cruelty to Animals Act, 301
Crystal lasers, 31
CT; *see* Computed tomography
Curettage, podiatric laser applications versus, 275
Curing composite, 156
Current Procedural Technology (CPT) codes, physician reimbursement and, 351
Custom packs, cost-efficiency and, 356, 357
Cutaneous lesions, 172-178
CW mode; *see* Continuous wave mode
Cyclophotocoagulation, transscleral, 120, 121
Cystitis, chronic, 235
Cysts
    ganglionic, 284
    pilonidal, 198
    plugged duct, 279
    podiatric laser applications and, 278-280, 283-286

D

Dacryocystorhinostomy (DCR), 138
Danazol (Danocrine)
    endometrial suppression and, 215
    endometriosis and, 210
DCR; *see* Dacryocystorhinostomy
Debulking of lasers, 34
Decorative tattoo, removal of, 178-179, 180-181
Decubitus ulcer, 285, 286
Defective laser equipment, 360-361
Delivery system of lasers, 32
Dental caries, detection of, 155
Dental spectroscopy, 156
Dentistry, laser applications in, 153-155
Depot leuprolide acetate, 215
Depth of penetration of laser beam, 18, 33-34
Dermabrasion with laser, 174-176
Dermatology
    laser, sample discharge instructions for, 395
    and plastic surgery laser applications
        for actinic cheilitis, 177-178
        for cutaneous lesions, 172-178
        dermabrasion with laser and, 174-176
        for keloids, 173-174
        laser blepharoplasty and, 182-185
        for pigmented lesions, 167-169
        for port-wine stain, 160, 161-167
        repair of pierced ear and, 184-185
        for scars, 173-174

Dermatology—cont'd
    and plastic surgery laser applications—cont'd
        for skin incisions, 172-173
        for tattoo removal, 178-182, 183
        for telangiectasia, 169-172
        for vascular lesions, 161-172
        for verruca, 177
32% Dextran 70 in dextrose (Hyskon), endometrial ablation and, 215-216
Diagnosis in Standards of Care, 410-411
Diagnosis-related group (DRG), facility reimbursement and, 352-353
Didactical session, laser conference and, 400-402
Diffuse reflection, laser-tissue interaction and, 14
Diffusional interception, filtration of surgical smoke and, 96, 98
Dilantin; *see* Phenytoin sodium
Diode laser, 55, 112, 113
Direct interception, filtration of surgical smoke and, 96, 97
Direct mail in marketing of laser program, 374
Discharge instructions, 340
Disposable fibers, Nd:YAG laser technology and, 45, 46
Documentation
    adminstration of laser program and, 360-362
    as responsibility of laser team, 331
Dolphins, laser surgery on, 309-313
Dopant, solid lasers and, 31
Dougherty, Thomas, 256
Drake, Ellet, 60
Dye-enhanced laser photocoagulation, 116
Dystrophy, reflex sympathetic, 295

E

Ear
    anatomy of, 132
    laser procedures for, 131-135
    nose, and throat (ENT) specialists, 131
    pierced, repair of, 184-185
Ebonization, reflected laser beam and, 86
Economics of laser program development, 350-353
    charges in, 350-351
    costs in, 350
    reimbursement in, 351-353
Ectopic pregnancy, 213
Education
    continuing, 357-358
    laser; *see* Laser education
    of laser safety officer and laser team, 327
    in Standards of Professional Performance, 413
Einstein, Albert, 3
Electrical hazards, 90
Electrocautery, comparison of, with laser, 19-25, 26, 27, 199
Electromagnetic spectrum, 4-5

Electrosurgery
  lasers versus, 19-25, 26, 27
  podiatric laser applications versus, 275
Electrosurgery large loop excision of the transformation zone (electrosurgery LLETZ) conization, 202
Electrosurgery unit (ESU), 19-25, 239
Elephants, laser surgery on, 308
Emergency laser procedures, laser team member available for, 330
Emphysema, bullous, thoracoscopy to treat, 245-246
Enamel replacement, 156
Endometrial ablation, 214-220
Endometrial cancer, diagnosis of, after endometrial ablation, 219-220
Endometriosis vaporization, 209-211, 221-222
Endorphins, floating, laser biostimulation and, 294
Endoscope, 355
  safety precautions with, 88-89
  spinal, laser discectomy and, 291-293
Endoscopic laser surgery, stereotactic, of brain, 298
Endoscopic urological laser applications; *see* Urology laser applications, endoscopic
Endoscopy, laser; *see* Laser endoscopy
Endotracheal (ET) tube, airway explosion and, 82-83, 140, 356
Energy, radiant, 4
ENT specialists; *see* Ear, nose, and throat specialists
Environmental controls, adminstration of laser program and, 362
Epinephrine, lidocaine with; *see* Lidocaine (Xylocaine) with epinephrine
Epistaxis, 138
Erbium laser, dental applications of, 154
Erbium:YAG laser
  cataract extraction and, 129
  dental applications and, 156
  ophthalmic procedures and, 109
  orthopedic procedures and, 288-290
Esophageal obstruction, laser treatment for, 189-191
Esophageal tumor vaporization, 190-191
ESU; *see* Electrosurgery unit
ET tube; *see* Endotracheal tube
Ethics
  laser program and, 333-334
  in Standards of Professional Performance, 413-414
Evaluation
  in business plan development, 322
  of laser conference, 406
  of marketing of laser program, 380-381
  in perioperative patient education, 390-393
  in procurement of laser systems, 343-345
  in Standards of Care, 412
Excimer laser, 55-56
  cataract extraction and, 129
  disadvantages of, 266

Excimer laser—cont'd
  laser thrombolysis and, 272
  photorefractive keratectomy and, 126
  photorefractive surgical procedures and, 126
Excision of carcinomas, laser microlaryngoscopy and, 139
Excitation source of lasers, 30
Executive summary, business plan development and, 321
Experimental laser procedures, laser education and, 387
Explosive tattoo, removal of, 179
External assessment
  of laser services, business plan development and, 321
  in marketing of laser program, 368-369
Eye, anatomy of, 110-111
Eye examination, baseline, 362
Eye filters, 71
Eye injuries, 67-68
Eye protection, 68-73, 217, 298, 355
Eye safety, 65-76
  baseline eye examination and, 74-76
  eye filter and, 71
  eye injuries and, 67-68
  eye protection and, 68-73
  patient eye protection and, 73, 74

F

Face, seborrheic keratoses of, 178
Facility reimbursement for laser procedure, 352-353
FDA; *see* Food and Drug Administration
Feasibility study, laser committee and, 342-343
Federal Food, Drug, and Cosmetic Act, 344
Feedback mechanism of laser light production, 31
Fiberoptics, 43
Fibers
  bare, fiber repair procedure for, 45
  disposable, 355
  Nd:YAG laser technology and, 43, 45
Fibroids, 213, 221, 222
Finances of laser program, 342-358
  cost containment and, 353-356
  laser economics and, 350-353
  maintaining adequate laser utilization and, 356-358
  procurement of laser systems and, 342-350
Finsen, Nils, 3
Fire, airway, emergency measures for, 145
Fire safety, 78-88
  airway explosion and, 82-86
  flammable materials and, 81-83
  halon fire extinguisher and, 79, 81
  methane gas explosion and, 82
  nonreflective instruments and, 86-88
  surgical drapes and, 80-81

Fissures, 198, 278-280
Fistulas, 194, 198
Flammable materials, fire safety and, 81-82
Flashlamp pulsed dye laser, 231
    biliary stones and, 255
    dermatology and, 181
    ureteral calculi and, 230
Flashlamp-pumped pulsed dye (FLPPD) laser, 54
Floating endorphins, laser biostimulation and, 294
FLPPD laser; *see* Flashlamp-pumped pulsed dye laser
Fluence, laser power and, 13
Fluorescein angiogram, 112, 113
Fluoroscopy, 267, 268
Focal length of beam, CO_2 laser and, 35, 36
Focal length of lens, 11
Food and Drug Administration (FDA), 58, 256, 344, 361
Foot pedals, 89-90, 91, 92
Fovea centralis, 110
Free electron laser, 56
Free flowing CO_2 laser, 34
Freestanding laser programs, 334, 335
Frequency, 6-7
Frequency doubled YAG laser, 50-51, 208
    adhesiolysis and, 220
    allergic rhinitis and, 136
    brain tumors and, 297
    cervical procedures and, 203
    condyloma acuminata and, 206
    dermatology and, 159
    ectopic pregnancy and, 213
    endometriosis and, 210
    fibroids and, 221
    gallbladder procedures and, 250
    laser microlaryngoscopy and, 145
    laser stapedectomy and, 132
    laser tonsillectomy and, 150
    laser-assisted uvula palatoplasty and, 152
    nasal conditions and, 137
    nasolacrimal duct surgery and, 137
    neurosurgical applications of, 296
    spider veins of legs and, 171
    urology applications of, 224
Fungus nail, 281, 282

G

Gamma rays, 7
Ganglionic cysts, 284
Gas, active medium of lasers and, 31
Gastroenterology and colorectal laser procedures, 186-199
    for fissures, 198
    for fistulas and abscesses, 198
    laser endoscopy; *see* Laser endoscopy
    laser hemorrhoidectomy, 195-198
    for pilonidal cysts and sinuses, 198-199
    for rectal and perianal conditions, 195-199

Gastrointestinal bleeding lesions, photocoagulation of, 191-193
Gastrointestinal tract, malformations in, 193-194
Gastrostomy, laser, sample discharge instructions for, 394
Gated CW mode, 13
General surgery and oncology, laser applications and, 239-260
    for abdominal organs, 248-255
    in breast procedures, 240-244
    in the chest, 246-247
    for head and neck dissection, 244-246
    photodynamic therapy and, 255-260
Genital warts, 94, 206
Gingival overgrowth, 155
Gingival toughening, 155
Glaucoma
    closed-angle, 120-121
    laser procedures for, 118-123
    open-angle, 118-119
Glycopyrrolate (Robinul), 215
Goldman, Leon, 60, 157
Grant Laser Center, 335
Granuloma
    laser microlaryngoscopy and, 139
    pyogenic, 151
Green-only argon laser, 159
Gynecological anatomy, 201
Gynecology laser applications, 200-223
    hysteroscopic, 214-220
    intraabdominal, for infertility, 220-222
        adhesiolysis, 220, 221
        myomectomy and endometriosis vaporization, 320-321
        reanastomosis, 220-221
        salpingoplasty, 220-221
        tubal reimplantation, 220-221
    laparoscopic, 206-213, 214
        endometrial vaporization, 209-211
        laser treatment of ectopic pregnancy, fibroids, and adhesions, 213, 214
        neosalpingostomy, 211
        ovarian procedures, 212
        presacral transection, 211-212
        uterosacral transection, 211-212
    lower tract, 200-206
        cervical conditions, 200-204
        condylomata acuminata vaporization, 206
        vaginal conditions, 205-205
        vulvar conditions, 205-206

H

Hair, flammability of, 81-82
Halon fire extinguisher, fire safety and, 79, 80
Harvey, William, 300
Head, laser, 30-31

Health care professional education; *see* Laser education, health care professional

Heel fissures, 280

Heel spurs, 284

Helium-neon laser, 61, 295

Hemangioma, 167
  cavernous, 168

Hematoma, subungual, 282, 283

Hemorrhoidectomy, laser, 195-198

HEPA filter; *see* High-efficiency particulate air filter

Hereditary hemorrhagic telangiectasia, 138, 193

Herpetic lesions, 153-154

Hexascanner, 51, 53, 160, 170

High-efficiency particulate air (HEPA) filter, 95, 96

Holmium laser, 288, 293
  adhesiolysis and, 220
  ankle joints and, 288
  biliary stones and, 255
  dental applications of, 154
  depth of penetration of, 33
  ectopic pregnancy and, 213
  fibroids and, 222
  internal sclerostomy and, 123
  laparoscopy and, 208
  laser discectomy and, 291
  laser thrombolysis and, 272
  neurosurgical applications of, 296
  oculoplastic surgery and, 129
  shoulder joints and, 288, 290
  soft tissues and, 293
  urology applications of, 224

Holmium:YAG laser, 127
  arthroscopic procedures and, 288
  laser angioplasty and, 266
  laser thrombolysis and, 272
  nasolacrimal duct surgery and, 138
  podiatric laser applications and, 275

Horses, laser surgery on, 309

Hospital commitment and permission, laser conference and, 399

Hospital policies and procedures, laser safety and, 60

HPV; *see* Human papilloma virus

Human papilloma virus (HPV), 94, 200, 206

Hydrosalpinx, chronic, 211

Hyperplasia of prostate gland, 232

Hypertrophic scars, 284-285

Hypogastric plexus, transection of, 211

Hypomenorrhea, 214

Hyskon; *see* 32% Dextran 70 in dextrose

Hysterectomy, 214, 219-220, 221

Hysteroscopic laser applications, 214-220

I

IACUCs; *see* Institutional animal care and use committees

Impact, laser education and, 391

Implants, exposure of, 155

Implementation
  in perioperative patient education, 387-390
  in Standards of Care, 411

Incisions, skin, 172-173

Incoherent laser light, 10

Incus, 131

Indirect ophthalmoscope, 115

Inertial impaction, filtration of surgical smoke and, 96, 97

Infertility, intraabdominal laser applications for, 220-222

Informational brochures
  in community education, 397
  in marketing of laser program, 378-380

Informed consent, 363-364, 391

Infrastructure of laser program, 317-341

In-line smoke filters, 100

Instant Ocean, 206

Institutional animal care and use committees (IACUCs), 301-302

Instruments, nonreflective, fire safety and, 86-88

Integrated laser programs, 334-335

Interdigital neuroma, 283-284

Internal assessment
  of laser services, business plan development and, 321
  in marketing of laser program, 368-369

Internal sclerostomy, 121, 122-123

International Laser Surgery Society, 60

Intraabdominal laser applications for infertility, 220-222

Intraocular lens (IOL), cataract extraction and, 129

Intravascular sealing, laser, 273

Intravascular ultrasonic imaging, laser angioplasty and, 267

Investigational Device Exemption, 58

IOL; *see* Intraocular lens

Ionizing radiation, 7

Iridectomy, laser, 121

Iris, anatomy of eye and, 109, 110

Irradiance, laser power and, 10

Ischemia-producing retinal conditions, 112

J

Jaegar plate, 183

Jako, Geza, 131

JCAHO; *see* Joint Commission on Accreditation of Healthcare Organizations

Jet ventilation, 86, 142

Joint Commission on Accreditation of Healthcare Organizations (JCAHO), 30, 59-60, 361, 365, 392

K

Kaplan, Isaac, 60

Keloids, 173-174, 284-285

Keratoses, seborrheic, of face, 178

Key storage for laser units, 79

Knee, arthroscopy of, 287
Krypton fluoride (KrF), 55
Krypton laser, 53, 159
Krypton rod laser, 113-114
KTP laser, 51, 159
  arteriovenous malformations and, 193
  excitation source of, 30
  hemorrhoids and, 196
  keloids and, 284
  laser discectomy and, 291
  podiatric laser applications and, 275
  prostatectomy and, 231
  soft tissues and, 293

L

Laboratories, ongoing physician training, 358, 402
Laboratory exercises, laser, 404-405
Laparoscopic cholecystectomy, 252, 253, 254
Laparoscopic gynecologic laser applications, 206-213, 214
Laparoscopic oophorectomy, 212
Laparoscopic uterine nerve ablation (LUNA), 211-212
Laparoscopy, 21-23, 239
Laryngeal stenosis, laser microlaryngoscopy and, 138
Laryngoscope, laser microlaryngoscopy and, 143, 146
LASER; *see* Light Amplification by the Stimulated Emission of Radiation
Laser angioplasty, 56, 270
  peripheral, 262-270
    diagnostic testing and, 262
    history of, 264
    intraoperative procedures and, 265-269
    patient selection criteria and, 264
    postoperative phase of, 269-270
    preoperative patient education and, 264-265
    surgical alternatives to, 262-263
  photoablative, 265, 266
  photothermal, 265-266
  thermal, 265
Laser applications, 107-314; *see also* specific specialty or body area
Laser benefits, 25-26
Laser biophysics, 3-27
  basic atomic physics and, 7-8
  laser benefits and, 25-26
  laser light characteristics and, 8-10
    coherent, 10
    collimated, 9-10
    monochromatic, 8-9
  laser power and, 10-13
    fluence and, 13
    power density and, 10-12
  laser versus electrosurgery and, 19-25, 26, 27

Laser biophysics—cont'd
  laser-tissue interaction and, 14-19
    absorption and, 15-19
    reflection and, 14
    scattering and, 15
    transmission and, 15, 16
  principles of light and, 4-7
    amplitude and, 6
    frequency and, 6-7
    velocity and, 6
    wavelength and, 4-6
Laser biostimulation, orthopedic laser applications and, 294-296
Laser blepharoplasty, 182-184
Laser bronchoscopy, 147-150, 247
  bronchoscope systems for, 148-149
  complications associated with, 149
  laser systems for, 147-148
  protocol for, 149-150
  safety during, 149
Laser charges, 356
Laser committee, 61-62, 317-321
  membership of, 317-318
  responsibilities of, 318-321
  structure of, 317-318
Laser conference in health care professional education, 398-406
Laser control panel, 403
Laser dermatology, sample discharge instructions for, 395
Laser director, 329, 330
Laser discectomy, 290-293
Laser education, 264-265, 383-408
  community, 393-397
    booth display in, 397
    informational brochures in, 397
    slide presentation in, 396-397
  health care professional, 397-407
    developing laser conference in, 398-406
    performance appraisals in, 397-398
    preceptorships in, 406-407
  laser laboratory exercises in, 404-405
  perioperative patient, 364-365, 383-393
    assessment of, 386
    benefits of, 385
    evaluation of, 390-393
  perioperative patient—cont'd
    implementation of, 387-390
    initiation of, 383-386
    planning in, 386-387
  postoperative, 340
  sample discharge instructions in, 394, 395
Laser endoscopy, 186-195
  for esophageal obstruction, 189-191
  laser colonoscopy and, 194-195

Laser endoscopy—cont'd
  lower, 189
  malformations in GI tract and, 193-194
  photocoagulation of GI bleeding lesions and, 191-193
  protocol for, 186-189
  upper, 188-189
Laser equipment, defective, 360-361
Laser gastrostomy, sample discharge instructions for, 394
Laser guiding bridge, 226
Laser hemorrhoidectomy, 195-198
Laser intravascular sealing, 273
Laser iridectomy, 120
Laser laboratory exercises, 404-405
Laser light, characteristics of, 8-10
Laser literature, 357
Laser log, sample, 333
Laser matrixectomy, 281
Laser microlaryngoscopy, 138-147
  indications for, 138-140
  safety precautions for, 140-145
Laser newsletter, 358
Laser nurse, 328-329, 331
Laser photocoagulation
  dye-enhanced, 116
  for trichiasis, 126
Laser plume, 91-103
  masks and, 102-103, 104
  research on, 91-95
  smoke evacuation and, 93-94, 95-102, 103, 188, 208
Laser power, 10-13
Laser program
  administration of, 315-408
    documentation of, 360-362
    environmental controls and, 362
    patient consent and education and, 363-365
    physician credentialing and, 362-363
    physician liability and, 365-366
    standards of care and, 359-360
    total quality management and, 363
  administrative support for, 358
  business plan development in, 321-323
  communication about, 358
  economics of; see Economics of laser program development
  education in; see Laser education
  ethics in, 333-334
  expanding laser services in, 334-341
  finances of; see Finances of laser program
  infrastructure of, 317-341
  laser committee and, 317-321
  legal aspects of, 359-366
  maintaining adequate utilization of, 356-358

Laser program—cont'd
  marketing of; see Marketing of laser program
  medical director of, 318
  multispecialty, 357
  physician credentialing in, 323-325
  position of, in marketing of laser program, 370
  staffing in, 325-333, 357
Laser repair of retinal tears and detachments, 118
Laser safety, 59-105
  in airway, 141, 145
  backstops and, 88
  checklist for, 65
  controlled treatment area and, 76-78
  electrical hazards and, 90
  endoscope precautions and, 88-89, 90
  eye safety and; see Eye safety
  fire safety and; see Fire safety
  foot pedals and, 89-90, 91, 92
  hospital policies and procedures and, 60
  laser classifications and, 61
  laser committee and, 61-62
  laser plume and; see Laser plume
  laser safety officer and, 62-64
  laser safety references and regulatory bodies and, 58-60
  laser team members and, 62-64
  mirrors and, 88
  policies for, 103-104
  state and local regulations and, 60
  transportation hazards and, 90-91, 92
Laser safety officer (LSO), 62-64, 327, 329
Laser safety reference sources, 319-320
Laser safety technician, 332
Laser stapedectomy, 131-135
Laser stone basket, ureteral calculi and, 230, 231
Laser systems, procurement of; see Procurement of laser systems
Laser team, 62-64, 357
Laser thyroidectomy, 245-246
Laser tips, 47-48, 49
Laser tonsillectomy, 150-151
Laser trabeculoplasty, 119
Laser training program, 323
Laser turbinectomy, 137
Laser welding of vessels, 272-273
Laser-assisted uvula palatoplasty (LAUP), 152
Lasers, 7, 28-57
  Alexandrite, 178
  ancillary components of, 31-32
  and animals; see Veterinary medicine, laser technology and
  argon; see Argon laser
  argon fluoride excimer, 126
  carbon dioxide; see Carbon dioxide laser
  chemical effects of, 19

Lasers—cont'd
  comparison of, with electrocautery, 199
  contact YAG, 171
  control panel of, 32, 64
  copper vapor, 55
  crystal, 31
  debulking of, 34
  delivery system of, 32
  depth of penetration of, 18, 33-34
  developments in technology of, 28
  diode, 55, 111
  versus electrosurgery, 19-25, 26, 27
  erbium:YAG; *see* Erbium:YAG laser
  excimer, 55-56
  excimer; *see* Excimer laser
  excitation source of, 30
  flashlamp pulsed dye; *see* Flashlamp pulsed dye laser
  flashlamp-pumped pulsed dye, 54
  free electron, 56
  frequency doubled YAG; *see* Frequency doubled YAG laser
  head of, 30-31
  helium-neon, 61, 295
  holmium; *see* Holmium laser
  holmium:YAG; *see* Holmium:YAG laser
  krypton, 53, 159
  krypton rod, 113-114
  KTP; *see* KTP laser
  laser wavelengths and colors and, 29
  liquid, 31
  mechanical effects of, 19
  mode-locked Nd:YAG, 124
  Nd:YLF, 127
  neodymium: yttrium-aluminum-garnet; *see* Neodymium: yttrium-aluminum-garnet laser
  parts of, 29-32
  Q-switched Alexandrite, 159
  Q-switched Nd:YAG, 124
  Q-switched ruby, 159
  Q-switched ruby laser, 54
  semiconductor diode, 31
  solid, 31
  temporal characteristics of, 13
  thermal effects of, 13, 15, 18, 19
  tunable dye, 31, 54
    skin tags and, 173
  wavelength of, 11-12
Laser-surgi centers, 335-341
Laser-tissue interaction, 14-19
LAUP; *see* Laser-assisted uvula palatoplasty
Leasing agreements, laser procurement and, 346-348
Legal aspects of laser program, 359-366
Leiomyoma, uterine, 221

Lens
  anatomy of eye and, 111
  intraocular, cataract extraction and, 129
Leukoplakia, 153
Lidocaine (Xylocaine), 311
  with epinephrine
    breast biopsy and, 240
    excision of verrucae plantaris and, 276
    wedge resection of tongue and, 153
Light, principles of, 4-7
Light Amplification by the Stimulated Emission of Radiation (LASER), 3
Limited partnership, laser procurement and, 348-349
Liquid laser, 31
Local and state regulations, laser safety and, 60
Lower bowel stenosis, 195
Lower endoscopy, 189
Low-pressure suction valve, smoke evacuation and, 101
LSO; *see* Laser safety officer
LUNA; *see* Laparoscopic uterine nerve ablation

M

Macula, 110
Maiman, Theodore H., 3
Malformations in GI tract, 193-194
Malfunctioning laser equipment, 360-361
Malignant leions of oral cavity, 153
Malignant melanoma, 129-130, 286
Malleus, 131
Mallory-Weiss syndrome, 193
Managed care, 334
Mark, William B., 60
Marketing of laser program, 358, 367-382
  advertising in, 371-374
  development of, 367-370
  establishing focus of, 369-370
  evaluation of, 380-381
  external and internal assessment in, 368-369
  implementation of, 370-380
  personal selling in, 374-375
  publicity in, 377-380
  sales promotion in, 376-377
Masks, 102-103, 104
Mastectomy, 242-244
Matrixectomy, 281
Maximum permissible exposure (MPE), eye protection and, 66
Mechanical effects of lasers, 19
Medical Device Amendments to Federal Food, Drug, and Cosmetic Act, 344
Medical director of laser program, 318
Medicare, physician reimbursement and, 352
MEDWatch, 361

Meetings, laser committee and, 318
Melanoma, 169
   malignant; *see* Malignant melanoma
Menorrhagia, endometrial ablation for, 214-220
Methane gas explosion, fire safety and, 82
Metrorrhagia, 214
Microendoscopes, 209
Microlaryngoscopy, laser; *see* Laser microlaryngoscopy
Microwaves, 7
Mirhoseini, Mahmood, 270
Mirrors
   adhesiolysis and, 220
   safety and, 88
Mission of laser committee, 318
Mode-locked Nd:YAG laser, 41-42, 124
Monochromatic laser light, 8-9
Monopolar electrosurgery unit, 21
Morton's neuroma, 283-284
MPE; *see* Maximum permissible exposure
Mucoceles, 153
Multispecialty laser systems, 357
Myomectomy and endometriosis vaporization, 221-222

N

Nail procedures, 281-282, 283
Nasolacrimal duct surgery, 138
National Institute for Occupational Safety and Health (NIOSH), 59
Nd:YAG laser; *see* Neodymium: yttrium-aluminum-garnet laser
Nd:YLF laser, 127
Neck, laser procedures of, 244-246
Neck dissection, radical, 244-245
Neodymium: yttrium-aluminum-garnet (Nd:YAG) laser, 6, 39-50, 61
   absorption of, 19
   backscattering of, 15
   bladder tumors and, 225
   characteristics of, 39-42
   closed-angle glaucoma and, 120
   condyloma acuminata and, 206
   contact; *see* Contact Nd:YAG laser
   contact fiber delivery system of, 47-50
   control panel of, 32
   dental applications and, 154
   depth of penetration of, 33
   endometrial ablation and, 217
   excitation source of, 30
   heel spurs and, 284
   hemorrhoids and, 196
   intravascular sealing and, 273
   laparoscopy and, 208

Neodymium: yttrium-aluminum-garnet (Nd:YAG) laser—cont'd
   laser angioplasty and, 264, 265
   laser bronchoscopy and, 147, 247
   laser endoscopy and, 186
   laser turbinectomy and, 137
   laser welding and, 272
   malformations in GI tract and, 193
   mastectomy and, 243
   mode-locked, 41-42
   neck procedures and, 244
   noncontact; *see* Noncontact Nd:YAG laser
   noncontact fiber delivery system of, 42-46
   ophthalmological applications of, 126
   pancreatic procedures and, 249
   penile carcinoma and, 237
   posterior capsulotomy and, 124
   prostatectomy and, 231, 233
   Q-switched, 41-42, 181
   scattering of, 148
   tattoo removal and, 179
   urethral strictures and, 229
   urological conditions and, 224
   veterinary medicine applications and, 302
   visual laser ablation of prostate and, 232
Neosalpingostomy, 211
Nephrectomy, partial, 238
Networking, laser committee and, 318-321
Neurectomy, presacral, 211
Neuroma
   acoustical, 297
   interdigital, 283-284
   Morton's, 283-284
Neuroma excision, 283-286
Neurosurgical laser applications, 296-298
   laser applications of brain and, 296-297
   laser procedures of spinal cord and, 297-298
   stereotactic endoscopic laser surgery of brain and, 298
Neurovascular corn, 280
Nevus, 169
Newsletter, laser, 358
Newspaper advertising in marketing of laser program, 372-373
Newsworthy information in marketing of laser program, 377
NHZ; *see* Nominal hazard zone
NIOSH; *see* National Institute for Occupational Safety and Health
Nodules, laser microlaryngoscopy and, 139
Nominal hazard zone (NHZ), eye protection and, 66
Noncontact Nd:YAG laser, 42-46
   bladder tumors and, 226
   brain tumors and, 298

Noncontact Nd:YAG laser—cont'd
  capillary hemangiomas and, 159, 168
  condylomata acuminata and, 236
  endometrial ablation and, 216
  fiber used for, 217
  hemorrhoids and, 196
  liver procedures and, 248
  neurosurgical applications of, 296
  penile carcinoma and, 237
  prostatectomy and, 232, 233
  sealing of blood vessels by, 240
  transurethral ultrasound-guided laser-induced
      prostatectomy and, 234
  urethral strictures and, 229
Nonionizing radiation, 7
Nonreflective instruments, fire safety and, 86-88
Norton metal endotracheal tube, 140
Nose
  anatomy of, 136
  laser procedures for, 135-138
Nosebleed, 138
Nurse, laser, 328-329, 331
Nursing/Allied Health Division of the American So-
      ciety for Laser Medicine and Surgery, 398,
      409

O

Obstructive sleep apnea, 152
Occupational Safety and Health Administration
      (OSHA), 59
On the Motion of the Heart and Blood, 300
Oncology; *see* General surgery and oncology, laser
      applications and
Ongoing physican training laboratories, 358
Onychomycosis, 281, 282
Oophorectomy, laparoscopic, 212
Open-angle glaucoma, 119-120
Operating life of sealed lasers, 34
Ophthalmic focusing lens, 117
Ophthalmological laser applications, 109-130
  capsule contraction syndrome and, 126
  cataract extraction and, 129
  laser photocoagulation for trichiasis and, 126
  laser procedures for glaucoma and, 118-123
  laser repair of retinal tears and detachments and,
      118
  oculoplastics and, 129
  photorefractive surgical procedures and, 126-129
  posterior capsulotomy and, 124-126
  recent, 126-130
  retinal photocoagulation for retinopathies and, 111-
      117
Ophthalmological laser applications, anatomy of eye
      and, 110-111
Ophthalmoscope, indirect, 115
Optic disc, 110

Oral cavity
  benign lesions of, 153
  laser procedures in, 153-154
Oral contraceptives, endometriosis and, 210
Orthopedic laser applications, 286-296
  arthroscopic procedures and, 287-290
  laser biostimulation and, 294-296
  laser discectomy and, 290-293
  laser use for soft tissues and, 293-294
  vaporization of polymethylmethacrylate and, 294
OSHA; *see* Occupational Safety and Health Adminis-
      tration
Otorhinolaryngology, 131-156
Otosclerosis, 131
Outcome identification in Standards of Care, 411
Outdoor advertising in marketing of laser program,
      374
Ovarian procedures, 212
Ownership method of laser procurement, 345-346

P

Pain
  cramping and, 390
  sympathetic maintained, 295
Pain gate blocking, laser biostimulation and, 294
Panretinal photocoagulation, 113, 114
Papillomatosis, laser microlaryngoscopy and, 139
Paralysis of vocal cords, 139
Partial nephrectomy, 238
Patient consent, 363-364, 391
Patient eye protection, 73, 74
PDT; *see* Photodynamic therapy
Peas, frozen, bag of, as ice compress, 184
Pedagogical method, laser education and, 386
Penile carcinoma, 237
Perez, Jim, 211-212
Performance appraisal
  in health care professional education, 397-398
  in Standards of Professional Performance, 412-413
Perianal conditions; *see* Rectal and perianal condi-
      tions
Perioperative clinical practice, standards of, in laser
      medicine and surgery, 409-414
Perioperative patient education; *see* Laser education,
      perioperative patient
Personal selling in marketing of laser program, 374-
      375
Phenytoin sodium (Dilantin), overgrowth of gum tis-
      sue and, 154
Photoablation, excimer laser and, 55
Photoablative laser angioplasty, 266
Photocoagulation
  of GI bleeding lesions, 191-193
  laser, for trichiasis, 126
  panretinal, 113, 114
  retinal, for retinopathies, 111-117

Photocoagulation, dye-enhanced, 116
Photodynamic therapy (PDT), 255-260
  laser bronchoscopy and, 147
  malignant melanoma of choroid and, 129-130
  patient instructions for, 259-260
  veterinary applications of, 308
Photons, 4, 8
Photorefractive keratectomy (PRK), 125-126
Photorefractive surgical procedures, 125-128
Photothermal laser angioplasty, 265-266
Physician credentialing, 323-325, 357, 362-363
Physician liability, legal aspects of laser surgery and, 365-366
Physician reimbursement for laser procedure, 351-353
Physician training laboratories, ongoing, 358
Physics, basic atomic, 7-8
Pierced ear, repair of, 184-185
Pigmented lesions, 167-169
Pilonidal cysts and sinuses, 198-199
Planning
  in perioperative patient education, 386-387
  in Standards of Care, 411
Plantar warts, excision of, 276-278
Plastic surgery; *see* Dermatology and plastic surgery laser applications
Plugged duct cyst, podiatric laser applications and, 279
Plume, laser; *see* Laser plume
Pockel's cell, Q-switched ruby laser and, 54
Podiatric laser applications, 275-286
  callus, cyst, corn, and fissure treatments and, 278-280
  excision of verrucae plantaris and, 276-278
  nail procedures and, 281-282, 283
  neuroma, cyst, and soft-tissue excisions and, 283-286
Podophyllin, condylomata acuminata and, 235
Polymethylmethacrylate, vaporization of, 294
Polyps, colon, 194, 195
Polyvinyl chloride (PVC) endotracheal tube, airway explosion and, 82-83
Population inversion, 31
Porokeratosis, podiatric laser applications and, 279
Port-wine stain, 160, 161-167
  discharge instructions for, 165
  eye protection and, 163
Posterior capsulotomy, 124-126
Postoperative education, 340
Power, wattage of, 10
Power density, laser power and, 10-12
Preceptorships in health care professional education, 406-407
Pregnancy, tubal, 213
Presacral neurectomy, 211
Presacral transection, 211-212
Principles of Humane Experimental Technique, The, 301

PRK; *see* Photorefractive keratectomy
Procurement of laser systems, 342-350
  acquisition of, 345-350
  evaluation of, 343-345
  justification of, 342-343
Progestins, endometrial suppression and, 215
Prograde technique of esophageal tumor vaporization, 190
Proliferative diabetic retinopathy, 112
Prostate
  transurethral incision of, 233, 234
  transurethral resection of, 231-232
  visual ablation of, 232, 234
Prostate gland, hyperplasia of, 232
Prostatectomy, 231-235, 234
Pseudo-Asherman's syndrome, 214
Pterygium, 130
Publicity in marketing of laser program, 377-380
Pulsed ruby laser, 179, 181
PVC endotracheal tube; *see* Polyvinyl chloride endotracheal tube
Pyogenic granulomas, 153

Q

Q-switched Alexandrite laser, 159, 181
Q-switched lasers, 13
Q-switched Nd:YAG laser, 41-42, 124, 181
Q-switched ruby laser, 54, 159, 181
Quality of care in Standards of Professional Performance, 412
Quartz fiberoptic delivery system, laser endoscopy and, 186
Quartz rods, 221, 355

R

Radial keratoplasty, 57
Radial keratotomy, 126
Radiant energy, 4
Radiation, ionizing, 7
Radical neck dissection, 244-245
Radio advertising in marketing of laser program, 373
Ranulas, 153
RBRVS system; *see* Resource-based relative-value scale system
Reanastomosis, 220-221
Reconstruction, laser education and, 391
Rectal and perianal conditions, 195-199
  fissures and, 198
  fistulas and abscesses and, 198
  laser hemorrhoidectomy and, 195-198
  pilonidal cysts and sinuses and, 198-199
Rectal polyps, 194, 195
Reflection, laser-tissue interaction and, 14
Reflex sympathetic dystrophy (RSD), 295
Regression, laser education and, 391
Regulatory bodies, laser safety and, 58-60

Reimbursement for laser procedure, 351-353

Relative value unit (RVU), physician reimbursement and, 352

Rentals, laser, 348, 349

Repetitive stress injury (RSI), 295-296

Reprofiling, corneal, 127

Research in Standards of Professional Performance, 414

Resident certification policy and procedure, 325

Resource utilization in Standards of Professional Performance, 414

Resource-based relative-value scale (RBRVS) system, physician reimbursement and, 352

Retin A; *see* Tretinoin

Retina, anatomy of, 110

Retinal detachments, laser repair of, 118

Retinal photocoagulation, 111-117

Retinal tears, laser repair of, 118

Retinoblastoma, 129

Retinopathy(ies)
    diabetic, 111-112
    retinal photocoagulation for, 111-117
    types of, 111-112

Retrograde technique of esophageal tumor vaporization, 190-191

Reusable fibers, Nd:YAG laser technology and, 43, 45, 46

Rhinitis, allergic, laser surgery for, 136-137

Rhinophyma, 175, 176

Robinul; *see* Glycopyrrolate

Rods, anatomy of eye and, 110

RSD; *see* Reflex sympathetic dystrophy

RSI; *see* Repetitive stress injury

Rubeosis iridis, 112

Ruby laser, 157
    dermatology and, 157
    pulsed, 179, 181
    Q-switched, 159, 181

RVU; *see* Relative value unit

S

Safe Medical Device Act (SMDA), 59, 361

Safety; *see* Laser safety

Sales promotion in marketing of laser program, 376-377

Salpingoplasty, 220-221

Salpingostomy, 220

Scalp, seborrheic keratoses of, 178

Scars
    hypertrophic, 284-285
    laser procedure versus electrocautery and, 390
    removal of, 173-174

Scatting, laser-tissue interaction and, 15

Schawlow, A.L., 3

Schlemm's canal, anatomy of eye and, 110-111

Scissors, bipolar, 21

Sclera, anatomy of eye and, 111

Sclerostomy, internal, 121, 122-123

Scrub technician, 329

Sealed tube CO_2 laser, 34

Seborrheic keratoses of face, 178

Selling, personal, in marketing of laser program, 374-375

Semiconductor diode laser, 31

Semifreestanding laser programs, 334, 335

Shelf life of sealed lasers, 34

Sinus
    anatomy of, 136
    laser procedures for, 135-138
    pilonidal, 198-199

Site of service differential, physician reimbursement and, 352

Skin incisions, 172-173

Sleep apnea, obstructive, 152

Slide presentation in community education, 396-397

SMDA; *see* Safe Medical Device Act

Smoke evacuation, 93-94, 95-102, 103, 188, 208, 356

Smoke evacuation tubing, 100, 101

Smoke evacuation unit, noise of, 98

Smoke wand, positioning of, smoke evacuation and, 100

Snoring, laser treatment for, 151-152

Soft palate, adenoma of, 153

Soft tissues
    orthopedic laser applications and, 293-294
    podiatric laser applications and, 283-286

Soft-tissue laser procedures of oral cavity, 154

Solid lasers, 31

Speakers, laser conference and, 400

Speaking engagements in marketing of laser program, 375

Spectroscopy, dental, 156

Specular reflection, laser-tissue interaction and, 14

Spider angiomas, 170-171

Spinal cord, laser procedures of, 297-298

Sponges, wet, 81

Spot size of laser beam, 11

Spurs, heel, 284

Squamous cell carcinoma in dolphin, 309-313

Staff of laser program, 325-333, 357

Standards
    of care, 359-360, 398, 410-412
    of clinical nursing practice, 409
    of perioperative clinical practice in laser medicine and surgery, 398, 409-414
    of perioperative professional performance, 409
    of professional performance, 398, 410, 412-414

Stapedectomy, laser, 131-135

Stapes, 131

State and local regulations, laser safety and, 60

Stenosis
    laryngeal, 139
    subglottic, 139
Stereotactic endoscopic laser surgery of brain, 298
Steroids following laser intervention for hemangioma, 168-169
Stimulated emission, 8
Straight fiber, fiberoptics and, 43
Strategic planning, laser committee and, 318
Strictures, urethral, 229-230
Subglottic stenosis, laser microlaryngoscopy and, 139
Subungual hematoma, 282, 283
Suggested State Regulations for the Control of Radiation, Volume II, Nonionizing Radiation, Lasers, 60
Superficial varicosities, 170-171
Superpulse CO_2 laser, facial chemical peel and, 178
Supply charges, 357
Surgical drapes, fire safety and, 80-81
Surgical technician, 329
Sympathetic maintained pain, 295

T

Target audience
    laser conference and, 399
    in marketing of laser program, 370
Tattoos, removal of, 178-182, 183
Teaching aids, laser education and, 387
Teeth, protection of, 143-144, 145
Telangiectasia, 169-172
Television advertising in marketing of laser program, 373-374
TEM; *see* Transverse electromagnetic mode
Temperature, increases in, tissue changes with, 17
Temporomandibular joint (TMJ), laser procedure for, 151
Tetracycline, laser angioplasty and, 270
Thermal effects of lasers, 13, 15, 18, 19
Thermal laser angioplasty, 265
Thermal tissue effect of lasers, 13
Thoracoscopy to treat bullous emphysema, 246-247
Thyroidectomy, laser, 245-246
Time pulsed mode, 13
Tissue changes with temperature increases, 17
TMJ; *see* Temporomandibular joint
TMR; *see* Transmyocardial revascularization
Tongue surgery, 152
Tonsillectomy, laser, 150-151
Torso, seborrheic keratoses of, 178
Total quality management, 363
Townes, C.H., 3
Trabeculoplasty, laser, 120
Trabeculotomy, argon laser, open-angle glaucoma and, 129
Transection
    of hypogastric plexus, 211

Transection—cont'd
    presacral, 211-212
    uterosacral, 211-212
Transmission, laser-tissue interaction and, 15, 16
Transmyocardial revascularization (TMR), 270-271
Transportation hazards, 90-91
Transscleral cyclophotocoagulation, 121, 122
Transurethral incision of prostate (TUIP), 233, 234
Transurethral resection of prostate (TURP), 231-232
Transurethral ultrasound-guided laser-induced prostatectomy (TULIP), 234
Transverse electromagnetic mode (TEM), 11-12
Traumatic tattoo, removal of, 179, 180
Tretinoin (Retin A), 180
Trichiasis, laser photocoagulation for, 126
t-shirts in marketing of laser program, 380, 381
Tubal pregnancy, 213
Tubal reimplantation, 220-221
TUIP; *see* Transurethral incision of prostate
TULIP; *see* Transurethral ultrasound-guided laser-induced prostatectomy
Tunable dye laser, 31, 53-54, 173
Turbinectomy, laser, 137
TURP; *see* Transurethral resection of prostate

U

Ulcer
    aphthous, 154
    bleeding, in stomach, 191-193
    decubitus, 285, 286
ULPA filter; *see* Ultra-low particulate air filter
Ultra-low particulate air (ULPA) filter, laser plume and, 95, 96
Ultrapulse CO_2 laser
    facial chemical peel and, 178
    hair transplants and, 178
Ultrasonic imaging, intravascular, laser angioplasty and, 267
United States Department of Agriculture (USDA), 302
Upper endoscopy, 188-189
Ureteral calculi, 230-231
Urethral condylomata, 235-237
Urethral strictures, 229-230
Urinary system, anatomy of, 225
Urology laser applications, 224-238
    circumcision and, 237, 238
    for condylomata acuminata and, 235-237
    endoscopic, 224-235
        for bladder tumors, 224-229
        for chronic cystitis, 235
        prostatectomy, 231-235
        for urethral calculi, 230-231
        for urethral strictures, 229-230
    external, 235-237
    open, 235-238

Urology laser applications—cont'd
    partial nephrectomy and, 238
    for penile carcinoma, 237
    vasectomy reversal and, 237-238
USDA; *see* United States Department of Agriculture
Uterine fibroid, 221
Uterine leiomyoma, 221
Uterosacral transection, 211-212
Uvea, 109-110

V

Vacuum pump, carbon dioxide lasers and, 32
Vaginal conditions, 204-205
Vaginal intraepithelial neoplasia (VAIN), 204-205
Vaporization
    of cervix, 202
    of polymethylmethacrylate, 294
Varicosities, superficial, 170-171
Vascular lesions, laser surgery for, 161-172
Vasectomy reversal, 237-238
Vasopressin
    cervical conization and, 202
    ectopic pregnancy and, 213
Veins, spider, 170-171
Velocity, 6
Vendor participation in health care professional edu-
    cation, 405-406
Venereal warts, 206
Ventilation methods, laser microlaryngoscopy and,
    141
Verruca, 177
Verrucae plantaris, excision of, 276-278
Vertigo, laser stapedectomy and, 133
Veterinary medicine, laser technology and, 300-314
    animal use in laser research and, 300-302
    on dolphins, 309-313
    elephants and, 308
    on horses, 309

VIN; *see* Vulvar intraepithelial neoplasia
Vinegar; *see* Acetic acid
Visual ablation of prostate (VLAP), 232, 234
Vitreous humor, 110
VLAP; *see* Visual ablation of prostate
Vocal cords, paralysis of, 139
Vulvar conditions, 205-206
Vulvar intraepithelial neoplasia (VIN), 205

W

Waffling technique, 282
Warts
    genital, 94, 206
    plantar, 276-278
    venereal, 206
Wattage of power, 10
Wavelength, 4-6, 7, 11, 29
Wedge resection of tongue, 153
Welding, laser, of vessels, 272-273
Wiggler, free electron laser and, 57
Written objectives, laser conference and, 399-400

X

XeCl; *see* Xenon chloride
XeF; *see* Xenon fluoride
Xenon chloride (XeCl), 56
Xenon fluoride (XeF), 56
X-rays, 7
Xylocaine; *see* Lidocaine

Y

YAG; *see* Yttrium-aluminum-garnet
YALO; *see* Yttrium-aluminum-oxide
Yellow light laser energy, 171
YLF; *see* Yttrium-lithium-fluoride
Yttrium-aluminum-garnet (YAG), 31
Yttrium-aluminum-oxide (YALO), 31
Yttrium-lithium-fluoride (YLF), 31